Melancholia

This book provides a comprehensive review of melancholia as a severe disorder of mood, associated with suicide, psychosis, and catatonia. The syndrome is defined with a clear diagnosis, prognosis, and range of management strategies, differentiated from other similar psychiatric, neurological, and general medical conditions. It challenges accepted doctrines in the classification and biology of the mood disorders and defines melancholia as a treatable mental illness. Described for millennia in medical texts and used as a term in literature and poetry, melancholia was included within early versions of the major diagnostic classification systems, but lost favor in later editions. This book updates the arguments for the diagnosis, describes its characteristics in detail, and promotes treatment and prevention. The book offers great hope to those with a disorder too often misdiagnosed and often fatal. It should be read by all those responsible for the management of patients with mood disorders.

Michael Alan Taylor is Professor of Psychiatry Emeritus at Rosalind Franklin University of Medicine and Science, North Chicago, IL and Adjunct Clinical Professor of Psychiatry at the University of Michigan School of Medicine, Ann Arbor, MI, USA.

Max Fink is Professor of Psychiatry and Neurology Emeritus at the State University of New York at Stony Brook, USA.

Melancholia

The diagnosis, pathophysiology, and treatment of depressive illness

Michael Alan Taylor, M.D.

Professor of Psychiatry Emeritus at Rosalind Franklin University of Medicine and Science, North Chicago, IL, and Adjunct Clinical Professor of Psychiatry at the University of Michigan School of Medicine, Ann Arbor, MI, USA

Max Fink, M.D.

Professor of Psychiatry and Neurology Emeritus, State University of New York at Stony Brook, USA

CAMBRIDGE
UNIVERSITY PRESS

CAMBRIDGE UNIVERSITY PRESS
Cambridge, New York, Melbourne, Madrid, Cape Town, Singapore, São Paulo

CAMBRIDGE UNIVERSITY PRESS
The Edinburgh Building, Cambridge CB2 2RU, UK
Published in the United States of America by Cambridge University Press, New York

www.cambridge.org
Information on this title: www.cambridge.org/9780521841511

First published 2006

Printed in the United Kingdom at the University Press, Cambridge

A catalog record for this publication is available from the British Library

ISBN-13 978-0-521-84151-1 hardback
ISBN-10 0-521-84151-8 hardback

Contents

	List of patient vignettes	*page* ix
	Preface	xi
	Acknowledgments	xv
1	**Melancholia: a conceptual history**	**1**
	Origins of the concept	2
	The psychodynamic interruption	6
	The recognition of melancholia in psychiatric classification	7
	Notes	10
2	**Melancholia defined**	**15**
	Melancholy	15
	Manic-depressive illness	18
	Psychotic depression is melancholia	24
	Depression with catatonia or stupor is severe melancholia	30
	Melancholia defined by a specific event	32
	Notes	37
3	**Defining melancholia by psychopathology**	**45**
	DSM depression categories and diagnostic criteria	46
	Consensus and empirical approaches defining a syndrome	51
	Psychopathology data supporting the validity of melancholia	53
	The nature of melancholia	56
	Conclusions	58
	Notes	59
4	**Defining melancholia: laboratory tests**	**62**
	Neuroendocrine measures in mood disorders	62
	The hypothalamic–pituitary–adrenal axis	64
	The hypothalamic–pituitary–thyroid axis	72
	Electrophysiologic measures	72

	Conclusions	76
	Notes	78
5	**Examination for melancholia**	**85**
	Examination strategy	86
	Examining mood	87
	Examining psychomotor functioning	88
	Examining for vegetative signs	88
	Examining for psychotic features	89
	Examining for suicidal thoughts	90
	Examining cognition	90
	Examining for personality disorder	91
	Rating scales of depression	91
	Notes	95
6	**The differential diagnosis of melancholia**	**97**
	Non-melancholic depressive mood disorders	97
	Melancholia in children and adolescents	103
	Melancholia in the elderly	104
	Melancholia in a patient with a psychotic disorder	106
	Distinguishing melancholia from anxiety and obsessive-compulsive disorders	108
	Distinguishing melancholia from drug-related depressive-like states	109
	Melancholia associated with general medical illnesses	110
	Avolitional, apathetic, and bradykinetic syndromes	112
	Neurologic disease associated with apathy and depression-like syndromes	113
	Notes	118
7	**Suicide in melancholia**	**125**
	Errors in suicide prevention	126
	Suicide risk assessment	134
	The effect of specific treatments on suicide rates	139
	Management of the suicidal melancholic patient	143
	Notes	146
8	**Electroconvulsive therapy for melancholia**	**153**
	ECT in melancholia	155
	ECT for psychotic depression	157
	ECT and suicide risk	159
	ECT for catatonia and depressive stupor	161
	ECT in pregnancy and postpartum depression	163
	ECT in children and adolescents	165
	ECT in the elderly	170
	ECT and characterological conditions	171

	ECT in unipolar and bipolar depression	172
	Conclusion	174
	Notes	174
9	**Achieving effective ECT**	**181**
	Patient selection	181
	Technical considerations	183
	Conclusions	190
	Notes	190
10	**The validity of the pharmacotherapy literature in melancholia**	**196**
	Industry influence undermines conclusions about newer agents	197
	Head-to-head comparisons are biased to favor newer drugs	199
	Antidepressant drug efficacy: TCA versus pure SSRI	201
	Antidepressant drug efficacy: pure SSRIs compared to non-TCA agents	204
	Conclusions	206
	Notes	207
11	**Basic pharmacotherapy for melancholic patients**	**211**
	Acute treatment	212
	Combining drugs and psychotherapy	218
	Continuation and maintenance treatment	219
	Pharmacotherapy for melancholia	220
	Treatment of severe melancholia	222
	Optimizing treatments for manic-depressive illness	229
	Notes	231
12	**Pharmacotherapy for melancholic patients in complicating circumstances**	**239**
	Melancholia in pregnancy and breast-feeding	239
	Melancholia in childhood and adolescence	244
	Melancholia in old age	250
	Melancholia with co-occurring alcohol or drug abuse	255
	Melancholia with co-occurring neurologic disease	257
	Melancholia co-occurring with general medical conditions	261
	Melancholia with co-occurring personality disorder	265
	Summary recommendations	266
	Treatment-resistant depression	268
	Notes	273
13	**Proposed treatments for melancholia**	**284**
	Light therapy	284
	Transcranial magnetic stimulation	286
	Magnetic seizure therapy (MST)	288
	Vagal nerve stimulation (VNS)	289

Glucocorticosteroid receptor agonists 289
Targeted neurotransmitter system agents 290
Hormones 291
Herbal remedies 292
Notes 294

14 The pathophysiology of melancholia 298
Genetic predisposition 299
Environmental factors 303
Abnormal stress response 307
Abnormal neurochemical functioning 311
Abnormal brain structure 317
Abnormal brain metabolism 318
Electrophysiologic abnormalities 320
Cognitive deficits 327
Why some melancholic patients have manic episodes 328
Conclusions 330
Notes 333

15 Future directions 346
Changing the DSM classification of depression 347
Changing the DSM diagnostic criteria for melancholia 348
Changing the standards of pharmacotherapy research 349
Changing treatment guidelines: endless drug trials elicit chronicity 351
Improving the education of medical practitioners in mood disorders 351
Studies of the mechanism of convulsive therapy 353
Preventive approaches to reduce the burden of melancholia 354
Pharmacogenetics 359
The pathophysiology of melancholia 360
Coda 364
Notes 365

References 371
Index 522

Patient vignettes

2.1	A woman with melancholia (Hopewell-Ash)	*page* 17
2.2	A woman with melancholia (Hopewell-Ash)	17
2.3	A man with melancholia (Hopewell-Ash)	17
2.4	A woman with melancholia (Hopewell-Ash)	17
2.5	A woman with cycloid psychosis (Hopewell-Ash)	22
2.6	A man with a psychotic melancholia (DSM-IV Casebook)	28
2.7	A man with psychotic melancholia (Fink)	28
2.8	A woman with Cotard syndrome (Hansen and Bolwig)	29
2.9	A woman with melancholia (Taylor)	30
2.10	A catatonic woman with psychotic melancholia (Kalhbaum)	31
2.11	A 15-year-old girl with psychotic melancholia and catatonia (Hoch)	32
2.12	A woman with a postpartum melancholia (Protheroe)	35
2.13	A woman with postpartum melancholia (Hamilton)	35
3.1	A man with an apathetic frontal lobe syndrome meeting criteria for major depression (Vaidya and Taylor)	49
5.1	A melancholic man with a psychotic depression (Taylor)	89
6.1	An epileptic man with brief depressions (Taylor)	116
7.1	An 87-year-old woman with a psychotic depression (Taylor)	128
7.2	A 44-year-old melancholic man misdiagnosed with PTSD who committed suicide (Taylor)	130
7.3	A hospitalized depressed woman with a suicide plan (Taylor)	131
7.4	A melancholic woman who received poor treatment (Taylor)	132
7.5	A 30-year-old man with a "postpartum" melancholia (Taylor)	133
7.6	A man who refused hospitalization and committed suicide (Taylor)	133
7.7	A 70-year-old man who hanged himself (Taylor)	137
7.8	A 21-year-old woman who made a suicide attempt following a psychodynamic interview (Taylor)	145
8.1	A 66-year-old woman with melancholia (Fink)	157
8.2	A professor of surgery describes his psychotic depression (Nuland)	158
8.3	A former medical school dean describes his depression (Rosenberg)	160
8.4	A 58-year-old woman with melancholia and catatonia misdiagnosed as having Alzheimer's disease (Fink)	162

8.5 A psychotically depressed mother who killed her five children (Ottosson and Fink) 164
8.6 A 16-year-old boy with melancholia unresponsive to medications and psychotherapy who responded to ECT (Fink) 168
8.7 A 17-year-old boy with manic delirium who responded to ECT (Fink) 168
8.8 An 8 1/2-year-old girl with melancholia and catatonia, unresponsive to medications, who responded to ECT (Cizadlo and Wheaton) 169
8.9 A 76-year-old melancholic man with a recent surgical repair of an aortic aneurysm who responded to ECT (Fink) 170
8.10 A 68-year-old man with Parkinson's disease and depression who responded to ECT (Fink) 171
8.11 A woman with hypochondriasis (Roueché) 171
8.12 A woman with manic-depressive illness (Sienaert and Peuskens) 173
11.1 A man with a psychotic depression (Taylor) 223
12.1 A pregnant woman with a psychotic depression (Taylor) 240
12.2 A 78-year-old depressed woman; antidepressant medication-associated status epilepticus (Taylor) 253
12.3 A 26-year-old woman with recurrent depression not adequately evaluated (Taylor) 269

Preface

O Lord, all my desire is before you;
From you my groaning is not hid.
My heart throbs; my strength forsakes me;
The very light of my eyes has failed me.
My friends and neighbors stand back
Because of my affliction;
My neighbors stand afar off. *Psalm 38*

At any point in time on this planet, almost two and a half times as many persons are depressed as are demented. Counting all variations on the theme, about 10% of men and 20% of women are at lifetime risk for experiencing a depressive illness. Based on numbers of persons affected, the World Health Organization estimates that depressive illnesses are the fourth highest cause of medical disability and premature death worldwide in years of illness, treatments required, lost productivity during episodes, and death rates.[1]

Ten to 15% of depressed persons die by suicide. This rate translates into about one million persons annually, worldwide, and 30000–90000 persons annually in the USA. The first figure is the accepted count and the latter figure is estimated from analyses that acknowledge underreporting. In the USA, suicide is the 11th leading cause of death. Most persons over age 50 have known at least one individual who has committed suicide. Among depressed persons, sufferers of melancholia have the highest suicide rates.

Depressive illness is increasing in frequency among persons born closer to the present (a period effect), and first episodes are occurring at younger ages (a cohort effect). These trends result in more ill persons with more years of illness.

Of the persons who kill themselves annually in the USA, nearly 50% (15000–45000 individuals) seek help from a physician within the 3 weeks before they commit suicide – a sad sign of a public health failure because suicide is preventable. In treating depressed patients, psychiatrists meet *minimal* standards of care about 80% of the time, whereas generalist physicians, who see most sufferers of depression, meet the standards of care only 20% of the time. Although the mood is often recognized, a depressive illness is frequently interpreted as disappointment, bereavement, or demoralization, and is ignored as the brain disease that it is. Although misfortune can precipitate a depressive episode, once the sequence of pathophysiologic events that become a depressive illness unfolds, the changes in brain functioning sustain the expression of the illness. Depressive illness is highly responsive to proper treatment, but more often than not, depressed persons are inadequately treated.

Many forms of depressive illness are recognized. The most prominent are identified as the mood disorders of major depression, dysthymia, bipolar depressive disorder, and depressive illnesses associated with a general medical condition. To this list are added specifiers of frequency (single or recurrent), severity, psychosis, catatonia, and pattern (typical or atypical). Other syndromes of depressive mood are found throughout the *Diagnostic and Statistical Manual* (DSM) classification system. This varied taxonomy lacks supporting psychopathological or pathophysiological evidence and, as a consequence, the taxonomy lacks validity. Reliable diagnosis, prognosis, selection of treatment, and outcomes for sufferers of depressive illness are often poor.[2] Decades of research, however, identify a central pathophysiology in the neuroendocrine system. This theme is *melancholia*, and identifying this syndrome clarifies diagnosis, prognosis, and treatment for more successful outcomes.

Melancholia is a severe disorder of mood, often fatal, that has been described for millennia in medical texts and by poets, novelists, and playwrights. Melancholia is definable by measurable signs and symptoms, characteristic neuroendocrine and neurophysiologic profiles, and its treatment-responsiveness to electroconvulsive therapy (ECT) and to pharmacodynamically broad-spectrum antidepressant drugs. Melancholia is often associated with stupor, catatonia, psychosis, suicide, and manic-depressive illness.[3] Melancholia is a lifelong process with a genetic risk.

Early *International Classification of Diseases* (ICD) editions and DSM-I and DSM-II classifications identified melancholia, but these classification systems were not helpful in prescribing newly introduced treatments (e.g., insulin coma, psychosurgery, convulsive therapy) that were found to be effective in schizophrenia and then in manic-depressive illness. The efficacy of psychotropic drugs was also weakly correlated with heterogeneous DSM categories, discouraging the search for treatment response as a feature of classification. The DSM-III and subsequent classifications, introduced as operationally defined and more "scientific," produced no better results. To achieve the approval of the largest segments of the diverse memberships of professional organizations, the DSM definition of mood disorder became overly broad and criteria for the diagnosis of major depression overly liberal. The "worried well" with characterological depressive moods were conflated with melancholia into the category of "major depression." The neuroendocrine, neurophysiologic, and psychopathologic delineators of melancholia were confounded, and discarded as diagnostic and prognostic clinical laboratory aids. Under the DSM-III system, the dexamethasone suppression test (DST) identified melancholia in 50% or more of depressed patients, but rather than concluding that the other 50% represented different forms of distress, the DST was discarded as a measure of melancholia.[4]

In the decades after the introduction of DSM-III, intrusive actions of the pharmaceutical industry encouraged a weakening of criteria to justify the use of antidepressant drugs in the largest number of persons. The safety and efficacy of the older, no longer patentable agents (tricyclic antidepressants, monoamine oxidase inhibitors, and lithium) were maligned through aggressive marketing that relied on unsound industry-sponsored comparison studies. Academic psychiatry went to the highest bidder.[5]

In response to weakened criteria and confusing classification, we reintroduce melancholia as the classic depressive illness with definable diagnostic criteria and effective treatment algorithms. We write this book for physicians and other health care professionals who treat severely ill depressed patients. It is intended to spur better modeling of disorders in psychiatric classification schemes.[6] Our approach is that of the clinician-scientist, not the bench researcher, although we detail the biology of depressive illness and the evidence that it is a brain disease.

We set the historical stage and describe the remarkably consistent conceptual image of melancholia over millennia. We describe the disorder and review studies that systematically delineate melancholia, mirroring the historical record, and validating melancholia as a definable syndrome. Laboratory findings that support the melancholia syndrome and its variations (e.g., psychotic depression) are presented. We offer a systematic examination for the classic psychopathology of melancholia.

A variety of labels have splintered the melancholia concept. We show these to be variations of melancholia. We offer criteria on how to separate melancholia from depressive-like syndromes that have been inappropriately attached to it, and from other conditions in which apathy and psychomotor slowing are features. Suicide is a principal risk in melancholia, and we discuss the recognition of suicide and suicide prevention. Convulsive therapy is the syndrome's most effective treatment and we discuss how to maximize its effect. We detail medication management of patients suffering from melancholia. Newly proposed treatments are critiqued. We review the evidence that depressive illness is a lifelong process, discuss its pathophysiology, and offer the evidence that melancholia is an expression of brain dysfunction. Finally, we offer our conclusions that melancholia is a syndrome that warrants separate classification in the mood disorders category. We present prevention strategies, and how research needs to be refocused to provide a better understanding of melancholia.

We come to this book after decades of treating depressed patients, often those so severely ill that their deaths seemed imminent. One of us, (MAT) has been a career-long student of descriptive psychopathology in the nineteenth-century tradition, detailing the characteristics of patients with mania, depression, psychosis, and catatonia. He has been a teacher of neuropsychiatry for medical students, psychiatric residents, neurologists, and psychologists. He prescribes and administers ECT. The other (MF) has encouraged the development and administration of modern ECT, which is recognized as the most powerful antidepressant treatment. He has an extensive experience in clinical and experimental psychopharmacology, in the electrophysiology of psychoactive drugs, and in psychopathology.

Together, we have witnessed the birth and infancy of the psychopharmacology era and experienced its promises to treat patients with mood disorders better. We are concerned about the effects on psychiatric practice, education, and research, as well as on popular culture that we see in the unhealthy relationships between academia and the pharmaceutical industry. Despite the escalation of new agents, remission rates are lower than ever and "treatment resistance" is said to be common.[7]

We write this book, however, with optimism because we know that when physicians "get it right" – the diagnosis and treatment – depressed patients have a good response and many achieve remission of their symptoms and return to productive lives. There is nothing more elating in clinical psychiatry than to see an animated and cheerful person who only a few short weeks before was immobilized with indecision and overwhelmed by apprehension, gloom, and thoughts of death.

To understand melancholia is to understand depressive illness and the care of patients with mood disorder. If we improve this understanding, we will have achieved our goal.

NOTES

1 Murray and Lopez (1996); Uston *et al.* (2004).

2 At a 2003 presentation of brain metabolic abnormalities in depressive illness to a large group of depression researchers, the chairperson opened the session by stating that the present DSM depression taxonomy was inconsistent with clinical evidence and unhelpful in research and clinical practice. The audience agreed. (University of Michigan Depression Center symposium series: M.A. Taylor, personal observation.)

3 We prefer the classic term "manic-depressive illness" to that of "bipolar disorder." It offers historical continuity and captures the essence of the disease better. Chapters 2 and 5 discuss manic-depressive disorder and its relationship to melancholia.

4 Chapter 4 provides a discussion of laboratory tests for melancholia.

5 Chapter 10 discusses industry influence on antidepressant treatment trials.

6 We have taken a similar approach in presenting the evidence for catatonia as a distinct syndrome (Fink and Taylor, 2003; Taylor and Fink, 2003).

7 Montes *et al.* (2004).

Acknowledgments

Documenting points of view is never easy, and gathering supporting citations is a daunting task. Toward that effort Georgette Pfeiffer tirelessly compiled and corrected our large list of citations. We are in her debt.

We are also grateful to Drs. Bernard Carroll and Edward Shorter who helped us understand the history of the melancholia concept and its pathophysiology.

1

Melancholia: a conceptual history

Depression, most people know, used to be termed "melancholia". . . Melancholia would still appear to be a far more apt and evocative word for the blacker forms of the disorder, but it was usurped by a noun with a bland tonality and lacking any magisterial presence, used indifferently to describe an economic decline or a rut in the ground, a true wimp of a word for such a major illness . . .

The Swiss-born psychiatrist Adolf Meyer had a tin ear for the finer rhythms of English and therefore was unaware of the semantic damage he had inflicted by offering "depression" as a descriptive noun for such a dreadful and raging disease. Nonetheless, for over seventy-five years the word has slithered innocuously through the language like a slug, leaving little trace of its intrinsic malevolence and preventing, by its very insipidity, a general awareness of the horrible intensity of the disease when out of control.[1]

A scientific classification of behavior disorders is still an unreachable goal. The efforts in the past two centuries are reminiscent of the many attempts to bring order into the universe of plants and animals before the singular rules of Linnaeus and Mendel allowed meaningful classifications to emerge. The maladaptive variations in human mood, thought, and motor behavior observed over the millennia offer a myriad of images that have captured the attention of one observer or another who attempted to formulate these observations into an understandable framework. More organized systems emerged at the end of the Eighteenth Century with the attentions of German and French physicians.[2] The classifications often lacked a central thesis and, for the most part, clinicians have been attracted by one aspect of behavior or another, allowing the behaviors to be classified by the dominant symptom or presumed etiology. Patients have been lumped or split into classes or described as categories or continua according to idiosyncratic opinions.[3]

Neurosyphilis is an interesting neuropsychiatric disorder that offered a potpourri of images and therapies. So varied were its presentations that clinicians dubbed it the "great imitator."[4] Descriptions filled volumes, but once the common cause was identified and a laboratory test developed, the variations assumed less significance. An effective treatment gave descriptive syphilology the *coup de grâce.*

The classification of mood disorders presents the same dilemma. Which disorders of mood are expressions of a common pathology and which are not? How many pathopathologies are represented in the mood disorders? How many disorders are derived from one cause? Acknowledging our limited understanding of human neurobiology, is it prudent to support the many disorders of mood characterized in the *Diagnostic and Statistical Manual* (DSM) classification or is it better to seek a simpler basis?

For a medical classification to be useful it should be precise in its criteria of differentiation, predict the probable course of an illness, and guide the selection of the most optimal intervention. It should also offer the scientist a lodestone for the selection of homogeneous populations for research study.[5]

The psychiatric classifications embodied in DSM-IV and the 10th *International Classfication of Diseases* (ICD-10) are not precise, and do not predict the course of illness nor effectively guide intervention. A simplified classification of depressive mood disorders under the rubric of "melancholia" achieves these aims better. "Melancholia" is recognized as a syndrome of gloom, apprehension, inhibited motor activity, slowed thoughts, homeostatic distress, and psychosis. Clinical criteria of the disorder are definable, laboratory tests offer support, and course of illness is predictable with the available therapeutic options. The burden of this report is to establish melancholia as a definable syndrome in psychiatric classification.[6]

Origins of the concept

Melancholia is a concept of depressive illness with an extensive literature and a detailed history. Its recognition as a form of "madness" with "bodily causes" has been consistent for 3000 years. Except for two periods in western history – the Middle Ages, when church teachings dominated western thought, and again in the twentieth century, particularly in the USA, when psychoanalytic notions dominated psychiatric thinking – melancholia was identified as a disorder in brain function. Modern writers who offer detailed histories of the syndrome are Hopewell-Ash (1934), Lewis (1934a), Schmidt-Degenhard (1983), Jackson (1986), Goodwin and Jamison (1990), and Parker and Hadzi-Pavlovic (1996). Discussions of melancholia are to be found in Hunter and Macalpine's *Three Hundred Years of Psychiatry* (1982), Berrios and Porter's *A History of Clinical Psychiatry* (1995), Shorter's *A History of Psychiatry* (1997), and Porter's *Madness* (2002). Literary writings are presented by Hefferman (1995) and Radden (2000). A review of the role of psychotherapies in the history of depression is offered in a special number of *Psychiatric Annals*.[7]

Melancholia was identified by Hippocrates in the fifth century BCE as a persistent sadness and morbid thoughts that had their source in a disorder of the brain. In '*The Sacred Disease*,' he wrote:

> And men ought to know that from nothing else but thence [from the brain] come joys, delights, laughter and sports, and sorrows, griefs, despondency, and lamentations. And by this, in an especial manner, we acquire wisdom and knowledge, and see and hear, and know what are foul and what are fair, what are bad and what are good, what are sweet and what are unsavory . . . And by the same organ we become mad and delirious, and fears and terrors assail us, some by night, and some by day, and dreams and untimely wanderings, and cares that are not suitable, and ignorance of present circumstances . . . All these things we endure from the

brain when it is not healthy, but is more hot, more cold, more moist, or more dry than natural . . . And we become mad from humidity [of the brain].[8]

Hippocrates described a specific syndrome, not a vague dysphoria or dourness of character. Although rooted in beliefs in the essential balance of four body humors for health, other early images of melancholia define the same syndrome. Galen and Arateus, both writing in the first century CE, considered melancholia as an affliction of the brain. Arateus described:

And yet in certain of these cases there is mere anger and grief and sad dejection of mind . . . they are suspicious of poisoning or flee to the desert from misanthropy or turn suspicious or contract a hatred of life. Or if at any time a relaxation takes place, in most cases hilarity supervenes. The patients are dull or stern, dejected or unreasonably torpid . . . they also become peevish, dispirited and start up from a disturbed sleep.[9]

Plutarch noted that when a man is melancholic:

Every little evil is magnified by the scaring spectres of his anxiety. He looks on himself as a man whom the gods hate and pursue with their anger . . . Awake, he makes no use of his reason; and asleep, he enjoys no respite from his alarms. His reason always slumbers; his fears are always awake. Nowhere can he find escape from his imaginary terrors.[10]

In western Europe from the tenth to the eighteenth centuries, mental disorders were often ascribed to demons and witchcraft.[11] Relief was theorized to come with exorcism. The medical teachings that psychiatric disorders resulted from aberrations in the brain were officially denied. Many physicians, however, continued to recognize melancholia as disease. Bright (1586) described a "natural" form of mental disorder that resulted from "the mind's apprehension" and an "unnatural" illness of the humors of the body. The "natural" is recognized today as "reactive depression", the "unnatural" as "major depression."[12] A similar division is presented by Robert Burton in *The Anatomy of Melancholy* (1621), the most detailed and poetic description of melancholia in the literature.[13] Another description is that of Richard Baxter (1716) (Hunter and Macalpine, 1982, p. 241):

Melancholy Persons are commonly exceedingly fearful . . . Their Fantasie most erreth in aggravating their Sin, or Dangers or Unhappiness . . . They are still addicted to Excess of Sadness, some weeping they know not why, and some thinking it ought to be so . . . They are continual Self-Accusers . . . They [apprehend] themselves forsaken of God . . . They are utterly unable to rejoyce in anything.

A great part of their Cure lieth in pleasing them, and avoiding all displeasing Things, as far as lawfully can be done . . . As much as you can, divert them from the Thoughts which are their Trouble.

If other means will not do, neglect not Physick; and tho' they will be averse to it . . . yet they must be perswaded or forced to it . . . I have known a Lady deep in Melancholy, who a long time would not speak, nor take Physick; nor endure her Husband to go out of the Room; and with the Restraint and Grief he Died, and she was Cured by Physick put down her Throat, with a Pipe by Force.[14]

In the nineteenth century melancholia was recognized as a core illness among many forms of insanity. One writer defined six classes of insanity: melancholia, mania, fatuitas, stupiditas, amentia, and oblivio".[15] Another offered five "species" of insanity: melancholia, mania with and without delirium, dementia, and idiocy.[16] Yet another author divided insanity into three orders, with mania and melancholia combined as one.[17] Mania was considered a higher form of melancholia or as the same illness in a different form. A specific view is expressed by the apothecary of London's Bethlem Hospital, John Haslam, in 1809 (Hunter and Macalpine, 1982, p. 580):

> As the terms Mania and Melancholia are in general use, and serve to distinguish the forms under which insanity is exhibited, there can be no objection to retain them; but I would strongly oppose their being considered as opposite diseases. In both there is an equal derangement.[18]

Other observers emphasized the connection between the mood disorders of depression and mania. Descriptions of a circular insanity were detailed by Falret (1854) and Baillerger (1854).[19] Falret described melancholia:

> At the commencement of this phase . . . the patients begin to withdraw and now speak only rarely. Sometimes they express remorse over their previous condition . . . the patients withdraw, remaining all alone and motionless . . . they are now meek, and their humility may go so far as for them to refuse treatment in the belief that they do not deserve it. This despondency becomes more pronounced daily . . . [and] the patient is transformed into a statue . . . were he not coaxed to eat, the patient would not bother to seek food . . .
>
> The thought processes are very slow; rarely this may result in complete cessation of all intellectual activity . . . his movements are sluggish or absent. The face is pale; the features sag, suggesting dejection rather than anxiety . . . Appetite is decreased, and the patient eats little; digestion is equally slow and defecation is laborious.
>
> Nevertheless, there are a certain number of patients who present with specific preoccupations, among which we have noticed ideas of humility, of ruin, of being poisoned, or of guilt.[20]

The lack of a coherent formulation of psychiatric disorders encouraged two camps to develop, one dividing the behaviors into many conditions and the other offering a single disorder of the brain as the basis for many forms of psychiatric illness.[21] The single cause for psychiatric disorders was formulated when anatomic studies showed diverse forms of mental illness to be associated with thickening of the brain's meninges, later seen as secondary to cerebral syphilis.[22] The brain diseases took various forms, one dissolving into another, and arguments ensued as to the relevance of a single brain disorder (*Einheitspsychose*) or multiple disorders.[23]

Of many attempts to develop a coherent nomenclature, Emil Kraepelin's formulation of melancholia as an abnormal mood state was widely accepted.[24] An active and agitated form of the illness was grouped with manias, and the periodicity of recurrences was highlighted. He recognized two forms of the psychoses – a progressive deteriorating illness of dementia praecox (*Verblödungsprocesse*) and a non-deteriorating form of periodic illnesses (*das periodische Irresein*). The latter term was replaced in his next edition by *das manisch-depressive Irresein* which established a condition of manic-depressive illness. Melancholia was retained as a separate depressive syndrome that occurred in a perceived "involutional period." In writings in the first half of the Twentieth Century it became the syndrome of *involutional melancholia.*

For mania, Kraepelin described a progression in severity from hypomania to mania to delirious mania. For melancholia, he described a parallel progression of simple retardation, retardation with delusions and hallucinations, and stuporous conditions.[25]

Various attempts to distinguish depressive mood disorders were made. One attempt divided depressed patients with anxiety as "reactive" to stress (psychoneurotic), and an autonomous form that had a systemic or biologic basis.[26] The arguments were of popular interest at the beginning of the twentieth century, with prominent British authors arguing for a unitary model.[27]

Melancholia was described as a specific disorder by Aubrey Lewis (1934b) in his detailed study of 61 melancholic patients:

> ***Melancholia*** is one of the great words in psychiatry. Suffering many mutations, at one time the tenacious guardian of outworn schemes or errant theories; presently misused, cavilled at, dispossessed, it has endured into our own times, a part of medical terminology no less than of common speech. It would seem profitable to consider the history of this word, and of the states of fear and distress with which it has from the beginning been associated.[28]

The concept of melancholia was brought to life in the description by Hopewell-Ash (1934).[29]

> MELANCHOLIA is a depressed state [meaning subdued, not a diagnostic category] of the entire personality reaction. Depression of spirits, psychomotor retardation and general torpidity of mind and body are its essential features. Invariably associated with these are insomnia, indigestion and constipation. It is true that morbid, restless anxiety often colours the depression, but in typical cases it is the general slowing up of the rhythm that characterizes the clinical picture. Mental depression may be due to many causes, both physical and mental; toxemia reflex irritation and physical fatigue on the one hand and psychological stress on the other are responsible for many instances. But in the melancholic state – using that term to indicate a particular clinical condition – there is a sluggishness of mind manifested by difficulty in thinking, poverty of ideas and loss of attentive control that is not found in any kind of simple nervous depression. In well-developed cases the "slow-motion" life of melancholia is extraordinarily characteristic; slow movements, retarded reaction and difficulty of ready response combine to present us with appearances that are familiar to all who have much to do with cases of mental disease. It is a clinical picture accentuated by the foetid breath, furred tongue and story of digestive troubles which express the inhibited gastro-intestinal functions. The lacklustre expression, lifeless hair and greasy complexion, which are equally common, complete a characteristic facies. In more severe degrees of melancholia one finds, as will be noted later, such symptoms as the above combined with hallucinations and delusions. The latter are usually concerned with ideas of wrong-doing, evil, disaster and death. The man who believes that he has committed the "unpardonable" sin and will not admit any doubt about it is always suffering from melancholia. No anxiety state representing a psychoneurosis ever produces a reaction of this kind.

A contemporary, Denis Hill (1968), found no merit in the subdivisions of the mood disorders, concluding that the treatments defined the condition:

> It is a striking fact that the antidepressant drugs and ECT have their profoundest therapeutic effect when the primary functional changes of depression are most in evidence and that, given

these, the secondary symptoms disappear as the primary functional changes are alleviated. To put the matter at its greatest simplicity there is little to contradict in the statement that biological therapeutic agents operate only on biological functional systems.[30]

The psychodynamic interruption

Kraepelin's formulation of melancholia as a core mental disorder had many critics. The strongest attacks came from Freud and his followers, who offered a "mental" or "psychological" basis for melancholia.[31] Their theory pictured active exchanges of energies within a tripartite mental apparatus defined as the *superego*, *ego*, and *id*. Mourning for the loss of a love object deranged the energetics so that melancholia emerged. The physical attributes of the illness resulted from a displacement of energies from the *ego* – the emotional part that related to the outside world – to the *id* – the hidden source of drives and emotions. When a loss could be associated with a specific subject or event in the subject's history, "reactive depression" ensued. When a loss was not identifiable and the condition seemed unrelated to history, a "psychotic depression" ensued.[32] As psychodynamic theory came to dominate American psychiatry, interest in the biological aspects of melancholia diminished.

Adolf Meyer, a leading professor of psychiatry in the USA, is described as:

> desirous of eliminating the term melancholia, which implied a knowledge of something that we did not possess, and which had been employed in different specific ways by different writers. If, instead of melancholia, we applied the term depression to the whole class, it would designate in an unassuming way exactly what was meant by the common use of the term melancholia; and nobody would doubt that for medical purposes the term would have to be amplified so as to denote the kind of depression . . . We might distinguish the pronounced types from the simple insufficiently differentiated depressions. Besides the manic-depressive depressions, the anxiety psychoses, the depressive deliria and depressive hallucinations, the depressive episodes of dementia praecox, the symptomatic depressions, non-differentiated depressions will occur.[33]

Meyer stated that depressive mood disorders were individualized "reactions":

> The conditions which we meet in psychopathology are more or less abnormal reaction types, which we want to learn to distinguish from one another, trace to the situation or condition under which they arise, and study for their modifiability.[34]

Meyer's formulations were adopted in the concept of "reactions" that became the basis for the American Psychiatric Association classification of psychiatric disorders (Table 1.1) in DSM-I (1952) and the revision of DSM-II (1968).[35]

The concepts of Freud or Meyer, or those of the adherents to their philosophies, would not have been so widely accepted had there been a competing biological model of psychiatric illness or effective treatments for psychiatric disorders. Neuroscience technologies and laboratory procedures were primitive and no somatic treatment was established. The introduction of malarial fevers (1917), insulin coma (1933), convulsive therapy (1934), and leucotomy (1935) challenged the psychodynamic model. The success of these treatments in quickly relieving the most severe psychiatric

Table 1.1. Diagnostic and statistical manual, 2nd edition (DSM-II) "depression" formulations

DISORDERS OF PSYCHOGENIC ORIGIN OR WITHOUT CLEARLY DEFINED PHYSICAL CAUSE OR STRUCTURAL CHANGE IN THE BRAIN
Psychotic disorders
Disorder due to disturbance of metabolism, growth, nutrition, or endocrine function
Involutional psychotic reaction
Disorders of psychogenic origin or without clearly defined tangible cause or structural change
Affective reactions
Manic-depressive reaction, manic type
Manic-depressive reaction, depressive type
Manic-depressive reaction, other
Psychotic depressive reaction
Schizophrenic reactions
Schizophrenic reaction, schizoaffective type
Psychoneurotic disorders
Disorders of psychogenic origin or without clearly defined tangible cause or structural change
Psychoneurotic reactions
Anxiety reaction
Depressive reaction

illnesses changed clinical psychiatric practice and once again directed attention to the brain as central to psychiatric disorders.[36] A new therapeutic optimism improved the tenor of psychiatric institutions.[37]

The recognition of melancholia in psychiatric classification

New typologies were envisioned as the basis for more effective prescription of the available treatments. Altered mood states were now labeled as *vital* or *personal, primary* or *secondary, atypical, vegetative, endogenomorphic depressions* and *anxious thymopathy.*[38]

In an unusual study, Klein and Fink (1962a, 1962b) randomly assigned patients of varying diagnoses (depression, mania, psychosis) referred for medication treatments in an inpatient hospital setting to one of three treatments – imipramine, chlorpromazine (combined with the antiparkinson agent, procyclidine), or placebo.[39] Imipramine relieved depressed mood in both the retarded and agitated forms. Chlorpromazine relieved psychosis but also relieved depressed mood. The labeling of the new psychoactive substances as either "antidepressant" or "antipsychotic" was challenged.

The diagnostic criteria of DSM-II served as poor guides in the prescription of the compounds.[40] Many psychopharmacologists described their frustration with DSM-II criteria for the selection of treatments.[41] They struggled with a confusion generated by the varying proposed causes of depression: being rooted in life events (*reactive depression*) or in body physiology (*endogenous, vital depression*), or dominated by neurotic symptoms (*neurotic depression, dysthymia*), psychosis (*psychotic depression*), or character pathology.

By the late 1960s it was no longer acceptable to treat all depressed patients as if they were suffering from a single condition because some treatments were effective for some patients and not for others. One group, for example, examined 33 studies that had assessed medication treatments of depression and could not find a diagnostic formulation that had predictive strength.[42] The DSM-II and ICD-8 classifications had poor reliability, best demonstrated in international studies.[43]

An operationally defined diagnostic scheme was offered in the Research Diagnostic Criteria (RDC).[44] Its usefulness encouraged the American Psychiatric Association to update the official classification in DSM-III of 1980.[45] Lacking a defined theory of psychiatric illness, however, the classes represented a consensus among observers who used different texts, idiosyncratic personal clinical experiences, and different psychological and pharmacologic theories as guidelines. For some disorders, a Kraepelinian template can be recognized (e.g., the schizophrenia criteria); for others, a psychological template is apparent (e.g., dissociative disorders). The committees represented diverse constituencies and the final formulations were designed to be accepted by the average psychiatrist who would vote it up or down in an American Psychiatric Association election.[46] Within a few years, dissatisfaction with the classification called for revisions (DSM-IIIR) in 1987 and in 1994 (DSM-IV).[47]

Melancholia was ignored as each revision added new categories in response to the needs of different practitioner groups. In the first DSM classification, four different depressive reactions were identified, with four subtypes for "affective reactions." In the 1968 version, two additional subtypes were added. By 1980, four major mood disorders were identified, with 10 subtypes. For major depression, an additional three subtypes were listed. "Melancholia" could still be specified as either present or absent for major depression but was not recognized as a specific disorder. As the core disorder of mood, the DSM-III commission offered a single concept of "major depression" (with descriptors of single episode or recurrent) and with the variant *bipolar depression* (with mixed, manic, and depressed variants). *Depressive disorder not otherwise specified* and *abnormal bereavement* were two additional entities. *Psychosis* became a specifier of mood disorders. A syndrome of "dysthymia" was revived.[48] The concepts of melancholia, melancholic depression, and involutional depression were discarded.[49]

Bipolar disorder was distinguished as a separate class by the occurrence of excitement, distractibility, agitation, and talkativeness in the patient's life history. Parallel to the subtyping in the DSM category of major depression, the bipolar disorders were divided into *bipolar I* with a *single manic episode* (with more recent episode *mixed* or *depressed* or *unspecified*), *bipolar II (with hypomanic but not manic episodes)*, and *cyclothymic disorder.*[50] The list of specifiers is similar to those in the major depressive category, with the addition of *rapid cycling.*

The new classification and specific criteria were quickly challenged by clinicians who could not fit their patients within the defined categories. In response, new diagnostic classes were included in the 1987 revision (DSM-IIIR) and again in the 1994 iteration (DSM-IV).[51] The number of recognized diagnostic entities dramatically increased. The episodic nature of emotional illnesses was recognized in the definition of *major depressive, manic, mixed,* and *hypomanic episodes* that were combined into *major depressive disorder* (either *single* or *recurrent*), and further divided by the specifiers of *chronic* and *severity/psychotic/remission* and by the features of *catatonia, melancholia, atypical,* or *postpartum onset.* To the recurrent disorders, two additional specifiers of *course* and *seasonal pattern* were offered.

This extended list of diagnoses was still considered insufficient. Clinicians labeled variations in the duration of the illness, its seasonal features, differential response to medication, and mixtures of psychopathology as *seasonal affective disorder, atypical depression, double depression, brief recurrent depression,* and *endogenomorphic depression.*[52] Mood disorders were separated by assumed precipitants and labeled major depression following childbirth (*postpartum depression*), in menopause (*invonal depression*), with aging (*geriatric depression*), and after the loss of a loved one (*abnormal bereavement*). The labels were offered as if the psychopathology, course, outcome, or treatment of the condition was differentiable from other depressive disorders. In clinical practice, however, these situational precipitants do not define the presentation of the illness, the response to treatments, or the endocrine markers.[53]

The limitations of the present DSM classification are well recognized. The DSM-V iteration planned for the years 2007–2010 seeks a basis in experimental studies of genetic, neuroanatomic, neuroimaging, developmental science, and family criteria.[54] Whether the neurosciences will offer sufficient data to define a more useful classification is unpredictable.

Instead of looking to an unsure future classification based on models and studies yet to be reported, there is merit in a simplified classification of the mood disorders based on the classical principles of clinically defined signs and symptoms and course of illness, as offered by nineteenth-century psychopathologists. The psychodynamic and psychopharmacologic interruptions are false trails, misjudgments in the development of a psychiatric science that were attractive for a time. In addition to clinical criteria, biological treatments are remarkably effective and they may be used to define diagnostic criteria. Some laboratory tests hold promise for supplementing treatment response. To redress the present false trail on which psychiatric classification is embarked, a single image of depressive mood disorders is parsimonious. *Melancholia,* recognized as a central theme of depressive illness throughout much of medical history, provides the standard on which to judge mood disorder.

NOTES

1 Styron (1990), pp. 36–7.
2 Wallace (1994); American Psychiatric Association (1980, 1994).
3 Parker (2000).
4 Osler, Wm. Cited among aphorisms. See: http://www.vh.org/adult/provider/history/osler/5.html.
5 Sadler *et al.* (1994).
6 The evidence for these conclusions is detailed in subsequent chapters.
7 Beck *et al.* (1977).
8 Adams (1939), *The Sacred Disease*, p. 344. Hippocrates describes a patient:

> In Thasus, a woman, of a melancholic turn of mind, from some accidental cause of sorrow, while still going about, became affected with loss of sleep, aversion of food and had thirst and nausea . . . On the first, at the commencement of night, frights, much talking, despondency, slight fever; in the morning frequent spasms, and when they ceased, she was incoherent and talked obscurely; pains frequent, great, and continued. On the second, in the same state; had no sleep; fever more acute. On the third, the spasms left her, but coma, and disposition to sleep, and again awaked, started up, and could not contain herself; much incoherence; acute fever; on that night a copious sweat all over; apyrexia, slept, quite collected; had a crisis. About the third day . . . a copious menstruation (*The Epidemics*, p. 346–7.)

Hippocrates offers treatments such as abstaining from all excesses, a vegetable diet, exercise short of fatigue, sexual abstinence, and bleeding, if necessary.

9 Mathews M. Theories of depression before the 20th century. http://www.priory.com/homol/dephist.htm
10 Zilboorg (1941).
11 Middle Eastern physicians such as Avicenna (980–1037 CE) recognized melancholia as a brain disease and not due to the influence of the supernatural (Jackson, 1986, pp. 62–4).
12 Bright (1586). See Hunter and Macalpine (1982), pp. 36–40.
13 Burton's scholarly work is encyclopedic, describing many forms of the illness. It was often reprinted and is now considered a literary classic. Burton was himself a sufferer. For a delightful frontispiece of Burton's fourth edition, see Hunter and Macalpine (1982), p. 99. A reprint of the three volumes, published in 1932, was recently published by the *New York Review of Books* and also a fully annotated six-volume series by Oxford University Press (Rosen, 2005).
14 Hunter and Macalpine (1982), pp. 241–3. For a detailed description of psychotherapy recommended for this condition, see Timothy Rogers (1691), *ibid.* pp. 248–51. For a description of the use of opium for melancholia, see George Young (1753), *ibid.* pp. 395–8.
15 Ascribed to Vogel (1772) by Lewis (1934a).
16 Pinel (1806).
17 Melancholia is "a chronic afebrile, brooding delirium fixed on a small number of objects" Boissier de Sauvages, quoted by Lewis, 1934a, p. 6.
18 From Haslam's *Observations on Madness and Melancholy*, quoted by Shorter (2005), pp. 36–7.
19 Portions of Falret's book are translated by Sedler (1983). Falret's description of *la folie circulaire* is acknowledged by Kraepelin in his formulation of manic-depressive insanity. A circular insanity was recognized by many authors, including Baillerger (*la folie à double*

forme), Neftel (periodical melancholia), Lange (periodic psychic depression), Kahlbaum (cyclothymia), and Hecker (cyclothymia). The separation of depressed and manic disorders is a feature of modern classification.

20 Sedler (1983), p. 1131.

21 Engstrom (2003).

22 Shorter (2005).

23 The concept of an *Einheitspsychose* became the basis for a popular school of psychiatric thought that was developed by writers such as Joseph Guislain and Wilhelm Griesinger. Ewald Hecker supported a more diverse classification based on course of the illness and Karl Kahlbaum elaborated a Linnean classification of disorders based on clinical description and course (van Renynghe de Voxvrie, 1993; Shorter, 1997; Engstrom, 2003).

24 Kraepelin (1896, 1921).

25 As quoted by Jackson (1986; pp. 191–2), Kraepelin divided the depressive states:

> *the mildest form of depression . . . without either hallucinations or prominent delusions. The onset is generally gradual . . . mental sluggishness, thought becomes difficult [as does] coming to a decision or expressing themselves. . . . The process of association of ideas is remarkably retarded . . . they have nothing to say; there is a dearth of ideas and a poverty of thought. . . It is hard to remember most commonplace things. They appear dull and sluggish, and explain that they really feel tired and exhausted. . . The patient only sees the dark side of life. They are unsuited to their environment; are a failure in their profession; have lost religious faith . . . express a desire to end their existence.*

26 Gillespie (1926, 1929).

27 Mapother (1926), Lewis (1934a).

28 Quotation is from page 1. In 1934 Lewis reviewed the records of 61 patients admitted to the Maudsley Hospital in 1928 and 1929 who met his understanding of melancholia (Lewis, 1934a). These "pure" examples of a well-defined illness met the professional consensus of that era as to diagnosis and course. Effective treatment was unavailable, and Lewis could not know that insulin coma and induced seizures had been described in Vienna and Budapest in 1933 and 1934. The phenomenology offered by Lewis is cited in Chapter 2.

29 Hopewell-Ash (1934), pp. 1–2. His descriptions of the many varieties of melancholia are discussed in Chapter 5.

30 Hill (1968). Quotation, p. 455.

31 The most dedicated followers of Freud writing about melancholia were Karl Abraham, Sandor Rado, Otto Fenichel, Grete Bibring, and Melanie Klein.

32 Abraham (1927); Freud (1984).

33 Quoted by Jackson (1986); pp. 197–8.

34 Quoted by Jackson (1986); p. 198.

35 American Psychiatric Association, 1952. The formulation was modified in 1965 as DSM-II.

36 Kraepelin (1918); Kraepelin (1896); Duffy (1995); Pressman (1998); Braslow (1997); Shorter (1997); Porter (2002).

37 The conflicts between the psychodynamic and the biological views of psychiatric disorders were outspoken. The attacks by the Group for the Advancement of Psychiatry on convulsive therapy set the stage for public stigmatization of the somatic treatments. For a detailed history of these conflicts see Ottosson and Fink (2004); Fink (1979, 1999a); and Shorter and Healy (in preparation).

38 *Vital depression* and *personal depression* were descriptive replacement terms for endogenous and reactive depression. The defining characteristic of vital depression was its inexplicable

onset. The patient may not necessarily feel sad, but rather physically dragged down. Vital depression was proposed as an endogenous illness, in contrast to a reactive form.

Shorter (2005) considers the term endogenous as borrowed from the eighth edition of Kraepelin's textbook in 1913, where it was used as a qualifier for dementia praecox (schizophrenia). Endogenous depression represented a disturbance of the body's "vital" feelings. "In such a feeling we grasp life itself, and in this feeling something is imparted to us: ascent, decline, health, illness, [and] danger." Endogenous depressions, therefore, were unprovoked or autonomous disorders of vital feelings; reactive depressions were mental disorders caused by situational problems. Endogenous depressions were characterized by disturbances of the body's physical functions, such as diurnal variation (feeling worse in the morning), loss of weight, and irregularities in menstruation. Vital depression and endogenous depression were synonymous.

"Primary vs. secondary" depression: dividing affective disorders (depression and mania) into primary and secondary forms – "primary" meaning patients with no previous history of psychiatric illness, and "secondary" patients who had "a preexisting, diagnosable psychiatric illness, other than a previous primary affective disorder"– was suggested by the Faculty of Washington University Department of Psychiatry in the 1970s (Robins and Guze, 1972; Woodruff *et al.*, 1974).

"Vegetative" depression associated affective disorders with autonomic disturbances characterized by an anxious-depressed mood and autonomic symptoms.

Atypical depression, a subset of depressive patients who responded to the drug iproniazid (Marsilid), an inhibitor of brain monoamine oxidase, was identified. The subset did not have the classic picture of endogenous depression, with self-reproaches and early-morning worsening, but rather were highly anxious, phobic, and greatly fatigued. These patients "may . . . have become bad tempered, irritable, hyperreactive and aggressive, quite unlike so many of the more endogenously depressed patients." Sargant's work represents one of the first attempts to identify a class of depression patients differentially responsive to a given medication. Marsilid was subsequently withdrawn from market as toxic and usage of the concept lapsed.

The concept of atypical depression was revived by a group at Columbia University. They described the patients as dysphoric, mood-reactive, with symptoms such as overeating, gaining weight, oversleeping, sensation of leaden fatigue, and taking rejection poorly. They were thought to respond to monoamine oxidase inhibitors. Atypical depression was accepted as an official psychiatric diagnosis ("atypical features specifier") in DSM-IV (American Psychiatirc Assocation, 1994).

Endogenomorphic depression was proposed by Klein (1974) to cut across the reactive versus endogenous distinction in depression nosology. Although the diagnosis was not adopted in DSM-III, the loss of interest and of pleasure were considered the core criteria of this depressive mood disorder and anhedonia was accepted as a mood state equivalent to depressed mood.

Anxious thymopathy was formulated by López Ibor (1950-: *La Angustia Vital*: (*Patologia General Psicosomatica*)), who argued that anxiety and anguish represented an autonomous disease of an "endogenous" nature; anxious thymopathy possessed deeply somatic roots and was not at all psychogenic.

39 It was early in the psychoactive drug era and the medicines were considered "research treatments." All patients referred for medication were randomly assigned to the three treatment regimens regardless of the dominant psychopathology. All medicines were administered in a liquid formulation that contained 75, 150, 225, or 300 mg imipramine;

300, 600, 900, or 1200 mg chlorpromazine with appropriate doses of the antiparkinson agent procyclidine, or no active psychoactive substance (placebo). Neither the patients nor the assessors knew which medication was being administered. Trials were for 6 weeks with weekly increments in dosing. The first study, completed in 1961, included 152 patients. Klein replicated the study in a second population (Klein, 1967).

40 The studies confirmed imipramine as an antidepressant and chlorpromazine as an antipsychotic (Klein and Fink, 1962a, b; Fink *et al.*, 1965; Klein, 1967). That phobia was relieved by imipramine was a specific finding that has encouraged the present use of selective serotonin reuptake inhibitors for this illness (Klein and Fink, 1962a ; Klein, 1964). The finding that chlorpromazine was an effective antidepressant heralded the recognition of psychotic depression (Klein and Fink, 1962b). Imipramine worsened the psychosis of adolescent psychotic patients (Klein and Fink, 1962a; Pollack *et al.*, 1965).

41 Klerman (1971), Klein (1974), and Paykel (1975) are a few of the active writers who offered different solutions to the diagnostic dilemmas. The frustrations among the psychopharmacologists are documented in their interviews, annotated by Healy (1996, 1998, 2000), also in his *The Anti-Depressant Era* (1997) and *The Creation of Psychopharmacology* (2002). Additional personal essays by psychopharmacologists are presented in the biennial volumes of the history of the Collegium Internationale Neuropsychopharmacologicum (CINP) published by Ban *et al.* in 1998, 2000, 2002, and 2004.

42 Nelson and Charney (1981).

43 Sandifer *et al.* (1969); Spitzer and Fleiss (1974); Robins and Barrett (1989).

44 Feighner *et al.* (1972); Spitzer *et al.* (1978); Meier (1979); Overall and Hollister (1979).

45 American Psychiatric Association (1980). DSM-III lists 265 disorders. The number is increased in DSM-IIIR to 292 and in DSM-IV to 295 (Shorter, 1997, p. 303).

46 The vote was taken by its membership prior to the May 1979 annual American Psychiatric Association meeting. As with many bills enacted in the USA congress, few of the voters had read the proposal in detail.

47 A planned revision of DSM-V is in progress.

48 DSM-III offers "major depression" as the principal depressive syndrome and revives "dysthymia" (1980). Among the many disorders to be reconfigured were the depression diagnoses ("affective disorders") in a manner sharply different from the RDC of 1978. DSM-III created three new disease labels in the mood area: (1) "major depression" (anticipated in 1978), which was a mixture of psychotic and non-psychotic depressive conditions; (2) "dysthymic disorder," which was a new label for what had been known as "neurotic depression"; and (3) "adjustment disorder with depressed mood" for minor depressions supposedly treatable with psychotherapy alone.

Manic-depressive illness, for which the DSM drafters adopted Karl Kleist's label "*bipolar disorder*": the Kahlbaum label "cyclothymic disorder" was adopted for less serious manic-depressive illness. To meet the criteria for major depressive episode, the patient had to have a dysphoric mood for a certain period of time plus four of a list of eight other criteria that included poor appetite, insomnia, and loss of pleasure in formerly pleasurable activities.

Dysthymia was a term devised as a replacement for melancholia by Carl F. Flemming in 1844. It was used by Kahlbaum to distinguish a systemic depressive disorder that seems to meet modern descriptions of endogenous depression (Shorter, 2005). Dysthymia was out of fashion until revived in DSM-III as equivalent for depressive neurosis, i.e., a low-grade chronic depressive illness.

49 The formulations are almost wholly based on the clinical experiences of committee members, not on experimental studies. The formulations are imprecise, the overlaps great, and the classification was not associated with any objective test. See Chapters 3, 6, and 15 for discussions of DSM criteria.

50 Clinicians have added additional varieties of bipolar disorder as bipolar spectrum prototypes I, II, III, and IV (Akiskal and Pinto, 1999).

51 American Psychiatric Association (1994).

52 *Double depression* is the overlapping of two depression categories in RDC – a major depressive disorder superimposed on an underlying chronic depression ("dysthymic disorder"). The prognosis for patients with double depression is considered worse than for those with major depression alone.

Seasonal affective disorder (SAD) (1984) was postulated as a depressive mood disorder that routinely worsened in the winter months. Treatment with bright light was proposed. The concept was incorporated in DSM-IIIR in 1987 as a "specifier" for major depression and for bipolar disorder defined as "a regular cyclic relationship between onset of the mood episodes and a particular 60-day period of the year," especially the time from early October to late November. It is retained in DSM-IV.

Recurrent, brief depression (1985). In the context of a longitudinal study of a cohort of young adults in Zurich, Angst realized that many of the patients suffered recurrent bouts of depression too brief to qualify as "major depression" or "dysthymia" in DSM terminology. Angst (1985). proposed the diagnosis of "recurrent, brief depression" (RBD) as a subtype of affective disorder. No characteristics were specified except the timing.

53 The number of published "expert" treatment algorithms have increased markedly in the past decade. The most frequently cited are the *Practice Guidelines* endorsed by committees of the American Psychiatric Association, the Texas Medication Algorithm Project (TMAP), and an expert consensus panel of the *Journal of Clinical Psychiatry.* These projects recognize two forms of depressive mood disorder (with or without psychosis) and bipolar disorder in adults. Individual guidelines have been formulated for other psychiatric disorders (schizophrenia, substance dependence, dementia, delirium, and panic disorder). The available evidence for treatment efficacy is reviewed and the guidelines formulated by consensus. The hierarchies of treatments are idiosyncratic. Four of the algorithms are under multisite studies under National Institute of Mental Health contracts.

54 Helzer and Hudziak (2002); Kupfer *et al.* (2002).

2

Melancholia defined

Melancholy

*(**n.**) - c.1303, "condition characterized by sullenness, gloom, irritability," from O.Fr. melancholie, from L. L. melancholia, from Gk. melankholia "sadness," lit. "black bile," from melas (gen. melanos) "black" (see melanin) + khole "bile."*

Medieval physiology attributed depression to excess of "black bile," a secretion of the spleen and one of the body's four "humors."

***Adj.** sense of "sullen, gloomy" is from 1526; sense of "deplorable" (of a fact or state of things) is from 1710.*[1]

The precision of medical diagnostic terms is essential to establish the reliability and validity of proposed disease states. While the term "depression" is widely used in society, its meaning varies with the user, an attitude best expressed by *Alice in Wonderland's* Humpty-Dumpty, "When I use a word, it means just what I choose it to mean – neither more nor less."[2] In psychology, depression represents a decrease in psychomotor activity or intellectual agility. Within neurophysiology, depression refers to a decrease in the brain's functioning, measured in electrical activity or cerebral blood flow. For the pharmacologist, depression means the decrease in body functions induced by sedatives, soporifics, and anesthetics. In clinical practice, depression describes a normal human emotion, a pathologic state if it is retained too long or too deeply, or a psychopathologic syndrome that may be mild or severe. A clinical depressive episode may be defined by its associated adverse life events or it may strike a subject without cause.[3] Accepting "depression" as a medical diagnosis is equivalent to accepting "infection" as a definitive diagnostic term in clinical medicine.[4]

"Melancholia" has a more precise meaning. As a central organizing model of mood disorder, melancholia is *a recurrent, debilitating, pervasive brain disorder that alters mood, motor functions, thinking, cognition, perception and many basic physiologic processes.*

Pathological mood is expressed as pervasive and unremitting apprehension and gloom that colors all cognitive processes, resulting in a loss of interest, decreased concentration, poor memory, slowed thinking, feelings of failure and low self-worth, and thoughts of suicide. Regardless of antecedent events, whether a personal loss or a

Table 2.1. Melancholia syndromes as commonly labeled in present classifications

Manic-depressive illness
Melancholic "major" depression (unipolar depression)
Manic-depressive depression (bipolar depression)
Psychotic depression
Catatonic and stuporous depression
Puerperal depression
Abnormal bereavement

general medical illness, a persistent and unrelieved feeling of gloom is essential to the diagnosis.

Psychomotor disturbance, either as retardation or agitation, is the second characteristic.[5] Retardation varies from a reluctance and hesitation to participate in daily activities, to prolonged inactivity that is so severe as to be labeled a stupor simulating death.[6] Agitation appears as restlessness, hand-wringing, and inability to remain still. It may be expressed as pacing and continuous movement progressing to purposeless activity so severe that it has been described as furor or frenzy.

Vegetative functions are severely affected. Sleep is disrupted, appetite and weight lost, sex no longer arouses interest, and the response to stress and chronobiologic functioning are disturbed. Patients describe these changes as beyond their understanding or control, or the signs of illness are obvious in a loss of weight, unkempt appearance, body odor, and haggard look. Neuroendocrine dysfunctions are identified in laboratory studies.[7]

Psychosis is recognized when the disorder is severe and occurs in over 30% of melancholic patients.[8] Like psychomotor dysfunction, it is an integral part of melancholia.[9] Melancholic patients are preoccupied with thoughts of guilt, worthlessness, and helplessness, often so severely distorted and exaggerated as to dominate daily living.

Melancholia is a well-defined clinical picture that can be honed by laboratory tests, course of illness, and treatment response.[10] Understanding the many putative mood disorders in the present classification as they relate to melancholia offers an opportunity to define a common biology and to simplify and improve therapeutics. A revival of the concept of a single manic-depressive illness with the depressed phase recognized as "melancholia" is also parsimonious and best fits the evidence. From this perspective, many of the disorders of mood that are described in psychiatric classifications can be considered melancholic illness (Table 2.1). The mood disorders that do not meet the definition of melancholia are discussed in Chapter 6.

Descriptions of individual patients with a depressive mood disorder offer rich imagery of the patients who meet the criteria for melancholia. The vignettes from Hopewell-Ash's *Melancholia in Everyday Practice* (1934) offer pictures before the present psychiatric classifications and modern therapies evolved.[11]

Patient 2.1

An unmarried woman, aged 38. Independent and socially well situated. Chief symptoms: Depression, insomnia, slowness of mental and physical reaction, with great reluctance to carry out even the simplest occupations, for example, writing letters. Associated obsessing and "anxious thoughts." Morbid ideas of unworthyness in regard to the man she had been going to marry; on account of this had broken off her engagement. There had been a previous attack of depression lasting some months. The severe depression, psychomotor retardation [were] completed on the physical side by indigestion, constipation and melancholic expression. Recovered.[12]

Patient 2.2

Unmarried woman, age 39. Independent. Very strict Calvinist religious training. History of several minor attacks of depression. Had become very depressed with onset of early menopausal symptoms associated with anxiety and some agitation; much obsessed by ideas of dereliction of duty, questions of conscience and religious salvation. On various occasions wrote: "I am not ungrateful for all the help you have given me; but there is nothing but blankness and darkness and less and less strength to meet it with. I wish I could end it all, but the fear of death and eternity would be still worse." . . . After several attacks of profound depression following quickly one on the other without definite recovery this patient returned to normality.[13]

Patient 2.3

A middle-aged clergyman. Crisis of depression; melancholia, "suicidal feelings." There was a history of some two years increasing mental depression. The present crisis arose because he had suddenly left home and travelled a long way to relatives with the object of "obtaining peace." Described himself as "an agonized atom through an utterly incomprehensible and torturing universe." There was some improvement under treatment [suggestion] and a few days later patient said he felt "like a person who has crawled out of a morass and is lying on the brink." . . . He appeared much brighter and better. He came to see me unaccompanied . . . but instead of going home he went to a station and took a train to –, where he wandered about and eventually gave himself up to the police. He had sent postcards to his friends and one to me which read: "I am tormented by evil spirits and must flee them. You will never see me again. Your most unfortunate patient." However, he was brought back by friends and found to be depressed. Recovery was slow.[14]

Patient 2.4

An acute crisis of melancholia, involutional type, is exemplified here, the patient suffering from a combination of agitated excitement with depression . . . although there was excitement the affective tone was depressive and . . . not the least elated or exalted. She was a married woman, aged 52, mentally depressed and very reticent. "What is really wrong with me is that I am mad." . . . Four days afterwards the patient became uncontrollable "bellowing like a bull, banging her head on the wall and generally uncontrollable." She was treated with hyoscine and Nembutal (pentobarbital) which resulted in a deep sleep of several hours duration with a subsequently calm night . . . The next day she was mildly excited, asking to be sent to a lunatic asylum and potentially suicidal.[15]

The recent literature has equally compelling descriptions. In a memoir of his illness, the novelist William Styron offers a poignant description of melancholia.[16] After depending on alcohol "as a conduit to fantasy and euphoria, and to the enhancement of the imagination" for more than 40 years, he was suddenly unable to drink without experiencing nausea, "wooziness," and epigastric distress. He slowly became melancholic. At first he experienced malaise; the shadows of nightfall seemed more somber, the mornings less buoyant. Insomnia and a host of bodily fears followed and everything "slowed down." He became suicidal, explaining that: "The pain of severe depression is quite unimaginable to those who have not suffered it, and it kills in many instances because its anguish can no longer be borne."[17] Frightened of these thoughts, he turned to a hospital for asylum. Its protection and the support of antidepressant medication and of friends allowed him to heal slowly; he avers that the protection served him well.

A physician describes his experience with melancholia:[18]

> Depressive illness is probably more unpleasant than any disease except rabies. There is constant mental pain and often psychogenic physical pain too. If one tries to get such a patient to titrate other pains against the pain of his depression one tends to end up with a description that would raise eyebrows even in a medieval torture chamber. Naturally, many of these patients commit suicide. They may not hope to get to heaven but they know they are leaving hell. Secondly, the patient is isolated from family and friends, because the depression itself reduces his affection for others and he may well have ideas that he is unworthy of their love or even that his friendship may harm them. Thirdly, he is rejected by others because they cannot stand the sight of his suffering . . . Fourthly, the patient tends to do a great cover-up . . . he does not tell others how bad he feels.

Additional vignettes of melancholic patients are to be found in Chapter 8 (patients 8.1, 8.3, 8.6–8.8).[19]

Manic-depressive illness

In psychiatric classifications today, mood disorders are divided along the faultline of the presence or absence of manic or hypomanic periods in the patient's personal history. The 1980 *Diagnostic and Statistical Manual* (DSM) classification recognized a disorder of depressed mood as a *major depression*. The presence of mania or hypomania, either in the examination or in the history, categorized the illness as a *bipolar disorder*.

In the seesaw of psychiatric history, the mood disorders were seen either as two disorders or as a single entity. Defining the intimate connection between depression and mania is usually ascribed to the French authors Falret (1854) and Baillerger (1854), who described patients with both disorders at different times in their illness.[20] Karl Kahlbaum (1882) applied the term *cyclothymia* to a syndrome of circular disorders of excitement and depression that did not end in dementia.[21] The concept was adopted by Kraepelin (1921) when he differentiated manic-depressive illness from that of dementia praecox. In Kraepelin's view, the moods in manic-depressive illness included:

certain slight and slightest colouring of *mood*, some of them periodic, some of them continuously morbid, which are to be regarded as the rudiment of more severe disorders . . . [or] pass without sharp boundary into *personal predisposition* . . . I have become more and more convinced that [manic-depressive] states represent manifestations of a *single morbid process*.[22]

The groundwork for splitting manic-depressive illness into bipolar and unipolar disorders was laid by Leonhard (1995). In family studies he described patients suffering an endogenous illness with a history of mania who had a higher than expected prevalence of relatives with mania (labeled *bipolar* illness). These patients were distinguished from patients and their families with depressive illnesses only (*monopolar* illness). The binary model was quickly supported by family history studies.[23] It was incorporated in the DSM-III classification.

This change in nosology encouraged the elaboration of new subtypes of bipolar disorder. Hospitalized depressed patients were divided into those with a history of mania and those who experienced hypomania into *bipolar I* and *bipolar II* groups.[24] Unipolar depressed patients were divided into *familial pure depressive disease, sporadic pure depressive disease*, and *depressive spectrum disease* based on the family history of alcoholism and antisocial personality.[25] Additional variants were proposed in studies of less severely ill patients using criteria of family histories and statistical analyses of rating-scale items.[26]

The argument to classify unipolar and bipolar depression separately was challenged by Taylor and Abrams, first in literature reviews and then in a prospective clinical study of hospitalized, acutely ill patients with mood disorders and their first-degree relatives.[27] The family illness patterns were not clearly dichotomous. The most common mood disorder in the first-degree relatives of patients with bipolar disorder was recurrent depressive illness (unipolar disorder). The morbid risk (age-corrected prevalence) for unipolar disorder in the families of the bipolar patients was greater than the morbid risks for unipolar depression in the families of unipolar patients. The authors reviewed reports of mixed concordance for the two forms of mood disorder in twins, concluding that they could not distinguish the unipolar and bipolar patients by any family, psychopathological, treatment response or laboratory variable *as long as depression was defined as melancholia*. They could not justify separating mood disorders by the presence of mania or hypomania, or by the clinical features of depression.

In another detailed analysis, Goodwin and Jamison (1990) examined the course, epidemiology, family history, physiological measures, and similar criteria for the unipolar and bipolar forms of depression. These are assessed as either "less" or "more," "younger" or "older," "lower" or "higher" and other descriptive, non-quantitative differences.[28] Similar qualitative factors assess the incidence of the clinical signs of anxiety, anger, psychomotor agitation, mood lability, sleep time, pain sensitivity with the items rated as unipolar > bipolar or unipolar < bipolar.[29] Even in the absence of defined criteria these authors conclude:[30]

Despite the heterogeneity in both the bipolar and unipolar groups, the breadth of reported bipolar–unipolar differences is impressive. They include four separate spheres of data – genetic, clinical, biological and pharmacological. Bipolar and recurrent unipolar disorders, nevertheless, appear to be very similar in some important respects (e.g., prophylactic response to lithium). Taken together, the data suggest that they are best considered as two subgroups of manic-depressive illness rather than separate and distinct illnesses. The available data also support a continuum model, with "pure" bipolar illness at one end and unipolar illness at the other.

Clinical studies of the bipolar–unipolar dichotomy

In the 15 years since the Goodwin and Jamison review, the separation of unipolar and bipolar depression has been increasingly questioned, and the difficulty in separating mood disorder patients into two clusters is exemplified by evidence of frequent misclassification. A review of the records of 48 patients identified as having bipolar disorder and 4 patients considered schizoaffective disorder (bipolar type) found that 40% (19/48) were previously diagnosed with a unipolar major depressive disorder.[31] An average of 7.5 years elapsed before the patients were relabeled as suffering from bipolar disorder. Over the course of illness, depression was the predominant mood disturbance found in a literature review assessing the incidence of depressive phases of patients with bipolar disorder.[32] The authors concluded that the label of bipolar disorder is more often associated with psychosis, melancholia, psychomotor retardation, "atypical" symptoms, and higher suicide rates, and that the depressed phase is the major contributor to the disability in this illness. This understanding follows the conclusion by Taylor and Abrams (1980; Taylor *et al.*, 1980) that mood disorders should be separated by the presence or absence of melancholia and not by the presence of mania or hypomania.

Psychopathologic studies of unipolar and bipolar disorder are rife, with overlaps in psychopathology, course of illness, and family illness. An examination of patients with rapid-cycling mood disorder found major depression in 85% and salient manic features were identified in at least half the patients with recurrent depression.[33] An assessment of depressive features in 36 patients with bipolar disorder and 37 patients with unipolar major depressive disorder was unable to separate the two groups.[34] The authors concluded that "bipolar disorder is characterized by some depressive features less likely to be found in unipolar depression," but that otherwise the two conditions are alike. In yet another study, a sample of 313 patients with bipolar I disorder with an index episode of depression, signs of agitated depression were readily identified in 61 (20%) as the only distinction from recurrent depressive illness.[35]

A prospective longitudinal study of 86 patients with the bipolar II designation re-examined patients at 6- and 12-month intervals over a mean course of 13.4 years.[36] The patients were symptomatic in 53.9% of all follow-up weeks. Depressive symptoms occurred in 50.3% of the weeks and dominated over hypomanic symptoms (1.3% of weeks) and over cycling or mixed symptoms (2.3% of weeks). The authors note that bipolar II, like bipolar I and unipolar depression, is a chronic longitudinal illness with the modal expression dominated by depressive symptoms. They conclude that "longitudinally, BP-II is a chronic affective disorder expressed within each patient as a fluctuating dimensional symptomatic continuum, which includes the full severity range of depressive and hypomanic symptoms, but dominated primarily by minor and subsyndromal depression."[37] Examining the impact of treatments on the course of the illness, the authors note:

> that symptomatic chronicity occurred even in the context of relatively more (rather than less) medication therapy leads us to conclude that we are describing the true naturalistic expression of BP-II as it unfolds across the life cycle.

The same conclusion of a singularity of manic-depressive illness is described in numerous reports by Angst, Benazzi, and Akiskal.[38] In one study, two distinct mixed types of mania and depression were identified in the more severely ill hospitalized patients.[39] Overlaps in criteria for the subtypes of bipolar disorder are reported. A distinct *bipolar II* disorder was not supported in a sample of 194 *bipolar II* outpatients.[40] Examining the criteria of psychomotor agitation or psychomotor retardation, agitation was more common in *bipolar II* patients and retardation more common in *bipolar I* outpatients, a distinction of weak significance.[41] Patients meeting criteria for *bipolar II* had more atypical features and more evidence of depressive mixed states than those meeting criteria for *major depressive disorder*, leading the author to conclude: "*finding no zones of rarity supports a continuity between BPII and MDD (meaning partly overlapping disorders without clear boundaries.)*" Other iterations of these failures to support a bimodal model are reported.[42]

In yet another study seeking to reinforce the image of a bipolar mixed state to encompass psychotic agitated depression, 336 outpatients with major depressive episodes without a history of mania were identified.[43] Based on evidence of hypomania, 206 were assigned to *bipolar II* and 130 to *major depressive disorder*. The investigators found numerous permutations of major depressive episodes in the bipolar I patients and concluded that bipolar depression is melancholia:

> Agitated depression is validated as a dysphorically excited form of melancholia, which should tip clinicians to think of such a patient belonging to or arising from a bipolar substrate. Our data support the Kraepelinian position . . .

Other investigators have had similar difficulties in supporting a mood disorder dichotomy. In a sample of 117 subjects with *recurrent unipolar depression* and 106 with *bipolar I* disorder, the authors of a large multisite Italian study identified those who had achieved partial or complete remission of their index episode.[44] They assessed 140 items in an extensive psychopathology interview and could not distinguish two groups in the distribution of the overall scores or in the number or severity of depressive or manic items. Paranoid ideation, auditory hallucinations, and suicide attempts were, however, more common in the lifetime experience of patients defined as *bipolar I*.[45] The authors discuss their experience:

> Cumulatively our empirical findings support a continuous view of the mood spectrum as a unitary phenomenon that is best understood from a longitudinal perspective. Our data suggest that unipolar disorder and bipolar disorder are not two discrete and dichotomous phenomena but that mood fluctuations – up and down – are common to both conditions . . .[46]

Considering the extent of the studies seeking a distinction between unipolar depression and the two subtypes of bipolar depression, the two disorders are best considered variations of a single disorder. Patient 2.5 meets criteria for bipolar disorder.

Patient 2.5[47]

A typical cyclical psychosis in a married woman aged about 55, with alternating phases of melancholia and excitement lasting approximately six months over a number of years. The story was always the same; after six months occupation in "having a really good time" which included an endless round of social engagements and great popularity, patient suddenly "felt ill" and then within a few days became "livery" and depressed. The crisis intensified . . . and the patient complains of indigestions and burning pains above the epigastrium, easily nauseated. Very depressed, especially in the mornings. Much worried about her "inside" . . . slow motion very conspicuous.

Antidepressant drug-induced mania[48]

The induction of mania by antidepressant treatments is often cited as support for a mood disorder dichotomy. When tricyclic antidepressants (TCAs) and monoamine oxidase inhibitors (MAOIs) were introduced, concepts of unipolar and bipolar depression were not in use, so that the treatment was offered to all patients who met criteria for a depressive episode. Manic episodes that appeared during the course of treatment were interpreted as a medication side-effect. The reports did not recognize a personal history of mania nor cycling into mania as natural features of a depressive mood disorder. No direct experimental studies of this effect were offered. After reviewing the literature of induced mania with antidepressant treatments, Goodwin and Jamison (1990) concluded:

> In summary, absolutely incontrovertible evidence of antidepressant induced mania and cyclic induction is still lacking . . . The available evidence strongly suggests, however, that antidepressant drugs can precipitate mania in some bipolar-I patients, especially those who respond to antidepressants, and that some bipolar-II patients appear to be vulnerable to hypomania while taking antidepressants. Although antidepressant-induced rapid cycling does occur in some patients, its frequency is not easy to determine, and therefore, the generalizability of the observation is unclear.[49]

Since that review, little new evidence has been published. Assessments of the incidence of manic episodes in patients with depression offer the conclusion that 10–15% will have a manic or hypomanic episode in the next decade.[50] The reports recognize that the patients most likely to do so have a history of depressive disorders early in life or an initial psychotic depression or melancholia.[51] Cross-sectional clinical features do not distinguish a first recurrent depression from the initial depression in a manic-depressive course.[52] A review of the databases of several pharmaceutical companies reported that the switch in unipolar patients was 11.2% for TCA, 3.7% for selective serotonin reuptake inhibitors (SSRIs), and 4.2% for placebo.[53]

The Stanley Foundation bipolar network assessed the spontaneous and treatment-associated switch rates in patients with bipolar depression.[54] In a group of 258 outpatients examined for 1 year, the number of days depressed was three times greater than the number of days manic. In a second study, 127 bipolar depressed patients were randomized to 10 weeks of augmentation of mood stabilizers with the non-TCAs bupropion, sertraline, or venlafaxine. They reported that 9.1% were associated with switches to hypomania. In 73 continuation-phase antidepressant trials, 16–19% were associated with manic and hypomanic switches. Despite the low switch rates that did not exceed natural switch rates in manic-depressive patients, the authors conclude that depression and depressive cycling are a substantial problem in intensively treated bipolar outpatients.

A consequence of the belief in the risks of antidepressant drugs is the intensive search for alternative treatments for bipolar depression. While the efficacy of lithium for the manic phase is established, its merits as an antidepressant received mixed reviews.[55] The introduction of carbamazepine for mania encouraged a belief that mania resulted from the kindling of abnormal seizure-like activity and started a search for anticonvulsants as treatments for bipolar disorder.[56] Several anticonvulsants are now recommended as "mood stabilizers" in the long-term management of bipolar depression.[57] The relatively weak therapeutic effect of anticonvulsants as mood stabilizers, however, is reflected in the recommended algorithms requiring a complex polypharmacy of mood stabilizers, SSRI antidepressants, antipsychotic agents, and benzodiazepine sedatives for reasonable efficacy. Another tactic has been to recommend the combination of newly introduced agents such as olanzapine–fluoxetine.[58] A more formal dependence on psychotherapy, now presented as *psychoeducation*, is also offered.[59] To optimize a treatment strategy for clinical practice, the National Institute for Mental Health has recently contracted with a consortium of medical centers to test a complex algorithm known as the STEP-BD.[60]

Despite the absence of experimental evidence, trials of antimanic agents among bipolar patients often cite drug-induced cycling, without accounting for natural cycling rates as a justification for the use of these agents.[61]

Bipolar and unipolar conditions genetically overlap

After the original studies by Leonhard and by Perris reported that familial differences between recurrent depressive illness and manic-depressive illness, subsequent family and genetic studies commonly reported an overlap between the two forms of mood disorder, supporting a unitary construct.[62] Both forms of illness occur with increased frequency in the families of patients with manic-depressive illness.[63] When recurrent depressive illness is defined as melancholia, families have an increased risk for manic depression.[64]

Twin studies show this overlap.[65] In an analysis of 30 monozygotic and 37 dizygotic twin pairs, the proband concordance was higher for monozygotic than for dizygotic twins, with heritability estimated at 89%.[66] In almost 29% of the monozygotic pairs, one twin had both manic and depressive episodes while the other had recurrent depressive illness. Among the dizygotic pairs 13.5% had a mixed concordance. The investigators tested several liability models and concluded that manic-depressive illness was not simply a more severe form of recurrent depressive illness, but that nevertheless, there was substantial genetic overlap between the two forms (about 30%) that may represent the risk for depressive illness.

Conclusion

The scientific evidence fails to distinguish unipolar and bipolar depressive disorders. About 10% of melancholic patients exhibit manic features. The overlap is clearly expressed in the many descriptions of "mixed" and "spectrum" depressive and manic conditions. Patients may exhibit depressive and manic features during the same episode or episodes may recur in cycles, changing from one to another within weeks, days, or even within hours. The depressive state that is identified in a patient with a history of a manic or hypomanic episode cannot be distinguished from the depressive state in a patient without such a history. Neither family history nor course of illness successfully separates the two conditions. Nor does the putative induction of mania by antidepressant drugs assure the separation as the incidence of manic switches is no greater than the natural switch rate; it is sufficiently uncommon as not to be useful as a diagnostic test.

The responses to lithium and to anticonvulsants are cited as justifications for bipolarity.[67] To support such a view, the evidence of the antidepressant efficacy of lithium is minimized, and the control of manic episodes by anticonvulsants maximized. Lithium is both an effective antidepressant, especially in maintenance therapy, and an effective control for mania. Anticonvulsants are weak mood stabilizers; the treatment algorithms commonly require the polypharmacy of mood stabilizers (often two), antipsychotic, and sedative agents. Yet patients in both the depressive and manic phases of the illness respond rapidly to electroconvulsive therapy (ECT).[68]

The neuroendocrine and sleep laboratory tests that demarcate severe depressive mood disorders from other psychiatric disorders are abnormal during both the manic and depressive phases of their illness.[69] The degree of abnormality is apparently less for patients in the manic phases but the difference is not sufficient to support the concept of bipolarity.

Bipolarity as a separate psychiatric disorder is not supported by psychopathology, family studies, laboratory tests, or treatment response. A single disorder of melancholia circumscribes the present knowledge and offers a better model for continuing scientific efforts.

Psychotic depression is melancholia

Approximately one-third of melancholic patients are psychotic.[70] Psychotic features in melancholia are reported at all ages, although the recognition of psychotic depression increases with the patient's age. In some reviews nearly all patients with psychotic depression are melancholic.[71]

Historical background

In nineteenth-century psychopathology, disorders of thought were identified in patients classified as manic-depressive insanity, involutional and melancholic depression, dementia praecox, and dementia paralytica (neurosyphilis). Psychosis was not pathognomonic for any condition. During the early and mid twentieth century, however, "first-rank" psychotic features (e.g., complete auditory hallucinations, experiences of alienation and control) were associated with the hereditary disorder of dementia praecox, later redefined as "schizophrenia." The presence of these signs was considered pathognomonic of schizophrenia regardless of the presence of a concurrent mood disorder.

The view that schizophrenia encompassed almost all episodes of psychosis was favored in the USA but not in Europe. Cross-Atlantic differences in the prevalence of schizophrenia and of manic-depressive psychosis were reported, and to assess the basis for the discrepancy, a cross-national group of investigators examined patients in the UK and in the USA. Differences in diagnostic perceptions, not national distinctions in populations, best explained the differences in prevalence of the disorders.[72] The broad definition of schizophrenia in the USA materially increased the numbers of patients who were labeled schizophrenic while reducing the numbers diagnosed with mood disorders.

The place of psychotic mood disorder in psychiatric classification remained unclear. Some considered these states to be more severe forms of manic-depressive illness while others preferred to define them as "schizoaffective" and to include them among the psychotic disorders.[73] One understanding of psychosis in patients with mood disorders derived from the clinical trials of TCAs. Among depressed hospitalized patients treated with imipramine with serum blood levels monitored to assure adequate dosing, some patients failed to respond to imipramine but did respond to ECT.[74] The presence of delusions discriminated the patients who had not improved with imipramine alone. A decade earlier, a large Italian study by De Carolis *et al.* (1964) had also reported that the psychotic depressed patients had not responded to imipramine but had recovered with ECT.[75] The association between depression, psychosis, poor response to TCAs, and rapid response to ECT was quickly confirmed and is now widely accepted.[76]

The DSM classifications of 1980 and 1994 still give preference to psychotic features as defining schizophrenia, and they primarily link catatonia with schizophrenia despite its strong association with mood disorder.[77] Psychotic features are recognized as a non-specific psychopathologic phenomenon, appearing within different diagnostic classes, and delusions in a mood disorder are considered signs of severity, not distinctions in pathophysiology, but this classification is only permitted when directly linked to a disturbed mood state. If the patient has delusions that last longer than the mood symptoms or the psychotic features are deemed more pronounced, the schizoaffective diagnosis is preferred and the patient assigned to the psychotic disorders, not mood disorder, category. Nevertheless, for each principal mood disorder – *major depressive disorder, bipolar I disorder,* and *bipolar II disorder, depressed type* – the presence of psychosis could be recognized by coding the *severity/psychotic/remission* specifier in the fifth digit.[78]

Once a condition of "psychotic depression" or "delusional depression" was recognized, attention was paid to its delineation from other depressive illnesses. Focusing on the motor aspects of melancholia, Parker and Hadzi-Pavlovic (1996) envisioned three forms of depressive illness – psychotic depression, non-psychotic melancholia, and non-melancholic depression.[79] They offered criteria of discrimination by age of onset,[80] degree of cognitive impairment,[81] and prominence of personality and life events.[82] Non-melancholic depression was characterized by early onset of illness, little cognitive impairment, deviant personality traits, and little psychomotor disturbance. Severity of psychomotor disturbance and cognitive impairment characterized psychotic melancholia.[83] Psychotically depressed patients exhibited more severe psychomotor disturbance, including facial immobility, slumped posture, slowed and limited movements and speech, poverty of associations, and poor responsiveness. Non-suppression on the dexamethasone suppression test was recorded in 72% of the patients. The mood was characterized as "non-reactive."[84] While the distinction was clear between non-melancholic depression and the other two forms of depressive illness, psychotic and non-psychotic melancholia were not shown to be different diseases.

Other authors focused on abnormalities in neuroendocrine and neurocognitive measures, course of illness, familial transmission, and response to treatment as distinguishing psychotic and non-psychotic depression.[85] Among the criteria were greater guilt feelings and psychomotor disturbances, biochemical differences in glucocorticoid activity, dopamine beta-hydroxylase activity, levels of dopamine and serotonin metabolites, severity of sleep measures, and ventricle-to-brain ratios. Neuropsychological deficits were found to be greater in degree among psychotic depressed patients than among the non-psychotic depressed.[86] None of these efforts identified a clearly distinguishing variable.

In a retrospective examination of patients in Denmark who had a diagnosis of a single depressive episode at their first ever discharge during the period 1994 through 1999, patients were identified as with or without the *International Classification of Diseases*, 10th edition (ICD-10) diagnosis of melancholia ($n = 248$ and 293 respectively), and with and without psychosis ($n = 1275$ and 1639, respectively).[87] Relapse rates were highest in the psychotic depression group. The groups did not differ in suicide rates or melancholic features. Compared to non-melancholic depressed patients, the melancholic patients were less likely to be diagnosed as having a personality disorder, stress-related disorder, or "nervous" disorder.

It is difficult to recognize the presence of psychosis in melancholic patients. The more severely ill depressed patients are common in referrals for ECT. In an analysis of ECT referrals, only 2/52 patients had been adequately treated for psychotic depression.[88] The authors assumed that, had the referring physicians recognized the presence of psychosis, the medications prescribed would have been more appropriate for psychotic depression.

Other than the recognition of psychosis, no measures distinguish the psychotic and non-psychotic forms of melancholic illness.

Mood-congruent and mood-incongruent delusions

In the 1980 DSM classification attention was directed to *mood congruence* of psychotic thoughts. If the patient's delusional content was deemed depressive (e.g., low self-worth, guilt), the delusion was defined as congruent with the mood state and the patient was deemed as most likely suffering from a mood disorder. If the delusional content was deemed "bizarre" (e.g., delusions of passivity), the delusion was defined as incongruent with the mood and the patient was considered to be schizoaffective or schizophrenic. Patients with an affective syndrome with mood-incongruent as well as mood-congruent delusions, however, were allowed within the class of major depression.

In a review of the writings that supported a concept of a mood-incongruent psychotic mood disorder, three hypotheses were considered: it was a form of depressive illness, a subtype of a schizoaffective disorder, or a subtype of schizophrenia.[89] After reviewing the evidence of demographic studies, degree of risk in families of probands, laboratory test data, and treatment response, Kendler concluded that mood-incongruent psychotic depression was best viewed as a subtype of mood disorder and not as a feature of schizophrenia or schizoaffective disorder.

In an examination of the clinical, genetic, and prognostic significance of mood-incongruent psychotic symptoms, Abrams and Taylor (1983) further concluded that mood-incongruent psychotic symptoms did not identify a unique subpopulation of melancholic patients. In another large clinical study, the authors were unable to define differences in the congruence of delusions among patients classified as schizophrenia, schizoaffective disorder, psychotic, or mixed mania.[90]

Neither a history of psychosis nor mood-incongruent delusions has prognostic significance for the treatment of bipolar depression.[91] It is reasonable to conclude that mood congruence of delusions does not distinguish patients with a mood disorder from those with a non-mood disorder psychotic illness. Delusions represent degrees of severity, not unique psychopathology.[92]

Psychotic depression meets criteria for melancholia

Patients who are depressed and who are also psychotic are best included within the concept of melancholia. The manifestations of depressed mood, family history and course of illness, laboratory test findings, and response to treatments are indistinguishable for those with and those without evidence of psychosis (Table 2.2).

Table 2.2. A comparison of psychotic depression and melancholia

	Psychotic depression	Non-psychotic melancholia
% ECT referrals	30%	70%
HPA tests abnormal	80%	60%
Sleep tests abnormal	Positive	Positive
Family illness	Positive	Positive
Treatment response		
TCA	20–30%	50–70%
ECT	90%	75–85%

Clinical vignettes are consistent with the view that psychotic depression is a severe form of melancholia and not a distinct entity.[93] An example of psychotic depression is described in Chapter 8, patient 8.2. Another representative vignette is abstracted from the DSM-IV casebook.[94]

Patient 2.6

Mr. D. O'M is a small, bent disheveled 63-year-old man, referred to a psychiatric clinic after telling his internist that he was hearing voices. A few weeks earlier he heard a stranger call him "an Irish fag." He said his mood was "lousy," "nervous" and "shaky". He lost interest in seeing friends or "doing anything" since his mood deteriorated. He had no appetite, lost weight, but his sleep was not disturbed. He denied thoughts of suicide "because, as a Catholic, I would not go to heaven if I committed suicide; but I would be better off if my heart stopped." A similar illness occurred 12 years earlier when he heard blaspheming voices and became preoccupied with religious "scruples." Treatment with medicines at that time was successful and he returned to work as a cab driver. He had retired five years earlier because of worsening diabetes and ulcerative colitis. He denied drinking alcohol in 30 years. His wife confirmed his history.

He was hospitalized and treated with antipsychotic medication. A few weeks later, when the voices diminished, the depressive mood and retardation became more obvious. Nortriptyline was prescribed and he left the hospital four weeks later, improved and less anxious, but still complaining of the voices. He recovered slowly in the next year.

The editors describe Mr. D. O'M as suffering from a major depressive disorder, recurrent, with mood-incongruent psychotic features.[95] Even a cursory reading of the literature will show that this patient's delusional thoughts are expressions of his depressed mood, are fully congruent, and are classic for melancholia. The discussant, however, agreed with the proffered diagnosis but suggested that had the patient been offered ECT, he might have had a better outcome and a shorter duration of illness.

The next patient with a psychotic depression was successfully treated to a full resolution of his illness.

Patient 2.7

A 69-year-old business executive had fretted about the sale of his company. His work had been the main interest in his life. When his wife become ill and was unable to manage their home, he grew despondent, slept during much of the day, was up much of the night, bathed irregularly, ate poorly, complained of constipation, and thought that his food was poisoned. He insisted, contrary to fact, that he had cancer and would soon die. He accused his wife of infidelity and refused to talk to her. He watched the street from behind curtained windows for hours at a time believing that his neighbors were spying on his home. After nine months he was hospitalized.

His wife reported a single episode of severely depressed mood when the patient was age 45, following business reversals and fears that he would lose his business. After the business difficulties resolved, he became well.

On examination he walked slowly, appeared emaciated, disheveled and unkempt, and had an unpleasant body odor. He refused to answer questions and was reluctant to be examined, yet insisting that he was physically ill, that his condition was hopeless, and that treatment would be of no avail. At times, he stared into space, listened as if hearing voices, and muttered inaudible responses.

Eczema and dermatitis resulting from poor skin care and impaired kidney functions were found, the latter resulting from drinking too little. Intravenous fluids and feeding were started. He refused medications, insisting that treatment was pointless, as death was imminent.

A diagnosis of psychotic depression was made and a course of ECT prescribed. After the fourth treatment he began to drink and eat, his sleep cycle normalized and he showered and shaved. After six treatments, he thought that he had been ill but denied the thoughts of infidelity and paranoia. After 10 treatments, he was sufficiently improved to return to his home. Continuation ECT every two weeks for two months resolved his illness.

Throughout his hospitalization he had been uninterested in ward events spending most of each day in his room, staring out the window, and rarely taking part in communal activities when directed. After his return home, he read the daily newspaper and watched television. One year later, he had maintained his weight, slept well, and his illness had not recurred.

Cotard syndrome as an example of psychotic depression

Delusions reported by patients are variable and often elaborate, enticing poets and scholars alike. An author's name has been applied as an eponym in descriptions of some dramatic delusions. Patients who avowed the nihilistic delusion of "being dead" or having "no brain, nerves, chest or entrails, and was just skin and bone" met criteria for the *délire de négation*, now recognized as the Cotard syndrome. Identified in the late nineteenth century, it is often reported among manic-depressive patients.[96] An analysis of 100 cases reported in the literature found 89% of the patients to be depressed, the others suffering from various brain disorders.[97] The most common nihilistic delusion concerned the body (86%), existence (69%), and immortality (55%). Co-occurring anxiety, guilt, and hypochondriacal delusions were frequent.

The appearance of delusions of negation even in the presence of a mood disorder syndrome does not preclude the possibility that the condition is the result of structural brain disease, and Cotard syndrome is also described in patients after brain injury.[98] The following vignette illustrates the delusion of negation in a patient with a melancholic depression.[99]

Patient 2.8

A 74-year-old widow, confused and dehydrated, was admitted to hospital from a nursing home. She claimed that she was dead, that the surroundings were mystical, that she was probably "up there," and that she was among dead people since they were wearing white coats that she considered shrouds. She did not display signs of depression but appeared resigned. She had lost considerable weight, slept little, and refused to eat or to drink, as unnecessary for a person already deceased. She was treated with 10 bilateral ECT, recovered, began eating and drinking, and asked for an appointment with a hairdresser. She was discharged to the nursing home and was well two years later.

ECT is considered an effective treatment of the syndrome,[100] as are antidepressants.[101] The syndrome is described in adolescents as well as adults.[102]

Other syndromes that are also associated with psychotic depression are the Capgras syndrome (illusion of doubles), de Clérambault syndrome (erotomania), Othello syndrome (delusion of infidelity in a spouse), and Ganser syndrome (approximate answers).[103] These syndromes have been described in patients with melancholia but are also associated with neurologic disease. Cotard and Capgras syndromes have been described to occur together more than by chance, consistent with the neurologic understanding of these states.[104] Recognizing these syndromes as most commonly associated with melancholia, however, offers the opportunity for specific effective treatment.

Depression with catatonia or stupor is severe melancholia[105]

When a depressive mood disorder is expressed in repetitive speech, repetitive movements, mutism, negativism, or other motor signs of catatonia, the differentiation from a structural dementia is difficult.[106] Catatonia in melancholic patients may be associated with such profound psychomotor retardation that it appears as stupor. Indeed, undiagnosed stupors (comas) that meet criteria for catatonia are an occasional feature of hospitalized patients on general medical and neurological services. Melancholic patients often exhibit catatonic features of prolonged fixed postures (catalepsy).[107] They pay little attention to their surroundings, stare into space, speak sluggishly or not at all, and look and move as if under the influence of sedatives. They are insensitive to painful stimuli and may be incontinent. The syndrome of catatonia is no longer considered a feature of schizophrenia alone, but is associated with depressive and manic mood disorders, and toxic and general medical disorders.[108]

The close association between melancholia and catatonia was described by Karl Kahlbaum.[109] In his patient descriptions, the motor signs of catatonia developed after melancholia had been fully expressed. Catatonia was also described in manic states, a finding that has been confirmed in the prominence of catatonia in the manic phases of manic-depressive disorders.[110] An example of catatonia in a patient with melancholia is presented by Kahlbaum.[111]

Patient 2.9

Baroness MB, a 45-year-old married woman with three children became psychotic during her menopause, convinced that she had been poisoned by matches left at her bedside. She reported a metallic taste in her mouth and showed an aversion to metals. She was preoccupied by religious ideas and practices and claimed to be in contact with the Almighty. Outbursts of anger and temper, for which she later attempted to atone for in the tenderest and loving manner, occurred. She developed cramps in her feet, arms and jaw, accompanied by sounds resembling the ticking of a clock, which were audible in her mouth. Fits of laughing and weeping were followed by agitation and imagination that she saw the coffin of her son (who was in active military service) and became manic. After admission to a psychiatric hospital, she became apathetic and presented "a pitiful appearance." She was transferred to Görlitz [a sanatorium in the city of Görlitz that Kahlbaum directed].

She appeared prematurely aged, cowering in an immobile position, her limbs folded close to her body. She refused to answer questions put to her and resisted attempts to move her limbs passively. This state alternated with marked talkativeness, to herself and to her surroundings and conjured up reminiscences that were, in part, coherent and sensible and, in part, veering off into fantasies that were puerile, lascivious, or haughty. She had a compulsion to alter the names of peoples around her, spoke of herself in the second person, and from time to time would recite lessons learned by heart that did not allow interruption. At first she maintained her hygiene and cleanliness, but later became slovenly. She behaved indecently, often undressing and walking about scantily clad. On one occasion, she tore out the hairs from her head, one by one, and had to be restrained to prevent her from becoming bald. She progressed to a stage of mutism and repeated twisting of pieces of cloth into the shape of sausages, a motor manifestation that persisted even when she was asleep. [Kahlbaum does not tell us of the further course of the illness.][112]

Depressed catatonic patients stop eating and drinking, lose weight, and become dehydrated. In recent times, these factors put them at risk for neuroleptic malignant syndrome, a form of malignant catatonia that can be elicited by many disorders and pharmaceuticals and is seen most commonly today in patients treated with antipsychotic agents. Younger patients with catatonia due to a mood disorder may be misdiagnosed as schizophrenic, particularly if delusions were expressed at the onset of the illness. The expression of persecutory hallucinated voices, however, is consistent with a depressive mood disorder, particularly when the voices are linked to delusions of self- blame and worthlessness.

The presence of catatonia may be confirmed by a challenge with an acute administration of a benzodiazepine.[113] The intravenous administration (e.g., 1–3 mg lorazepam) often relieves mutism and rigidity of the catatonic patient permitting further examination. Demented and delirious patients become further sedated with such doses.[114] The benefit of the test is illustrated.

Patient 2.10

In the course of a week, a 28-year-old woman became progressively mute and mostly unresponsive. At first she looked frightened, but then just stared into space, speaking few words in a low slow voice, but only when prompted. She sat awake all night, not sleeping. She stopped eating and drinking. She showed automatic obedience.[115] Catatonia was diagnosed.

Because of the rapid onset of her condition, a brain scan (MRI) was requested to rule out an emergent neurologic process. Hospital policy required all psychiatric patients to be sedated in the MRI suite.[116] The psychiatrists caring for the patient accompanied her to the imaging suit and an IV line was established. The patient was unresponsive to the needle. Two mg of midazolam was given. The patient immediately sat up, looked around the basement-like area outside the MRI suite, and said "You are going to put me in the incinerator where I belong. I deserve to die. I'm no good." She then became fully sedated. The MRI was normal. Catatonia was treated with lorazepam and resolved fully within 72 hours.

A melancholic patient with benign stupor, psychosis, catatonia, and a manic-depressive course unaffected by medications or physical treatments is described by August Hoch.[117]

Patient 2.11

A 15-year-old girl was admitted to hospital with a three-week history of abnormal behavior that began with thoughts that a girl at her shop was making remarks about the patient's red hair. She was distressed and asked to change her place of work. Her mother kept her at home. She became mute, crying at times, expressing the wish that she were dead and her wish to join her dead father. Four days before admission, she became immobile, lay in bed, did not speak, eat or drink. She became febrile.

On admission she was constrained, stared fixedly into space, mute, required to be dressed and fed. For five months she presented a marked stupor, rarely blinking so that her conjunctiva became dry. She did not swallow, held her saliva. She did not react to pinpricks or feinting motions before her eyes. Sometimes she retained her urine, again wet and soiled the bed. Often there was marked catalepsy, and the retention of very awkward positions. As a rule she was quite stiff, offering passive resistance towards any interference. She had to be tube-fed. During the first month, the stupor was interrupted for short periods by a little freer action: she walked to a chair, sat down, smiled a little, fanned herself very naturally when a fan was given her, though even then did not speak.

She menstruated on admission but then not again until she was well. Several times she had rises of temperature to 103° F [39° C] with a high pulse and respiration.

Over the next year, she vacillated between stupor and periods when she was able to care for herself, respond appropriately to simple questions and commands. The apathy cleared up and she was talkative. She recalled the events of the latter few months of her illness, recalling being stuck by a pin and tube-feeding. When she was ready to return home, she became more elated. She was talkative, conversed with strangers on the street, and now told her mother that "she wanted a fellow." She became overly elated and was returned to the hospital. Dr. Hoch describes a manic-depressive course over the next few years. Another hospitalization with a similar stupor (immobility, mutism, catalepsy, rigidity) followed a period of depression, inability to concentrate, and fears that another attack would come on. That episode was "immediately preceded by a seizure in which the whole body jerked." In recalling the onset of her illness, the patient claimed that she had felt "queer," "nervous," "depressed," and sleepless. She recalled that she had the thought that she was dying and that her father's picture was calling her.

Melancholia is often associated with catatonia and one or the other syndrome may dominate at any one time. The overlap of syndromes suggests a commonality in the sites of brain dysfunction.

Melancholia defined by a specific event

Clinicians often ascribe etiologic significance to a special event preceding an episode of mood disorder, but the causal association is not established and the depressive illnesses that occur under such circumstances do not differ from classical melancholia.

Descriptions of *postpartum* melancholia, *vascular or late-life depression, abnormal bereavement*, and *seasonal* depression are examples of disorders labeled according to the presence of hypothecated precipitants.

The circumstances assumed to be precipitants do not alter the typical features of the melancholic syndrome, the characteristic laboratory findings, or the treatment response. The melancholic syndromes are indistinguishable in characteristics and to the extent known, in their biology. It is confusing for clinicians and inhibiting of scientific assessments to separate patients with episodes of illness that meet the criteria for melancholia simply because the episodes are associated with a specific circumstance. Adverse events are commonly associated with emerging disease, but a myocardial infarction is no less a heart attack for occurring amidst personal turmoil, and neither is depressive illness.

Pregnancy-related mood disorders (puerperal depression)

Depressive illnesses that occur during pregnancy and immediately postpartum, defined in the literature as puerperal major depression, are examples of melancholia. Postpartum depressive illness occurs in 5–10% of women during the weeks after delivery.[118] When accompanied by suicidal feelings, these ruminations warrant hospitalization.[119] The psychopathology of postpartum depression does not differ from melancholia at other times,[120] although treatment considerations may differ.[121]

The dramatic hormonal changes of pregnancy and delivery are the probable precipitants.[122] For example, cortisol, corticotropin-releasing hormone, and adrenocorticotropic hormone are increased manifold during pregnancy and 80–90% of non-depressed women are non-suppressors to dexamethasone in the first week postpartum.[123] These abnormalities in the hypothalamic–pituitary axis (also characteristic of melancholia) rapidly normalize by the third postpartum week.[124] The stresses of parenting, however, might equally be considered in depressive illness following the birth of a child, as seen in patient 7.5. Following the birth of a son and his eating and sleeping difficulties, the father who had a history of depressive illness became melancholic.

Postpartum blues are so commonly associated with delivery, occurring in up to 50% of women, that they may be considered a normal response to the delivery process.[125] They have been associated with elevated progesterone metabolites[126] and low levels of oxytocin.[127] However, postpartum depressive illness occurs more often in women with a personal or family history of mood disorder, suggesting that if these risk factors are present, the emergence of postpartum blues may signal the unfolding of depressive illness triggered by the hormonal and environmental stresses of childbirth.[128]

A *puerperal psychotic depressive illness* is indistinguishable from a psychotic depressive illness that occurs at other times. Three studies used rating scale items to examine patients in the postpartum period. The items that discriminated puerperal and non-puerperal psychosis are differences in severity, not uniqueness, except for a greater incidence of "confusion."[129] At the conclusion of the review, the authors note:

> If the concept of manic depression were extended to include cycloid patients, there would be no problem in recognizing puerperal psychosis as typical manic depressive insanity.[130]

Puerperal psychotic depression is, however, more likely to present as a mixed affective state characterized by the sudden onset of mania, delirium, confusion, delusions, hallucinations, excitement, and depressed mood.[131] Manic and depressive forms of the syndrome are well described, with the manic form the most common in the older literature.[132] In some series, up to 18 times as many women were admitted to a psychiatric hospital in the first month postpartum as in each month of the pregnancy.[133]

A similar syndrome has been described as oneirophrenia.[134] Despite the temporal relationship to pregnancy, the sudden appearance of delirium drives clinicians to search for causes other than mood disorder.[135]

Postpartum non-psychotic melancholia is defined as a depressive illness during the first 6 months after delivery. The patient becomes despondent, feels inadequate as a parent, sleeps poorly, loses weight, and is unable to concentrate her thoughts or actions to organize the care of the infant. Thoughts of harming the child (or other children) dominate daily life.[136] The syndrome occurs more often in women with prior episodes of depressive mood disorder, premenstrual dysphoric disorder, or undue psychosocial stress.[137]

The records of all female admissions over a 35-year period to an English hospital were examined and 134 patients were identified who satisfied criteria for puerperal psychosis.[138] The average age of the patients was 28.3 years, 125/134 were married, and 60% were primiparous. The psychopathology of the patients was described as affective in 68% (79% depressed and 21% mania), 28% as schizophrenia, and 4% as due to general medical illness.

> Some patients became obviously depressed and apathetic and gradually lapsed into stupor and had the usual appearance associated with the depressive syndrome of manic depressive psychosis; others became elated, with the usual features of the manic syndrome. However, a number . . . rapidly alternated in mood between depression and mania, sometimes within the same day[139]

The onset of the psychosis was within the week after delivery in 31%, within 2 weeks in 65% and within 4 weeks in 94% of cases.

> Little or no treatment other than general medical and nursing care and a little sedation was given these patients prior to 1943. From 1944 onwards, physical treatments were used, first ECT, then insulin from 1947 up to 1956, and from 1956 onwards chlorpromazine and other drugs.[140]

In summarizing his experience, the author wrote:

> Two only of 52 women admitted before 1942 received treatment other than general care. Twenty-five percent of those women died in hospital, mainly from diseases attributable to general medical conditions . . . The last death occurred in a patient admitted in 1943. The introduction of physical treatments has lessened the period of in-patient stay for patients with affective states (from 8 months to 2.4 months average) and even more so for schizophrenics (4 years to 3.8 months).[141]

He presents a clinical vignette.

Patient 2.12

A married woman of 32 years was admitted to hospital under a certificate in April 1938. Three to four weeks after the birth of her seventh child she had become depressed and sleepless. At admission, "tears were trickling down her face" and she was auditorily hallucinated, the voices saying that she was bad and was to be burnt alive. She remained apathetic, retarded and asocial. A little improvement was noticed in November 1944. In August 1945 she was given a course of ECT and at the end of this was greatly improved, mixing on the wards, talking freely, etc. She was discharged in December 1945. Since then she has had two further children with no psychiatric complications. When interviewed in 1962, she could remember little of her stay in hospital during the 7 years prior to being given ECT, but much of the few months following.

A decade later, another detailed review of puerperal psychosis reports the onset of puerperal psychoses to vary from 0.8 to 2.5/1000 deliveries and to be acute with a course up to 6 months of illness.[142] About 50% of women diagnosed with postpartum psychosis are primiparous. Recovery occurs in 60–80% of patients, although before the introduction of modern somatic treatments, about 9% of patients died from "exhaustion" or by suicide. Infanticide is a persistent risk.[143] An interesting historical example is cited.[144]

Patient 2.13

In 1847 MP gave birth to a baby boy in the UK. A few days later, neighboring ladies got word to the physician who had delivered her that she was not doing well. At a house call the next day, the physician diagnosed postpartum psychosis. He ordered the baby kept apart from the mother and advised round-the-clock surveillance and nursing by the neighboring ladies. Four days later there was a lapse in the availability of neighbors and the patient's daughter, age 13, was left in charge. MP, exercising her maternal authority, ordered her daughter to bring in the baby. A little later she complained of a hard callous on her hand and demanded a razor to pare it. The inevitable happened.[145]

Another analysis of a sample of 250 women admitted to a Rotterdam psychiatric hospital between 1967 and 1989 reported that 72% were admitted within 2 weeks of delivery. Although the symptoms met a range of Research Diagnostic Criteria affective diagnoses, the European classification of a continuum of psychosis (*Einheitspsychose*) and cycloid psychosis served to describe the sample best.[146]

No family, genetic, or environmental precipitant of postpartum melancholia has been identified, although the incidence is higher in women who experience miscarriage or stillbirth.[147] For women with a prior history of depressive illness, the risk of recurrence after miscarriage appears double the risk of recurrence after delivering a live infant. Prior history of depressive mood disorder increases the risk, whereas women without prior mood disorder are at no greater risk than are women at other times.[148] A history of manic-depressive illness dramatically increases the likelihood of a postpartum mood disorder.[149] Other risk factors include premenstrual dysphoric disorder, obstetric complications, environmental stress, inadequate social support, and depressive symptoms during pregnancy.[150] The presence of unrealistic thoughts of death or dying from pregnancy complications is associated with an unfolding depression.[151]

The outcomes of the illness were dramatically changed with the introduction of ECT, with almost all patients responding within 3 weeks to 4–10 treatments.[152] The first reports appeared within 3 years of the introduction of ECT. In one study, mothers with postpartum psychosis were randomly assigned to either ECT (20 treatments) or chlorpromazine (300–1200 mg/day). ECT was more effective than chlorpromazine alone, with the best results achieved in a second trial of chlorpromazine combined with ECT.[153]

A reasonable inference from the sudden appearance of puerperal psychosis immediately after delivery brought attention to the massive changes in the concentrations of sex hormones, especially the sharp fall in progesterone. The experience with hormone replacement therapy in either ameliorating the psychosis or preventing another episode in future pregnancies is unclear.[154]

Puerperal mood disorders are examples of melancholia. As with melancholias at other times, puerperal depressive illness can be non-psychotic or psychotic, with pseudodementia or catatonia, and with or without associated mania. From a heuristic standpoint, the search for specific precipitants will be useful but identifying the illnesses and treating the patients as melancholia is clinically the most favorable option.

Abnormal bereavement is melancholia

The DSM psychiatric classification includes *abnormal bereavement* as a specified form of depressive mood disorder. The dying and death of a loved one is traumatic. About half of women and 10% of men over age 65 have had a spouse die. By age 85, over 80% of women and 40% of men have had a spouse die.[155] Although grief may persist for several years and one-third of widowed older persons initially meet DSM criteria for major depression, the common signs of depression rarely last beyond several weeks.[156] Features persisting past 1 month after the death are associated with continuing mood disorder.[157] Suicide remains a persistent risk.[158] The clinical dilemma is the uncertainty of whether these prolonged symptoms reflect the circumstances and the patient's personality, or are signs of an illness that requires treatment.

Abnormal bereavement is not distinguishable from melancholia, and the DSM criteria for it could easily be used as descriptors of melancholia (Table 2.3). Sleep architecture and immune functions are disturbed in the normal bereaved, and their morbidity and mortality rates are high.[159]

While disturbances in general medical health do not distinguish melancholia, the dexamethasone suppression test may be helpful as normal grieving is not associated with high cortisol levels and non-suppression.[160] Four weeks following the death of a parent, children and adolescents have normal cortisol functioning. In one study of bereavement, however, 39% were non-suppressors. These patients had many melancholic features and were suicidal, clinically meeting criteria for melancholia as well as abnormal bereavement.[161]

Table 2.3. Features of abnormal bereavement

Sustained and non-reactive mood disturbance
Psychosis
Marked psychomotor impairment
Failure to regain level of pre-death social functioning within 2 months
Preoccupation with worthlessness and desire to die
Suicide attempt

Identifying a syndrome of abnormal bereavement is unnecessary. The literature offers no defining characteristics that would distinguish this form of melancholia from any other. When bereavement is followed by a severe depressive illness and the illness meets criteria for melancholia, the illness warrants treatment for melancholia.

NOTES

1 From http://www.etymonline.com/m4etym.htm.
2 Carroll (2002); p. 186.
3 Shorter (2005) describes many terms that are equivalent to the modern term "depression." He includes "vapours" and "hysteric fits." By the mid eighteenth century, spleen and "hyp" [-ochondria] had become fashionable diagnoses. Indeed, a nervous illness of Britain's Queen Anne in the late eighteenth century was ascribed to "spleen and hyp" as she was "frequently subject to depression of spirits."
4 Parker (2004).
5 Psychomotor change is considered essential to melancholia in the studies of Parker and Hadzi-Pavlovic (1996) and the review by Rush and Weissenburger (1994).
6 An excellent description of *benign stupor* is by August Hoch (1921). In a posthumous volume he described patients with stupor who were severely depressed and delusional, and often exhibited diverse motor signs, now defined as signs of catatonia. Many patients met criteria for catatonia, and the syndrome is considered an alternate face of catatonia (Fink and Taylor, 2001, 2003). The overlap of catatonia and melancholia is not limited to patients in stupor but careful examination of patients with melancholia often finds multiple signs of catatonia; and among patients with retarded catatonia, other signs of melancholia are often described (Abrams and Taylor, 1976; Fink and Taylor, 2003.)
7 Chapter 4. Patients with the eating disorders of anorexia and bulimia exhibit many of the elements of melancholia; the connection has yet to be explored.
8 There was a European tradition of treating serious depressions as "psychotic." In Kahlbaum's description of catatonia, he described patients with catatonia who were depressed and psychotic. For many decades, the presence of psychosis was considered so pathognomonic of a schizophrenic disorder that the co-occurrence of depression or mania was rejected as a diagnostic feature. In the 1970s, a syndrome of psychotic depression was demarcated from schizophrenia and established as a diagnostic entity in its own right, based on the failure of depressed patients with psychosis to respond to adequate trials with imipramine (Glassman

et al., 1975; Avery and Lubrano, 1979; Glassman and Roose, 1981; Kroessler, 1985). The syndrome was recommended as a separate entity in classification by Schatzberg and Rothschild (1992).

9 Considerable confusion exists with regard to the role of psychosis in melancholia. Does the presence of psychosis mark a different psychopathological disorder? Such a distinction is made by Parker, Hadzi-Pavlovic and their associates (Parker and Hadzi-Pavlovic, 1996; Parker *et al.*, 1992a, b, 1995a–c, 1997, 1998a, b, 1999a–c, 2001). They offer algorithms to distinguish melancholia from other varieties of depression and then distinguish three classes of illness, defined as psychotic depression, non-psychotic melancholia, and non-melancholic depression. These groups are differentiated by rating-scale scores of observable psychopathology without reference to other clinical aspects. In the absence of characteristic differences in treatments, treatment response, vegetative signs, or neuroendocrine measures, the justification for the differences in classification is obscure.

10 See supporting discussions in Chapters 2, 4, and 14.

11 Hopewell-Ash (1934). These patients were treated by suggestion, hospital protection, nursing care, and sedation.

12 *Ibid.*, patient I, p. 9.

13 *Ibid.*, patient V, p. 10.

14 *Ibid.*, patient VIII, p. 11.

15 *Ibid.*, patient XXI, pp. 19–20.

16 Styron (1990), p. 40.

17 *Ibid.*, p. 33.

18 Price (1978).

19 For non-psychotic melancholia, also see patient MA, pp. 33–4 in Fink (1999a).

20 Wallace (1994); Shorter (1997, 2005).

21 Kahlbaum's essay is translated into English (Baethge *et al.*, 2003a). The elaboration by Ewald Hecker is translated into English and his work reviewed (Baethge *et al.*, 2003b).

22 Kraepelin (1921).

23 Winokur *et al.* (1969); Angst and Perris (1972). Goodwin and Jamison (1990) assessed the family data (p. 62): "Some family history studies are consistent with a model in which bipolar and unipolar are variants of the same fundamental disorder, with bipolar representing the more severe end of the spectrum."

24 Dunner *et al.* (1976). A non-severe form of hypomania was also recognized in separating the two syndromes.

25 Winokur (1979).

26 Angst (1978), Akiskal (1981, 1999), Endicott *et al.* (1985), and Coryell *et al.* (1985a), Akiskal and Katona (2001).

27 Taylor and Abrams (1973, 1980), Abrams and Taylor (1980). Also see Mitchell and Malhi (2004).

28 Table 3-1, p. 63.

29 *Ibid.*, Goodwin and Jamison (1990); p. 67.

30 *Ibid.*, p. 65.

31 Ghaemi *et al.* (1999b).

32 Mitchell and Malhi (2004).

33 Goldberg *et al.* (2004).

34 Ghaemi *et al.* (2004a, b).

35 Maj *et al.* (2003).
36 Judd *et al.* (2003).
37 Vieta *et al.* (1997); Akiskal and Pinto (1999); Baldessarini *et al.* (2000); Benazzi, (2001, 2003a, b; Benazzi and Akiskal (2001).
38 Angst and Marneros, 2001; Akiskal and Benazzi, (2003); Benazzi (2004a); Akiskal *et al.* (2005); Angst *et al.* (2005).
39 Akiskal and Benazzi (2004).
40 Benazzi (2004b) used criteria developed by Akiskal and Benazzi (2003) in this study.
41 Benazzi (2004c, d).
42 Benazzi and Akiskal (2001, 2003b); Benazzi *et al.* (2004).
43 Benazzi (2003b); Benazzi *et al.* (2004a).
44 Cassano *et al.* (2004).
45 The principal distinction is the degree to which psychosis is recognized in the patients initially labeled as bipolar depressed.
46 Cassano *et al.* (2004), p. 1268.
47 Hopewell-Ash (1934); patient XXVII, p. 36.
48 The experience with mania following the treatment of depression with antidepressant medications is also discussed in Chapter 12.
49 Goodwin and Jamison (1990), p. 651.
50 Angst (1987); Angst *et al.* (2005); Johnson *et al.* (1991); Akiskal *et al.* (1995); Coryell *et al.* (1995b); DelBello *et al.* (2003).
51 Ghaemi *et al.* (2000).
52 Dorz *et al.* (2003).
53 Peet (1994).
54 Post *et al.* (2003).
55 In Chapters 11 and 12 we discuss the use of lithium to treat recurrent depressive illness with and without associated mania or hypomania.
56 Post (1988); Post and Weiss (1989).
57 Hirschfeld *et al.* (2002a).
58 Calabrese *et al.* (2005); Malhi *et al.* (2003); Calabrese (2004); Keck (2004). Another example of the turmoil in such recommendations, an industry-sponsored, multisite study now reports olanzapine to be more effective than placebo and olanzapine–fluoxetine combination more effective than olanzapine or placebo in bipolar I depression (Tohen *et al.*, 2003).
59 Perry *et al.* (1999); Frank *et al.* (2000); Miklowitz *et al.* (2000); Otto *et al.* (2003); Vieta and Colom (2004).
60 Sachs *et al.* (2003); Sachs (2004); Simon *et al.* (2004). A multisite naturalistic study comparing algorithm-based treatment with "treatment as usual" in which the assessments are compromised by the distance between the investigators and the patients or the therapists.
61 Calabrese *et al.* (1999a); Ghaemi *et al.* (2001, 2004b); Baldessano *et al.* (2003); Das *et al.* (2005) are some examples. The Das *et al.* study is interesting because it is a screening study for bipolar disorder in a primary care practice, finding 10% of the subjects to meet criteria for bipolar disorder. They state: "Current guidelines for bipolar disorders (American Psychiatric Association, 2002) caution against monotherapy with antidepressants since these agents may induce a hypomanic, manic, or mixed depressive/manic episode (Boerlin *et al.*, 1998; Howland, 1996). In our study, almost two thirds of participants with lifetime manic symptoms who received medication in the past month reported

taking antidepressant monotherapy." If the risks of induced mania were high, would these authors not have observed such manic episodes in their survey?

62 Taylor and Abrams (1980); McGuffin and Katz (1989); Duffy *et al.* (2000).

63 Jones *et al.* (2002a).

64 Taylor and Abrams (1980).

65 Bertelsen *et al.* (1977); McGuffin *et al.* (2003).

66 McGuffin *et al.* (2003).

67 Chapter 12.

68 The clinical evidence is cited in Chapter 8.

69 Chapter 6.

70 Among referrals for ECT, about 30% of the patients meet criteria for psychotic depression: Mulsant *et al.* (1997); Petrides *et al.* (2001).

71 Rush and Weissenburger (1994). These authors examined the psychiatric literature to assess the relevance of melancholic symptom features for DSM-IV. They found melancholic symptom features to be predictive of a positive response to ECT and tricyclic antidepressants in the severely ill. They noted that: "Melancholic features are not uniquely associated with a positive family history *per se*, but they may be especially associated with a family history of severe depression" (p. 489).

72 Cooper *et al.* (1972). Samples varied from 3 to 40 patients from populations in nine New York state hospitals for a total of 192 patients. These were compared to 174 patients derived from 22 psychiatric hospitals in London.

73 Taylor (1984, 1986).

74 Glassman *et al.* (1975); Kantor and Glassman (1977); Glassman and Roose (1981).

75 Avery and Lubrano (1979) cite the 1964 study of De Carolis and associates.

76 Dunn and Quinlan (1978); Charney and Nelson (1981); Coryell and Zimmerman (1984); Kroessler (1985); Spiker *et al.* (1985); Hickie *et al.* (1986); Buchan *et al.* (1992); Parker *et al.* (1992b); Vega *et al.* (2000); Petrides *et al.* (2001); Birkenhäger *et al.* (2003); Husain *et al.* (2004); Kho *et al.* (2003). The details as to the response to treatments are discussed in Chapter 10.

77 The criteria permit the diagnosis of schizophrenia if the patient experiences a sustained hallucinated voice or delusions of experience of alienation or control. Although mood disorder is many times more likely than is schizophrenia to be the cause of a catatonic episode, the criteria for catatonia remain in the schizophrenia category. See Fink and Taylor (2003) for a presentation of the data linking catatonia to mood disorder.

78 APA (1994).

79 Parker and Hadzi-Pavlovic (1996), pp. 179–201.

80 Parker *et al.* (1995a, b, 1997, 2001); Brodaty *et al.* (1997).

81 Austin *et al.* (1999).

82 Parker *et al.* (1998a, b).

83 Parker *et al.* (1991).

84 Parker *et al.* (1995b). "Non-reactivity" in the distinction between a melancholic and a non-melancholic depression does not refer to the absence of a preceding stressful event, but to the unchanging nature of the patient's mood. Melancholic patients cannot forget their worries and their moods do not "react" to circumstances.

85 Charney and Nelson (1981); Rihmer *et al.* (1984); Brown *et al.* (1988); Schatzberg and Rothschild (1986, 1992); Belanoff *et al.* (2001a).

86 Schatzberg *et al.* (2000).

87 Kessing (2003).
88 Mulsant *et al.* (1997).
89 Kendler (1991); Abrams and Taylor (1983).
90 Pini *et al.* (2004).
91 Keck *et al.* (2003a).
92 Bellini *et al.* (1992).
93 In Fink (1999a), see RB, pp. 37–38. A description of Rickie, an adolescent with a psychotic depression, is abstracted on pp. 49–51. Adult patients with psychotic mania are described as SF, pp. 54–5, and DG, pp. 56–7; a manic adolescent, PH, is described on pp. 58–60.
94 Spitzer *et al.* (2004); pp. 112 *ff.*
95 The editors cite DSM-IV-TR, p. 413, for the basis for this diagnosis.
96 Enoch *et al.* (1967); Berrios and Luque (1995a). Cotard syndrome is also described in patients with non-dominant parietal lobe and thalamic stroke (Critchley, 1953).
97 Berrios and Luque (1995b).
98 Young *et al.* (1992). As with all patients with evidence of a severe affective illness, systemic medical causes must be excluded by examination.
99 Hansen and Bolwig (1998); case 3, p. 462.
100 Lohmann *et al.* (1996); Mahgoub and Hossain (2004).
101 Hashioka *et al.* (2002); Soultanian *et al.* (2005).
102 Soultanian *et al.* (2005) found 17 cases in the literature, with 12 girls and 5 boys. Nine of the 17 have been successfully treated with ECT. Bipolar disorder was commonly diagnosed in follow-up.
103 Enoch *et al.* (1967).
104 Young *et al.* (1994). Also see Taylor (1999).
105 For a detailed discussion of catatonia, see Fink and Taylor (2003).
106 Chapter 6.
107 It is a common misconception that catatonic patients must be mute and posturing, and that the mutism must be total. Many manics exhibit substantial catatonic features while still having pressured speech. Depressed catatonic patients can be fully mute, selectively mute, or limited to a few occasional utterances (Fink and Taylor, 2003).
108 Mania is the most common underlying disorder when catatonia is identified in an adult patient. In children and adolescents, which condition is most common depends on the clinical setting, but catatonia is found in patients suffering from a mood disorder, antipsychotic drug toxicity, developmental disorder, seizure disorder, psychotic disorder, or illicit drug toxicities.
109 Kahlbaum first described catatonia in a treatise published in 1874. In an English translation (1973; p. 26), Kahlbaum writes:

> the psychiatric disorder described till now as atonic melancholia cannot be regarded as a separate disease entity . . . this phenomenon represents a temporary stage or a part of a complex picture . . . we recognize that the disease [catatonia] manifests itself in the first stage with an easily recognizable clinical picture of melancholia; very often the stage of melancholia is preceded by true manic states. . .

110 Bräunig *et al.* (1998, 1999); Fink and Taylor (2003).
111 Kahlbaum (Mora translation 1973), case history #3, pp. 17–20.
112 Another example of catatonia in a patient with severe depression from Kahlbaum's series is his patient Benjamin L (Mora translation, pp. 9–14), annotated in Fink and Taylor (2003) as patient 3.1 (p. 39).

113 For details on the benzodiazepine test and treatments for catatonia, see Fink and Taylor (2003).

114 The presence and severity of signs of catatonia are measured using a catatonia-rating scale. An intravenous line is established and 1 mg lorazepam is injected. The patient's response is noted. If no change in motor signs is observed a second bolus is administered and catatonia signs recorded. A 50% reduction in the catatonia-rating scale is a positive test that augurs well for the successful treatment of catatonia with oral high doses of benzodiazepines (Fink and Taylor, 2003).

115 Automatic obedience is elicited by the examiner telling the patient not to let the examiner move the patient's limbs. Despite these repeated instructions the patient cannot resist the examiner's light touch, permitting the movement. See Fink and Taylor (2003) for a full discussion of the examination for catatonia.

116 The belief that psychotic patients are at risk for violence or panic illustrates the widespread lack of understanding of psychiatric illness, even by health care professionals who should know better. Careful explanation of the procedure, to even the most psychotic patient, will usually achieve cooperation.

117 Hoch (1921); case 1, pp. 6–11.

118 Josefsson *et al.* (2001); Bloch *et al.* (2003).

119 Jennings *et al.* (1999); Spinelli (2003).

120 Affonso *et al.* (1990); Seyfried and Marcus (2003); Wisner *et al.* (1993, 1995); Beck (1996); Hendrick *et al.* (2000).

121 Chapter 12 details treatment of melancholia in complicating circumstances and chapters 8 and 9 discuss ECT.

122 Brockington and Kumar (1982); Brockington *et al.* (1982); Hamilton (1982, 1989); Stein (1982); Bloch *et al.* (2000); Freeman *et al.* (2002).

123 The dysphoria of postpartum blues may reflect hypothalamic–pituitary–adrenal (HPA) hyperactivity and high cortisol levels now unopposed by progesterone in the rapid decline of HPA hormones postpartum. In women with few risk factors for depressive illness, the "blues" resolve with hormonal normalization. In women with risk factors for psychiatric illness, the hormonal changes precipitate illness and "blues" becomes a depressive mood disorder.

124 Magiakou *et al.* (1996); Wisner and Stowe (1997).

125 For most women, no medical intervention is needed.

126 Nappi *et al.* (2001).

127 Miller and Rukstalis (1999).

128 Hapgood *et al.* (1988); Fossey *et al.* (1997); Bloch *et al.* (2003).

129 Brockington *et al.* (1982); tables 2–4, pp. 46–9.

130 *Ibid.*, p. 51. Cycloid psychosis is a European concept developed by Karl Leonhard to describe patients with a phasic psychosis with good clinical outcome. The descriptions best fit those of manic-depressive disorders. The term has been applied to patients with puerperal psychosis (Pfuhlmann *et al.*, 1998).

131 The syndrome is characterized in European literature as *oneirophrenia* (Meduna, 1950; Fink, 1999b).

132 Brockington *et al.* (1982) cite the reports of Esquirol, Connolly, and Marcé. More than half the patients with puerperal psychosis were manic, a lesser number were melancholic, and a smaller number demented. The dementia syndrome is described as "transitory intellectual enfeeblement" – a description of pseudodementia?

133 Paffenberger and McCabe (1966); Paffenberger (1982).

134 Oneirophrenia is an acute delirium that is indistinguishable from delirious mania. The syndrome is uniquely responsive to convulsive therapy (Meduna, 1950; Fink, 1999b; Fink and Taylor, 2003).

135 Thyroiditis, hypothyroidism, vitamin B_{12} deficiency, and toxicity to bromocriptine, metronidazole, and to hallucinogens such as LSD, PCP, and ecstasy are specifically cited by Miller (2002). These causes are likely to be exceedingly rare.

136 Miller (2002) cites these thoughts as ego-dystonic, "obsessional in quality," and at variance with the patients' actual statements or behaviors. If the mother becomes suicidal, the infant and other children become the target of attack. For a description of such a tragic event, see Andrea Yates (patient 8.5).

137 Hamilton, J. A. (1982, 1989); Robling *et al.* (2000); Freeman *et al.* (2002); Miller (2002).

138 Protheroe (1969).

139 *Ibid.*, p. 12.

140 *Ibid.*, p. 13.

141 *Ibid.*, p 17. Considering the differences in styles of diagnosis, it is probable that many of the patients classified as schizophrenic were manic psychotic.

142 Brockington *et al.* (1982). Confirmation is found in Ndosi and Mtawali (2002), with an incidence of 3.2/1000 births.

143 Spinelli (2004).

144 Hamilton, J. A. (1982); p. 11.

145 At the trial for murder, the jury returned a verdict of "not guilty by reason of insanity." Hamilton offers another vignette of a similar patient in California in 1976 in which the jury verdict was "guilty of second-degree murder" and the patient spent 6 months in prison. Compare this result also with that of Andrea Yates, patient 8.5, who murdered five children, was deemed psychotic and yet was committed to prison for life in Texas.

146 Klompenhouwer and van Hulst (1991). The authors called for a separate status for puerperal psychosis within modern classification systems.

147 Miller (2002). It may be that the miscarriage is an early sign of the depressive illness, and not a precipitating factor.

148 Eberhard-Gran *et al.* (2002); Janssen *et al.* (1996).

149 Jones and Craddock (2001a); Freeman *et al.* (2002).

150 O'Hara *et al.* (1991); Steiner and Tam (1999); Josefsson *et al.* (2001); Johnstone *et al.* (2001); Verdoux *et al.* (2002).

151 Chaudron *et al.* (2001a).

152 Miller (1994); Reed *et al.* (1999); Tabbane *et al.* (1999).

153 Baker *et al.* (1961).

154 An interesting experiment to simulate the postpartum state was undertaken in 16 women, 8 with and 8 without a history of postpartum depression. The gonadotropin-releasing hormone agonist leuprolide acetate was administered to simulate the postpartum hypogonadal state. Supraphysiologic doses of estradiol and progesterone were added for 8 weeks and then withdrawn under double-blind conditions. Five of the 8 women with a history of postpartum depression (62.5%) and none of the 8 women in the comparison group developed "significant mood symptoms." The authors interpret their experiment as direct evidence of the involvement of reproductive hormones in postpartum depression (Granger and Underwood, 2001).

On the other hand, different regimens of reproductive hormones failed to relieve postpartum depression (Pfuhlmann *et al.*, 2002; Kumar *et al.*, 2003). The experimental literature is weak. In a recent report, Ahokas *et al.* (2000) found low levels of estradiol in 2 patients with puerperal psychosis and treatment to raise serum levels was accompanied by reduction in psychosis.

155 Rosenzweig *et al.* (1997).

156 Bonanno and Kaltman (2001).

157 Zisook and Shuchter (1993); Brent *et al.* (1994).

158 Latham and Prigerson (2004).

159 Rosenzweig *et al.* (1997).

160 Kosaten *et al.* (1984); Shuchter *et al.* (1986).

161 Weller *et al.* (1990).

3

Defining melancholia by psychopathology

And the mind's canker in its savage mood,
When the impatient thirst of light and air
Parches the heart; and the abhorred grate,
Marring the sunbeams with its hideous shade,
Works through the throbbing eyeball to the brain
With a hot sense of heaviness and pain[1]

The descriptions of melancholia over millennia by medical authorities, writers, and public figures have face validity. The recognition led to the inclusion of "melancholia" in some form in all psychiatric classification systems.[2] This heritage regards melancholia as a disorder in mood accompanied by perturbations in circadian and ultradian rhythms. Psychomotor disturbance is always present, expressed as agitation or inactivity, slowness of movement and speech, catatonia, or stupor. Ruminations of despondency and death dominate the sufferer's waking thoughts. Suicide is all too frequent.

Melancholia is the classic depressive mood disorder. Psychotic depression, manic-depressive depression, puerperal depressions, and abnormal bereavement are part of the melancholia picture. Diverse disease processes, such as endocrinopathies and seizure disorder, induce it. It is recognized worldwide and at all ages, becoming most prominent in older adults. Melancholia is less recognized in young children, but that omission may be a distortion of classification.

Despite its long history, the position of melancholia in psychiatric taxonomy is unclear. Traditionally it was considered a distinct illness.[3] More recently it has been viewed as a stage of illness, not fundamentally different in pathophysiology from other depressive illnesses.[4] Which view is correct?

The historical record clearly presents melancholia as a distinct disorder of mood that is present from its onset. *Simple retardation* was considered a mild form.[5]

There appears gradually a sort of mental sluggishness; thought becomes difficult; the patients find difficulty in coming to a decision and in expressing themselves. It is hard for them to follow the thought in reading or ordinary conversation. They fail to find the usual interest in their surroundings.

> The process of association of ideas is remarkably retarded . . . they have nothing to say; there is a dearth of ideas and a poverty of thought . . . It is hard to remember the most commonplace things. They appear dull and sluggish, and explain that they really feel tired and exhausted . . .

Melancholia was viewed as a distinct disease, not a stage of illness. The milder features occurring at the onset of an episode were considered as typical of melancholia as were its most severe symptoms. By contrast, the historical record does not recognize most of the depression syndromes in the present classifications, although some diagnoses, such as abnormal bereavement and postpartum depression, can be seen as variants of melancholia. Other *Diagnostic and Statistical Manual* (DSM) depression options, such as dysthymia and adjustment disorder, have unclear meaning or validity.[6]

Depressive-like states are classified by severity or episode duration into major and minor categories on the assumption that all have the same pathophysiology. This assumption lacks proof and the mixing of the variations in depressive illnesses, like the mixing of apples and oranges in discussing fruits, clouds the traditional face of melancholia.

DSM depression categories and diagnostic criteria[7]

Classification difficulties

The image of depressive illness dramatically changed between 1960 and 1980. Instead of "depressive reactions" and "manic-depressive illness" the disorders in mood were divided by their association with mania or hypomania into *bipolar* (with) and *unipolar* (without) categories.[8] The authors of the recent classification took the theoretical position that most depressive illnesses are on the same continuum of severity. Melancholia became a specifier for the presence of defined signs deemed to characterize a form of depressive illness of high severity.[9] Melancholia was merged into a category that includes any sustained episode of sad mood that substantially affects behavior and functioning. The specifiers *psychotic*, *catatonic*, and *seasonal* were also added to the major depression category as variations of illnesses, rather than as traditional aspects of melancholia.

Other depressive illnesses, such as *postpsychotic depression*, *major depression superimposed upon delusional disorder or schizophrenia*, and *postpartum depression*, were listed separately as if distinct from melancholia. The boundaries between melancholia as a recognizable entity and other depressive states were blurred.

Milder depressive disorders (*dysthymia*, *premenstrual dysphoria*, *minor depression*, and *brief depression*) were described, based on epidemiologic surveys that reported their presence to be associated with depressive illnesses later in life.[10] A "subsyndromal" depression[11] and a "characterological" depression[12] were offered as part of a depression spectrum. *Substance-induced mood disorder* and *mood disorder due to a general medical condition and* "not otherwise specified" are other options.

Other forms of mood disorders were recognized in different DSM sections.[13] *Bereavement* became a form of major depression if symptoms persisted longer than

2 months after a loss or the following symptoms were present: guilt "about things other than actions taken or not taken by the survivor at the time of death," "thoughts of death other than the survivor feeling that he or she would be better off dead or should have died with the deceased person," "morbid preoccupation with worthlessness," "marked psychomotor retardation," "prolonged and marked functional impairment," and "more than transitory hallucinations of the deceased person." These features are consistent with melancholia, however, and do not warrant a separate classification.

Adjustment disorder with depressed mood is separately listed.[14] It is described as the presence of "a depressed mood, tearfulness, or feelings of hopelessness" that is so severe as to cause "marked distress" and "significant social or occupational impairment" occurring within 3 months of an identifiable stressor other than the loss of a loved one (i.e., bereavement). The condition is described as "chronic" if the symptoms persist 6 months after the stressor or its consequences have abated. Severe depressive illness, however, often follows stress and may abate spontaneously by 6 months, and in less time with treatment. Other than not meeting the list criterion for major depression and probably meeting the list, but not the duration, criterion for dysthymia, no justification is offered for separating adjustment disorder from the same spectrum that includes major depression at one end and dysthymia at the other.

Table 3.1 displays the DSM classification choices that are best viewed as forms of melancholia or that can be distinguished from melancholia.

In clinical practice, however, the DSM classification choices for depression are mostly ignored. Patients are diagnosed as having a major depression, dysthymia, or both. Polarity is then determined. The number of Medline citations for each choice is an indication of interest in each condition. Each of the terms "melancholia" and "endogenous depression" generates over 43 000 citations with substantial overlap dating from 1966 to 2003. "Major depression" generates about 11 000 citations. "Psychotic depression" generates about 4100, while none of the remaining terms produces more than 1800 responses, with many producing fewer than 1000 citations each.

In the DSM system, the pathophysiology is assumed to be the same for the mild and severe forms of depressive illnesses. This perspective leads to treatment homogenization, which reasons that more severe episodes warrant higher doses, but not different classes of medication or different forms of treatment. If heterogeneity exists, however, many patients will receive suboptimal treatment, and efforts to understand the pathophysiology of depressive illnesses will be hampered by the lumping of different conditions under the umbrella term "major depression." One explanation for the number of patients considered "treatment-resistant" and who are referred for ECT is the failure to recognize that psychotic depression is not just severe depression, but a form of depression requiring more specific treatment.[15]

Treatment algorithms for depressive mood disorders that are offered by expert panels ignore the DSM choices. Exceptions are made for psychotic depression and depressive phases of manic-depressive illness. The incorporation of patients with

Table 3.1. *Diagnostic and statistical manual* (DSM) depression choices

Melancholic "major" depressions	Heterogeneous "mixed bag", mostly non-melancholias
Melancholic	Superimposed on psychotic disorder
Psychotic	Substance-induced
Catatonic	Secondary to general medical condition
Postpartum	Postpsychotic
Abnormal bereavement	Major depression without any modifier
	Dysthymia
	Brief
	Minor
	Premenstrual dysphoria
	Adjustment disorder
	Atypical, seasonal

the many forms of depressed mood into the major depression category encourages antidepressant medication trials to ignore melancholic features or treat them as a marker of severity.[16] Study designs, especially the choices to include patients with different forms and severities of depressive symptoms, markedly affect the outcome assessments in clinical antidepressant medication trials.[17] In one study, the failure to differentiate the efficacy of citalopram and placebo in a large sample of very old unipolar depressed patients was explained by the heterogeneity of the sample. A benefit for citalopram was discerned, however, when its impact on the more severely depressed patients was separately assessed.[18]

Diagnostic criteria limitations

Boundaries have been blurred between melancholia and other conditions that share depressive features (e.g., the apathy and motor slowing in some neurologic disease, and low energy, shyness, and anxiety in some personality deviations). This difficulty arises from the vagueness and non-specificity of the diagnostic criteria. All are cross-sectional and course of illness is ignored. For example, the diagnosis of major depression requires five or more items in any combination.[19] "Fatigue or loss of energy" and "diminished ability to think or concentrate" are two choices. Severity of the difficulty is not defined; nor is a method of scoring offered. Surprisingly, depressed mood need *not* be present for the diagnosis of the depressive illness, as a loss of interest or the ability to experience pleasure is an acceptable alternative. These criteria are also not operationally defined. In the quest for diagnostic reliability, the criteria are oversimplified, thereby lowering the bar for admission into the category of depression. Taken literally (which is necessary to obtain reliability), the following patient meets DSM-IV criteria for major depression.

Patient 3.1

For almost a year a 51 year old man experienced a substantial loss of interest and anhedonia. He was sleeping 10 or more hours daily [hypersomnia is a criterion choice], and his movements and thinking became moderately slowed [psychomotor retardation is a criterion choice]. He had difficulty in concentrating his thoughts, and had no energy. He was pessimistic about the future. Although he did not want to kill himself, he did not want to be in his present state. If he could not get better he would just as soon go to sleep and not wake up. His symptoms caused "clinically significant distress [and] impairment in social functioning." His condition could not be explained as the "direct physiological effects of a substance . . . or a general medical condition." The neurologic examination was normal, except for slowness of movement and thought. His symptoms began after his trailer home burned, destroying all his possessions. He was not burned. Post traumatic stress disorder was ruled out because he did not experience nightmares and was neither anxious nor ruminating about the event. Major depression was diagnosed by several clinicians and antidepressant medications were prescribed without improvement.

During the examination, however, the man's mood was reactive, and although subdued, he showed mildly diminished emotional expression rather than sadness or apprehension. A frontal lobe avolitional syndrome[20] was diagnosed and carbon monoxide poisoning hypothesized as the cause of his behavioral change. CT-scan showed bilateral basal ganglia calcifications, a finding consistent with the diagnosis of carbon monoxide exposure. Methylphenidate treatment improved his condition. (Vignette based on case in Valdya and Taylor, 2004.)

The validity of the DSM depression criteria has been questioned. In an examination of comorbidity in twins and the occurrence of future episodes to validate externally the DSM depression criteria, the number of symptoms (the hallmark of the criteria), their duration, and resulting impairment did not predict the presence of depressive illness in a co-twin or future episodes in the proband.[21] Another study found DSM criteria to have poor agreement with core features of melancholia derived from cluster analytic and similar techniques.[22]

A consequence of the non-specificity of the diagnostic criteria is seen in prevalence figures for depression which have increased from a population lifetime base rate in the 1960s of about 6–8% to present estimates of over 10% for men and 20% for women.[23] In both periods investigators actively sought and evaluated community samples and used similar methodology, making unlikely the explanations that the increase is based on better identification procedures or a postulated greater willingness of sufferers to seek help. Cohort and period effects (respectively, earlier onset ages for first depression and more new depressions in persons born closer to the present)[24] may account for some of the change, but not to the extent indicated by marked increase in base rates. In another example in a Swedish population cohort study of 2612 persons, the lifetime cumulative probability of suffering from depression was estimated to be almost 27% for men and a staggering 45% for women, but only 8 men and 9 women were identified as having a "serious" depressive illness.[25]

The recent surveys rely on inexperienced clinicians using highly sensitive but less specific criteria in a more structured way. Two examples illustrate this problem. Using the structured instrument of the Schedule for Affective Disorders and Schizophrenia (SADS) lifetime version in an 18-month test–retest analysis, researchers found inconsistent reporting about age at illness onset and inconsistent details and number of episodes.[26] In a European multicenter epidemiologic study, using the Beck Depression Inventory, mostly non-specialists in five countries assessed persons in the community for the presence of a major depression, adjustment disorder, or dysthymia. Prevalence rates varied dramatically across countries, in some cases over threefold for men and 10-fold for women.[27] This study also accepted a Beck depression scale score of 12 and higher as reflecting a depressive disorder. Scores below 20, however, do not indicate a depressive illness identified by other rating scales or by standard clinical assessment. This depression scale score correlates only weakly with scales that better identify melancholia.[28]

Industry influence

The concept of "depression" has been broadened by targeting tendencies to shyness, social anxiety, and moodiness to justify medication treatment.[29] The rise in the number of approved antidepressant drugs parallels the increase in the variations of depression categories and in the numbers of persons diagnosed as depressed. In the early 1960s two tricyclic antidepressants (TCAs) (imipramine and amitriptyline) and three monoamine oxidase inhibitors (phenelzine, iproniazid, tranylcypromine) were marketed. In 2002, 17 antidepressants were in use in the USA, and several anticonvulsants, atypical antipsychotic agents, and lithium were described as having antidepressant properties. Additional agents are available in Europe and more are in the pipeline.[30]

In the 1990s prescriptions for antidepressant drugs increased severalfold in industrialized countries, mostly due to the prescribing of selective serotonin reuptake inhibitors.[31] Intensive industry marketing has been argued as a primary factor in this increase.[32] One example of this usage comes from an 8-month survey of 20000 French households. Three percent of persons over age 15 were taking an antidepressant during a 4-week assessment period. Although 62% were diagnosed as depressed by their treating physician, 90% of whom were non-specialists, 46% of those receiving a medication did not meet authorized indications and 25% had no diagnosis.[33]

The influence of industry is illustrated by the creation of an epidemic of "depression" in pursuit of the sale of the antidepressant Paxil in Japan.[34] Until the late Twentieth Century, "depression" in Japan mostly referred to melancholia and treatment was characterized by lengthy hospital care. Aggressive industry marketing publicizing "mild depression" prompted the government Ministry of Health to create a committee to help educate the public about depression. Celebrities talked openly about their depression and in July 2004 the Imperial Household Agency acknowledged that the Crown Princess was being treated with antidepressants and counseling for depression and an adjustment disorder. "Depression" has gone from a bad word to a buzzword. An interesting aspect of the story is a quotation from the Harvard anthropologist Arthur Kleinman, co-editor of *Culture and Depression*[35]:

> I could take you all over the world, and you would have no difficulty recognizing severely depressed people in completely different settings. But mild depression is a totally different kettle of fish. It allows us to re-label as depression an enormous number of things.

Industry marketing practices also influence clinical practice by asserting that all antidepressants have similar efficacy for all types of depressive illnesses, and by claims that the newer, more expensive agents are safer and less likely to elicit side-effects.[36] Encouraging the use of "the newest" agent, combinations of agents, and multiple sequential treatment trials for the widest market homogenizes diagnosis and treatment.

Although most patients with a diagnosis of major depression receive prescriptions for antidepressants, the decisions to treat and the antidepressant selected are not based on clinical features of the episode. The choices are based on characteristics of the patient (age, gender, race, educational level), the prescriber (generalist, specialist, geographic location of the practice), and health care insurance coverage (health management organization, non-insured).[37]

The return of a concept of melancholia as a distinct entity within the depression "scheme of things" has treatment and scientific implications. Defining melancholia as a distinct entity encourages more focused treatments that differ from those prescribed for other forms of depressive disorders. Higher doses of the same treatments alone would not be adequate. An analogy is the diagnosis and treatment of cancer. The clinical features of breast and prostate cancer may suggest each to be a homogeneous condition, but staging and identifying specific cell lines affect treatment choice and outcome.[38] Is a similar, individualized approach useful for depressive illness? Does empirical psychopathology delineate melancholia as a distinct form or stage of depression?

Consensus and empirical approaches defining a syndrome

Expert consensus

Psychiatric nosology rests on the writings of nineteenth-century European psychopathologists. Present-day classifications, including the DSM and International Classification of Diseases (ICD), are based on expert consensus. The Feighner criteria[39] and the Research Diagnostic Criteria (RDC)[40] are examples of consensus among researchers. Syndromes familiar to clinicians are identified in the classification, and agreement is reached on the main features of each syndrome. The features are then offered as diagnostic criteria. Diagnostic reliability is sought to improve the identification of proposed syndromes and to guide research. Validation of diagnostic categories is sought through laboratory testing, treatment response, and genetic investigation.

Consensus requires participants to be grounded in the clinical characteristics of the syndromes. As the different versions of DSM and ICD emerged, each consensus was restructured to account for new experiences.

Empirical definition

Diagnostic consensus should reflect empirically derived data as well as experience. In the former effort, syndromes are identified as they seem to occur naturally among large groups of patients or in community samples. Rather than assigning each patient to a category predetermined by expert consensus, the sample's inherent groupings (if any) are determined by statistical modeling and then given descriptive names.[41] Psychopathology and other clinical features expressed by each subject are systematically recorded and that database subjected to statistical analyses designed to reveal "patterns" of signs and symptoms. A well-defined pattern is assumed to represent a coherent condition when it is supported by mathematical and logical assumptions. The validity of the pattern, however, must be tested against external variables not used to generate the patterns.

Different statistical techniques have been used.[42] Factor, discriminant function, cluster, and latent class analyses are among the strategies employed.[43] The identified groups are observed for treatment response, laboratory findings, family history, and other independent criteria to determine if the groups remain distinct.

Such an empirical process begins, however, with preconceptions. The patient groups are typically hospitalized psychiatric patients who were first clinically diagnosed by the expert consensus system. The starting point is almost always the "psychiatric patient," and the search for patterns of depressive illness typically begins with patients labeled "depressed" by other systems. Examining non-patient community samples partially overcomes this bias, but these studies are few and have their own limitations (see below). Thus, the empirical strategy is a refinement of the expert consensus, not a distinctly different approach.

The empirical technique also has methodological limitations. The quality of psychopathology rating scales is uneven. The items to be measured and their ranges are arbitrary. The degree of interrater reliability and the raters' clinical skills influence results. In community sample studies, the training of the assessors is often poor compared to the quality and training of raters of hospital-based patients. The instruments used in community studies, while psychometrically sophisticated, are phenomenologically simplistic. They ignore the duration, sequence of appearance, and severity relationships among symptoms.[44]

Ascertainment bias influences results. Psychotic features are more commonly recognized in hospitalized depressed patients than in outpatients. A study of outpatients might not identify psychotic depression as readily as an analysis of inpatients. Differences in samples and sampling, clinical instruments used, the skills of the examiners, and the statistical methods employed are better explanations for differences in patterns identified across studies than any inherent differences in psychopathology in the samples.

Psychopathology data supporting the validity of melancholia

Pre-1980 literature

The strongest attack on the concept of melancholia and endogenous depression as distinct from other depressive illnesses was made by Kendell (1968, 1976). He divided the records of patients admitted between 1949 and 1963 to the teaching services of London's Maudsley Hospital into two samples ($n = 696$ and 334), the first for analysis and the second for validation. Patients clinically diagnosed as melancholic, psychotic depressed, involutional depressed, and neurotic or reactive depressed were included. Trainee psychiatrists recorded discharge information on to data sheets designed for the clinical purposes of that era. Using 60 items deemed related to depression, Kendell performed factor and discriminant analyses looking at the distribution of individual patient scores. He anticipated that a bimodal distribution would indicate two different types of depressive illnesses, while a single distribution would indicate a continuum of illness. Kendell reported a single distribution. Factor scores did not predict diagnoses, nor did they relate to any external validating variable.

Kendell acknowledged several limitations of this study. The classic features of melancholia were not included in the data collection form. Quality and reactivity of the depressed mood, non-delusional ideas of guilt or suspiciousness, diurnal mood swing, different patterns of insomnia (e.g., problems falling asleep and staying asleep), anorexia and weight loss, and slowing and poverty of speech were omitted. Omitting these items undermines the analysis, much as seeking to discriminate men from women without assessing external gender characteristics. The trainee recorders' thoroughness to assess items from the written records and their interrater reliability are also unknown.

Despite his rejection of the two-depression concept, Kendell's factor analyses revealed two factors consistent with "neurotic" and "psychotic" forms of depression (Table 3.2). The clinical features that statistically load on each factor are instructive. The neurotic features are longitudinal or historical items suggesting personality traits playing a major role in the hospitalization of those patients. The features in the psychotic depression factor are cross-sectional, indicating symptoms in immediate relation to the illness.

Because the definition of bimodality in the distribution of factor scores depends on influences beyond the existence of two different conditions, the failure to identify bimodality, Kendell's main argument, cannot resolve the relationship among depressive syndromes.[45] Other analyses, like cluster and latent class analysis, are better suited to evaluate clinical heterogeneity.[46]

Although challenged by some authors prior to 1979, such statistical investigations identified between 15% and 50% of each sample of severely depressed patients as having features of melancholia.[47] Psychomotor retardation was the most consistent melancholic feature observed across these studies,[48] a factor that is also emphasized by the experimental studies of melancholia by Parker and Hadzi-Pavlovic.[49]

Studies by Paykel (1971; Paykel *et al.*, 1973; Paykel and Henderson, 1977) illustrate the earlier efforts. In 1971 the researchers applied cluster analysis to examine the history, stress events, symptoms, treatment, and premorbid personality characteristics in 165

Table 3.2. Kendell's two depression factors

Neurotic depression	Psychotic depression
Previous anxiety symptoms	Gross disturbance in food intake
Previous subjective tension	Gross disturbance in weight
Brief duration before admission	Delusions (guilt, self-reproach, unworthiness)
Previous "hysterical" symptoms	Abnormal quantity of speech
Childhood neurotic traits	Ideas of reference
Suicidal feelings	Retarded activity
Previous obsessional symptoms	Suspiciousness
	Persecutory delusions
	Severe insomnia
	Social withdrawal

depressed patients. Four groups were identified: (1) psychotic depression with good premorbid personality (an older age group with melancholic features); (2) anxious depression with abnormal premorbid personality (a younger age group); (3) irritable depression (mixed features); and (4) mild depression with abnormal personality. In a second study, they examined the response to amitriptyline of a different sample of 85 depressed women clustered statistically into the four groups. The most severely ill psychotic patients improved most and the anxious depressed patients with abnormal personality traits improved the least. The differences in treatment response implied different pathophysiologies.

In a third report they again found depressive disorders to be clinically heterogeneous. This sample clustered into three groups: (1) older-age psychotic depressives; (2) younger-age anxious depressives with abnormal personality; and (3) younger-age mild depressives, also with abnormal personality traits. The psychotic depressive patients again responded best to amitriptyline while the other groups did poorly.[50]

The literature since 1980

With few exceptions, the many studies since 1980 using similar statistical techniques support a patient group best labeled *melancholia* (the studies use the term *endogenous depression*). The remaining patients in these samples are less easily delineated, but two subtypes emerge: atypical depression and a non-melancholic depressive illness without atypical features.[51] The consistency of these studies is striking. Despite the diversity of clinical instruments, raters, rating criteria, and patient samples spanning over two decades, when classic melancholic features are included in the assessment, a group emerges with a common distinguishing pattern (Table 3.3).

Studies examining the heterogeneity of depressive disorders that reveal a melancholic syndrome also identify a group as anxious depressed, often with somatic concerns.[52] When cross-sectional features are linked to normal premorbid function, the patients appear apprehensive and melancholic. When cross-sectional features are linked to personality traits, the patients are distinguished from those with melancholia. These findings echo Kendell's factors and support the two-depression model of "neurotic" and "melancholic."

Melancholic patients are often psychotic.[53] Others identify a separate psychotic group with melancholic features,[54] but these different views likely reflect differences in study populations and not meaningful clinical distinctions. All psychotically depressed patients are best considered as melancholic. Many melancholic patients who are not overtly delusional are suspicious and have unshakeable ideas about their low self-worth, poor health, and past unworthy actions. These ideas are also best considered the *forme fruste* of delusions.

Despite empirical support for a melancholic syndrome, not all studies have clearly separated depressed patients into melancholic and non-melancholic groups.[55] Some observers report depressed patients to differ in severity of illness, not in the quality of their depressive signs.[56]

In a sample of over 700 depressed patients from a collaborative study who met the RDC criteria for depression, latent class analysis was applied to SADS ratings.[57] They could not establish a dichotomy of melancholia and non-melancholia from the quality of mood or other DSM-III melancholia criteria. They did, however, identify two dimensions according to the presence or absence of anhedonia and vegetative signs. Vegetative signs were associated with anhedonic patients, a combination suggestive of melancholia.

A Danish study of first-ever hospital-discharged patients with the ICD-8-defined diagnosis of endogenous, reactive, or neurotic depression between the years 1970 and 1994 with follow-up to 1999 reported low diagnostic stability and poor validity for the concepts of reactive (pre-illness stressful event) and neurotic forms (the severity of symptoms is out of proportion to the assumed provoking experience). The author concludes that a classification of depression into different forms is unwarranted.[58] On re-examination, however, the endogenous form was associated with a re-diagnosis of manic-depressive illness and had substantial stability.

Using logistical regression, Benazzi could not distinguish melancholia from atypical depression, but melancholic patients with psychomotor retardation were distinguished from patients with atypical depression.[59] Psychomotor disturbance is an identifying feature of melancholia.[60] It is probable that Benazzi also found a syndrome akin to melancholia, but did not label it so. Both these studies considered cross-sectional psychopathology only. Omitting assessment of premorbid personality and laboratory measures of hypothalamic–pituitary activity limits the ability to identify melancholia.[61]

A long-standing concern is that the categorical cross-sectional approach of the DSM misses important classification information.[62] The argument asks whether cross-sectional features alone are sufficient to delineate subgroups or whether longitudinal features, such as speed and manner of emergence, the course of the episode, and personality traits should also be included. Clinical course is influenced by biologic, social, and quality of care factors, but personality, once developed, is considered stable

Table 3.3. Distinguishing features of melancholia

Matussek *et al.* (1981)	Grove *et al.* (1987)	Maes *et al.* (1990a, b)
Distinct quality of mood Loss of mood reactivity Withdrawal from social contact Inhibition (cognitive, motivation, emotional, movement) Circadian rhythm disturbance Vegetative signs	Severity of depressed mood Terminal insomnia Poor appetite and weight loss or gain Loss of interest and pleasure Agitation	Distinct quality of mood Loss of mood reactivity Loss of interest Anorexia with weight loss Sleep disorder Psychomotor retardation Loss of energy Early-morning wakening Suicidal Cognitive disturbance
Parker *et al.* (1994)	**Sullivan *et al.* (2002)**	**Ambrosini *et al.* (2002)**
Non-interactive Facial immobility Postural slumping Non-reactivity Delayed responsiveness Paucity of speech Body immobility Poverty of associations Reduced spontaneity	Distinct quality of mood Anhedonia Anorexia with weight loss Insomnia Psychomotor agitation Fatigue Cognitive disturbance Feelings of guilt and worthlessness Suicidal thoughts	Distinct quality of mood Irritability Anhedonia Diurnal mood Fatigue Cognitive disturbance Psychomotor retardation Anhedonia Hopelessness and helplessness Social avoidance

unless distorted by brain disease. Several investigators suggest that using standardized methods of personality assessment usefully distinguishes depressive illness from anxiety disorder with depression.[63] Personality disorder is more often considered in the concepts of atypical depression and non-melancholic syndromes.

The nature of melancholia

Some studies identify a melancholia subtype as a severe form on a continuum of depressive illness.[64] Others regard melancholia as a distinct disease.[65] Another view is that melancholia is a unique stage of depressive illness that only develops when a physiologic threshold is crossed. This last interpretation combines the first two models, arguing that depressive mood disorders begin in a continuum of severity but at some point develop a qualitative change in pathophysiology.

Statistical cluster analyses of depressed patients in the National Institute of Mental Health collaborative study addresses this question.[66] Using depression items of the SADS in 150 patients, they identified three depressive clusters: one with vegetative signs and a non-reactive mood; one characterized by emotional lability, reactivity, irritability, and alcohol abuse; and a third characterized by reduced interest, anhedonia, and a non-reactive mood. The first and the third clusters were similar to each other, with the first the more severe. These two clusters differed from the second cluster, indicating a distinction among the groups. The investigators interpreted their results as representing both quantitative and qualitative differences among depressed patients. An alternative interpretation is that the first and the third clusters represent severities of melancholia and the second cluster represents a non-melancholic mood disorder.

In a second (1982) sample of 228 patients, the investigators identified four clusters: (1) a severe endogenous type; (2) a mild depressive illness; (3) a mood disorder associated with mania; and (4) a severe psychotic depressive form. Each group had a strong familial loading for depression. These findings are similar to the first sample but with more severely ill patients and the inclusion of depressed patients with manic-depressive illness.

In an extension of this sample (1982, 1987), data from 569 patients were divided into "nuclear" and "non-nuclear" depressive forms. The nuclear depression group overlapped with the endogenous concept; the patients were less responsive to antidepressant medications and had a more severe course than the non-nuclear group. The non-nuclear group were less well defined but overlapped with the reactive depression concept. The investigators interpreted their findings to represent both a continuum and a qualitative change at a point along that continuum.

The threshold model suggests that the simple addition of symptoms (a characteristic of the recent DSM editions) is insufficient to capture the melancholia syndrome because most depressed patients share many symptoms. For example, in a latent class analysis that identified a melancholia group, few individual symptoms distinguished melancholic patients from other depressed patients.[67] Most item loadings (sleep, appetite, anhedonia) were similar in both groups. The signs of psychomotor disturbance, however, clearly distinguished the two patient groups (Table 3.3). These investigators previously reported that the psychomotor disturbance in depressed patients represents three factors: retardation, agitation, and "non-interactiveness."[68] These factors occur independently, confirming the clinical experience that a patient can be agitated and simultaneously have psychomotor retardation. When patients had high scores on only one factor, distinguishing subgroups was poor. Melancholia was best identified with high scores on all three factors. The presence of several clinical dimensions, not the number of motor features or vegetative signs, identified melancholia.

Psychomotor disturbance is as fundamental to melancholia as are vegetative signs.[69] In a review of factor and cluster analytic studies of depression, Nelson and Charney (1981) concluded that psychomotor change was the clearest and most consistent feature associated with melancholia. Among nine operational definitions of melancholia, Rush and Weissenburger (1994) reported psychomotor retardation to be the single feature common to all. Five of the nine definitions also included agitation. Indeed, the presence of psychomotor change is the most recognized feature in almost all studies that identify melancholia as a form of depression.[70]

Conclusions

Melancholia is a distinct syndrome

In severely ill depressed patients, melancholia has been reliably identified by clinical examination and sophisticated statistical techniques. The few studies that do not delineate this form of depressive disorder do identify clusters of cross-sectional psychopathology that are consistent with the classic concept of melancholia. The separation of melancholia from other depressive conditions is based on qualitative clinical signs of non-reactive mood, psychomotor disturbance, vegetative signs, and psychotic features (Table 3.4). Such a systematic recognition of melancholia is consistent with centuries of descriptions by psychopathologists. Some clinical features, however, are shared by other mood disorders (e.g., all depressive disorders are associated with mood and sleep disturbance) and several studies report a general depression factor shared by all depressive illnesses.[71] This shared factor, however, does not address the relationship of melancholia to other depressive disorders. Many distinct diseases have common features (e.g., fever and weakness in systemic infections, weakness and shortness of breath in heart failure and anemia, pain and anorexia in various neoplasmic disorders).

Melancholia is a specific depressive disorder:

Although a distinctive syndrome, psychopathology alone does fully define melancholia's pathophysiology. In the unique stage formulation, when specific clusters of psychopathology coalesce, they represent a qualitative change in underlying pathophysiology. The depressed patient has passed over a threshold and the nature of the illness has changed. Classic psychopathologists, however, would argue that these specific features are present in mild form at the onset of an episode and so melancholia is best seen as a distinct form of depressive disorder. Studies that assess patients from wellness through onset of illness may best resolve this issue. Laboratory studies of the pathophysiology of melancholia, discussed in Chapters 4 and 6, offer further clarification.

Additional indication that melancholia is a specific form of depression comes from the review of analytic studies that have tried to resolve the question of whether there is one depression (the continuum hypothesis) or two: melancholia/endogenous or neurotic/reactive.[72] Most of these studies report that they identified melancholia/endogenous depression. These studies often fail to define adequately any other form of depressive illness, however, other than as a "general illness" factor. Some have interpreted the failure to identify several forms of depressive illness as proof that the melancholia/endogenous versus neurotic/reactive concept has no merit and that there is only one depressive illness. The logic of "Occam's razor" suggests that this illness is melancholia.

Melancholia offers a specific paradigm

Identifying a severe depressive illness with a defined psychopathology, laboratory evidence, and a predictable response to known interventions as "melancholia" offers

Table 3.4. Behavioral characteristics of melancholia

Unchanging abnormal mood autonomous from circumstances
(often with anxiety and apprehension)
Psychomotor disturbance
(retardation, agitation, reduced responsiveness)
Vegetative signs
(anorexia, weight loss, sleep disturbance)
Psychotic features
Normal premorbid personality

a paradigm shift in thinking about mood disorder. Separating melancholia from other mood disorders for which the psychopathology and treatment response are varied and without specific laboratory tests offers clinicians a way to organize their perceptions so that treatments are optimized and population samples for research are more homogeneous.[73]

NOTES

1 Byron (1970); p. 367.
2 Rush and Weissenburger (1994); Paykel (2002).
3 Angst (1966).
4 Lewis (1934a); Ascher (1951/1952); Hamilton (1967).
5 The description of melancholia by Defendorf in his 1902 textbook, as cited by Jackson (1986); p. 191.
6 Chapter 6.
7 See below and Chapter 15 for suggested modifications to present DSM criteria to identify melancholia as a defined clinical entity, as the nosology recognizes delirium, dementia, and catatonia (Taylor and Fink, 2003).
8 To understand the thinking that led to the unipolar and bipolar concept, see Perris (1966, 1969, 1992).
9 Major depression may also be diagnosed as "major depression with melancholic features" when the patient also has three of six features: (1) distinct quality of depressed mood that feels different from bereavement; (2) symptoms worse in the morning; (3) early-morning awakening; (4) marked psychomotor retardation or agitation; (5) significant anorexia or weight loss; and (6) excessive or inappropriate guilt (DSM-IV, p. 384).
10 Kessler *et al.* (2003a, b); Pezawas *et al.* (2003).
11 Solomon *et al.* (2001); Lavretsky and Kumar (2002).
12 Akiskal *et al.* (1980).
13 DSM-IV, pp. 684–5 and discussion in Chapter 5.
14 DSM-IV, pp. 623–7 and discussion in Chapter 6.
15 Mulsant *et al.* (1997); Fink (2003a, b).
16 Chapter 6.
17 Khan *et al.* (2004).

18 Roose *et al.* (2004).
19 DSM-IV, p. 327; also see Shankman and Klein (2002).
20 There are several frontal lobe syndromes, some of which have signs that overlap with mood disorder. See Taylor (1999), Chapter 1.
21 Kendler and Gardner (1998).
22 Joyce *et al.* (2002).
23 Silverman (1968); Blazer *et al.* (1988; 1994); Maier *et al.* (1992a,b); Olsson and von Knorring (1999); Dowrick *et al.* (2001); Kessler *et al.* (2003a); Malhi *et al.* (2005).
24 Cross-National Collaborative Group (1992); Kessler and Walter (1998).
25 Rorsman *et al.* (1990).
26 Bromet *et al.* (1986).
27 Ayuso-Mateos *et al.* (2001).
28 Chapter 5.
29 Healy and Sheehan (2001).
30 Hirschfeld and Vornik (2004).
31 Norris (2001); Sleath and Shih (2003).
32 Healy and Thase (2003).
33 Olie *et al.* (2002).
34 Shulz (2004).
35 Kleinman and Good (1985).
36 Chapter 10.
37 Sleath and Shih (2003).
38 Abuzallouf *et al.* (2004); Schelfout *et al.* (2004).
39 Feighner *et al.* (1972).
40 Spitzer *et al.* (1975).
41 Overall and Hollister (1980).
42 A technical discussion of these methods is presented by Fleiss (1972).
43 Kendler *et al.* (1996).
44 Eaton and Kessler (1985).
45 Murphy (1964); Everitt (1981).
46 Cluster analysis, although considered a superior technique to factor analysis, may be distorted by variations in the choice of subjects, calculations, assumptions and hierarchies in the analysis, selection of criteria, and in the number of predetermined clusters forcing a solution that is spurious. Conclusions should not be drawn from a single analysis, but need to depend on consistencies across studies.
47 MacFadyen (1975a, b).
48 Blashfield and Morey (1979).
49 Parker and Hadzi-Pavlovic (1996).
50 Prusoff and Paykel (1977). The identification of different numbers of subgroups in these studies by the same investigator or among different investigators should not be disconcerting. The variability across clinical samples and the multitude of factors that influence symptoms guarantee studies will vary in the number of subgroups identified. The Paykel studies demonstrate the similarities of the findings, and the consistent identification of melancholia.
51 Overall and Hollister (1980); Matussek *et al.* (1981); Andreasen and Grove (1982); Feinberg and Carroll (1982); Copeland (1985); Petho (1986); Grove *et al.* (1987); Miller and Nelson (1987); Blazer *et al.* (1988); Biro and Till (1989); Eaton *et al.* (1989); Nurcombe *et al.*

(1989); Maes *et al.* (1990a, b); Furukawa and Sumita (1992); Haslam and Beck (1993); Parker and Hadzi-Pavlovic (1993); Maes *et al.* (1994); Staner *et al.* (1994); Parker *et al.* (1995a, 1999a, b 2000a, 2002, 2003); Kendler *et al.* (1996) Robertson *et al.* (1996); Carmanico *et al.* (1998); Serretti *et al.* (1998b); Sullivan *et al.* (1998, 2002); Fountoulakis *et al.* (1999); Olsson and von Knorring (1999); Tylee *et al.* (1999) Chen *et al.* (2000); Solomon *et al.* (2001); Ambrosini *et al.* (2002); Benazzi (2002); Lavretsky and Kumar (2002); Ohaeri and Otote (2002).

52 Overall and Hollister (1980); Blazer *et al.* (1988); Biro and Till (1989).

53 Copeland (1985); Maes *et al.* (1990a, b).

54 Biro and Till (1989); Parker and Hadzi-Pavlovic (1993); Parker *et al.* (1995b).

55 Young *et al.* (1986).

56 Sullivan *et al.* (1998, 2002).

57 Young *et al.* (1986).

58 Kessing (2004b).

59 Benazzi (2002).

60 Parker and Hadzi-Pavlovic (1996).

61 Miller and Nelson (1987).

62 McHugh and Slavney (1982); Eysenck *et al.* (1983); Klein and Riso (1993).

63 Clark and Watson (1991); Watson *et al.* (1995); Brown *et al.* (1998).

64 Sullivan *et al.* (1998, 2002).

65 Parker and Hadzi-Pavlovic (1996); Parker (2000).

66 Andreasen *et al.* (1980); Andreasen and Grove (1982); Grove *et al.* (1987).

67 Parker *et al.* (1994).

68 Parker *et al.* (1993).

69 Lewis (1934).

70 Benazzi (2002b). He identified a melancholia subtype in almost 18% of his patients, but could not demonstrate psychomotor disturbance as a core feature of the syndrome. On the other hand, the extensive studies by Parker and Hadzi-Pavolvic, summarized in their monograph *Melancholia: A Disorder of Movement and Mood* (1996), emphasize psychomotor disturbance as the classic sign of the syndrome.

71 Biro and Till (1989); Serretti *et al.* (1998b).

72 MacFadyen (1975a). The term "reactive" was originally used to define the quality of the depressed mood and its changeability within the depression episode, i.e,. under some circumstances the mood improved or worsened. It did not mean that the depression was a reaction to stress. "Endogenous" depression was also recognized as being precipitated by stressful events, but the mood was unshakeable (Blinder, 1969).

73 Modern psychology recognizes perception as socially constructed through mental models or mind sets (paradigms) that frame our experience. Clinical diagnosis is not based on percepts that are in a blank state but on the focusing, selection, and organization of percepts to fit within a learned mind set (Senge, 1990; Gorman, 1992; Werhane, 1999). Clinicians develop models to which an individual's complaints, history, and examination are compared. Clinical diagnosis is the recognition of dysfunction that predicts cause and response to interventions. Melancholia is a mental model that is heuristically useful.

4

Defining melancholia: laboratory tests

The lesson of the history of psychiatry is that progress is inevitable and irrevocable from psychology to neurology, from mind to brain, never the other way round. Every medical advance adds to the list of diseases which may cause mental derangement. The abnormal mental state is not the disease, nor its essence or its determinant, but an epiphenomenon. This is why psychological theories and therapies, which held out such promise at the turn of the century when so much less was known of localization of function in the brain, have added so little to understanding and treatment of mental illness, despite all the time and effort devoted to them.[1]

The serological identification of syphilis is the model of a specific laboratory test for a general medical disorder. The test separates the behavioral syndrome of neurosyphilis from phenotypically similar but etiologically diverse conditions of mood and psychotic disorders. No such assessment exists for psychiatric disorders, despite more than a century of effort. A major hurdle in this quest has been the inability to define syndromes with biological homogeneity, thus confounding samples and eliciting conflicting findings. The dexamethasone suppression test (DST) was positive (non-suppression) in about 50% of depressed patients but was deemed unsuitable as a laboratory test in depressive illness, despite the evidence that samples of depressed patients were heterogeneous.[2] Severely depressed patients, however, have substantial perturbations in their neuroendocrine functioning and measures of the endocrine system remain the best laboratory-based opportunity to demarcate mood disorders.[3]

Neuroendocrine measures in mood disorders

Nineteenth-century descriptions of the clinical effects of atrophy of the adrenal glands and adrenalectomy opened the door to the study of the endocrine glands.[4] Definition of the physiology of the adrenal extracts, isolation of epinephrine (adrenaline), descriptions of Cushing's syndrome, demonstration of chemical neurotransmission by Otto Loewi, and demonstrations of hypothalamic control of the pituitary gland by Geoffrey Harris established the science of endocrinology. Of particular interest was the association of hyperadrenalism with insomnia, loss of mental concentration, and "fits of unnatural irritability (alternating with periods of depression)."[5] The injection of thyroid extract to relieve myxedema showed the benefit of replacement hormone therapeutics. The discovery of insulin and its use in insulin coma therapy established another connection between hormones and behavior.[6] The effects of acute and chronic stress on body metabolism, especially on functions of the adrenal glands, were recognized by Walter Cannon and by Hans Selye.[7] More recently, abnormalities in inflammatory markers and cytokines have been identified in patients with severe depression.[8]

Brain cellular aggregates dispatching chemical messengers into the blood to affect structures in the body, the release of hormones with multisystem effects, and specific chemical and hormonal feedback responses became the defining model of reciprocal relations between the brain and other organs. Among these, the principal relationships of interest for psychiatric disorders today are the hypothalamic–pituitary–adrenal (HPA) and hypothalamic–pituitary–thyroid (HPT) systems. Other systems, like the hypothalamic–pituitary–growth hormone (HPGH) system, also surely affect human behavior.[9]

Neuroendocrine abnormalities were initially hailed as indices of an abnormal mental state, particularly as measures of the severity of a depressive mood disorder. But some patients who met *Diagnostic and Statistical Manual* (DSM) criteria for depressive disorder did not exhibit the abnormalities, and patients with diagnoses other than major depression and manic-depression exhibited abnormal findings. Abnormalities also occurred during the third trimester in pregnancy and in cachectic and starved patients. The value of the DST as a specific diagnostic test was questioned.[10]

Rather than challenging the classification criteria, however, tests of neuroendocrine function were deemed diagnostically not specific, and were discarded.[11] To recognize the tests as diagnostic criteria would implicitly have accepted the criticism that the DSM definitions for major depression were seriously flawed.[12] The decision to discard a measurable and safe index of systemic dysfunction and to rely solely on phenotypic non-objective classification also blunted interest in laboratory tests as indices of diagnosis.[13] The re-examination of tests of neuroendocrine function in mood disorder is, however, warranted because of the heterogeneity repeatedly found in samples of depressed patients and the problems with DSM diagnostic criteria for mood disorder.[14]

This re-examination addresses the validity of neuroendocrine abnormalities as valid markers of mood disorder, and the evidence indicates that such functions are abnormal when the patients are severely depressed. These abnormalities resolve with remission, become abnormal again with recurrence, and vary with the severity of mood disorder. They are state markers of a disorder in mood. Neuroendocrine tests tap into a dimension that is not visible in clinical assessments or family histories, offering useful diagnostic and treatment information. Does such information identify the melancholic syndrome, aid in treatment selection and care, and predict future illness?

Present methodology focuses attention on the DST, its modification in the DEX/CRH test (see below), and on tests of thyroid function. Electroencephalogram (EEG) studies, especially studies of sleep EEG which are associated with neuroendocrine abnormalities, may also have a role in the identification of melancholia and the treatment of the illness.[15]

The hypothalamic–pituitary–adrenal axis[16]

The association between elevated plasma levels of 17-hydroxycorticosteroids and severe mood disorder was a defining observation.[17] While patients with Cushing's syndrome exhibited hypercortisolemia and severe disorders of mood, the same phenomena were also found in severely depressed patients who did not have adrenal or pituitary lesions characteristic of Cushing's syndrome. A diurnal variation in cortisol was described, as was its fall with the administration of exogenous corticosteroids. These observations set the stage for the development of the DST as a standardized test of the HPA system.

The HPA axis refers to the indirect negative-feedback system of interacting hormonal discharges between the hypothalamus, pituitary, and adrenal cortex. Central nervous system control over the axis comes from inhibitory circuitry involving the hippocampus and fornix, and from excitatory circuits involving the amygdala. Stress circuitry involves the amygdala and brainstem centers, while circadian organization is mediated primarily through the suprachiasmatic nucleus. The controlling chemical cascade begins with the corticotrophin-releasing hormone (CRH) of the hypothalamus stimulating the release of adrenocorticotropic hormone (ACTH) of the pituitary.[18] ACTH stimulates the release of cortisol from the adrenal cortex and the feedback cycle is completed when increasing levels of cortisol inhibit the functions of the hypothalamus and the anterior pituitary.[19] The HPA axis has both circadian and ultradian periodicity. The glandular products not only modify the actions of the endocrine glands but also affect the functions of all cells in the body.[20]

In normal subjects, cortisol is released in bursts in a diurnal cycle with peaks in the morning and troughs in the early night. The release of CRH, then ACTH, then eventually cortisol is inhibited by synthetic glucocorticoids such as dexamethasone and prednisolone. In severely depressed patients the cortisol levels are elevated, diurnal rhythmicity is shallow, and the response to synthetic glucocorticoids is lost.

Much credit for the development of our understanding of the HPA axis and the DST is due to the work of Bernard Carroll and his associates at Universities of Melbourne and Michigan.[21] Beginning in 1967, they studied cortisol release and the effects of glucocorticoid administration. They varied the time and dosage of glucocorticoid administration and the number and times of sampling; examined plasma, urine, and cerebrospinal fluid levels of cortisol; and sought to optimize the statistical handling of these complex measures.[22]

They explored the differences between severely depressed and non-depressed psychiatric patients and normal subjects. They found abnormal cortisol regulation in the more severely depressed patients. Weight loss, agitation, and duration of illness were associated with dexamethasone non-suppression.[23]

Elevated plasma cortisol levels fell with successful antidepressant treatment, exhibiting posttreatment values similar to those of normal subjects. In 5 depressed patients treated with electroconvulsive therapy (ECT), for example, the abnormal cortisol levels and response to dexamethasone normalized when substantial improvement in their clinical condition occurred.[24] Of the depressed patients studied over

4 years, 7 patients persisted in an abnormal response to dexamethasone despite treatment. All persistently exhibited physiological symptoms of depression and active outpatient treatments were required to prevent relapse and re-hospitalization. Carroll concluded that: "The suppression test distinguished clearly between the depressed and the control patients who could not be distinguished simply on the basis of their diurnal plasma cortisol levels."[25]

At the time of these studies (1968–1972), psychoanalytic theories and concepts of stress dominated psychiatric thinking. The significance of abnormal plasma cortisol levels in relation to anxiety and psychological defense mechanisms was explored. One author concluded that elevations of steroid products in the urine were associated with the "breakdown of psychological defenses."[26] In a detailed study of cortisol in severely depressed patients treated with ECT, writers concluded that adrenal activation was related "not to the depressive illness per se, but rather to the more universal ego phenomena, such as . . . neurotic 'signal anxiety' or psychotic 'disintegrative anxiety'."[27] As a test of these hypotheses, Carroll examined groups of depressed, schizophrenic, and manic patients, finding: "a psychoendocrine distinction between primary depressive behavior and secondary depressive symptomatology . . . [complementing] the same distinction which can be made on clinical grounds, in terms of response to treatment, and in terms of factor analysis of the Hamilton [depression rating] scale."[28] Alternative ways to measure the HPA axis, including intravenous ACTH infusion, lysine vasopressin, insulin-induced hypoglycemia, and measures of plasma growth hormone, were explored.[29]

Attempts to suppress HPA axis function with exogenous steroids developed rapidly in the early 1960s.[30] The use of the synthetic dexamethasone as a test of endogenous cortisol suppression evolved into the "dexamethasone suppression test."[31] In its present form, plasma cortisol is measured at anticipated peak and trough times (0800 and 2300 h), and at additional times to increase samples for study (usually 1200 and 1600 h). A single oral dose of steroid, usually 1–2 mg dexamethasone, is administered orally at 2300 h to exert maximum effect on morning cortisol levels. In the "standard" DST, a post-dexamethasone serum cortisol level of 5 μg/dl is a recommended cutoff.[32] Normal persons exhibit diurnal cortisol periodicity (although the values may vary within "normal" ranges). Post-dexamethasone, the levels fall. In melancholic patients cortisol levels are higher than 5 μg/dl, rhythmicity is lost, and post-dexamethasone levels do not fall.[33]

The principles of the test were established in a 1968 study reporting that plasma 11-hydroxycorticosteroid did not undergo its normal fall after dexamethasone in 14 of 27 hospitalized severely melancholic patients. Following recovery from depression, normal responsiveness returned.[34] The details of the test were established by 1976.[35] In 42 patients with "endogenous depression" compared to 42 patients with other psychiatric disorders, the patients with endogenous depression had greater HPA activity before dexamethasone and less complete HPA suppression after dexamethasone. Patients with two or more abnormal cortisol values after dexamethasone were correctly identified as being endogenously depressed.[36] A 1981 study validated the DST in 438 patients using a cutoff level of 5 μg/dl plasma cortisol after 1 mg dexamethasone administration "as a test for the diagnosis of melancholia (endogenous depression)."[37] Two blood samples taken at 1600 and 2100 h after dexamethasone "detected 98% of the abnormal test results. This version of the DST identified melancholic patients with a sensitivity of 67% and a specificity of 96%."[38]

Technical difficulties, however, plague the DST and account for much of the variability in findings. Chemical assays of steroids are difficult to standardize so that laboratories differ in the levels of cortisol in normal subjects. Carroll concludes that, although the chemical assays "lack specificity in varying degree . . . they are quite adequate for detection of change in the plasma cortisol level, e.g. diurnal variation, stimulation and suppression."[39] Each center, however, must establish its own laboratory normal values for a proper interpretation of the DST.

While modern assays depend on plasma levels, urinary measures provide complementary information about steroid levels.[40] Lately, salivary levels offer a simplified and non-stressful measure of cortisol.[41]

After accounting for the variations in test administration and chemical assays, the overriding conclusion was that plasma cortisol levels are elevated in severely depressed patients. Cortisol rhythmicity and response to dexamethasone are also lost. The degree of abnormality was correlated with the severity of the mood disorder and, where assessed, was seen as a measure of endogeneity of the mood disorder or of melancholia. Cortisol measures normalize with successful antidepressant treatment.[42] Higher cortisol values and greater changes were found in hospitalized patients, especially those referred for ECT. Cortisol levels were also found to be higher in older depressed patients.[43]

In the 1980s, the DST was examined widely and the conclusions published by Carroll were, for the most part, confirmed. Hypercortisolemia was identified as a state marker of depressive mood disorder. The system measured differences between hospitalized and non-hospitalized populations. The more severe the mood disorder, the more likely the test would be abnormal. The more the patients met criteria for endogenous illness, the higher the percentage with abnormality. But several investigations, while confirming that endogenous/melancholic patients were more likely to be non-suppressors than other patients, also found non-suppression in patients with other illnesses. Unlike the framers of the DSM, however, these investigators generally concluded that the test was helpful and that the classification was problematic.[44]

The identification of patients with abnormal HPA functioning by clinical features is complicated. A study using four different sets of diagnostic criteria that relied solely on unweighted clinical features to identify endogenous depression found small differences in the DST. The range of non-suppression in the DST for endogenous depressed patients was 36–48%, while the range for non-endogenous depressed patients was 28–33%.[45] Another study examining the same four sets of criteria found the sensitivity of the DST to range from 39% to 48% and the specificity to range from 80% to 100%.[46] Diagnostic confidence ranged from 66% to 100%. The DSM-III showed the lowest specificity and lowest predictive value.

When depressed patients are divided into melancholic and non-melancholic groups using the classic formulation for melancholia, high serum cortisol levels and non-suppression to DST are mainly found in the melancholic group. Only half the patients identified as melancholic by different diagnostic systems exhibit non-suppression in the DST. An interesting example is the analysis of the DST in samples divided using the concept of "endogenomorphic depression."[47] Baseline measures of plasma cortisol and urinary free cortisol were higher in 40% of 42 patients with endogenomorphic depression compared to elevated levels in 12% of the 42 patients with depressive neuroses. The probability of a patient with a high value being an endogenomorphic depressive was calculated to be 77%.[48]

An explanation for the above findings is the assumption that varying numbers of features in any combination are adequate to identify melancholia. Such an assumption assesses features that are not specific to melancholia ("add noise") and do not add discriminating power to the system. In a study of 220 depressed inpatients using cluster analytic and similar strategies, both melancholic (39% of the sample) and non-melancholic clusters were identified.[49] Only quality and non-reactivity of mood, diurnal mood variation, early-morning awakening, psychotic features, and psychomotor disturbance were substantially helpful in this delineation.[50]

In another study of 95 depressed inpatients, initial insomnia, agitation, loss of libido, and weight loss correlated positively with DST non-suppression. The investigators combined their data with a literature review and concluded that non-suppression was associated with vegetative signs but not with the symptoms of loss of interest, anhedonia, guilt, worthlessness, helplessness, hopelessness, or suicidal ideation that are considered the "psychological" features common to many forms of mood disorder. Psychomotor disturbance was the most commonly reported feature and sleep disturbance was the next most common feature to correlate with non-suppression.[51] Others have reached similar conclusions.[52]

The severity of the melancholic episode increases the likelihood of high serum cortisol levels and DST non-suppression.[53] This is best seen in the high specificity of the DST in patients with delusional (psychotic) depression.[54] Detailed studies find high plasma and 24-hour urinary free cortisol levels both before and after dexamethasone in psychotic depressed patients.[55] Psychotic schizophrenic patients typically do not show abnormal cortisol levels, arguing that the high levels are not a characteristic of the psychosis, but of mood disorder.[56] A meta-analysis of 14 studies comparing DST results in psychotic and non-psychotic depressed patients found the non-suppression rate to be substantially higher in psychotic depressed patients.[57]

A study not included in the meta-analysis assessed 131 consecutive hospital admissions and 356 adult outpatients with depressive illness for their response to the DST.[58] Of these, 422 were labeled unipolar depressed and 65 bipolar depressed. Non-suppression occurred in 27% of all patients with major depression and 43% of those identified as bipolar depressed. In the outpatients, non-suppression was found in 35% of the endogenous depressed and 9% of the non-endogenous depressed. In the inpatients, non-suppression was found in 62% of the endogenous subjects and 19% of the non-endogenous depressed. For the inpatient and outpatient total sample, the DST exhibited a sensitivity of 46% and a specificity of 90%. Weight loss, gender, and severity added little to the differences between groups. The authors conclude that the Research Diagnostic Criteria (RDC) endogenous/non-endogenous dichotomy was validated by the DST.

A detailed study of hourly cortisol and ACTH levels also reported distinct differences between non-psychotic depressed and psychotic depressed patients with distinct profiles of HPA axis dysregulation.[59] In extensive studies of melancholia by Parker and his associates, psychotic melancholia was characterized by severity of psychomotor disturbance.[60] DST non-suppression was recorded in 72% of the psychotic depressed patients. The mood was characterized as "non-reactive."[61]

In an outpatient study, a single measure of cortisol correctly identified 40% of patients diagnosed as endogenous depression by RDC criteria but was weaker in identifying those who met criteria for major depressive disorder.[62]

The change in DST from non-suppression to suppression after a course of ECT was first described by Carroll (1972c) in 5 severely depressed patients. In the next decade, both DST suppressors and non-suppressors were treated and both groups experienced immediate clinical benefits of ECT. In the non-suppressors, however, the failure to reverse to suppression was considered a harbinger of early relapse.[63] In an early study of DST in hospitalized male veterans with unipolar depression, 17 of 20 patients exhibited hypercortisolemia and 14 failed to suppress after dexamethasone. Normalization of cortisol function occurred after successful courses of ECT.[64]

An unexpected finding in some patients treated with ECT was the development of cortisol non-suppression after initial cortisol suppression. The reversal of the DST results was not associated with an immediate worsening of the clinical condition. This apparent anomaly arises as the stimulus of the seizure stimulates the hypothalamus to release CRH and increase ACTH. Serum cortisol levels increase up to fivefold in the first seizure. After the last seizure, the increase is twofold.[65] In tests weeks after the last ECT, the CRH–ACTH–cortisol levels have returned to normal levels.[66] Should melancholia recur, however, cortisol levels are again elevated and the DST abnormal, reflecting the hormonal changes inherent in the relapse.

The admission DST values have prognostic value for the long-term course of depressive illness.[67] In the initial DST of 29 severely depressed hospitalized patients, 16 were non-suppressors and 13 suppressors. In the follow-up period of 5–7 years with continuing treatment, 8/16 DST non-suppressors and 2/13 DST suppressors were readmitted to hospital.

Depressed patients with abnormal DST have a higher risk for suicide.[68] In one 15-year follow-up study the suicide risk was 27% compared to 3% among patients with a normal DST.[69] A review of 101 patients followed for 2 years confirmed the higher risk for suicide and higher risk for hospitalization for suicidality in those with abnormal DST.[70] Patients with abnormal cortisol metabolism are more likely to make suicide attempts.[71] Yet, other studies do not find the association.[72]

Although described as a state marker for depressive mood disorder, the DST was examined as a screening diagnostic test. When applied in patients with diagnoses other than depressive mood, the incidence of abnormal DST was considerably lower than that found in depressed patients. The examination of the DST in patients with manic-depressive illness, however, is complicated by the presence of depressive moods and symptoms in these patients and the relationship of manic-depressive illness to melancholia.[73] The frequency of non-suppression in manic patients varies from 0% to 70%.[74] The highest frequency of abnormal tests is seen in mixed bipolar disorder, even higher than in psychotic unipolar depression.

The incidence of DST non-suppression varies greatly in patients with dysthymic disorder, posttraumatic stress disorder, and schizophrenia. Non-suppression is more frequent in the schizophrenic patients with high scores on the negative symptom scale.[75] Suicide is also common in patients with schizophrenia, accounting for 10% of the deaths among these patients.[76] The same variability in cortisol non-suppression is reported in patients with obsessive-compulsive disorder, panic disorder, and anxiety states.[77] The DST is reported to be abnormal in patients with chronic fatigue syndrome.[78] These studies, and many other similar assessments of the DST, do not assess the patients for concurrence of mood disorder, but nevertheless conclude that the DST is not a useful DSM diagnostic criterion.

Carroll was cognizant of the limitations of the early forms of the test when applied to diagnosis. Summarizing his experiences, he concluded: "that there is no all-or-none HPA suppression response to dexamethasone. Rather a *graded series* of abnormal responses can be identified. An observation period of 24 hr is needed for the adequate assessment of this HPA response."[79] Despite this caution, the DST was widely used and the test engendered controversy.[80]

One study examined 231 psychiatric inpatients with either 1 or 1.5 mg dexamethasone at 2300 h. Blood samples were taken at 0900, 1600, and 2300 h and there was a cutoff threshold of 5 μg/dl.[81] Comparing the two forms of DST, the authors concluded: "Neither test significantly separated endogenous depressed patients from patients with other depressive and non-depressive psychiatric disorders." They reported 12% non-suppressors in 75% normal healthy subjects.

Another assessment concluded that the DST "has not proved to reflect pathophysiologic changes at the level of the central nervous system or pituitary, and tissue availability of dexamethasone may contribute to test outcome. The sensitivity of the DST in major depression is limited (about 44% in over 5000 cases) but is higher in psychotic affective disorders and mixed manic-depressive states (67% to 78%). The high specificity of the DST vs control subjects (over 90%) is not maintained vs other psychiatric disorders (77% specificity overall), and acute 'distress' may contribute to nonsuppression of cortisol."[82] Despite these negative conclusions of the test's clinical utility, the authors conclude: "The test may have power in differentiating severe melancholic depression, mania, or acute psychosis from chronic psychosis (8% specificity) or dysthymia (77% specificity)." With regard to prediction of treatment response: "The DST adds about 11% to the prediction of short-term antidepressant response." And: "Uncritical enthusiasm or excessive skepticism regarding the DST are unwarranted."

As an indicator of endogenous depression the DST was examined in 187 consecutively admitted unipolar depressed patients.[83] The results "strongly support the construct validity of the DST as a marker of endogenous depression."

In 166 consecutive admissions to a general psychiatric hospital unit the percentage of abnormal DST results progressed with severity as the diagnoses changed "from 'depressive symptoms' to major depression without melancholia to major depression with melancholia to major depression with psychosis . . . Patients with the most severe subtypes of major depression (melancholia and psychosis) showed both the highest rate of serum cortisol non-suppression and the highest post-DST serum cortisol concentrations."[84]

The discussions of the DST as a laboratory test of psychiatric significance encouraged the National Institute of Mental Health to call together a Workshop to review the various claims of clinical significance. The reporters focused their interest on the diagnostic use of the test, concluding that "at this time there are no clear indications for routine use of the DST in the diagnosis or clinical management of depression, although it is a useful research tool" (Hirschfeld *et al.*, 1983). A volume of the proceedings in 1985 again emphasized the limits of the test for diagnostic purposes, as a predictor of treatment response to antidepressant treatments, and as a predictor of relapse, and focused attention on the technical issues that limited the test's usefulness. They did recommend further research. (Hirschfeld *et al.*, 1985).

A committee of the American Psychiatric Association was convened to examine the DST as a laboratory test.[85] Reports published to the end of 1986 were reviewed and the authors concluded: "The sensitivity of the DST (rate of positive outcome, or nonsuppression of cortisol) in major depression is modest (about 40% – 50%) but is higher in very severe, especially psychotic, affective disorders, including major depression with psychotic as well as melancholic features, mania and schizoaffective disorder." As to the findings in normal subjects: "The specificity (true negative outcome) of the DST in normal control subjects is above 90%, but it varies from less than 70% to more than 90% in psychiatric conditions that often need to be separated from major affective disorders." With regard to prediction of treatment response the committee wrote: "Positive initial DST status in major depression does not add significantly to the likelihood of antidepressant response, and a negative test is not an indication for withholding antidepressant treatment." Further, they noted: "Some recent data suggest that DST-positive depressions (cortisol nonsuppression) are less likely than DST-negative cases (cortisol suppression) to respond to placebo." Finally, in considering prognosis, the committee concluded: "Failure to convert to normal suppression of cortisol with apparent recovery from depression suggests an increased risk for relapse into depression or suicidal behavior." They ended: "Although the clinical utility of the DST as currently understood is limited, in certain specific situations its thoughtful use may aid clinical decision making."

Carroll (1989a) responded to these assessments: "Modest and reasonable proposals for the dexamethasone suppression test (DST) and sleep electroencephalogram (EEG) became exaggerated; methodological, conceptual, and interpretive caveats were ignored; and some clinicians adopted these tests uncritically with the enthusiasm of magical, absolutist thinking . . . An unfortunate consequence of such positive and negative absolutist thinking has been the tendency to hold laboratory measures to a higher standard than other external validators of diagnosis."[86] In another venue Carroll (1989b) recalled that the greatest challenge to the test was "the arbitrary, data-free change in the clinical diagnostic criteria for depression and melancholia introduced by the American Psychiatric Association in 1980 with the DSM. This change had the effect of creating a nonvalidated 'gold standard' against which the DST inevitably was compared."[87]

Among the early studies of the clinical usefulness was a report by Brown *et al.* (1979) that found the test useful in identifying melancholic patients, their response to treatment, and their relapse. A decade later, the report was cited as a "citation classic" by the editors of *Current Contents* and Brown (1990) was asked to consider what had happened to the DST. He offered a cogent explanation of the initial enthusiasm since the test offered a laboratory procedure sorely lacking in psychiatry. But as the test was used, the populations were less critically appraised for severity of illness and the specificity of the test plummeted. Psychiatrists felt betrayed and the test was spurned with a vengeance. Brown concluded that the question had been confused; it should have been: "What can an endocrine abnormality . . . tell us about the pathophysiology, prognosis, and treatment of depressive illness?"

A few years later, another detailed analysis of the DST as a predictor of outcome in depression, concluded that "Baseline DST results may be devoid of prognostic value, but posttreatment nonsuppression . . . is strongly associated with poor outcome" (Ribiero *et al.*, 1993).

After this cascade of variable assessments, the DST was rejected as a clinical measure of interest. The recent literature is dominated by variations in the test assessment, the use in estimating suicide risk, correlations with diagnoses of post-traumatic stress disorder and character pathology, and laboratory animal studies of physiology. Research interest has waned, although some stalwart researchers still report findings that are consistent with the original reports.[88] There is now a consensus that the metabolism of dexamethasone is a major source of variance in the DST, and that measurement of plasma dexamethasone concentrations is needed for valid interpretation of the test results. This additional laboratory burden is an important reason for the clinical disuse of the test.[89]

Alternative tests of the HPA axis have been proposed.[90] An elegant but more complex test is the combined dexamethasone and CRH (DEX/CRH) test.[91] Overall, the findings confirm those with the DST, although a higher sensitivity is offered as the basis for its use.[92] An interesting example is a study in which DEX/CRH tests were administered on admission and on discharge in 74 depressed patients.[93] Treatments were not controlled so that the patients received a variety of antidepressant regimens (other than ECT). During a 6-month aftercare, 61 remained stable and 13 relapsed. At admission, the two groups did not differ in DEX/CRH test values but at discharge, the patients who relapsed showed higher ACTH and cortisol values. This study confirmed the predictive value of the test of the HPA axis functions as a predictor of relapse.

Like the DST, the DEX/CRH test is sensitive to the hormonal changes in women, is more abnormal in patients with high usage of tobacco, and is interfered with by carbamazepine through its effects on liver enzymes.[94] The DEX/CRH test is also affected by plasma dexamethasone concentration. This confound has not been systematically controlled in the psychiatric studies to date.

The hypothalamic–pituitary–thyroid axis[95]

The considerations of the HPT axis are similar to those of the HPA axis.[96] Thyroid functions are modulated by the hypothalamus and pituitary in a negative-feedback system that parallels the HPA axis. The principal hormones released by the thyroid gland are thyroxine (T_4) and triiodothyronine (T_3). The release and biosynthesis of T_4 and T_3 are controlled by the anterior pituitary hormone thyrotropin (thyroid-stimulating-hormone (TSH)) which, in turn, is controlled by the tripeptide thyrotropin-releasing hormone (TRH). Although a TSH response to TRH is a functional test that parallels the DST, it is less well established. Measurement of thyroid products is a central feature of the assessments of thyroid function and behavior.

The intactness of the HPT axis is normally evaluated by measuring the concentrations of serum thyroid hormones. Abnormal values are measured in 6–49% of psychiatric hospital admissions.[97] Hypothyroidism has long been associated with anergia, constipation, appetite loss, weight increase, and depressed mood.[98] The syndrome of hypothyroidism is not an all-or-none phenomenon, but gradations in abnormality are recognized. Overt hypothyroidism is associated with decreased T_4, elevated TSH, and increased response of TSH to injected TRH.[99]

Varied responses are reported in psychiatric patients. Most depressed patients are euthyroid with normal T_3 and T_4 serum levels, although T_4 levels may be in the upper range. In several large studies of depressed outpatients the incidence of abnormal findings was found to be too low to warrant routine thyroid testing. Yet, in numerous studies of the change in thyroid functions with remission of depression, the serum T_4 levels were seen to fall. In respect to the TSH response to TRH test, it is not uncommon to find a blunted ΔTSH, abnormal circadian TSH rhythm, elevated basal TSH concentrations, and elevated titers of antithyroid antibodies. But the tests are abnormal in less than 20% of the patients studied, lowering the acceptance of the assay as a measure of severity of depressed mood or of response to treatment. It is likely, however, that the same problems that identify melancholic patients for DST studies also plague the studies of the HPT axis.

Electrophysiologic measures

The discovery in 1929 that electrical potentials could be measured from the scalp of human subjects set off a flurry of interest that the electroencephalogram (EEG) could be related to psychiatric illnesses. Although Berger, a clinical neuropsychiatrist, showed that the EEG changed with age, alertness and sleep, medications, and structural brain pathology, he was unable to define relationships with the psychiatric states that were defined at the time. In the interim, the EEG has been shown to have diagnostic relations with seizures. The changes associated with sleep have been found useful as a measure of the severity of melancholia.

The findings in the resting EEG and, activated EEG, including the averaged evoked potential, that are of interest to the pathophysiology of melancholia are discussed in Chapter 14. In this chapter we describe the applications of the sleep EEG for the diagnosis of melancholia.

Sleep EEG

Induction of sleep activates the EEG and elicits different brain patterns that have been related to diagnosis (e.g., epilepsy).[100] As sleep difficulties are ubiquitous among psychiatric patients, the sleep EEG commonly exhibits abnormalities in depressed patients. These are considered signs of the severity of illness rather than biological markers of depressive illness.[101]

Insomnia with early-morning awakening, numerous sleep interruptions, and shortened periods of sleep are common findings in patients with mood disorders. Sleep onset is delayed, deep sleep and total sleep time are reduced, and awakenings are frequent.[102] Rapid eye movement (REM) latency (the time to the first REM EEG period) is the sleep parameter that relates best to the presence of depressive mood disorder. Patients who have an endogenous, melancholic, or psychotic depressive illness differ the most from controls. The findings in over 1400 depressed patients are summarized in Table 4.1.

The greater the sleep disturbance, the greater is the likelihood of relapse.[103] A comparison of 83 elderly depressed patients with 48 age- and gender-matched controls reported that longer durations of depressive episodes were associated with greater sleep discontinuity and greater REM abnormalities.[104] In another study, the sleep EEG characteristics of 44 depressed inpatients, 44 matched normal subjects, and 181 outpatient depressed patients were examined.[105] A discriminant index score (based on reduced REM latency, increased REM density (frequency of eye movements per unit REM time), and decreased sleep efficiency (percentage of time in bed spent asleep)) differentiated the three groups and identified a subset of depressed outpatients who were older, exhibited a broader array of EEG sleep disturbances, and were less responsive to psychotherapies. The authors considered that the empirically developed sleep analyses offered predictors for the choice of medication treatment.[106] While such speculation has not been validated, the clinical features associated with the most sleep disturbances are consistent with melancholia.

The sleep EEG records of patients with a single depressive episode were compared to the records of patients with a recurrent depressive illness before and after medication treatment. Disturbances in sleep continuity, REM sleep, and slow-wave sleep were greater in the recurrent depressed patients.[107]

Comparing the sleep macroarchitecture and EEG temporal coherence in outpatients with depressive illness with those in healthy normal controls, age and gender differences were reported to be greater than disease-dependent components.[108] Low temporal coherence, one of many EEG variables, reflected "a disruption in the fundamental basic rest–activity cycle of arousal and organization in the brain strongly

Table 4.1. Sleep disturbances in depressed patients

Total sleep time reduced
Sleep "efficiency" reduced (percentage bed-time asleep)
Sleep latency prolonged (time to fall asleep)
Slow-wave sleep (SWS) and NREM percentage time reduced
REM latency shortened (time from sleep to first REM period)
Percentage time in REM increased
First REM period length increased

influenced by gender." Another study from the same laboratory examined non-ill patients with a history of a parent or grandparent treated for a depressive mood disorder.[109] Period analysis of the sleep EEG showed lower beta-delta coherence in male subjects (considered high-risk for mood disorder because of a positive family history for mood disorder). The group next compared the EEG delta activity in 8 symptomatic but unmedicated females with depressive illness with gender-matched healthy controls, reporting significantly lower delta amplitude and power in the first non-REM (NREM) sleep period.[110] From these findings the authors concluded that "the maturational time course of sleep EEG disturbance may differ for males and females with depression."

A study seeking sleep EEG differences for 14 unipolar, 14 bipolar I, and 14 bipolar II depressed patients reported remarkable similarity in the clinical and sleep EEG characteristics.[111] An earlier study examining the EEG sleep characteristics of 47 patients with primary (endogenous) depression and 48 patients with secondary (non-endogenous) depression reported that measures of REM latency and REM activity differed on discriminant function analysis.[112] Sleep efficiency, percentage time in slow-wave sleep, and percentage REM sleep separated psychotic from non-psychotic depressed patients in those initially identified as suffering from primary depression. Increased wakefulness, decreased REM sleep percentage, and decreased REM activity were next reported as characteristics of EEG sleep patterns in psychotic depression.[113] The authors concluded that psychotic depression was a distinct form of depressive illness. Lastly, shortened REM latency was considered a biological marker for psychotic depression in a study of the EEG sleep characteristics of 44 patients with psychotic depressive illness compared with the findings in 44 non-psychotic depressed patients matched for gender, age, and polarity of illness.[114]

Sleep and neuroendocrine variables

Many studies seek to correlate sleep and neuroendocrine measures but these are often unsuccessful as almost all depressed patients have sleep difficulties, while even in the best of hands only about 50% of melancholic patients have abnormalities in HPA function tests. Multivariate analyses, however, find strong associations between these markers of endogenous depression and the diagnosis of melancholia.[115] To assure correlations of test findings and diagnosis, Feinberg and Carroll (1984) recommended the use of both DST and sleep EEG parameters. After identifying melancholic patients by clinical features, they suggested that the DST be applied. In patients with a normal DST response, the sleep EEG is next assessed. This method of assessment maximized the identification of melancholic patients. Others also favor the combination of assessing HPA and HPT axes for distinguishing melancholic from non-melancholic depressed patients.[116]

The need to combine laboratory measures is highlighted by a study of 160 patients with depressive illness.[117] Among those considered "endogenous," 46% were DST non-suppressors compared to 15% of the non-endogenous patients. Fifty-six percent of depressed bipolar patients were also DST non-suppressors. A blunted TRH stimulation test was found in 25% of patients with endogenous depression, 10% of those with non-endogenous depression, and 44% of the bipolar depressed patients. Reduced REM latency was found in 65% of the endogenous depressed patients, 34% of the non-endogenous depressed patients, and 53% of the bipolar depressed patients. When the endogenous depressed and bipolar depressed patients were combined, 72% had an abnormal laboratory finding, and 50% of the patients with reduced REM latency were DST non-suppressors.[118]

In 280 inpatients with recurrent depressive illness, the TSH response to TRH was blunted in 28%.[119] Sleep parameters (percentage time awake, percentage stage II sleep, REM sleep, and REM latency) were more disturbed in the endogenous (psychotic) depressed patients. Confounds of age, gender, and severity of illness led to multiple regression analyses that found no relationship of TSH values with sleep values. A few years later the group reported the relationship between the DST and sleep EEG parameters in 300 patients with depressive illness.[120] After confirming the relationships of DST to age, weight loss, and depression scale scores, they reported positive relationships with percentage of awakenings and percentage stage I sleep, and negatively with percentage stage II, slow-wave, and REM sleep. Again, multiple regression analyses were done and DST findings were positively associated with amount of wake and stage I sleep times, and negatively with slow-wave sleep. But another report found no relationship between neuroendocrine test measures and sleep EEG disturbances.[121]

The group's latest study examines the neuroendocrine and sleep EEG findings in 113 patients diagnosed with depressive illness.[122] After recording the typical changes in neuroendocrine measures, they introduced sleep measures into principal component statistical analyses. Controlling for the effects of age and gender, three clusters of patients were identified with varying associations of sleep and neuroendocrine measures. No clinical criteria differentiated the three clusters. Similar associations of limited clinical and diagnostic significance are reported by others.[123]

Overall, assessments of EEG sleep characteristics report abnormalities in sleep continuity, slow-wave sleep, and REM in psychiatric patients with mood disorders. Shortened REM latency is considered an identifying feature in psychotic depressed and in elderly depressed patients.[124] Yet, few macro architectural EEG characteristics distinguish depressed patients and controls.[125]

A comparison of slow-wave activity during NREM sleep in 76 depressed outpatients with 55 healthy subjects found lower amplitudes in patients as a discriminating variable.[126] The findings were sensitive to gender and to age.[127] The same research group considered slow-wave sleep deficiencies characteristic of men but not women and were affected by age.[128] To examine the microstructure of sleep EEG, the records were digitized at 100 Hz from a single scalp derivation and the power subdivided into conventional EEG frequency bands. The frequencies of periods labeled REM and NREM differed significantly. They compared their findings to the changes in REM and NREM frequency bands after treatment with antidepressant medications and concluded that the NREM sleep cycle is the more sensitive measure of sleep EEG. Shortened REM latency is consistently observed in adult and adolescent depressed patients. It is an inconsistent finding in children.[129]

Sleep EEG measures are influenced by gender-related neuroendocrine findings. Low estrogen levels are inversely related to sleep disturbance.[130] Depressed women have more marked disturbances than depressed men.[131] While depressed men (particularly those 20–40 years of age) have reduced slow-wave sleep, there is no similar evidence in depressed women.[132] The sleep EEG findings of depressed patients are strongly influenced by age, gender, hormone levels, and cortisol activity.[133] In adults, alpha and beta fast-frequency amplitudes and power are increased while delta slow-frequency amplitudes and power are decreased.[134] Synchronization of ultradian (90-min) rhythms in the sleep EEG is disturbed, with poor temporal coherence between hemispheres.[135] Low coherence is reported in depressed women, whereas depressed men have reduced slow-wave activity, particularly in the first NREM sleep period.[136] Low coherence is reported in depressed adolescent girls, particularly after puberty.[137]

An association of slow sleep EEG coherence between hemispheres is reported in depressed girls.[138] Among children with a family history of depressive illness who had never been depressed, 23% exhibited low coherence. After comparing the sleep EEG rhythms in 41 adolescent girls with a maternal history of depressive illness to 40 healthy controls in a sample that was clinically assessed every 6 months for 2 years, the sleep phase coherence between hemispheres was lower in the high-risk girls and regression analysis correctly classified 70% of the high-risk group with a 5% false-positive rate among the controls.[139] Forty-one percent of the girls with the most abnormally low EEG sleep phase coherence developed depressive features during follow-up and 6 became depressed. Only one control participant became depressed. In a follow-up, 50% of the girls with low hemispheric EEG coherence had their first episode of depressive illness within 3–5 years from the study's onset.[140] Estrogen and progesterone effects on EEG and sleep have been proposed as an explanation for the gender difference in coherence.[141]

Conclusions

There are no laboratory tests that define psychiatric disorders with the specificity and sensitivity of methods that are used to identify infectious illnesses. Measures of the HPA axis, however, offer the best tests for the definition of melancholia. The findings are clinically relevant as they offer information for treatment choice, identify outcome, and warn of relapse.

Hypercortisolemia is evidence of an abnormal stress response state that is characteristic of melancholia, especially when the patient is psychotic. Hypercortisolemia is also found in manic patients (meeting criteria for bipolar disorder), patients in depressive or catatonic stupor, and demented patients when depressed (as in pseudodementia). To a lesser extent it is observed in patients meeting criteria for schizophrenia. These findings caution the clinician to examine such patients more thoroughly so that those with mood disorder can be identified and appropriate treatments applied.

Many observers consider hypercortisolemia to be a non-specific response to stress and of little meaning for psychiatric classification, claiming that many stressors affect human behavior and neuroendocrine responses.[142] Such an attitude is founded on the belief that the phenotypic descriptions of abnormal behaviors begun by nineteenth-century psychopathologists and codified in the DSM and ICD classification systems are sufficient for diagnosis and treatment. Such a belief is unwarranted. The present classification fails to identify phenomenologically the different forms of mood disorder.[143] It is weakly associated with biological markers of mood disorder, prediction of treatment response, or long-term outcome. The measurable functions of the neuroendocrine system, however, do separate melancholic patients from other patients and from non-ill persons. When these abnormalities are tested against the artificial classification of the DSM, the tests are found wanting. Rather than discarding the neuroendocrine measures, the evidence encourages the use of these tests to delineate populations of patients from among the greater number of patients with mood and psychotic disorders. The identified patients will be the most seriously ill and the most likely to respond to broad pharmacodynamic spectrum antidepressant drugs, benefit from lithium when a mood stabilizer is needed, and commonly achieve remission with ECT.[144]

The value of neuroendocrine tests in identifying melancholia can be compared with the role of the EEG in clinical neurologic practice. In the clinical situation, the EEG is a state marker of brain electrophysiology and neurochemistry at the time of examination. It offers information about brain physiology that is not available by observation or clinical examination. It is replicable, repeatable, and reliable. It has a defined role in clinical diagnosis. Among patients with confirmed seizure disorders, a single examination is positive in 56%. Repeated second and third samples increase the incidence of abnormal recordings by 26%, for an overall success rate of 82%. In normal samples, the likelihood of finding a dysrhythmic EEG is less than 2%.[145] This discrimination assures the examining neurologist of information that is invaluable for diagnosis and treatment.

Similarly, neuroendocrine assessments offer physiological information that is not otherwise measurable. The measures define characteristics that separate normal and abnormal psychiatric states. Tests for these dysfunctions are replicable, repeatable, and reliable. Their discard from psychiatric practice and from designed research has been premature. The DST has a place in identifying melancholia from other mood disorders, and is a practical tool in differential diagnosis and treatment.[146]

Activated EEG measures, including the sleep EEG, are potential measures of physiology that relate to psychiatric states. The sleep EEG, despite its technical difficulties, measures the severity and degree of sleep abnormalities that are ubiquitous in severely depressed patients. Prolonged sleep latency, shortened REM latency, and decreased slow-wave sleep characterize adult melancholic patients. About 50% of such patients have HPA abnormalities and are DST non-suppressors. Measures of HPA function combined with sleep EEG provide laboratory diagnostic criteria that should be incorporated into classification systems. Measures of HPA activity also provide guidelines for treatment.

NOTES

1 Macalpine and Hunter (1974); pp 256–7.
2 Chapter 3.
3 Chapter 14 details the pathophysiology of neuroendocrine systems in melancholia. The details of the dysfunctions that are the basis for laboratory tests of melancholia are described here.
4 Lindley and Schatzberg (2003).
5 Cushing (1932) (quotation cited by Rothschild (2003b); p. 139).
6 Sakel (1938); Shorter (1997); Fink (2003a).
7 Cannon (1929, 1939); Selye (1950); Selye and Stone (1950).
8 Rothermundt *et al.* (2001 a, b). The authors find different immune patterns in melancholic depressed patients compared to non-melancholic depressed.
9 Carroll and Mendels (1978); Carroll (1977).
10 APA Task Force on Laboratory Tests in Psychiatry (1987).
11 Not only were tests of neuroendocrine dysfunction discarded, but so were serum blood levels of psychoactive drugs, particularly lithium and tricyclic antidepressant medications, which are part of clinical practice. Electroencephalogram (EEG) recordings to identify brain disorders were also rejected.
12 At a conference of the American Psychopathological Association, the relations of different laboratory tests to the DSM-III diagnostic scheme were discussed (Fink, 1978). After psychological tests and EEG response strategies were presented, the discussion centered on whether tests could be included in classification schemes. Fink argued that the laboratory tests already in hand, although imprecise, offered better criteria for classification – possible genotypic measures – than the clinical criteria, even with potential family study reinforcement (pp. 332–3). In response, Spitzer noted:

> One of the problems . . . is that the purpose of diagnosis is to help you have a plan for action, to make a prediction about what is likely to happen in the future, and to suggest a course of treatment that might be successful. In making that judgment . . . the whole purpose of diagnosis would be confused if one were to use external validating criteria . . . (Spitzer and Klein, 1968, p. 333).

Sadly, this point of view rejects the merits of the available tests (e.g., serology for syphilis, EEG for seizure disorders, serum drug levels for drug toxicity) in psychiatric classification.

It rejects tests, such as measures of cortisol and other hormones that may be offered to demarcate patients within a psychiatric class. The present low level of clinical success and high incidence of "therapy resistance" in medication treatment trials are products of this point of view that dominates DSM classification philosophy.

13 The rejection of laboratory tests as markers of psychiatric states is the principal impediment to the development of an evidence-based psychiatric psychopathology.

14 Chapters 2 and 3.

15 The contributions from experimental psychiatry and neuropsychology focused on the use of the sedation threshold and denial tests to amobarbital, the use of Rorschach and other projective tests as predictors of outcome, the blood pressure responses to adrenergic and cholinergic drugs. These experiences are, at present, of historical interest. The findings of these early studies are to be found in Fink (1979).

16 The HPA axis has been the subject of numerous symposia and texts. A reasonable assessment of the progress can be found in de Wied and Weijnen (1970), Davies *et al.* (1972); Sachar (1976); Nemeroff and Loosen (1987); Schatzberg and Nemeroff (1988); and Wolkowitz and Rothschild (2003).

17 See Carroll (1972a, 1977; Carroll *et al.*, 1968).

18 Guillemin (2005).

19 For a detailed description of the negative feedback and potential positive feedback mechanisms, see Carroll (1972a).

20 Cortisol mobilizes body defenses to resist infection; regulates blood pressure and cardiovascular function; and modulates metabolism by regulating gluconeogenesis, liver metabolism, and protein catabolism. Excess glucocorticoids initially elicit euphoria but with prolonged exposure, irritability, emotional lability, and depression are fostered. Cognitive functions are impaired (Schatzberg *et al.*, 2000). With persistent high levels appetite increases, libido decreases, and insomnia becomes prominent. Excess glucocorticoid thyroid-stimulating hormone (TSH) synthesis and release are inhibited, limiting TSH response to thyrotropin-releasing hormone. Serum total thyroxine (T_4) concentrations are low secondary to a decrease in thyroxine-binding globulin. "Free" T_4 levels are normal. Total and free triiodothyronine (T_3) concentration may be low, as glucocorticoid excess decreases the conversion rate of T_4 to T_3. Despite these alterations, clinical manifestations of hypothyroidism are not manifest.

21 For historical roots, see Carroll (1972a, 1977, 1982a).

22 Carroll (1972c).

23 High plasma cortisol levels and non-suppression to dexamethasone was also accompanied by higher than normal cerebrospinal fluid cortisol levels.

24 Carroll (1972c).

25 *Ibid.*, p. 104.

26 Carroll (1972c), p. 137, citing Wolff *et al.* (1964). The psychological formulation was revised after findings of hypersecretion of cortisol in apathetic, non-anxious depressed patients as well as those with affective arousal (Carroll, 1977).

27 Carroll (1972c), p. 140.

28 Carroll (1972c), p. 145.

29 Carroll 1972d.

30 Carroll (1977). Davies *et al.* (1972) describe the studies undertaken in Melbourne, Australia, that laid the foundation for the clinical test (Carroll 1972a–1972d). Followers varied time of assessment and times and dosage of administration of dexamethasone, methods of

chemical analysis, and criteria for "normal" and "abnormal" cortisol levels and for "suppression" and "non-suppression." Much of the difficulty in usage and understanding of the DST is that there is no accepted single "DST."

31 Dexamethasone is a potent synthetic adrenal steroid hormone that acts on the pituitary to suppress secretion of ACTH. Under normal conditions the suppression is complete and relatively long-lasting.

32 Carroll *et al.* (1981 a, b). The cutoff criterion defining abnormality depends on the method of assay. Different criteria are recommended by different authors, varying with the "normal" values determined according to the method of assessment (Rothschild (2003b), p. 140).

33 Assay methods of cortisol vary across laboratories and at different points during the day. The 5 μg/dl figure is used here as it is the most widely cited cutoff. When used clinically, normal cortisol levels and DST cutoffs will reflect the laboratory being used. The principles described in this section, however, apply universally.

34 Carroll *et al.* (1968). Samples were collected at 0830 and 1630 h and then again the next day at 0830 h after 2 mg dexamethasone phosphate given at midnight.

35 Carroll *et al.* (1976a, b).

36 Carroll *et al.* (1976a) summarize their findings:

> By using an observation period of 24 hours postadministration of dexamethasone, a graded series of abnormal test responses was identified. Depressed patients show abnormal early escape from suppression rather than absolute resistance to HPA suppression by dexamethasone . . . . The essential disturbance of neuroendocrine regulation in depression is a failure of the normal brain inhibitory influence on the HPA system (p. 1039).

37 Carroll *et al.* (1981a); quotation p. 15.

38 While the formal test is based on multiple samples, assuring a more stable test, single samples, usually taken at 1600 h (4 p.m.), were also used in testing outpatients (Carroll *et al.*, 1980a).

39 Carroll (1972a), p. 50.

40 Multiple urinary steroids have been examined (Carroll (1972a), p. 52ff).

41 Bolwig and Rafaelson (1972); Kirschbaum and Hellhammer (1994).

42 Carroll (1972b). Much emphasis in the initial studies was on the impact of the stress of hospitalization on cortisol levels, a condition that was successfully challenged by Carroll (p. 75). Another concern was the impact of the stress of awaiting ECT. Again, the impact of the anticipated stress of a treatment day compared to a non-treatment day was negligible (p. 76).

43 Carroll's studies found no connection between cortisol elevation and complaints of diurnal mood variation, level of retardation, sleep disturbance, suicide attempt in the present illness, or level of anxiety, but did find severity of illness, especially the components related to physiological function (as measured by Hamilton and by Zung depression rating scales) related to cortisol levels.

44 Lu *et al.* (1988).

45 Zimmerman *et al.* (1985).

46 Davidson *et al.* (1984a).

47 Klein (1974); Carroll (1977).

48 Carroll (1977) concludes that: "only one-half the endogenomorphic patients can be identified by this laboratory procedure and a normal suppression response to dexamethasone will

not exclude a diagnosis of endogenomorphic depression which would otherwise have been made on clinical grounds."

49 Schotte *et al.* (1997).
50 The studies detailed in Chapter 3 define melancholia with similar features.
51 Miller and Nelson (1987).
52 Kumar *et al.* (1986); Rush *et al.* (1996); Gold *et al.* (2002).
53 Kumar *et al.* (1986).
54 Schatzberg *et al.* (1984), Rothschild *et al.* (1989); Posener *et al.* (2000, 2004).
55 Brown and Shuey (1980); Schatzberg *et al.* (1983); Schatzberg and Rothschild (1992).
56 Rothschild *et al.* (1982).
57 Nelson and Davis (1997).
58 Rush *et al.* (1996).
59 Posener *et al.* (2000).
60 Parker *et al.* (1991).
61 Parker *et al.* (1995a). "Non-reactivity" in the distinction between a melancholic and a non-melancholic depression does not refer to the absence of a preceding stressful event, but to the unchanging nature of the patient's mood. Melancholic patients cannot forget their worries and their moods do not "react" to circumstances.
62 Carroll *et al.* (1980a).
63 The principal early studies are by Papakostas *et al.* (1980); Albala *et al.* (1981); Coryell (1982); Coryell and Zimmerman (1983); Coryell (1986); Grunhaus *et al.* (1987). These, and other studies, are summarized in Fink (1987b).
64 Papakostas *et al.* (1980).
65 Swartz and Chen (1985); Swartz (1992).
66 Devanand *et al.* (1987, 1991).
67 Unden and Aperia (1994).
68 Chapter 7.
69 Coryell and Schlesser (2001).
70 Yerevanian *et al.* (2004a).
71 Targum *et al.* (1983); Banki *et al.* (1984); López-Ibor *et al.* (1985); Coryell (1990); Pfeffer *et al.* (1991); Pfennig *et al.* (2005).
72 Brown *et al.* (1986); Secunda *et al.* (1986); Ayuso-Gutierrez *et al.* (1987); Schmidtke *et al.* (1989); Norman *et al.* (1990); Roy (1992); Black *et al.* (2002).
73 The classification separation of bipolar disorder and major depression is inconsistent with the clinical reality of a single mood disorder (Chapter 2). The incidence of abnormal DST findings varies with the severity of the depressed mood. Another confounding factor is the difficulty in diagnostically separating patients with mania and psychosis and those with excited forms of schizophrenia.
74 Evans and Nemeroff (1983); Godwin (1984); Krishnan *et al.* (1983); Swann *et al.* (1992); Cassidy *et al.* (1998); Watson and Young (2002).
75 Rothschild (2003b).
76 Miles (1977).
77 Chapter 6.
78 Gaab *et al.* (2002).
79 Carroll (1977).
80 Carroll (1982b).
81 Berger *et al.* (1984).

82 Arana *et al.* (1985).
83 Zimmerman *et al.* (1986c).
84 Evans and Nemeroff (1987).
85 APA Task Force on Laboratory Tests in Psychiatry (1987).
86 Carroll (1989a) offers 10 "rules of the game" as criteria to establish the validity of tests in diagnosis. The main criterion is the clinical validity of a diagnostic class. In this study of melancholia, we suggest that the clinical criteria described identify a large population of mood-disordered patients with a high concentration of HPA axis abnormality. For this population, reassessment of the DST against the criteria for melancholia is warranted, with the expectation that the correlation of diagnosis and test-finding will be better than the examinations of the past quarter century in which the diagnostic criterion has been poorly defined and unreliable.
87 The test was developed in Australia with the International Classification of Diseases, 9th edition (ICD-9) clinical diagnostic system. In a review of his experience, Carroll (1989a) also notes:

> The subgroup of depressed patients with abnormal DST results resembles the classic melancholic clinical profile, has a high rate of recurrence and a strong family history, has a poor prognosis if the test does not normalize during treatment, and has the highest rate of response to antidepressant drugs. Abnormal DST results are strongly associated with suicide or violent suicide attempts . . . this group of patients will fail to respond to psychosocial treatment of their depressions

(At the time, the standard antidepressant treatments were tricyclic antidepressants and ECT.)
88 In developing the four-hospital collaborative study of continuation treatments (continuation lithium/nortriptyline combination or continuation ECT) after ECT, the opportunity to assess the merits of the DST as a predictor of outcome for ECT and as a test of relapse in continuation was included in the original request for funding support. The National Institute of Mental Health review committees deleted funding for this part of the study as of limited interest, despite the opportunity to assess the test findings in a very large sample.
89 Personal communication, Bernard Carroll, May 31, 2005. Also Devanand *et al.* (1987, 1991).
90 The commonest variations are in sampling times, methods of assay of cortisol, dosage of dexamethasone, and measurement of other hypothalamic-releasing factors and pituitary hormones. How these variations improve the specificity or reliability of the test is unclear; what is clear is that these variations, as well as small samples, poorly defined populations, and high variability in treatments have added much noise to the assessment of the DST.
91 Patients are pretreated with an oral dose of 1.5 mg dexamethasone at 2300 h and the next afternoon, through an intravenous catheter, a blood sample is withdrawn, 100 μg of human CRH is injected, and blood samples are withdrawn every 15 min for five additional samples. The blood samples are assayed for cortisol and ACTH using radioimmunoassay methods. The reported findings are mainly for cortisol. (Holsboer *et al.*, 1987; Amsterdan *et al.*, 1988; Heuser *et al.*, 1994; Zobel *et al.*, 2001; Künzel *et al.*, 2003a).
92 Zobel *et al.* (1999).
93 Zobel *et al.* (2001).
94 Künzel *et al.* (2003a).
95 Compendia on thyroid function and behavior are Prange (1974); Gold and Pottash (1986); Nemeroff and Loosen (1987); Joffe and Levitt (1993); Wolkowitz and Rothschild (2003).

96 O'Connor *et al.* (2003a).
97 Kronig and Gold (1986); O'Connor *et al.* (2003a).
98 Kronig and Gold (1986).
99 The TSH response to TRH is a parallel test to the DST. After a nighttime fast, an intravenous line is established and blood is drawn for baseline values of TSH, T_4, and T_3. A standardized dose of TRH (protirelin), usually 0.5 mg, is injected and samples are taken at 15-min intervals for 60 or 90 min. Various measures are made but the commonest is the increase in TSH (ΔTSH) at 30 min. In normal subjects the ΔTSH is 7–15 μIU/ml. Hypothyroid patients are supersensitive to TRH and therefore exhibit an increased ΔTSH. Hyperthyroid patients are subsensitive and exhibit a blunted ΔTSH (Kronig and Gold, 1986; Loosen, 1987).
100 Among the plethora of books on sleep and sleep EEG, the classical studies are those of Kleitman (1939); Oswald (1962); Kety *et al.* (1967); Mendelson (1987); and Kryger *et al.* (2000).
101 Morehouse *et al.* (2002).
102 Benca *et al.* (1992); Jindal *et al.* (2002).
103 Benca *et al.* (1992); Nofzinger *et al.* (1999a).
104 Dew *et al.* (1996).
105 Thase *et al.* (1997c).
106 The findings are for group data. The authors offer no evidence that the sleep EEG measures are applicable in individual patients.
107 Jindal *et al.* (2002). We believe that the recurrent depressive group represented a more homogeneous, seriously ill sample, and were more likely to have melancholia.
108 Armitage *et al.* (2000a).
109 Fulton *et al.* (2000).
110 Armitage *et al.* (2001).
111 Fossion *et al.* (1998).
112 Kupfer *et al.* (1978).
113 Thase *et al.* (1986).
114 Stefos et al. (1998).
115 Feinberg and Carroll (1984).
116 Staner *et al.* (1994).
117 Rush *et al.* (1997).
118 Chapter 2 discusses the literature that indicates bipolar depression is melancholia.
119 Hubain *et al.* (1994).
120 Hubain *et al.* (1998).
121 Staner *et al.* (2001). The patients, while hospitalized, were not assessed as to the presence of psychosis.
122 Staner *et al.* (2003).
123 Rao *et al.* (1996b, 2004); Hatzinger *et al.* (2004).
124 Kupfer *et al.* (1986); Roschke and Mann (2002).
125 Armitage *et al.* (1999).
126 Usually NREM is dominated by slow-wave sleep (SWS).
127 Armitage *et al.* (2000b).
128 Armitage *et al.* (2000c).
129 Birmaher *et al.* (1996a, b); Rao *et al.* (1996b). The failure to find the same effect in children is thought to result from lack of maturation.

130 Antonijevic *et al.* (2000a, b).
131 Liscombe *et al.* (2002).
132 Armitage *et al.* (2000b, c, d).
133 Antonijevic *et al.* (2000a, b, 2003).
134 The findings are interpreted as indicating increased "arousal" (Borbely *et al.*, 1984; Kupfer and Reynolds, 1992).
135 Coherence in quantitative EEG refers to the degree of correlation of EEG parameters within and among brain regions. In the sleep EEG literature assessing phases of sleep, the term is used to describe the degree of phase correlation between the left and right hemispheres.
136 Armitage *et al.* (1999).
137 Armitage *et al.* (2000c, d).
138 Fulton *et al.* (2000).
139 Morehouse *et al.* (2002).
140 Armitage, R. Grand rounds presentation, University of Michigan Medical School, Ann Arbor, 2003. Also see Armitage *et al.* (2002).
141 Driver *et al.* (1996). Gender differences are also observed in evoked potentials, with women having shorter latencies and larger amplitudes than men (Kaneda *et al.*, 1996).
142 See Paykel (2001a) for a review of stress responses in humans. Greater attention needs to be paid to the conditions that offer false positives, such as pregnancy, starvation, influence of medications, and serum protein abnormalities that affect steroid availability.
143 Chapters 2 and 3.
144 Chapters 9, 11, 12, and 13 provide a discussion of the evidence for the response of melancholic patients to different treatments.
145 Fink (2005, p. 1148).
146 Chapters 6–8.

5

Examination for melancholia

I began to sense the onset of the symptoms at mid afternoon or a little later – gloom crowding in on me, a sense of dread and alienation and, above all, stifling anxiety. Rational thought was usually absent from my mind at such times, hence trance.

I can think of no more appropriate word for this state of being, a condition of helpless stupor in which cognition was replaced by that positive and active anguish.[1]

The bedrock of psychiatric clinical research is the structured interview. It is designed to collect large amounts of information in a form suitable for multivariate analysis. To achieve reliability, questions are asked in a specific form and sequence. The opportunity for follow-up questioning, clarification, and discussion with the patient is limited. Experienced clinicians recognize the artificial nature of these instruments. Kendell commented on the exaggerated value given to structured interviews and rating scales, and the tendency to disregard the validity of a well-done clinical examination.

For most of medical history, syndromes have been identified intuitively by gifted physicians on the basis of their experience. They saw a pattern where others saw only confusion, or they saw a different pattern than had their predecessors.[2]

The art of the medical examination is learned at the bedside. It is not taught from books alone. It remains the bedrock of clinical psychiatric diagnosis.

Clinical diagnosis, however, is simplified when depressive mood disorders are considered a single state differing only in severity. Obtain the patient's endorsement of a sufficient number of the features associated with an illness, and the patient's condition meets diagnostic criteria. Standard rating scales for depression (see below) are comprised of these well-known features. When different forms of depressive illness are recognized, structured interviews are even more problematic and diagnosis becomes more difficult. Rating-scale items at best are guides to regions of useful inquiry, and rating-scale item scores are measures of change in the course of the illness that aid in treatment decision-making. The limitations of such measures for individual patient care, however, are recognized. Thus, careful inquiry into the patient's complaints and gathering "the story" of the illness by following clues that warrant more detail and probing are essential parts of clinical examination.

Examination strategy

The examination that best delineates a clinical condition is like a conversation, not an interrogation. Questioning a patient using a checklist, as if the sufferer were standing before an immigration official applying for a visa, is poor technique. A systematic structure cloaked in informality is the compromise between the need to obtain information about critical items and the need to put an anxious or despondent patient at ease so that the patient will confide in the examiner. Comforting comments and statements that verbalize the patient's subjective experiences facilitate the examination. The goal, however, is not a psychotherapy interaction, but to elicit the

Table 5.1. Techniques for examining melancholic patients

Problem	Technique
Psychomotor retardation	Slow down and give the patient extra time to respond
Agitation	Divide the examination into several short interactions. Do not directly face the patient. Speak clearly and deliberately in the lower voice register.[a] Low-dose benzodiazepine 30 min before the examination is helpful for severe agitation
Catatonia and stupor	In addition to a paucity of speech or mutism and prolonged immobility or catalepsy, there are many other catatonic features and associated behaviors that require specific exam techniques[b]
Cognitive problems	Speak deliberately and in short, uncomplicated sentences. Do not offer opposing choices, such as: "have you lost or gained weight?" Ask questions whose answers do not require complex decision-making, such as: "Are you having trouble remaining asleep?"
Diurnal mood swing	Break the examination into morning and afternoon segments
Psychosis	Do not challenge delusions or hallucinations. The goal is to get "the story" of the experiences from the patient's perspective

Notes:

[a] Such strategies reduce the patient's anxiety. Agitation usually reflects an intense mood. The faster and the higher the tone of the examiner's speech, the more it appears to reflect anxiety. A patient's perception of examiner anxiety will heighten his anxiety.

[b] For a detailed discussion of catatonia, how to examine for it, and its relationship to mood disorder, see Fink and Taylor (2003).

symptoms and course of the illness that lead to a correct diagnosis. Table 5.1 displays some techniques that are helpful when examining melancholic patients.

Examining mood

Examining a patient's mood requires observational skills and the ability to facilitate the patient to reveal his or her subjective experiences.[3] Melancholic patients look despondent. They may exhibit the classic signs of a sad face: a furrowed brow that looks like the Greek letter omega (the omega sign) or sunken eyes beneath downward-drooping upper eyelid folds (Veraguth's folds).

"Screening" questions are helpful: "Have you been feeling blue, or down in the dumps? Have you felt like crying more than usual? You look depressed, do you feel that way?" Indicating an understanding of the subjective experience of depression may gain the patient's confidence, permitting him or her to reveal feelings. "We have all been saddened by the loss of a friend or relative, but that feeling ends. Do you feel like that now?"

If the patient endorses the screening questions, subsequent statements begin with: "Persons who are depressed often feel overcome by worry . . . uncertainty . . . remorse – have you been feeling that way?"

Or, "Persons who are depressed are often very anxious. You look anxious, do you feel that way?"

Sometimes melancholic patients experience a loss of emotion: "Do you feel numb – as if you want to cry, but can't?"

The examiner determines duration, intensity, and the remitting nature and degree of reactivity of the mood: "Can anything cheer you up or make you forget your worries? Have you been feeling this way continuously, without any let-up?"

The quality of the experience is also assessed: "Is what you are feeling now similar to when you hear sad news or when you miss out on something?"

Mood fluctuation during the day is also tested: "Is there any time of the day when your mood is at its worst? Do you feel slowed and foggy-headed during the day and more clear-headed in the evening?"

Melancholic patients are often overwhelmed by anxiety and worry and should be asked about this experience: "Persons who are depressed often feel at their wits' end – as if the smallest thing is too much for them." Is your depression that bad?

"Do you have times when you suddenly feel very frightened?"

"Since your mood changed, have you been feeling anxious or apprehensive or frightened of the littlest things?"

Giving the patient a personal "yardstick" against which to measure present symptoms helps: "Compared to your worst feelings of depression, how bad is this one? If 10 is the worst you've ever felt, what score would you have now?"

Melancholic patients cannot be cheered by good humor: their mood is said to be "non-reactive." The response to humor during the examination assesses change in reactivity. A hearty laugh from a patient is the best indication that the depression is resolving, or that the depression is not melancholic.

Examining psychomotor functioning

Disturbances in motor behavior that characterize melancholia are observed during the examination. Agitation (increased repetitive and non-goal-directed movement) appears as fidgeting or coarse "pill-rolling" hand movements. Some patients do not sit quietly, but pace the hallways. When required to sit, these patients rock, wring their hands, and look as if danger lurked everywhere.

Melancholic patients may appear delirious. Perseverative rubbing of the face, hands, and other body parts can result in skin abrasion. One patient rubbed the flesh away from her fingertip, exposing bone. Self-injury (e.g., hitting, pinching, cutting, burning) may be perseverative or in response to delusions or hallucinations.[4]

Slow movements (bradykinesia) and slowed thinking (bradyphrenia) occur. These symptoms may be mild and limited to hesitancy in speech and delayed reaction time, or so severe that the patient may be mute or in a stupor. The greater the psychomotor retardation, the greater is the patient's lack of response.

Catatonia, a motor syndrome characterized by motor rigidity and posturing, stereotypy, negativism, mutism, and echophenomena, is associated with melancholia.[5] Table 5.2 displays the observable features of melancholia.

Table 5.2. Observable features of melancholia

Psychomotor disturbance	Disturbed mood
Bradykinesia	Sighing, groaning, moaning, and screaming
Delayed response	Omega sign and Veraguth's folds
Slowed speech	Crying and sobbing (often tearless)
Tremor	**Social withdrawal**
Shaking	Reduced eye contact
Perseverative head-, face-, and mouth-touching or rubbing	Inattentiveness and stupor
Sagging posture	Indifference to hygiene and grooming
Catatonia	**Other features**
Restlessness and pacing	Sweating
	Evidence of self-injury
	Evidence of weight loss

Examining for vegetative signs

"Vegetative signs" refer to perturbations in the homeostatic functions of sleep and digestion, and appetitive drives such as hunger and libido. Changes in circadian and ultradian rhythms, stress-response physiologic functioning, and autonomic nervous system activity mold the behavioral picture of melancholia. Sleep is disrupted and fatigue severe. Hypertension, tachycardia, and arrhythmias occur.[6] Appetite, motivation, and libido are reduced. Bowel motility slows and constipation and fecal impaction are common in older patients.

Questions begin broadly: "Has your depression affected your sleep . . . appetite . . . or general medical health?"

Specific questions follow: "Do you have trouble staying asleep?"

"About what time do you wake up?"

"Is your sleep restful?"

"Do your worries keep you awake?"

"Do you wake up sweating? And, do you notice your heart beating faster than usual when you wake up?"

"Have you lost your appetite? Is there any food that you now enjoy eating?"

"How has your weight been since your depression started? How much weight do you think you have lost?"

And, "Do you find yourself unable to enjoy things you once found pleasurable/fun? Has your depression affected your interest in sex?"

"Has your depression affected your menstrual periods?"

Examining for psychotic features

The association between psychotic depression and suicide risk compels examination about hallucinations and delusions. Melancholic patients may experience hallucinated voices that are derogatory and accusatory, encourage guilt, or command the patient to suicide: the risk for self-injury is high. Hallucinated odors are less common, but are described as unpleasant bodily emissions or poisons. Gustatory experiences are of foul or metallic tastes. Visions of demons or other frightening images occur. Delusions are of self-blame, deadly disease not appreciated by physicians, or of persecution.

Questioning begins with: "When a person is depressed, the world sometimes looks or seems different. Has this happened to you?"

"Have you heard unpleasant things said to you or about you when no one is near?"

"Have you noticed unpleasant smells?"

"Have you seen things that are frightening or unusual?"

Follow-up questions focus on the form of the psychopathology.[7] Asking patients' opinions about their health, the future, and what others think of them may reveal their delusions.

Patient 5.1

A 68-year-old man was hospitalized for depression. Retired, he had enjoyed classes at a community college. Several months before admission, his mood became depressed. He believed people were trying to kill him and was grateful for the protection of the hospital. Hallucinated voices said that he was evil, and that he would be punished. He believed that his brain waves had killed the Pope and the President, among many others. He could clearly and repeatedly hear his victims screaming and moaning in agony in the street below. He thought he was responsible for terrible world events, that he deserved to die and would kill himself had he the chance. His beliefs were unshakeable.

He had no appetite and had lost 10–15 pounds in the prior month. He could not sleep for fear he would be attacked. He reported unremitting apprehension.

On examination he fidgeted in his chair and appeared frightened. His breathing was rapid and shallow. His responses were delayed, but his speech was of normal rate and well organized. He said his thoughts were not clear. He had mild problems with concentration and in new learning. He said: "Things were going so well. I had a very good year. I don't understand what happened. I can't go on like this." His general medical and neurologic health could not explain his condition. He was diagnosed as having a psychotic depression. He received a course of bilateral ECT and had a full recovery.

Examining for suicidal thoughts[8]

Because suicide is the principal cause of premature death in persons with mood disorder, every depressed patient must be asked directly about self-destructive thoughts and actions. Patients often recognize the concern in the mildest questions and express their intent:

"Have you been feeling so badly that you'd just as soon go to sleep and not wake up? Would others be better off if you were dead? Have you been thinking a lot lately about death?"

Sometimes depressed patients will deny suicidal preoccupation, even to the most direct questions:

"Have you thought of harming yourself? Have you made a plan to kill yourself? If you had the chance, would you kill yourself now?" Suicide risk, prevention, and the treatment of the suicidal depressed patient are discussed in Chapters 7 and 8.

Examining cognition

Thinking, concentration, recent memory and recall, and new learning are often severely impaired in melancholia. The deficits may be profound, debilitating, widespread, and readily mistaken for degenerative brain disease. The syndrome is reversible and has been termed *pseudodementia*.[9] A detailed diagnostic evaluation is often needed to distinguish these patients from those whose dementias are of degenerative brain processes that are less readily treatable.

Cognitive assessment needs to be done in all depressed patients for both the differential diagnosis and to establish a baseline to monitor any cognitive changes associated with treatment. It is also needed in the assessment of suicide risk, and to guide rehabilitation once the acute illness is relieved.[10]

Patients' ability to relate the "story" of their illness is one indication of their executive functioning and memory. Biographical information and general fund of knowledge are obtained to establish a baseline in assessing the effects of medications and electroconvulsive therapy.

Questions about family and recent personal events are useful:

"Tell me about your children (or parents). What are their names? Their ages?"
"When did you last see them? Was there a family gathering last Thanksgiving (Christmas, or other holiday)? Where did the family meet and who was there?"
"What was the name of your high school (college)? Do you recall the names of classmates? When did you last see them?"
Cognitive function is also widely assessed using the Mini Mental State Examination.[11] The maximum score is 30, and a score of 22 or less is suggestive of dementia. For persons 75 and older, the age norm is about 27. To be a valid indicator, the patient must be alert (to eliminate poor performance due to delirium), cooperative, speak the language in which the test is administered, and not be aphasic. The assessment takes up to 20 min and can be administered by nursing staff. If the patient does well and there is no other clinical concern about cognition, no further testing is usually done.

Examining for personality disorder

Personality traits are habitual behaviors that characterize a person's tendencies to repeatedly think, feel, and act under specific circumstances. Impulsiveness, fearfulness, persistence, and assertiveness are examples. A trait is a dimension of behavior that can be scored along a continuum with high and low poles. Traits develop independently of each other, and being high on one trait does not predict the strength of other traits. Most "normal" persons are in the middle range on most traits. Personality traits are highly heritable and are usually fully formed by early adulthood.
Abnormal personality traits are not features of melancholia. They are more often associated with non-melancholic illnesses. The older literature refers to the personality traits associated with mood disorder as "neurotic" or "anxiety-laden." Impulsiveness is a trait associated with increased suicide risk, and lack of openness about one's feelings makes the assessment of suicide risk more difficult.[12]
Melancholia distorts a patient's self-perception and self-report in response to questions about personality. Questions referring to times when the patient was not depressed or to how the patient typically reacts, may capture the characteristics of the trait being assessed:
"When you are not depressed and you are feeling more like yourself, how would you then describe your personality?"
"Are you usually, or most of the time, [aggressive] [passive and shy] [outgoing]?"
Standardized tests of personality also provide clinically helpful information.[13] Table 5.3 displays some descriptors that help patients to recognize their trait behaviors.

Rating scales of depression

The Hamilton Rating Scale for Depression

Although various rating scales were in use before, it was the Hamilton Rating Scale for Depression (HAMD) that quickly dominated depression research.[14] In its various forms it is the most widely used instrument and has been applied in studies of

Table 5.3. Descriptors of trait behavior

Trait	Descriptors	Implications
Anxious-fearful	"Worry-wart," pessimist, shy, inhibited; uncomfortable in new situations; likes routine; overplans, not spontaneous; prefers others to make decisions	Non-melancholic depression Anxiety disorders
Impulsive	Easily bored; likes to take action and risks; likes novelty, "leaps before he looks;" messy and disorganized	Increased suicide risk when depressed Substance and alcohol abuse
Dramatic-emotional	Outgoing, easily upset, likes the limelight, exaggerates	Increased frequency of suicide attempts
Low openness	Aloof, private person; self-conscious, unemotional; not sentimental	Less likely to confide in the examiner

depressed patients worldwide.[15] The clinically administered (HAMD) is reliable.[16] It is enhanced by structured interviewing.[17]

Factor analytic and related studies find the HAMD a measure of severity at the time of assessment rather than an indicator of symptom change or diagnosis.[18] Published versions include 17, 21, and 24 items. Scores of 13, 17, and 21 and higher are respectively consistent with a diagnosis of depressive mood disorder. Factors derived from the scale are considered stable and are characterized as dimensions of *somatic anxiety/somatization*, *psychic anxiety*, *core depression*, and *anorexia*.[19] The somatic anxiety/somatization factor is influenced by co-occurring general medical illness[20] but the core depression dimension (mood disturbance, psychomotor disturbance) is not.[21] This limits the HAMD's usefulness in assessing depression in hospitalized general medical and neurologic patients who will commonly endorse the somatic anxiety/somatization items (e.g., sleep problems, weight loss, palpitations). A score > 13 on the 17-item version is a reasonable screening threshold for depressive illness in these patients.[22] In many studies, remission is defined as a persistent score of 10 or less for the 24-item scale and 5 and 7 or less on the shorter version. A score of zero can be achieved in patients who are adequately treated.

The *Depression Interview and Structured Hamilton* is an effort to diagnose depression in medically ill patents. It has been used in the Enhancing Recovery in Coronary Heart Disease (ENRICHD) study of depression in heart patients.[23] Using the HAMD as a clinical diagnostic tool, however, merges different mood disorders and fails to distinguish melancholia.[24] A score greater than 28 in the 17-item version, however, identifies a severe depressive illness.[25] In persons over 65, a score > 16 is consistent with mood disorder.[26]

Table 5.4. A short version of the Hamilton Rating Scale for Depression

Depressed mood
Guilt
Suicide
Work and interests
Agitation
Psychic anxiety
Somatic anxiety
Loss of libido

The HAMD has shorter "clones" that are practical in any clinical setting. One version has good specificity and sensitivity (0.89 and 0.96 respectively, based on 1.00 as perfect).[27] Predictive power is also good (96%). Items covered are listed in Table 5.4. Items are rated from 0 to 3 or 4, with 0 indicating absent and 4 the most severe. Guilty delusions are rated 4. These scales are used to track changes in severity of depression during the course of treatment.

The Montgomery–Asberg Depression Rating Scale (MADRS)

The MADRS, like the HAMD, is an observer-rated instrument designed to assess response to antidepressant treatment.[28] The MADRS has acceptable reliability.[29] A score > 35 identifies severe depression,[30] while a score < 10 is consistent with remission.[31] In persons over age 65 a score greater than 21 is evidence for a mood disorder.[32] Comparison studies of the HAMD and MADRS find them similar in usefulness.[33] A self-rating version of the MADRS is equivalent to the Beck Depression Inventory, but is less influenced by personality traits and more focused on core depression features.[34]

The Beck Depression Inventory (BDI)

The BDI is widely used as a self-rating scale of depressive illness.[35] The BDI correlates weakly with the HAMD, with younger persons with more years of education, and with atypical or non-melancholic illnesses scoring higher on the BDI relative to HAMD observer ratings. A "psychological/cognitive" factor derived from the BDI reflects its origin as an instrument in psychotherapy. Higher scores on this factor identify persons with personality disorder.[36] A "somatic/vegetative" factor includes some features of mild to moderate melancholia and is associated with dexamethasone non-suppression of cortisol. The BDI is designed as a measure of severity, not as a diagnostic instrument.[37] Its use in persons with co-occurring general medical or neurologic disease, or for patients with cognitive problems, is limited by its poor specificity in these patient groups.[38] The BDI is not useful in assessing melancholia, or in assessing the severity of depressive illness in patients in hospital settings. It may, however, be sensitive as a screening instrument for outpatient samples.[39]

Other rating scales

Two other self-rating scales are in occasional use. The *Zung Self-rating Depression Scale* (ZSDS) has good reliability and is useful as a screening instrument.[40]

The *Carroll Rating Scale* (CRS) was designed to match the HAMD in content. It has good reliability and predicts HAMD scores better than the BDI.[41] The CRS is used as a screening instrument in general medical settings.[42]

The Bech–Rafaelsen Melancholia Scale (BRMS) was developed as a self-rating scale based on the HAMD but focused on identifying melancholia.[43] Its more structured version has good reliability and good construct validity. It correlates highly with the HAMD.[44] The BRMS includes a mania scale, making it useful in assessment of manic-depressive patients.[45] One report finds it more sensitive at identifying relapse than either the HAMD or the MADRS.[46]

The *Newcastle Endogenous Depression Diagnostic Index* (NEDDI) has good reliability and construct validity with the HAMD and the MADRS. It separates endogenous from non-endogenous depression, identifying endogenous depressive illnesses, identifying the endogenous form by both cross-sectional (e.g., distinct quality of mood disturbance, psychomotor disturbance) and longitudinal (e.g., normal personality, previous depression) features.[47]

The *Edinburgh Postnatal Depression Scale* has high sensitivity and specificity and correlates with the MADRS. It is designed to screen for postpartum depression, but correlates highly with the MADRS.[48] The *Glasgow Depression Scale* is an instrument administered by an observer. It is designed to assess depression in persons with learning disability.[49] The *Geriatric Depression Scale* has several versions of assessing depression in community, hospitalized, and nursing-home older patients.[50]

Using rating scales

Whether applied to clinical assessment or in research, a scale's designed purpose should determine its use. Self-rating scales are designed to make evaluations with minimal use of professional time, and thereby, expense. They do not replace the skilled examination. The CRS and the BRMS are most helpful in screening for melancholia. The expanded version of the BRMS is particularly useful when assessing manic-depressive patients. The BDI is a psychotherapy assessment instrument that does not have adequate specificity when used in the care or study of melancholic patients. All self-rating scales are of little use when the patient is severely ill, a child, or cognitively impaired.

The HAMD is not a diagnostic scale. It is an instrument that measures severity of illness. While useful in gathering data from a large sample of depressed patients that can then be subjected to statistical search for forms of depression, it does not replace clinical examination in bedside subtyping. Without interpretation and modification its specificity is weak in general medical patients. Although the HAMD is widely used in drug trials, the MADRS was specifically designed to assess behavioral change in pharmacotherapy trials.

In interpreting changes in HAMD scores, initial severity must be accounted for. Drops in score from 32 to 16 and from 14 to 7 are both a 50% change, but the initial severities are markedly different. An endpoint score of 16 indicates continuing illness whereas the 7 endpoint is accepted as evidence of remission.

Observer-administered rating scales are also helpful in clinical practice. When patient assessment depends on several clinicians and staff, their systematic use of a scale over the course of acute and continuation treatment provides the most reliable information of behavioral change. HAMD scoring is routinely used in electroconvulsive therapy research programs.

There is no obvious advantage in using the other "boutique" scales. For example, postpartum melancholia is not different in signs and symptoms from melancholia at other periods in a patient's life, making a specific postpartum depression scale superfluous.

NOTES

1 William Stryon, W. (1990). *Darkness Visible: A Memoir of Madness.* New York: Random House, pp. 12, 17–18.
2 Kendell (1990) p. 308.
3 The terms "mood" and "affect" are often confused. Mood refers to the subjective experience of emotion that is also expressed in observable facial and other motor signs. The primary moods of anger, sadness, happiness, and anxiety in normal persons are transient and contextually appropriate. Mood is the content of emotional life. Affect is the form of emotional life and, regardless of any specific mood, can be assessed for intensity, lability, and appropriateness.
4 Schelde (1998a, b).
5 Fink and Taylor (2003).
6 In patients with co-occurring cardiovascular disease, heart-related morbidity and mortality are increased.
7 Separating the form of psychopathology from its content is important for diagnosis. Content is what the voices are saying, their gender, etc. Content of a delusion may be of guilt, persecution, etc. Content does not discriminate illnesses. Depressed, manic, and schizophrenic patients exhibit delusions of persecution and the content is not diagnostic. Content typically reflects the patient's life experiences and personality. The form of the psychopathology reflects the disease process. It is much more important diagnostically that a person hears things that are not there than what is heard. For further discussion of this phenomenological principle, see Taylor (1999).
8 Chapter 7.
9 Chapter 6 delineates the dementia accompanying melancholia from the dementias associated with degenerative brain disease.
10 The depressed elderly with mild to moderate impairment are at greater risk for suicide than are those without impairment (no added subjective burden) or with severe impairment (unable to plan and carry out the suicide, despite the desire to do so).
11 Mini Mental LLC, Boston, MA. For a review of this instrument, see Tombaugh and McIntryre (1992).
12 Chapter 7.
13 For more information about personality assessment, see Taylor (1999).

14 Hamilton (1960).
15 Leung *et al.* (1999); Akdemir *et al.* (2001).
16 Baca-Garcia *et al.* (2001).
17 Moberg *et al.* (2001); Freedland *et al.* (2002).
18 Gibbons *et al.* (1993).
19 Pancheri *et al.* (2002).
20 Linden *et al.* (1995).
21 Fleck *et al.* (1995).
22 Leentjens *et al.* (2000a).
23 Freedland *et al.* (2002).
24 Demyttenaere and De Fruyt (2003).
25 Muller *et al.* (2000).
26 Mottram *et al.* (2000).
27 Gibbon's *et al.* (1993).
28 Montgomery and Asberg (1979); Demyttenaere and De Fruyt (2003).
29 Davidson *et al.* (1986).
30 Muller *et al.* (2000).
31 Hawley *et al.* (2002).
32 Mottram *et al.* (2000); Zimmerman *et al.* (2004).
33 Senra (1996); Senra Rivera *et al.* (2000).
34 Svanborg and Asberg (2001).
35 Beck *et al.* (1961); Demyttenaere and De Fruyt (2003).
36 Enns *et al.* (2000).
37 Schotte *et al.* (1997a).
38 Leentjens *et al.* (2000b); Aben *et al.* (2002).
39 Viinamaki *et al.* (2004).
40 Lee *et al.* (1994); Passik *et al.* (2000); Thurber *et al.* (2002).
41 Carroll *et al.* (1981b); Feinberg *et al.* (1981a, b).
42 Golden *et al.* (1991); Koenig *et al.* (1992).
43 Bech and Rafaelsen (1980).
44 Bent-Hansen *et al.* (1995).
45 Rossi *et al.* (2001).
46 Bent-Hansen *et al.* (2003).
47 Davidson *et al.* (1984b).
48 Eberhard-Gran *et al.* (2001).
49 Cuthill *et al.* (2003).
50 Rinaldi *et al.* (2003).

6

The differential diagnosis of melancholia

But when the melancholy fit shall fall
Sudden from heaven like a weeping cloud,
That fosters the droop-headed flowers all,
And hides the green hill in an April shroud;
Then glut thy sorrow on a morning rose,
Or on the rainbow of salt sand-wave,
Or on the wreath of globed peonies,
Or if thy mistress some rich anger shows
Imprison her soft hand, and let her rave,
And feed deep, deep upon her peerless eyes[1]

We have defined melancholia as a depressive mood disorder characterized by psychomotor retardation and agitation, disturbances in vegetative functions, loss of interest, impaired concentration and memory, delusional thoughts, and preoccupation with suicide. Psychotic depression, depression that is part of a manic-depressive course, depression with catatonia, puerperal depression, and abnormal bereavement are melancholic illnesses. The evidence for including these conditions as melancholic disorders is discussed in Chapter 2.

Many other depressive disorders are delineated in psychiatric classifications that may or may not meet the criteria for melancholia. Atypical depression, dysthymia, seasonal affective disorder (SAD), adjustment disorder with depression, and similar syndromes are poorly defined. They encompass heterogeneous samples of patients who are best considered as having a non-melancholic mood disorder (Table 6.1).

Non-melancholic depressive mood disorders

Non-melancholic "major depression"

Cluster and latent class analyses identify depressed patients who do not exhibit melancholic features (Table 6.2). The studies do not indicate whether this group can be divided further. Such patients, however, are unlikely to exhibit vegetative dysfunction and associated neuroendocrine abnormalities, and they are thought to respond differently to antidepressant drugs than do melancholic patients. They are

Table 6.1. Non-melancholic depressive mood disorders

Non-melancholic "major depression"
Atypical depression
Dysthymia/minor/brief depression
Seasonal affective disorder
Adjustment disorder, depressed type
Premenstrual dysphoric disorder

Table 6.2. Characteristics of non-melancholic major depression

Reactivity of mood (mood fluctuates with circumstances)
Normal vegetative and circadian function
Tearfulness
Anticipatory anhedonia, but able to experience some pleasure
Blaming others or circumstances, not self
Minimal or absent psychomotor dysfunction
Abnormal premorbid personality (anxious-fearful)
Absence of history of manic-depressive illness

more likely to be associated with personality disorder and the abuse of illicit drugs that complicate treatment.

Atypical depression

Atypical depression is represented as a reactive mood state with hypersomnia, hyperphagia, weight gain, leaden paralysis, and sensitivity to interpersonal rejection (Table 6.3).[2] An important facet of the definition is the belief that such patients do not improve with tricyclic antidepressants (TCAs) or with electroconvulsive therapy (ECT), but do respond to monoamine oxidase inhibitor (MAOI) antidepressants.[3] The concept is controversial, and the differentiating characteristics and the importance of the treatment response in the definition are unclear.

In factor, cluster, and latent class analyses of patients with depressive mood disorders, an atypical depressed group represents 5–10% of the samples.[4] Clinical surveys of private practice outpatients[5] and of community samples[6] support the recognition of an atypical depressive class. A recent systematic assessment of 579 outpatients with major depression identified 22% as meeting the authors' criteria for atypical depression.[7]

Atypical depression is associated with generalized anxiety, phobias, and "hysterical" personality traits.[8] Age of onset for the first atypical depressive episode is in adolescence and substantially earlier than the typical age for melancholia.[9] Quitkin, Klein, and their associates argue that atypical depression overlaps with their concept of "hysteroid dysphoria."[10] This term incorporates, along with the atypical features

Table 6.3. Characteristic features of atypical depression

Mood reactivity
Reversed vegetative signs (hypersomnia, hyperphagia)
Leaden paralysis
Sensitivity to rejection

cited in Table 6.3, a premorbid histrionic personality disorder. When under stress or rejection these patients "respond' with a brief depressive episode.

Other authors fail to find evidence of an atypical depression, or question the usefulness of the reactivity of mood feature, or question the stability of the reversed vegetative signs feature, the hallmarks of the atypical concept.[11] The bulk of the evidence finds that patients with signs and symptoms of atypical depression do not have a melancholic illness.[12]

Atypical depression that occurs in the winter months is labeled "seasonal affective disorder." It is modestly associated with manic-depressive illness, particularly with its bipolar II variation.[13] Patients with atypical depressions are more likely to have seasonality of mood fluctuations with elevations in the spring and summer and dips in the fall and winter. They also exhibit lability of mood, with interpersonal "storms" that meet criteria for borderline personality disorder. Histrionic and borderline personality disorders are in the same *Diagnostic and Statistical Manual* (DSM) category and share several important trait behaviors that overlap with mood disorder, further confounding the separation of state from trait problems in these patients.

Although the studies are few, patients with atypical depression are said to respond more specifically to MAOIs than to other medications.[14] The first recognition of atypical depression was based on the examination of patients who did relatively poorly with TCAs but who responded well to MAOIs.[15] A recent multicenter study of the treatment-responsiveness of patients with atypical depression found that mood reactivity and reversed vegetative signs predicted a poor response to imipramine, but leaden paralysis and sensitivity to rejection did not.[16]

Atypical depression is not sufficiently well defined to include it in the syndrome of melancholia.

Seasonal affective disorder

Seasonal variations in mood, especially recurrent symptoms of depression during the winter months that subside during spring and summer, are recognized.[17] Interest in the biology of this phenomenon led to the formulation of SAD.[18] The interest in seasonality encouraged studies of chronobiology, the metabolism of melatonin, and imaginative treatment trials of increasing hours of exposure to simulated daylight. The concept became fashionable as clinicians adopted the treatment for chronically depressed non-hospitalized patients. Manufacturers offered light boxes with a range of light frequencies. The concept of SAD was adopted in DSM-IV as a "seasonal pattern specifier" for major depressive episodes in bipolar I or bipolar II disorder, or major depressive disorder, recurrent.[19] Epidemiologic studies report that 1–10% of depressed patients meet criteria for SAD.[20]

SAD patients who meet the DSM specifier criteria exhibit recurrent episodes (at least two are required). Atypical depressive symptoms of hypersomnia, hyperphagia, and weight gain dominate the clinical picture of SAD patients more frequently than non-SAD patients.[21] But not all investigators find this association.[22] The genetic loading for SAD, however, does not distinguish these patients from persons with other mood disorders, although alcoholism is more prominent in SAD families. High seasonality scores are reported in 63% of patients with atypical depression.[23] But the rates of onset of major depressive disorder were not higher in the spring and fall, nor were the rates of atypical depression higher in the winter. Higher rates of suicide were not found in the spring, as suggested from descriptions of SAD.[24] A comparison of the symptomatology of SAD patients with major depressed patients who attempted suicide found the SAD patients to have high scores, mainly in self-reported items in depression-rating scales.[25]

If the hypothesis is correct that SAD is precipitated by fewer hours of daylight during the winter, then the incidence of the illness should increase in populations in polar regions. Such a difference is not found.[26] The efficacy of light therapy is not related to wavelengths of energy, whether they simulate sunlight or not.[27] Light visors, antidepressant medications, and psychotherapy have limited benefit.[28]

The SAD concept does not describe patients with melancholia, and recognizing seasonality does not enhance the ability of clinicians to relieve the more serious forms of melancholia. The merit of recognizing a seasonal component to mood disorders is largely of research interest. Like atypical depression, the patients with these characteristics do not meet the criteria for melancholia.

Dysthymia/minor/brief depression

Several DSM diagnostic options among the mood disorders are defined by their duration and severity. Such delineation lacks validity, and many such patients experience severe depressive illness.[29]

Dysthymia is defined as a 2-year or longer period of almost daily low-grade depressive mood with sadness or irritability.[30] Accompanying features can be typical or atypical (most commonly non-melancholic). By definition, dysthymia is a unipolar mood disorder as it is not diagnosed if the patient has a manic-depressive course.[31] Patients who have the onset of dysthymia in their adolescent years may also have major depressions in adulthood – so-called "double depression."

Dysthymic patients with co-occurring anxious-fearful personality disorder, hypochondriasis, somatoform disorders, social phobia, anxiety disorders, or alcohol abuse are more likely to be suffering a non-melancholic illness.[32] Dysthymic patients with pre-existing personality disorder respond less well to antidepressant drug treatment than do those without an associated personality disorder.[33]

The more than one-third of dysthymic patients who do not fully meet DSM criteria for a major depression but have a family history of mood disorder and have made a suicide attempt are more likely to suffer from melancholia, to have been inadequately treated, or both.[34] The presence of vegetative signs or psychomotor disturbance or a past episode of melancholia strongly points to melancholia. The high frequency of the diagnosis of dysthymia likely results from the low threshold for the diagnosis of illness, and the overinclusiveness of patients with character pathology within the present diagnostic system of depressive disorders. Inadequate treatment that prolongs an episode of depression is a contributing factor. In a study of 410 patients with dysthymia, many of whom also experienced major depressions, only 45% had ever been treated with medication.[35] In a study of older dysthymic patients, a third had received no treatment and none had received ECT.[36] On the other hand, 50% of dysthymic patients are reported to improve with either imipramine or desipramine.[37]

Minor depression is a variation of the dysthymia concept. It is characterized by indistinct signs of a depressed mood that affects social functioning, but with duration of less than two years but more than two weeks. Depressive mood that is less than 2 weeks in duration and is recurrent is labeled " brief depression." Family history data do not support the category.[38] The duration criterion is best ignored, and with evidence of melancholia, the patient should be treated for melancholia.

Double depression is pictured as dysthymia with superimposed major depression.[39] It is often labeled *chronic depression* when it is applied to patients with lifelong symptoms that do not respond to single antidepressant drug therapy.[40] These patients are usually in outpatient care and in medication trials, recruited by advertisement for individuals with persistent depressed mood. The trials also assess novel methods of psychotherapy combined with the latest antidepressant medications.

Considering the descriptions offered in the studies, the patients do not meet criteria for melancholia. Many are labeled "therapy-resistant" according to algorithms that define adequate and inadequate medication trials.[41] When such patients are referred for ECT, the responses of those labeled therapy-resistant and those not so labeled are equivalent.[42]

The patients who are now labeled as meeting criteria for dysthymia, minor depression, double depression, and brief episodic depression most often do not meet criteria for melancholia.

Adjustment disorder, depressed type

A person so sensitive to stress as to develop depressed mood with social dysfunction when faced with mild to moderate stress is labeled as having an adjustment disorder of depressed type.[43] The patient's symptoms cannot be explained by another illness.[44] Implied in the concept is that the depressed mood will resolve within six months with guidance and stress reduction rather than medical treatment.[45] Data supporting this category are sparse.

Other than being younger and less ill than other patients with depressive illness, these patients are not distinguishable from those with mild to moderate depressive mood disorders.[46] In general medical settings its features may be associated with a pre-existing personality disorder or cognitive impairment.[47]

The depressive episodes that are common among adolescents are often classified as an adjustment disorder. Depressive symptoms in adolescence, however, are frequently followed by more severe mood disorders, suggesting that the "adjustment" episodes are stages of the more severe illness rather than difficulties dealing with stressful situations (such patients are reported to respond to antidepressants.)[48] Not to recognize these early episodes as depressive illness risks chronicity from a prolonged episode that is inadequately treated. The failure to identify accurately these early stress-associated episodes as depressive illness also inaccurately reduces the estimated number of actual depressive episodes a patient has had, information needed in planning long-term treatment.

The notion of adjustment disorder as a mild depressive mood state causally linked to stress is also conceptually problematic as no such linkage has been demonstrated.[49] Because an illness is preceded by a stressful event does not assure causality, nor does it assure that the illness does not have the same pathophysiology as an episode that occurs independently of a stressful event. A cerebral stroke with its subsequent pathophysiology is a stroke, regardless of whether or not it is preceded by a stressful situation.

Many persons who are diagnosed as suffering from an adjustment disorder are also likely to be suicidal.[50] The application of this label, with its suggestion of being benign, dangerously lowers clinical sensitivity to suicide risk.

Patients who meet criteria for adjustment disorder with depressed mood, however, are unlikely to meet criteria for melancholia.

Premenstrual dysphoric disorder (PDD)[51]

Some 3–8% of premenopausal women experience premenstrual dysphoria that may be mistaken for melancholia. Symptoms occurring in the four days before the onset of menses (late luteal phase) include irritability and sadness (dysphoria), apprehension, crying spells, reversed vegetative signs, sensitivity to rejection, cognitive difficulties, breast tenderness, abdominal bloating, headache, back, joint, and muscle aches, edema, and weight gain. Impulsivity with aggression occurs. Work and social functioning are impaired.

Women with PDD have cyclic hormonal changes similar to women without the syndrome. It is probable that PDD is triggered by these changes, but other vulnerability must also be present.[52] Thyroid dysfunction is not a factor in its expression.[53] Cortisol levels are normal in women with PDD, although some patients have delayed peak levels in cortisol secretion.[54] Along with the short duration of symptoms and the clear periodicity of PDD, a normal serum cortisol blood level also distinguishes this illness from melancholia.

PDD is considered modestly familial in inheritance. The concordance among monozygotic twins is twice that of dizygotic twins, suggesting a heritability of 30–40%.[55] PDD is associated with both manic-depressive illness[56] and recurrent depressive illness.[57] Some investigators find a link to anxiety disorder and offer selective serotonin reuptake inhibitor (SSRI) agents as treatment.[58] Whether PPD is a variant of mood and anxiety disorders or is a distinct condition is unclear.

Some investigators suggest serotonin dysregulation as a factor in the development of PDD,[59] and encourage treatment with intermittent SSRI antidepressant therapy.[60] The patients with a clear history of past episodes of melancholia or manic-depressive illness would likely fare better with treatments for those conditions.

Melancholia in children and adolescents

Melancholia occurs in children and in adolescents, although it may be less common than melancholia in older age groups. In community samples, depending on the age group and diagnostic criteria used, prevalence for depressive illness in children and adolescents ranges from 2% to 20%.[61] In clinical samples, rates are about 60% in teens and 40% in children.[62] Children do not fully express their subjective mood, so the illness is best identified by observation of the features of melancholia and caretaker information. Depression inventories offer structure to collecting information.[63]

Melancholia has been identified in young children with severe behavioral conditions.[64] These investigations criticize the DSM-IV classification of depressive disorders for children and adolescents. Large samples of young children with depressive symptoms or with "disruptive" behaviors were compared with a "healthy" group without psychiatric disorder.[65] Of 156 participants, the researchers identified 54 depressed children, with 57% being anhedonic. The more severe depressive mood in these children was accompanied by a lack of mood reactivity, alterations in cortisol reactivity, increased family history of major depressive disorder, and increased frequency of psychomotor retardation. This pattern is consistent with melancholic depression.

Depressed children and adolescents, however, have higher rates of co-occurring illness than do adult depressed patients. Pre-existing anxiety disorder, conduct disorder, and developmental disorder confound the clinical picture of depression in younger children.[66] Mild forms of manic-depressive illness may be misdiagnosed as hyperactivity or attention-deficit disorders.[67] Substance abuse and continuous, rather than episodic, manic-depressive alterations make the diagnosis more difficult in adolescents.[68] Only a few systematic studies of the characteristic laboratory variables found in adult melancholic patients have been reported in prepubertal children to define melancholia in this age group. The results are inconsistent, suggesting clinical heterogeneity in pattern of symptoms and perhaps in neuroendocrine development.[69]

The high rates of co-occurring conditions in depressed children also explain the reports that depressed children do not respond to medication treatments, including TCAs.[70] Depressed patients with these co-occurring conditions are difficult to treat at any age. Among teens with manic-depression the switch rate from depression to mania may be higher (28% versus 3%) than that seen in adults, further complicating treatment.[71] The use of overly broad diagnostic criteria for depressive disorder leads to sample heterogeneity that masks the therapeutic effect of TCAs in melancholic children. Using more structured instruments for assessing depressive features and careful history-taking from caregivers, however, identifies melancholia in children.

Melancholia in adolescents is more readily identified than in young children. Severe depression in teens is similar in signs and symptoms to severe depression in other age groups. No meaningful gender differences are reported in presentation, although girls are at twice the risk as boys. Unlike older adults, however, there is less stability in symptom pattern across episodes in adolescents and young adults.[72] Among adolescents with persistent depressive mood disorder, a serum cortisol at 2000h is often elevated, suggestive of melancholia.[73] Even in studies with large samples, however, characterizing different forms of depression is not done.[74] The most parsimonious conclusion is that depressed children and adolescents who have melancholic features and abnormal cortisol laboratory findings are melancholic and warrant treatment for melancholia.

Melancholia in persons with autism

Persons with autism and with Asperger syndrome present a special diagnostic challenge as they are at increased risk for a mood disorder.[75] Depressive mood disorder is the most common psychiatric condition among adolescents with Asperger syndrome.[76] The diagnosis of a depressive illness, however, is complicated because these patients typically have a restricted range of affect and reduced facial expression that are disconnected from subjective mood.[77] Communication difficulties and paucity of speech increase the diagnostic dilemma.[78] Among high-functioning autistic persons, a recent change in autistic obsessions and preoccupations, social withdrawal, crying spells, sleep and appetite disturbances, and loss of interest should raise suspicions of melancholia.[79] Among low-functioning autistic persons, vegetative signs, increased aggressive behavior, and loss of skills suggest the presence of depressive illness. Psychotic or catatonic features are signs of melancholia.[80]

Although more difficult to recognize, melancholia occurs in persons with autism. Those patients who meet criteria should receive treatments for melancholia. Treatment options are unfortunately restricted as antidepressant drug trials are few and limited to anecdotal or uncontrolled studies.[81] One report cautions that there is some association between the prescription of SSRI agents and extrapyramidal symptoms in this patient group.[82] The experience with ECT in these patients is limited to case reports.

Melancholia in the elderly

Melancholia must be considered when an older person with a history of recurrent depressive illness has a recent change in behavior and functioning. Depressed elderly persons are more anxious, have more somatic complaints, and are more cognitively impaired than are younger depressed patients, but otherwise their depressive features are similar to those in other age groups.[83] When cognitive impairment is severe, these depressed patients are difficult to distinguish from patients with degenerative brain disease.

The frequency of depressive illness in the elderly is about the same as in the rest of the population, although depressed older persons are more likely to be melancholic.

It is youth's vanity to think that depressed mood in older persons is a natural response to being old. Misinterpreting signs of melancholia in an old person as the result of aging or general medical comorbidity can be a fatal error.[84]

For some persons, however, depressive illness is not expressed until late in life. These first-time depressions occurring after age 60 have been termed *vascular depression* or *late-life depression.*[85] The belief that these conditions represent distinct forms of depressive disorders is unsupported.[86] More likely, the aging process and its associated social, interpersonal, endocrine, and general medical difficulties reduce the threshold for depression in a vulnerable person. Melancholia in a patient with brain microvascular brain disease or that occurs for the first time in the elderly is no different from melancholia without such brain changes or that occurs in other age groups.

The term "vascular depression" represents the belief that the expression of depressive illness for some persons requires substantial microvascular brain change. Although other neurologic conditions are associated with depression (e.g., Parkinson's disease), and traumatic brain injury to frontal limbic structures elicits depressive mood disorders,[87] the most common depression-inducing process is a cerebrovascular stroke. The concept of "vascular depression," as opposed to depression associated with stroke, is that the strokes underlying vascular depression are small, largely go unnoticed, and tip the balance to illness. The presence of vascular brain disease is necessary, but not sufficient for the depressive illness to unfold.[88] For most persons the adverse vascular process begins later in life and takes time to reach a critical density. "Vascular depression" is indistinguishable from "late-life depression," but neither of these depressive categories justifies their separation from other mood disorders.[89] They are best considered as melancholic depression when they meet the criteria for melancholia.

Persons with a first episode of depressive mood disorder late in life who do not have vascular risk factors are said to have experienced a recent severe stress.[90] Of these patients, 10–30% have a premorbid personality disorder and a three- to fourfold higher prevalence of alcohol abuse than the non-depressed elderly.[91] Other than less anxiety, no difference in symptoms is reported between persons with a first depressive episode later in life compared to those who develop depressive illness earlier in life.[92] The prevalence in the elderly of a first severe depression after age 60 is about 2–3%.[93]

Elderly persons with high risk factors for cerebrovascular disease are more likely than are those with low risk to develop a depressive illness. The typical magnetic resonance imaging (MRI) finding in these patients is deep white matter hyperintensities.[94] Also cited are greater left than right white matter involvement and more severe subcortical gray matter involvement, particularly in the putamen.[95] Increased lesion density in medial orbital frontal regions is also reported.[96] Such MRI changes are associated with poorer general functioning in the elderly, independent of the presence of depressive mood.[97] A correlation between the presence of white matter hyperintensities and poor cognitive function on executive and time-dependent tasks is reported.[98] While these brain changes are considered risk factors, they do not represent a unique pathophysiology of depressive illness.

A genetic vulnerability to vascular disease has also been postulated to predispose to a first episode of depression later in life.[99] The apolipoprotein E_4 gene linked to Alzheimer's disease has been associated with the deep white matter changes seen in first episodes of depression late in life in some studies.[100] The finding is not supported in other studies.[101] Persons with a first episode of depressive illness late in life do not have neuropathological changes characteristic of Alzheimer's disease.[102] A meta-analysis of risk for depressive mood disorders in a community sample of elderly persons identified general medical disability, bereavement, and prior depressive episodes as risk factors for a depressive illness later in life.[103]

While vascular and other brain changes may lower the threshold for depression in older persons, they are not causal, and the depressive mood disorder that occurs is not pathophysiologically or phenomenologically distinct from depressive disorders that occur at other times in life. This conclusion, and the fact that melancholia is the typical depression in older patients, warrants the clinical position that a depressive illness in the elderly is best considered melancholia until proven otherwise.

Melancholia in a patient with a psychotic disorder

Psychotic depression is a form of melancholia.[104] Psychiatric classifications also recognize depression in other psychotic disorders. The *International Classification of Diseases*, 10th edition (ICD-10) classification includes *postschizophrenia depression*, a depressive illness occurring within 12 months of an ICD-defined schizophrenic illness with "schizophrenic features" persisting during that year.[105] DSM-IV includes *postpsychotic depression* and "*superimposed*" depression in a category "for further study." The depressive episode must occur during the residual phase of schizophrenia and must meet DSM criteria for major depression with a depressed mood rather than exhibiting anhedonia alone.

Depressive states occur with sufficiently high frequency to be found by chance in some schizophrenic patients, but the reported co-occurrence is beyond a chance finding.[106] The proposed explanations for such findings are beyond the focus of this book.[107]

How can melancholia be identified in patients who meet diagnostic criteria for schizophrenia so that appropriate antidepressant treatments can be prescribed and chronicity avoided? Although the psychotic features that define schizophrenia and other non-mood disorder psychoses are often dramatic, they are not specific and do not discriminate schizophrenia from psychotic mood disorders.[108] The "positive" symptoms of psychoses not associated with mood disorders are indistinguishable from the symptoms of psychotic depression.[109] Somatic and guilty delusions are seen more often in patients with psychotic depression than in patients with schizophrenia, but they are an insufficient discriminator.[110] The presence of severe agitation or suicidal ruminations also suggests psychotic depression rather than schizophrenia.[111]

"Negative" symptoms that are considered characteristic of schizophrenia are infrequently associated with psychotic depression. Their presence discriminates the two

Table 6.4. Affective and mood features distinguishing schizophrenia from melancholia

Schizophrenic emotional blunting	Melancholic intense narrow mood range
Expressionless face without stupor	Sad face, often with omega sign and Veraguth's folds
Monotone voice (motor aprosodia[114])	Appears frightened or confused
Reduced hand-gesturing	Voice plaintive, whining, high-pitched
Apathy or irritability	Overly concerned about present situation
Indifference to present situation unless concerned about delusional content	
Prolonged inactivity and reduced interests without concern	Episodic inactivity and reduced interests with related guilt feelings
Minimizes problems or relates problems to delusional ideas	Maximizes problems and underrates performance on cognitive tests
No realistic future plans	Despite hopelessness, may reluctantly express what he/she would do if better

syndromes best. In a factor analytic study, the patient's concern about anhedonia was associated with the diagnosis of major depression rather than with schizophrenia.[112] In another factor analysis, emotional blunting was represented by two factors: avolition and loss of emotional expression. Schizophrenic patients had both factors while melancholic patients were avolitional when depressed, but not emotionally flat. Their emotional expression was intense, but narrowed to the moods of apprehension, dysphoria, and gloom, characteristic of melancholia.[113] A psychotic patient who complains about loss of ability to experience pleasure, and who also expresses the moods of melancholia, is best identified as being depressed. Recent sleep and appetite disturbance also indicate depressive disorder. Table 6.4 displays affect and mood features helpful in distinguishing schizophrenia from melancholia.

A more difficult challenge is the young male patient in an oneiroid (dreamlike) state who expresses vague persecutory ideas. Such patients may also exhibit catatonic motor features. Because many schizophrenic patients experience an associated depressive syndrome in their first psychotic episode, the discrimination is further confounded. Course of illness is helpful. Patients with schizophrenia, particularly those with their first psychotic episode in adolescence or early adulthood, are more likely than are melancholic patients to have early childhood neuromotor abnormalities (delayed developmental milestones, awkwardness, poor visual–motor coordination), cognitive difficulties (attention and working memory difficulties, difficulty shifting set), and abnormalities of affect, including emotional aloofness, lack of warmth, and hypersensitivity.

The dexamethasone suppression test (DST) has been examined for its ability to discriminate schizophrenic patients from patients with psychotic depression. The results are variable, reflecting heterogeneity across samples.[115] Some studies find that DST non-suppression poorly distinguishes melancholia from a psychosis with negative symptoms.[116] Season of the year has been offered as an explanation for differences in findings, as a greater rate of non-suppression is reported among schizophrenic patients in the winter.[117] An association between non-suppression in patients with schizophrenia and the likelihood of a suicide attempt is cited.[118]

Assessing corticotropin-releasing hormone stimulation of cortisol and adrenocorticotropic hormone (ACTH) levels along with the DST adds to the discrimination of schizophrenic patients from non-patient groups.[119] Rapid eye movement (REM) latency also appears to be shorter in schizophrenic patients who also have abnormal DST.[120]

The course of illness following the first psychotic episode may also identify schizophrenic patients who respond best to treatments for mood disorder. In a 6-year follow-up study, Winokur and associates (1996) observed that schizophrenic patients who received different diagnoses at different times in their illness course (e.g., schizophrenia at one time, schizoaffective on another occasion) were likely to have a mood disorder and to have DST non-suppression when depressed.

In sum, the data and clinical experience suggest that a psychotic patient with features of a major depression should be treated for melancholia, rather than for psychosis alone. Evidence of abnormal hypothalamic–pituitary functioning and perturbed sleep parameters identifies these patients, but alone these are not conclusive. Lack of the developmental problems is also helpful, but not pathognomonic. Taken together, the presence of a depressive mood and its associated physiologic features in patients diagnosed as schizophrenic identifies patients who respond to antidepressant drugs and to ECT.[121]

Distinguishing melancholia from anxiety and obsessive-compulsive disorders

Obsessive-compulsive disorder (OCD)

Patients with OCD often become depressed and many melancholic patients ruminate about the "bad" things (imagined and exaggerated) that they have done or are likely to do. When these intrusive thoughts are not obviously delusional (e.g., causing foreign wars and natural disasters), they can be mistaken for OCD. Melancholic patients may also say that their thoughts are "unreasonable" but that they cannot stop thinking them, and are frightened that they will act upon them. Because the suicide risk in melancholia is high, depressive features should take precedence over obsessions in deciding treatments. The obsessions should be considered to be ruminations and the patient treated for melancholia, not for OCD.

The usefulness of the DST or other hypothalamic–pituitary axis tests is unclear in distinguishing patients with OCD from melancholic patients. The few studies offer small samples with inconsistent results. Some investigators find 17–37% of OCD patients to be non-suppressors, with some non-suppressors having concurrent depression, but male non-suppressors need not be simultaneously depressed.[122] Some investigators rarely find non-suppression among patients with OCD and see the test as a useful discriminant.[123]

Anxiety disorders

Patients with panic disorder and other anxiety disorders also experience episodes of depression.[124] Melancholic patients are typically apprehensive and may be extremely frightened. Factor analytic studies identify a substantial anxiety component in severely depressed patients,[125] and the nature of an "anxious depression" has been debated.[126] Does anxious depression represent a mood disorder, an anxiety disorder, or does it reflect a common vulnerability? How these concerns are resolved has implications for long-term management. The acute question in differential diagnosis is more focused. Is the present episode of anxiety the expression of melancholia or an exacerbation of an anxiety disorder, particularly a cluster of panic attacks? Factor analytic studies suggest that the presence of depressive features should take precedence. The more depressive symptoms the patient experiences (i.e., the higher the score on a rating scale for depression), the more likely the patient is depressed and will respond to treatments for melancholia. The presence of catatonic features or psychosis supports the diagnosis of melancholia. An onset of illness after age 35 and a course that is episodic with anxiety or panic attacks limited to the episodes is also consistent with mood disorder. Family illness pattern is less helpful because depressive and anxiety disorders co-occur in the same pedigrees. The DST is also of limited use because comparison studies find a substantial proportion of patients with panic disorder or agoraphobia (25–40%) to be non-suppressors.[127] A high depression-rating scale score, episodes associated with psychomotor disturbance or psychotic features, first illness onset after age 35, and an episodic course warrant the diagnosis of mood disorder. Because melancholia is associated with a high suicide risk, particularly when the patient is anxious, and has an excellent outcome when appropriately treated, it is safest to consider a depressed, anxious patient ill with melancholia until proven otherwise.

Distinguishing melancholia from drug-related depressive-like states

Melancholic patients, like other persons, may use illicit drugs and drink alcohol to excess. Alcohol use may precipitate an episode of melancholia, complicating its treatment.[128] Patients become depressed after overuse. These patients often have risk factors for mood disorder and their overuse may be "the last straw." Such depressive illnesses respond to antidepressant treatment.[129] Still other patients experience depressive-like episodes or non-melancholic depressions associated with illicit drug use.[130]

Cocaine withdrawal

A depressive state often follows a prolonged binge and the sudden cessation of cocaine use. The syndrome develops rapidly, over hours or a few days, and is characterized by profound fatigue, hypersomnia, increased appetite, psychomotor retardation, vivid and unpleasant dreams, and dysphoria.[131] The co-occurrence of a *dramatic-emotional personality disorder* with a history of having non-melancholic depressive illness and other substance abuse is often elicited.[132] Patients seek hospitalization by feigning suicidal feelings or psychosis. Permitting the patient to sleep as needed and offering a high-carbohydrate diet allows these episodes to resolve within a few days without further intervention. The use of dopaminergic replacement agents has no proven effect.[133]

Abuse of organic solvents

The inhalation of volatile solvents is associated with avolition, apathy, loss of emotional expression, and low activity levels. Users are typically men 30–50 years old. They commonly have cognitive problems consistent with frontal lobe dysfunction. Unlike melancholic patients, they are not apprehensive or express thoughts of gloom. They have a paucity of thought and do not describe depressive ruminations. A lack of motivation to seek and prepare food leads to weight loss, but they are not anorectic. Sleep is undisturbed. They may be psychotic and, if prodded by their hallucinations or believing they are threatened, they may become briefly violent.[134] Antipsychotic medication may help.[135]

Overuse of prescription and over-the-counter drugs

Many medications are associated with changes in mood. Medication-induced mood changes vary in pattern, but rarely appear as melancholia (reserpine is the oft-cited exception). Apathy, lethargy, and low energy are prominent features. The most common offending medications are listed in Table 6.5. Until proven otherwise, a depressive mood state should be considered medication-related if the patient is using a known offender and the depressive-like state unfolded shortly after the drug was introduced or its dosing or pharmacokinetics changed. If discontinuing the medication does not improve the mood state within five times the drug's half-life (the time to reach steady state), the depression should be treated as a primary depressive illness.[136]

Table 6.5. Medications associated with induced mood disorder

Class	Some examples
Antiarrhythmics	Quinidine, procainamide, lidocaine
Antihypertensives	Reserpine. propranolol, methyldopa, hydralazine, nifedipine
Antibiotics	Penicillins, mycins
Anticonvulsants	Phenytoin, barbiturates, ethosuximide
Antineoplastics	Vincristine
H^2-blockers	Cimetidine, ranitidine
Hormonal agents	Corticosteroids, progestational agents, estrogen
Sedative-hypnotics	Benzodiazepines, chloral hydrate, alcohol
Others	Interferon-B, baclofen, cyproheptadine, disulfiram, methysergide

Melancholia associated with general medical illnesses

Many general medical conditions are associated with an increased prevalence of depressive mood disorder. These episodes are often odd. The mood may be apathetic or neutral rather than the intense apprehension and gloom characteristic of melancholia. Patients express the words that are associated with depressed mood (statements about decreased energy, loss of interest, pessimism about the future, helplessness) but not the mood or "music" of the syndrome. Perceptual disturbances may be present, but are not characteristic (e.g., seeing odd colors or only one end of the color spectrum, experiencing multiple hallucinatory phenomena in multiple sensory modalities). In melancholia, the patient typically has had previous episodes of depression or has the risk factors associated with depression.

Endocrinopathies

Thyroid disease, hyperparathyroidism, Cushing's and Addison's diseases are associated with a depressed mood that is linked to a hormone imbalance or its metabolic consequences. The endocrinopathy appears to be the "last straw" for a person vulnerable for depression. In cross-section, these depressive mood disorders are not easily distinguished from melancholia.

Thyroid disease interferes with antidepressant treatment, and every depressed patient warrants evaluation of thyroid dysfunction. On rare occasions, hyperthyroidism is associated with apathy. The condition is more likely to occur in elderly patients and is characterized by apathy, lethargy, cognitive impairment, loss of appetite, and non-restorative sleep. High-output heart failure may occur. The syndrome is resistant to antidepressant drugs but does respond to correction of the thyroid dysfunction.[137]

A history of calcified renal stones and severe fatigue suggests hyperparathyroidism. Physical examination for a chronic hypercortisol state indicates Cushing's disease. Cortisol levels in melancholia are not as high or as prolonged as in Cushing's disease and so do not produce these signs. Chronic fatigue even when not depressed, weakness, and tan-like skin pigmentation in an otherwise light-skinned person suggest Addison's disease. Men receiving androgen deprivation therapy for prostate cancer also appear to be at higher risk for depressive symptoms.[138]

Other general medical conditions

Lupus erythematosus is associated with an increased prevalence of mood disorder.[139] Up to two-thirds of patients with Lyme disease develop symptoms of depression. The current rates of depression in persons with syphilis are unknown but historically patients with syphilis have been identified as suffering from mood disorders.[140] Pancreatic carcinoma has classically been associated with depression, but there are only a few reports documenting this association.[141] The same is true for Crohn's disease.[142]

Although folate deficiency,[143] cancers of all types,[144] chronic renal disease,[145] and rheumatoid arthritis[146] are assumed to increase the risk for depressed mood, the actual rates of depressive mood disorders are not higher than in controls. Patients with acute myocardial infarction have increased rates of depressive symptoms but the actual rate of severe depression is unclear, although likely modestly elevated. The mechanism for this increased risk is unknown.[147]

Chronic fatigue syndrome (CFS) is characterized by chronic fatigue that waxes and wanes, unrelieved by rest.[148] Onset is acute or subacute and is described as following a viral infection with low-grade fever, sore throat, tender and periodically enlarged lymph nodes, muscle and joint pain, headache, sleep disturbances, anxiety, irritability and weepiness, and visual scotomata and photophobia. Cognitive impairment, particularly in attention and new learning, and work difficulties occur. CFS is distinguished from melancholia by its onset and course, and signs of infection. Fatigue is present in the absence of the profound apprehension and gloom of melancholia.[149] Abnormal cortisol metabolism has been reported in some patients with CFS,[150] but most do not have the neuroendocrine abnormalities observed in melancholia.[151]

The features of CFS overlap with those of generalized anxiety disorder (neurasthenia), somatoform disorder, and non-melancholic depression. Half or more of patients with CFS are said to have mood disturbances, but data from twins in which one suffered from CFS do not support a relationship between CFS and depressive illness.[152] Also, while low-dose TCAs combined with non-steroidal anti-inflammatory agents have been reported to be helpful in controlled studies,[153] CFS patients do not substantially benefit from pharmacotherapy for depression.[154]

Persistent pain

Persistent pain is a feature of somatoform disorder, CFS, fibromyalgia, and irritable bowel syndrome, but also occurs independently. One-third to a half of chronic pain patients fulfill the criteria for major depression – almost all are non-melancholic. Complaints of pain are common in melancholia, however, but these are acute or episodic, and resolve with successful antidepressant treatment. Hypothalamic–pituitary–adrenal abnormality is also a common finding, making the DST unhelpful in distinguishing these patients from those with melancholia.[155]

Obstructive sleep apnea

Sleep apnea affects about 10% of middle-aged persons and is characterized by daytime fatigue and sleepiness. Irritability, mild cognitive impairment, and depressive thought content may be present, triggering the consideration of a depressive illness.[156] The greater the fatigue, the more likely that features of depressed mood will be present.[157] Obesity, heavy and thick jowls, and a history of snoring identify these patients. Treating these patients for a depressive mood disorder does not benefit most sufferers.[158]

Avolitional, apathetic, and bradykinetic syndromes

Many conditions are associated with apathy severe enough to be mistaken for a depressive mood disorder.[159] Apathy is characterized by a loss of motivation leading to reduced activities, thoughts, interests, social interactions, and productivity, with increased dependence on others and lack of concern for the change in behavior.[160] Avolition and loss of emotional expression are part of the syndrome. Motor slowing is common, but not essential to the diagnosis. Although melancholic patients are avolitional, they are typically distraught by the change in their behavior and feel guilty about it. Melancholic patients exaggerate their loss of function whereas persons with apathetic syndromes minimize their dysfunction. Family members are usually more concerned about the situation than are the patients. Melancholic patients typically look upset, anxious, worried, and sad. Patients with an apathetic syndrome appear emotionally blunted. Other features of depression are usually absent. Some conditions associated with apathy that can be mistaken for melancholia are listed in Table 6.6.

Table 6.6. Conditions associated with apathy

Frontotemporal dementia
Basal forebrain trauma or stroke
Thalamic ablating disease
Bilateral amygdala ablating disease
Basal ganglia disease
(Parkinson's, Huntington's, carbon monoxide poisoning)
Demyelinating disease
(multiple sclerosis, HIV [human immunodeficiency virus] microvascular disease)
Myotonic dystrophy
Endocrinopathies
(hypothyroidism, hyperthyroidism, hyperparathyroidism, Addison's, Cushing's disease, androgen deficiencies)
Late-stage diabetes mellitus
Lyme disease
Chronic organ failure (heart, kidney, liver)
Chronic obstructive pulmonary disease
Nutritional deficiencies
Anemia and blood dyscrasia
Cancer and paraneoplastic processes
Chronic fatigue syndrome
Obstructive sleep apnea
Schizophrenia
Past chronic and heavy stimulant drug use
Psychotropic drug overdose
Chronic and severe stress
Autism

Neurologic disease associated with apathy and depression-like syndromes

Frontal lobe disease

Early in their illness, patients with pathology in the frontal lobe dorsolateral prefrontal cortex circuit (DLPC) are apathetic and appear to have become lazy and inefficient. Their personality coarsens and they become ill-mannered. Disinhibition may ensue, with silly shallow attempts at humor (*Witzelsucht*) and impulsiveness.[161] A marked change in personality after age 35 is almost always the result of brain disease. When severe, these patients are emotionally blunted, and become disheveled and unclean. Speech and thought content are repetitive. Bradykinesia is common. Basal ganglia motor signs of rigidity and resting tremor, or balance and arousal difficulties occur. Cognitive impairment is commonly observed. (Table 6.7)[162] Frontal-lobe apathy is associated with frontotemporal dementia, progressive supranuclear palsy, hydrocephalus, cerebellopontine myelinolysis,[164] and traumatic brain injury with axon shearing.

Table 6.7. The apathetic frontal lobe syndrome

Feature	Assessment[163]
Paucity of ideas	Generating a list of animals
Poor working memory	Digit span backwards/serial sevens
Poor cognitive flexibility	Trail-making test B
Poor planning and other executive functioning difficulties	Solving other tasks and problems
Problems with reciprocal and alternating motor tasks	Sequential hand movement
Behavioral avolition	History of recent interests and activities/typical day/future plans
Loss of emotional expression	Observation of facial and vocal expressions and hand gestures

Cerebrovascular stroke[165]

Over 10% of stroke patients who are not depressed are apathetic. Poststroke apathy is characterized by reduced activity, effort, and interest not explained by other neurologic deficits (e.g., motor weakness), dementia, or reduced level of arousal. Patients may be unconcerned about or indifferent to their disabilities and altered circumstances. Unlike depressed patients, they do not complain or maximize their difficulties. They may be pessimistic about the future, and believe that they are helpless to change their situation, but these statements are made with little conviction and no obvious altered mood. They are usually not agitated. They have difficulty initiating actions, including responses to questions, but once they start, they move and speak at normal speed. DST results in stroke patients have not been well studied. Apathetic, non-depressed patients appear to be normal suppressors with normal cortisol levels.[166] In one report, an abnormal DST at one week poststroke was associated with symptoms of depression at three weeks, although no patient met diagnostic criteria for depressive illness.[167]

Traumatic brain injury (TBI)

When TBI is substantial, 20–50% of victims experience mood disturbances. They are more likely to have co-occurring anxiety, aggressive behavior, and a history of mood disorder compared to TBI patients who do not develop depressive illness. They have more cognitive impairment than patients with TBI who are not depressed.[168]

In the *postconcussion syndrome* that quickly follows many head injuries, anxiety and moodiness are associated with headache, dizziness, and concentration and memory problems that are readily mistaken for depressive illness. Electroencephalogram (EEG) slowing may be present. Apathy is also an early posttrauma feature. A depressed mood after TBI may reflect "the last straw" phenomenon in a person vulnerable for depressive illness.[169]

Basal ganglia disease

Depressive features and basal ganglia disease co-occur.[170] These depressive features do not reflect demoralization, but result from disruption in frontal lobe basal ganglia circuits.[171] When the depression is "major" or melancholic in pattern, the patient typically reports pre-existing depressive illness or risk factors for depression.

Parkinson's disease (PD)

Half or more of patients with PD develop depressive mood disorders.[172] Depressive features may be the first signs of PD, and patients with PD appear more depressed than do patients with comparable impairment. The severity of the depressive mood disorder and motor impairment does not correlate. The treatments of PD aimed at enhancing brain dopamine levels have little effect on the mood disturbance.[173]

Persons who develop PD before age 65 and women with PD appear at greatest risk for comorbid depressive illness.[174] When the illness is melancholic, the diagnosis will depend on features other than psychomotor retardation.[175] Cog-wheeling and resting tremor indicate PD, although melancholic patients are often tremulous and catatonic. When rigidity is the primary motor feature of PD and apathy the primary behavioral feature, the combination can be misinterpreted as depressive illness, particularly as a depressed mood is an expected comorbidity of PD. Lack of ruminations about self-blame and guilt, no great apprehension, and the preservation of humor assist in this discrimination. The use of depression-rating scales is also helpful.[176]

The DST is helpful. Among PD patients with major depression, up to 75% are non-suppressors with high cortisol levels, whereas among non-depressed PD patients, only 25% are non-suppressors. PD patients who are also demented may be non-suppressors, so the presence of substantial cognitive impairment in a patient with PD confounds the interpretation of DST non-suppression.[177]

Huntington's disease

Perhaps 50% of patients with Huntington's disease become depressed, often before the motor features of the disease are fully expressed.[178] Apathy and irritability are often more prominent than the typical melancholic moods of unremitting gloom and apprehension, and the patient may already have noticed some increased clumsiness or trouble with coordination.[179] A family history for movement disorder with cognitive decline is almost always present, and laboratory identification of the number of CAG repeats in gene IT15 on chromosome 4 is considered diagnostic.

Wilson's disease

Patients with Wilson's disease (hepatolenticular degeneration) also develop depressive mood disorders, often before other features of the degenerative disease are prominent. Patients with onset after age 40 and who are also depressed or who have an apathetic syndrome are diagnostic challenges. Their motor features are subtle and their behavioral symptoms result in psychiatric hospitalization. The recent trend in using antipsychotic agents as enhancers of antidepressant medication in the non-psychotic patient confounds even the most careful motor examination. When Wilson's disease is suspected, 24-h urine copper assay is the most definitive laboratory test. Kayser–Fleischer rings (copper deposition around the outside of the corneas) are present in over 90% of patients with central nervous system involvement.

Demyelinating disease

White matter disease is associated with apathetic and depressive symptoms. While apathy and fatigue are common complaints in persons with *multiple sclerosis (MS)*, depressive mood disorder is also frequent.[180] MS is the second most common cause of neurologic disability in young and middle-aged adults and point prevalence for depressive symptoms in these patients may be as high as 50%.[181]

Melancholia is not common. Emotional lability and *pathological crying* and *laughing* occur. Pathological crying is confused with depressive mood disorder as these patients will endorse questions about tearfulness and crying spells. Pathological crying, however, is short-lived, explosive, with an absence of statements of subjective experience of sadness. In *emotional incontinence*, the subjective feeling of sadness is present but is substantially less than the outward severity of the tearful state.[182]

Epilepsy

About 40% of epileptic patients become depressed.[183] As with patient 6.1 below, when the depressed mood is directly linked to the seizure, seizure control is the best prevention. Telltale prodromal, ictal, postictal, and interictal symptoms reveal the seizure disorder. Clinical suspicion increases that a depressive disorder is seizure-related when it is of short duration and associated with brief anxiety attacks, an atypical mood, psychosensory features, and brief periods of altered arousal or "fuzzy" thinking.

Patient 6.1

A middle-aged man became profoundly gloomy and pessimistic, and unable to work. He whined and tearlessly cried, pleading for help, and needed constant reassurance. He was

Table 6.8. Differences between pseudodementia and Alzheimer's disease

Distinguishing feature	Pseudodementia of depression	Alzheimer's dementia
Awareness of illness	Exaggerates symptoms and problems	Minimizes symptoms and problems
Depressive symptoms	More symptoms and more melancholic features	Fewer symptoms and more avolition than sadness
Neurologic features	Bradykinesia and bradyphrenia	Early-onset form associated with rigidity and transcortical sensory aphasia; poor olfactory discrimination is an early sign, as is a pre-dementia period of mild cognitive impairment
Personal history	Previous mood disorder more likely	May have no previous psychiatric history
Family history	Mood disorders more likely	Alzheimer's disease more likely
Laboratory tests	1. Decreased metabolism on functional imaging more frontal or diffuse 2. MRI normal or mild atrophy without progression	1. Decreased metabolism on functional imaging biparietal and temporal early in illness 2. MRI shows more temporal lobe atrophy and ventricular enlargement

anxious and paced continuously. He made several serious suicide attempts. The depressive episodes typically began suddenly in the late afternoon and slowly resolved by evening. They occurred daily. On several occasions a depressive episode lasted for a week or more. Because of the unusual timing and duration of the moods a seizure disorder was suspected and confirmed. His depressive episodes ended when seizure control was achieved.

Depressive illness among epileptic patients, even of substantial severity, is often unrecognized.[184] Epileptic patients whose depressive illness preceded their seizure disorder are at higher risk for additional depressive illness.[185]

Partial complex seizures with temporal or frontal lobe foci are a common source of seizure-related depression MRI (reduced temporal lobe volume on the side of primary focus). Functional imaging (reduced interictal and increased ictal perfusion at the site of focus), and continuous EEG monitoring are helpful laboratory aids. Serum prolactin levels drawn 20 min after the suspected seizure are elevated in 40–60% of patients with partial complex fits.

Dementia

Annually, 10–30% of demented patients meet diagnostic criteria for major depression.[186] For the most part, these depressive disorders are not demoralization, bereavement reactions, or misdiagnosed apathetic syndromes. They are substantial clinical depressive mood disorders, often melancholic, and are associated with severe and rapid deterioration in functioning that presents as dementia.[187] Treating the depressive mood disorder, however, substantially improves the patient's quality of life and caretaker satisfaction.

Distinguishing the early stages of a structural brain disorder that meets criteria for Alzheimer's disease from a severe depressive mood disorder is challenging.[188] The elderly commonly exhibit modest cognitive decline with aging. Depressive mood disorder is also associated with cognitive impairment, particularly in frontal executive functioning, working memory, and sustained attention.[189] The cognitive decline in a depressive mood disorder, particularly in elderly persons, is the basis for a reversible dementia, referred to as *pseudodementia.* These patients respond well to antidepressant treatments, whereas misidentification as having Alzheimer's disease and failure to alleviate the mood disorder adequately leads to high mortality rates. An unusual example is reported of a patient with recurrent depressive illness who was misdiagnosed as suffering from Alzheimer's disease for 9 years before antidepressant treatment resolved the dementia and the depression.[190] There are distinct clinical advantages in questioning every diagnosis of Alzheimer's disease when accompanied by depressed mood, and in offering antidepressant treatment before consigning the patient to chronic nursing care.[191]

Table 6.8 displays some features distinguishing pseudodementia from Alzheimer's dementia.[192]

NOTES

1 *Ode to Melancholy*, John Keats, in Stillinger (1978/1982), pp. 283–4.
2 Stewart *et al.* (1993); Lam and Steward (1996); Rabkin *et al.* (1996); Sotksy and Simmens (1999).
3 Sargant and Slater (1946); West and Dally (1959).
4 Robertson *et al.* (1996); Serretti *et al.* (1998b); Sullivan *et al.* (1998, 2002); Fountoulakis *et al.* (1999); Parker *et al.* (1999a, b, 2000a); Tylee *et al.* (1999); Angst *et al.* (2002).
5 Benazzi (1999a, 2000).
6 Horwath *et al.* (1992); Levitan *et al.* (1997).
7 Posternak and Zimmerman (2002a).
8 Paykel *et al.* (1983).
9 Stewart *et al.* (1993).
10 Klein and Liebowitz (1982); Quitkin *et al.* (1989, 1991, 1993); Stewart *et al.* (1993).
11 Spitzer and Williams (1982); Paykel *et al.* (1983); Thase *et al.* (1991a); McGinn *et al.* (1996); Parker *et al.* (2002).
12 Lam and Steward (1996).
13 Perugi *et al.* (1998); Benazzi (1999a); Benazzi and Rihmer (2000).
14 Davidson *et al.* (1989); Quitkin *et al.* (1989, 1991, 1993); Stewart *et al.* (1997).
15 McGrath *et al.* (1992).
16 Sotsky and Simmens (1999).

17 Wehr (1989).
18 Rosenthal *et al.* (1984).
19 American Psychiatric Association (1994).
20 Magnusson and Boivin (2003).
21 Stewart *et al.* (1990); Allen *et al.* (1993).
22 Tam *et al.* (1997).
23 Pande *et al.* (1992).
24 Posternak and Zimmerman (2002b).
25 Pendse *et al.* (2004).
26 Booker and Hellekson (1992); Faedda *et al.* (1993).
27 Bielski *et al.* (1992); Lam *et al.* (1992).
28 Eastman *et al.* (1992); Rosenthal *et al.* (1993); Pjrek *et al.* (2004); Rohan *et al.* (2004).
29 Kessler *et al.* (2003b).
30 In children, the duration may be only 1 year.
31 DSM-IV, pp. 345–8.
32 Akiskal (1983a, b); Versiani and Nardi (1997).
33 Akiskal (1990); Ravindran and Lapierre (1997).
34 Schrader (1995).
35 Shelton *et al.* (1997).
36 Devanand *et al.* (1994).
37 Kocsis (1997).
38 Angst (1997); Kessler and Walters (1998); Rapaport *et al.* (2002).
39 Goldney and Fisher (2004).
40 Klein *et al.* (1996); Keller *et al.* (1998); Thase *et al.* (2002); Kocsis *et al.* (2003).
41 Quitkin *et al.* (1984); Prudic *et al.* (1990).
42 Husain *et al.* (2004).
43 The *International Classification of Diseases*, 10th edition (ICD-10) uses the descriptors "Usually interfering with social functioning and performance" and "some degree of disability in the performance of daily routines" while DSM-IV uses the descriptor "marked distress that is in excess of what would be expected given the nature of the stressor or by significant impairment in social or occupational (academic) functioning."
44 Greenberg (1997); Jones *et al.* (1999b).
45 Casey *et al.* (2001).
46 Jones *et al.* (1999b. 2002b); Lewinsohn *et al.* (1999).
47 Strain *et al.* (1998).
48 Lewinsohn *et al.* (1999); Aalto-Setala *et al.* (2002).
49 The relationship of stress to depressive illness is discussed in Chapter 8 on suicide.
50 Kryzhanovskaya and Canterbury (2001).
51 PDD is classified in the depressive disorder, in the not otherwise specified (NOS) section of the DSM. It is not the *premenstrual syndrome*, which is a time of varying discomfort experienced by many women.
52 Mortola *et al.* (2002).
53 Korzekwa *et al.* (1996).
54 Parry *et al.* (2000).
55 Kendler *et al.* (1992); Condon (1993).
56 Yonkers (1997); Hendrick and Altshuler (1998).
57 Warner *et al.* (1991); Severino and Yonkers (1993); Critchlow *et al.* (2001).

58 Freeman (2004); Perkonigg *et al.* (2004); Vickers and McNally (2004).
59 Elliott (2002); Steiner and Pearlstein (2000).
60 Steiner and Born (2000).
61 Costello *et al.* (1998).
62 Carlson and Cantwell (1980a); Kolvin *et al.* (1991); and Carlson (unpublished 1991 data in a personal communication, 2004).
63 Timbremont *et al.* (2004).
64 Luby *et al.* (2002, 2003a, b, c, 2004).
65 Luby *et al.* (2004).
66 Radke-Yarrow *et al.* (1992).
67 Carlson (1998); Wozniak *et al.* (2004).
68 Carlson and Cantwell (1980b); Costello *et al.* (1998); Kessler (1998).
69 DeBellis *et al.* (1996).
70 Ryan (2003).
71 Johnson *et al.* (1991); Strober *et al.* (1993).
72 Masi *et al.* (2001); Lewinsohn *et al.* (2003).
73 Goodyer *et al.* (2001, 2003); Forbes *et al.* (2005).
74 Lewinsohn *et al.* (2003).
75 Ghaziuddin *et al.* (2002a).
76 Ghaziuddin *et al.* (1998); Tantam (1988).
77 Macdonald *et al.* (1989); Capps *et al.* (1993).
78 Attwood *et al.* (1988).
79 Jolliffe *et al.* (1992); Ghaziuddin *et al.* (2002b).
80 Ghaziuddin *et al.* (2002b).
81 Ghaziuddin *et al.* (2002b).
82 King *et al.* (1991); Sokolski *et al.* (2004).
83 Baldwin and Tomenson (1995); Alexopoulos *et al.* (2002). Baldwin and O'Brien (2002); Baldwin (2005).
84 Alexopoulos *et al.* (2002); Schwenk (2002).
85 Benazzi (1999c); Baldwin and O'Brien (2002).
86 Stewart *et al.* (2001).
87 Mollica *et al.* (2002).
88 Hickie and Scott (1998); Lyness *et al.* (1999).
89 Thomas *et al.* (2001, 2003).
90 Van den Berg *et al.* (2001); Bruce (2002).
91 Devanand (2002).
92 Baldwin and Tomenson (1995).
93 Blazer *et al.* (1988, 1994); Beekman *et al.* (1999); Baldwin and O'Brien (2002); Baldwin (2005).
94 Simpson *et al.* (2000); Nebes *et al.* (2001); Krishnan (2002); Miller *et al.* (2002b).
95 Tupler *et al.* (2002).
96 MacFall *et al.* (2001).
97 Steffens *et al.* (2002).
98 Austin *et al.* (2001); Lockwood *et al.* (2002).
99 Hickie *et al.* (2001).
100 Nebes *et al.* (2001).
101 Hickie *et al.* (2001); Rigaud *et al.* (2002); Steffens *et al.* (2003).

102 O'Brien *et al.* (2001).
103 Cole and Dendukuri (2003).
104 Chapter 5.
105 Birchwood *et al.* (2000).
106 Candido and Romney (2002); Bressan *et al.* (2003).
107 Somnath *et al.* (2002); Taylor (1992).
108 Schizophrenia, schizophreniform disorder, and brief psychotic disorder, as defined in DSM-IV, differ mainly in duration criteria. Their hallmark is auditory hallucinations of voices and "passivity" delusions that were once characterized as "first-rank," in the mistaken belief that they were pathognomonic of schizophrenia. Delusional disorder requires the patient to believe an elaborate delusional story.
109 Taylor (1999); Chapters 7–9.
110 Schatzberg and Rothschild (1992).
111 Schatzberg (2003).
112 Romney and Candido (2001).
113 Berenbaum *et al.* (1987).
114 Aprosodia is the absence of the normal variations of pitch, rhythm, and stress in speech.
115 Yeragani (1990); Ismail *et al.* (1998).
116 Addington and Addington (1990); Tandon *et al.* (1991).
117 Rybakowski and Plocka (1992); Monteleone *et al.* (1994).
118 Plocka-Lewandowska *et al.* (2001).
119 Lammers *et al.* (1996).
120 Tandon *et al.* (1996). An abnormal DST and reduced REM latency are laboratory hallmarks of melancholia. When both findings are present in a patient diagnosed as suffering from schizophrenia, they should raise suspicions of misdiagnosis, with psychotic depression the most likely condition. Treatment for melancholia should be favored.
121 Siris *et al.* (1982); Kirli and Caliskan (1998); Mazeh *et al.* (1999); Addington *et al.* (2002).
122 Insel *et al.* (1982); Cameron *et al.* (1986); Jenike *et al.* (1987); Catapano *et al.* (1990).
123 Schlesser *et al.* (1980); Lieberman *et al.* (1985); Monteiro *et al.* (1986); Coryell *et al.* (1989a).
124 Gulley and Nemeroff (1993).
125 Mullaney (1984).
126 Downing and Rickels (1974); Mountjoy and Roth (1982); Whiteford and Evans (1984); Breier *et al.* (1985).
127 Coryell *et al.* (1985b, 1989b); Heuser *et al.* (1994); Schreiber *et al.* (1996).
128 Chapter 13 discusses these comorbidities.
129 Chapter 13.
130 Reports of. an apathetic syndrome associated with chronic and heavy use of cannabis are not substantial, although an association between chronic cannabis use and psychosis is suggested (Hall and Solowij, 1998; Stefanis *et al.*, 2004). Chronic use is also associated with cognitive impairment in new learning that may be reversible following abstinence (Pope *et al.*, 2001).
131 Sofuoglu *et al.* (2003).
132 Helmus *et al.* (2001).
133 Eiler *et al.* (1995).
134 Brain metabolic imaging may show general decreased frontal lobe metabolism similar to that seen in some depressed patients. MRI, however, may show white matter hyperintensities not typical of young depressed patients.

135 Ozaki and Wada (2001).

136 When a medication's half-life is 24 h, a constant daily dose will reach steady state in about 5 days. Once the prescription is discontinued, it will also take about 5 days for most of that dose to be eliminated from the body. Unless there is compelling evidence that the patient's ability to eliminate the medication has been compromised, no behavioral improvement after 5 days following the discontinuation of a medication with a 24-h half-life suggests that the behavioral syndrome is not directly due to the substance prescribed.

137 Brenner (1978).

138 Pirl *et al.* (2002); Wilhelm *et al.* (2004).

139 Iverson (2002).

140 Fallon and Nields (1994).

141 Fras *et al.* (1968).

142 Elsehety and Bertorini (1997).

143 Lee *et al.* (1998).

144 Akechi *et al.* (2001). The rates of depressive *symptoms* are higher in cancer patients than in controls. The rates of patients meeting criteria for major depression vary widely and reflect multiple factors such as degree of pain, premorbid personality and social factors, type of cancer, and treatments used. There is no direct evidence that cancer *per se* induces a pathophysiological process that leads to depression (Sutor *et al.*, 1998).

145 Kimmel (2002).

146 Dickens *et al.* (2002).

147 Sutor *et al.* (1998).

148 Two historical reviews of CFS describe its roots in the older, largely discredited psychosomatic literature (Shorter, 1992; Trimble, 2004).

149 In one brain metabolism study patients with CFS showed bilateral thalamic hyperperfusion whereas depressed patients showed right thalamic hyperperfusion and left prefrontal cortex hypoperfusion (MacHale *et al.*, 2000). This finding requires confirmation.

150 Greenberg (1997).

151 Demitrack (1997).

152 Roy-Byrne *et al.* (2002).

153 Wesely (1993).

154 Vercoulen *et al.* (1996); Weardon *et al.* (1998). Neural-mediated hypotension demonstrated with positional changes in blood pressure has also been implicated in some patients with CFS and these patients are reported to benefit from treatments like atenolol and disopyramide (Rowe *et al.*, 1995).

155 Campbell *et al.* (2003b). TCAs are superior to SSRIs in treating depressed mood and chronic pain (Fishbain, 2000; O'Malley *et al.*, 2000; Lynch, 2001; Jackson *et al.*, 2002).

156 Baran and Richert (2003).

157 Bardwell *et al.* (2003).

158 Bardwell *et al.* (2003). Weight loss, avoidance of alcohol consumption, and continuous positive-pressure air delivery at night are recommended interventions for obstructive sleep apnea (Sanchez *et al.*, 2001).

159 In the discussion in Chapter 13 of "treatment-resistant depression," 10–15% of these patients were misdiagnosed as depressed, but were suffering from other diseases with depressive features.

160 Marin (1991).

161 *Witzelsucht* means searching for humor. Some patients with frontal lobe disease become silly and repeatedly try to make light of even the most serious matter. They make inane and vulgar jokes and ignore the resulting discomfort of others.

Personality is highly heritable and typically fully formed by the time a person reaches young adulthood. For a full discussion, see Taylor (1999), Chapter 6.

162 Levy *et al.* (1998).

163 For a detailed discussion of these and other bedside cognitive tests see Taylor (1999), Chapter 4.

164 Cerebellopontine disease is associated with "frontal lobe" syndromes because these structures are connected to the frontal circuits through the thalamus. The frontal circuits, the anterior limbic system, and the cerebellar pons comprise a functional brain system. For further discussion, see Taylor (1999), Chapter 1.

165 Starkstein and Manes (2000).

166 Marchesi *et al.* (1996).

167 Harney *et al.* (1993); Harvey and Black (1996).

168 One study found them to have reduced left frontal gray matter volume on MRI (Jorge *et al.*, 2004).

169 Brown *et al.* (1994); Silver *et al.* (1994).

170 Lamberg (2001).

171 The data supporting this relationship are substantial (Taylor, 1999) Also see Slavney (1999) for a discussion of the identification of demoralization in general medical patients.

172 Slaughter *et al.* (2001b).

173 When the PD patient is also melancholic, ECT relieves both the mood disorder and the motor features. See Chapters 8 and 9 on ECT.

174 Zesiewicz *et al.* (1999); Slaughter *et al.* (2001b).

175 Rogers *et al.* (2000).

176 Leentjens *et al.* (2003).

177 Kostic *et al.* (1990); Rabey *et al.* (1990). Functional brain imaging may also distinguish PD patients with and without depressed mood, the depressed patients showing lower metabolic activity in the caudate and orbitofrontal cortex (Bissessur *et al.*, 1997).

178 Kirkwood *et al.* (2001); Slaughter *et al.* (2001a).

179 Craufurd *et al.* (2001).

180 Schiffer (2002).

181 Joffe *et al.* (1987). TBI is the most common cause of neurologic disability in this age group.

182 Feinstein and Feinstein (2001). Treatments for MS are also associated with mood disturbances. High-dose corticosteroids may induce hypomania or mania. Interferon beta-1B, used to ameliorate the relapsing-remitting form of MS, is associated with depressed mood and elevated suicide risk (Lublin *et al.*, 1996). Pretreatment with antidepressant drugs is reported to reduce the likelihood of the depressed mood. Desipramine is the only antidepressant systematically studied in the treatment of depression in MS, although other drugs are used (Schiffer and Wineman, 1990). It is effective and tolerated. Low-dose TCAs are the treatment for pathological crying (Schiffer *et al.*, 1985).

183 Victoroff *et al.* (1994); Taylor (1999), Chapter 10; Kanner and Balabanov (2002).

184 Wiegartz *et al.* (1999); Kanner *et al.* (2000). Epileptic patients with low or low-normal serum folate levels (below 7.5 ng/ml) associated with elevated total plasma homocysteine levels are reported to be most at risk for depressive mood disorder. Folate supplementation is recommended to reduce the risk (Rosche *et al.*, 2003).

185 Kanner and Balabanov (2002).
186 Nilsson *et al.* (2002).
187 Ballard *et al.* (1996).
188 O'Brien *et al.* (1997, 2000).
189 Royall (1999).
190 Bright-Long and Fink (1993).
191 Fink (1999a).
192 The use of putative markers of Alzheimer's disease to distinguish these patients from older depressed patients is preliminary (Buerger *et al.*, 2003).

7

Suicide in melancholia

I want to die. I can't believe I feel like this. But it's the strongest feeling I know right now, stronger than hope or faith or even love. The aching relentlessness of this depression is becoming unbearable. The thoughts of suicide are becoming intrusive. It's not that I want to die. It's that I'm not sure I can live like this anymore.[1]

Persons with mood disorders are at the greatest risk for suicide, with 50–70% of persons who kill themselves doing so during an episode of depressive illness.[2] Melancholic patients who are agitated and anxious, psychotic, or who have been hypomanic are at the greatest risk. Studies of suicide, however, do not typically identify the melancholic patients in their samples, and so the evidence for risk is mostly indirect. Patients who are severely depressed,[3] or who have abnormal hypothalamic–pituitary–adrenal functioning[4] are likely to be melancholic, but studies associating these factors of increased risk rarely define the form of depressive illness.[5] An exception is a study that compared suicide attempts in a large sample of melancholic and non-melancholic patients.[6] After controlling for severity and baseline characteristics as covariates, the melancholic patients were more likely to have had prior serious suicide attempts and to make more attempts during the follow-up period. Although the cited studies refer to severe depression, it is likely that the majority of patients meet criteria for melancholia.

In early estimates of suicide risk, 15–19% of depressed patients committed suicide.[7] Recent assessments report rates of about 9% for those ever hospitalized and a lifetime risk of 2–4% for all persons with depressive illness. The lower figures are still four to eight times greater than the rates from other causes.[8]

Worldwide estimates of suicide rates range from 3.4 per 100 000 (sub-Saharan Africa) to over 30 per 100 000 (China). Between 750 000 and 1 000 000 persons commit suicide annually worldwide. Although more than 60% are male, the gender ratio varies by geographic region, with the greatest differences in sub-Saharan Africa and the USA. In China more women than men kill themselves.[9]

Persons over age 70 have the highest rate, even in countries that pride themselves on valuing the elderly.[10] Euro-American elderly men in the USA commit suicide at six times the national average and typically when depressed.[11]

Gunshot is the leading cause of death by suicide for all ages and both genders in developed countries. Gun accessibility and increased alcohol use are the main explanations for higher worldwide rates among males.[12]

For most of the twentieth century, suicide rates in the USA remained steady, with about 30 000 documented and an additional 30 000–60 000 suspected suicide deaths annually. Recent figures suggest rates in the USA to have dropped by 10–15% during the 1990s.[13] During this same period, rates among the young rose, with an increased use of guns. In the USA about 4000 teenage persons kill themselves yearly, making suicide the third leading cause of death in that age group.[14] Substance abuse, family turmoil, and involvement in criminal or civil legal proceedings play more of a role in suicide in the young than in elderly patients, but other risk factors are similar to those for other age groups.[15] The most recent review of the trends in suicide ideation, plans, gestures, and attempts in the USA during the 1990s finds no decrease despite a dramatic increase in treatment.[16]

In England and Wales[17] and in Australia[18] suicide rates among the young have also increased. Although suicide rates in the elderly have decreased modestly, they are still the highest of all age groups. Suicide rates are also increasing in middle-aged persons.[19]

Suicide is reported to have dropped from the eighth to the 11th leading cause of death in the USA.[20] The ethnic differences in suicide annual rates relative to the prevalence of depression are reported highest in Euro-Americans followed by African-Americans, and lowest in Americans of Puerto Rican or Mexican decent. The risk in all ethnic groups is many times higher in men than in women.[21] Female adolescents, but not adults, have higher rates of attempts than males of comparable age.[22]

Errors in suicide prevention

Suicide is preventable. About 40–50% of persons who kill themselves each year seek help from their primary medical caregiver and about 20% have contact with a mental health service within the month prior to the suicide.[23] "Psychological autopsies" – detailed investigations of the events leading to suicide – are valid illustrations of the errors that led to a patient's suicide.[24] Table 7.1 lists these errors.

Table 7.1. Errors in failing to prevent suicide

Errors
Not recognizing a depressive illness
Attributing depressive symptoms to stress, not illness
Not adequately assessing suicide risk
Inadequate pharmacotherapy
Inadequate outpatient follow-up
Failure to protect patients adequately (hospitalize or involuntarily commit)
Failure to administer ECT

Not recognizing a depressive illness

A depressive mood disorder is often unrecognized, especially by primary medical caregivers.[25] In patients over age 65 who had made a suicide attempt, despite signs and symptoms of depressive mood, the prescribed treatments were focused on the relief of anxiety and of sleep disturbances. The diagnostic implications of the psychiatric features were not recognized.[26] Among elderly depressed patients who were seen by their primary physician shortly before their suicide, only 40% were prescribed antidepressant treatments.[27] In yet another study of suicide attempters who met *Diagnostic and Statistical Manual* (DSM) diagnostic criteria for major depression, only 39% were classified as depressed by a psychiatric consultant *after* the suicide attempt.[28]

In an experimental study, one of two clinical vignettes of a suicidal, depressed patient was mailed to over 200 primary care physicians.[29] The vignettes were identical except for the subject's age (38 or 78 years) and employment (working or retired). Depression and suicide risk were recognized in both vignettes by the respondents, but those receiving the "older" vignette were less willing to treat, gave the patient a poorer prognosis, and attributed the depressed mood and suicidal ideas to a rational response to aging.

Clinical ambiguity is another explanation for the underdiagnosis of depressive mood disorder. Among older patients, a change in mood can be overlooked when it is associated with increased somatic complaints. Poor sleep and appetite and loss of energy and interest are attributed to concurrent general medical or neurologic problems. Some examples are:

When depressed, a woman belched uncontrollably, leading her physicians to focus on her incapacitating abdominal discomfort. Elaborate gastrointestinal evaluations were unrewarding, delaying the recognition of melancholia and effective treatment with electroconvulsive therapy.

A depressed woman reported severe headaches, forcing her to stay in bed throughout the day. She was referred to a pain clinic rather than given antidepressant treatment. Interim treatments for pain were not helpful. Effective antidepressant treatment ultimately resolved both the depressive illness and the headaches.

When depressed, a woman suffered from dizziness that interfered with walking. When she was adequately treated for depression, these difficulties resolved.

Despite an increased risk of suicide associated with several neurologic disorders, depression and suicidal ideas in such patients are often interpreted as reasonable responses to decreased capacity.[30] When patients are hospitalized for medical reasons, diagnosis is further complicated by the complaints of poor sleep and appetite, loss of weight and of energy that characterize general medical disorders. These symptoms also characterize depressive mood disorders. When melancholia is expressed primarily by anxiety, the mood state is attributed as a reaction to the general medical illness or to adverse financial, social, and interpersonal problems that face elderly persons. Patient 7.1 illustrates the difficulty in diagnosis under complex circumstances.

Patient 7.1

An 87-year-old woman, living with her daughter, had been taking Triavil 75 mg daily for many years for symptoms of anxiety and depression.[31] She was functioning well. She developed oral–buccal dyskinesia and the prescription was changed to sertraline and risperidone. She became progressively depressed, however, experiencing loss of interest and energy, anhedonia, poor concentration, and feelings of hopelessness and worthlessness. She reported hearing God's and the Devil's voices, and of seeing the Devil and demons. The prescription was changed to paroxetine, with no benefit. Trazodone and mirtazepine were added, also with little benefit. Her complaints continued. She either remained in bed or wandered about the house, appearing confused. Several times daily she unnecessarily changed her clothes and took repeated showers. She wandered into the woods, and stopped eating and drinking at the command of the voices, telling her she was "evil." She threw away her credit card and diamond ring, lost 8 pounds in weight in two weeks, and began pinching herself and twisting her arms to punish herself. She wanted to die.

The patient was hospitalized and received overlapping prescriptions of mirtazepine and risperidone, nortriptyline and olanzapine, haloperidol for agitation, and benztropine. Several different benzodiazepines were prescribed to relieve insomnia and agitation. She required tube-feeding and an endoscopic gastrostomy for nutrition and hydration. She developed urinary retention, was catheterized, a urinary tract infection followed, and an antibiotic was given. Hyponatremia developed. Left lower lobe pneumonia followed with a transfer to another hospital for psychiatric care.

On admission she was agitated, disoriented, made little eye contact, and her speech was sparse. When responding, she mumbled "incoherently." When understood, she complained about auditory and visual hallucinations. Because of her earlier depression and a history of successful ECT 30 years before, two consultants evaluated her for ECT. She had an omega sign and Veraguth's folds, facial features consistent with melancholia. Her expressed moods, however, were either blunted or anxious. She said she was evil and was being punished. She was stiff, postured, and exhibited a grasp reflex and Gegenhalten. She was not febrile, but the lack of physiologic response was attributed to her age. A psychotic depression and an incipient neuroleptic malignant syndrome (NMS)/malignant catatonia were diagnosed and ECT was recommended.

Rising creatinine phosphokinase and falling serum iron levels were consistent with the NMS diagnosis. Her medications were discontinued. Decreased breath sounds and rhonchi bilaterally, a systolic ejection murmur, the hyponatremic and hyperreflexic state, and "confusion" led to the diagnosis of a delirium secondary to infection, and not psychotic depression or malignant catatonia. Her vital signs fluctuated. When she suddenly began to scream about mid sternal chest pain and began hitting her chest, a myocardial infarction or pulmonary embolism was suspected and she was transferred to a critical care medical unit. Neither heart disease nor embolism was found and she was transferred back to the psychiatry unit. A second episode of screaming and chest-beating led to another transfer to critical care, but again nothing emergent was found and she was transferred back to the psychiatric unit.

A week had passed. ECT was again recommended; the chest pain was attributed to her psychotic depression. Delirium, however, remained the working diagnosis and further evaluation for its cause proceeded without success. Her condition deteriorated. She remained bed-ridden, posturing and stiff, refusing food and drink. The ECT team again examined her. A bedside electroencephalogram (EEG) was done and read as normal and inconsistent with a delirium.

Over the next two weeks she received six bilateral ECT and had a full recovery.[32] She was animated, ambulatory but weak, eating and drinking and gaining weight. She was discharged back to her daughter's home where she continued to do well.

Attributing depressive symptoms to stress, not illness

Severe stress may trigger illness.[33] This is as true for depressive mood disorders as it is for cardiovascular disease, hyperthyroidism, and infection.[34] Stressful events linked to depression, however, do not distinguish melancholia from other depressive illnesses. About three-quarters of melancholic patients associate their episode with a stressful event or situation.[35]

A depressive illness is often discussed as a psychological consequence of stress and that removing the stress, understanding its underlying psychology, or adjusting to it will relieve the illness. This stress-and-reaction interpretation may account for some patients, even the melancholic at suicidal risk, not being prescribed medical treatment.[36] The presence of stressful events before an illness, however, does not mean that the patient does not have the illness. If stress precedes a myocardial infarction documented with electrocardiogram and enzyme changes, the stress in the patient's life may ultimately be addressed, but the myocardial infarction warrants immediate treatment. The same reasoning applies to a depressive illness.

The assumption that stress triggers a depressive illness may not be correct. Many studies that report the association do not demonstrate that the stress occurred first, questioning the causality theory.[37] Not considering pre-existing illness is the major confound. In one study, for example, the prevalence of depressive mood disorders during wartime was related to the degree of exposure to war events, but the strongest predictor of the wartime depressive illness was a pre-war depressive illness.[38] As this literature is retrospective, the recollection of past events may be biased to exaggerate events experienced as stressful. Depressed patients attach greater negative impact to life events than do healthy controls.[39] An assessment of the predictive potential of a stress-diathesis model for suicidal behavior found the most effective predictors of suicidal acts to be the history of prior suicide attempts, subjective ratings of severity of mood disorder, and cigarette smoking, each of which had an additive effect on future risk. Pessimism and aggression/impulsivity factors predicted suicidal acts.[40]

Even when they are not depressed, persons with a history of depression consider events as more stressful than do comparison groups, so the occurrence of stress before a depression may be coincidental.[41] Patients also become depressed when life is wonderful, but few would argue that the pleasant period in the patient's life triggered the depression.

A depressive illness may elicit events that are deemed stressful.[42] Living in an environment of increased stress is modestly heritable, in that personality (which is highly heritable) influences the choice of a person's environment and may also change that environment. Thus, a person's trait behavior affects decisions about where he or she lives and the degree of turmoil in that situation.[43] Lastly, increasing anxiety and dysphoria of an emerging melancholic episode disrupt interpersonal functioning and work performance. Stressful situations are followed by the unfolding of the full depressive illness, creating the impression that the turmoil led to the disorder in mood when, in fact, the early phases of the illness or the person's personality trait behavior led to the turmoil. Patient 7.2 tragically illustrates the danger of attributing a depressive illness to stress.

Patient 7.2

A 44-year-old retired military chaplain was hospitalized on a psychiatric treatment facility dedicated to patients suffering from posttraumatic stress disorder (PTSD). He was ruminating about his failures to minister better to enlisted personnel during the Vietnam War and he was unable to carry out his responsibilities in civilian life. A colleague questioned the diagnosis of PTSD and arranged for a visit with a consultant.

The patient had been functioning poorly for about a year. Sleeping was impaired. When very young, he had periods of depressed mood, but received no treatment and had functioned well. Other than a recent increase in alcohol use, he was not suffering from alcohol dependence nor was he an illicit substance abuser. The consultant observed the patient's general medical and neurologic health to be unremarkable.

On examination, the man was subdued, slowed in thinking and movement, but not agitated. His mood was of unremitting apprehension and anxiety. The faces of people he had not helped haunted him. Despite a highly praised career on active military duty, he thought of himself as a failure. He remained awake most nights ruminating on his failures, ate poorly, and had lost substantial weight. He often thought of death, but had no plan to kill himself.

The consultant concluded the patient was suffering from melancholia and recommended treatment. The patient was attending several therapy groups and "milieu" therapy, but was not receiving antidepressant medication. The consultant recommended transfer within the same hospital to a general psychiatric unit, and discussed the option of ECT.

The patient had confidence in his therapists and allowed them to make the decision. The consultant called the head of the PTSD unit and told him of his findings, emphasizing that he considered the patient a high suicide risk and recommended immediate transfer to the locked inpatient unit. The head of the PTSD unit said he and his team considered the patient's present condition to be stress-related and not a primary mood disorder, refusing transfer. A week later the patient fatally hanged himself.

Not adequately assessing suicide risk

Assessing suicide risk is difficult. In one study, 5-year outcomes for 4800 psychiatric inpatients were examined after suicide risk had been evaluated by a psychiatrist. Of the patients who were thought to be at risk, 30% did not make an attempt (false positives) while 44% of patients who did make an attempt were originally considered to be at relatively low risk (false negatives). Predictive suicide scales are of limited help and are rarely used by clinicians in suicide assessment.[44]

Despite the difficulty, suicide risk must be repeatedly evaluated in every depressed patient throughout the illness and for at least the year into recovery, when suicide risk is at its highest.[45] Among patients under psychiatric care who subsequently kill themselves, the intent to commit suicide is expressed about 60% of the time. About 20% of patients who kill themselves in general medical settings communicate their intent.[46] Among young persons who kill themselves, 78% had previously made attempts or communicated suicidal thoughts and 40% communicated intent shortly before killing themselves.[47]

Expressed suicidal thoughts must be taken seriously. If a depressed patient, however, does not express suicidal thoughts, the patient must still be asked about them. Not asking is poor practice. Asking does not increase the likelihood of suicide. It is the first step in suicide prevention.[48]

Patients often feel ashamed about their suicidal thoughts and hesitate to reveal them, for fear the examiner will think poorly of them. The examiner's manner should reflect the message that the illness is not the patient's fault. Detailed questions can be perceived as efforts to help, and not as accusatory. The experience of patient 7.3 is illustrative.

Patient 7.3

A 43-year-old woman was hospitalized for the recurrence of a depressive illness that had previously been successfully treated with ECT. After six months of being well with continuation ECT, she stopped treatments on the urging of her family because of problems with her memory. The depressive mood returned and for the next six months was treated unsuccessfully with medications. She was unable to meet her responsibilities and reported hearing voices saying "bad" things about her and urging her to kill herself. After taking several "pills" and repeatedly expressing the fear that she would kill herself, she was readmitted to the hospital.

In the admitting area she was assessed for suicide, her belongings were searched, and she was brought to the locked psychiatric unit (on a Friday afternoon). On the unit a nurse and an aide again assessed her symptoms and checked her belongings. A resident physician examined her, followed by an attending physician from the ECT team. Like the other assessors, he also asked about suicide. When she told him about her previous plans to overdose, he asked, "Where are the pills now?" After a long pause she tearfully told him she had the pills with her and that she was planning to take them that night. She then retrieved a bag of assorted antidepressant and antipsychotic pills from the lining of her coat. As the attending psychiatrist was leaving her room, she asked him if he thought badly of her for what she did. He told her that her feelings of suicide were part of her illness and that he and the staff did not get upset with a patient's symptoms of illness. They treated the illness.

The patient received her first bilateral ECT the following Monday morning. The ECT attending physician next saw her that noon while she was in the dining room eating lunch. As he approached, she smiled, and thanked him, saying that for the first time in months she was not having any suicidal thoughts.

Inadequate pharmacotherapy

Inadequate pharmacotherapy for mood disorder is the rule rather than the exception. One-third or less of depressed suicide completers received any antidepressant treatment. Fewer still are offered adequate doses of medication.[49] An example illustrates the problem.

Patient 7.4

A melancholic woman was referred to a university-sponsored mood disorders program. Paroxetine (20 mg daily) was prescribed. After several months at that dose her mood remained unchanged. She was unable to work and spent most of the time at home in bed, overwhelmed by the smallest decisions of daily living. Psychomotor retardation was severe. She ate little and lost substantial weight. Paroxetine dosage was increased to 50 mg daily only after the repeated insistence of a consultant. After several more months of unchanged symptoms and again through the insistence of the consultant, mirtazepine was added. The depression quickly resolved. The elapsed time of her dysfunctional state was 8 months.

Recognizing suicide risk does not guarantee improvement in quality of care. A comprehensive assessment of 43 patients with recurrent depressive illness living in Helsinki documented their care before and after each had made a suicide attempt.[50] Sixty percent had been previously hospitalized for depression and 27% had attempted suicide. Before the index attempt, only 16% had received antidepressant treatments at adequate doses, 16% had received psychotherapy alone, and none had been given ECT. One month after the attempt, 17% were receiving antidepressant medications in adequate doses, 22% were receiving psychotherapy, and none had received ECT. In another Helsinki study of manic-depressive patients who killed themselves, 74% were receiving psychiatric care at the time of the suicide and 39% had explicitly communicated their intent to health care givers within 3 months of the suicide.[51] Only 11%, however, had received adequate doses of antidepressant medications, 32% had been prescribed lithium, and none ECT.

In a survey of persons in New York City who had killed themselves, 84% had not received any medication.[52]

Antidepressant treatment of suicidal patients was studied in a sample of 180 depressed patients admitted to two US university hospitals.[53] During the 90 days prior to hospitalization only 21% had received the prescription of antidepressant medication in adequate doses. Patients with a history of a suicide attempt were no more likely than those without such a history to receive better care. In reexaminations of 136 of these patients at 3, 12, and 24 months, each previous attempt increased the likelihood of more attempts but not of adequate treatment.[54]

Inadequate outpatient follow-up

Making the correct diagnosis and prescribing the most likely effective medication for a patient is necessary, but not sufficient, to prevent suicide. Daily contact by phone rounds for the first several days of treatment and regular contacts during the weeks of treatment reassure the patient, monitor side-effects, and assess suicide risk.

Weekly office visits are needed until recovery is clearly defined. Discussions with family members are essential to evaluate suicide intent and changes in the patient's symptoms during this critical treatment period.[55]

Insisting on the removal of any firearms from the household is essential in suicide prevention. Unfortunately, one study of compliance with this request found that most families resist the effort. Non-compliance increases with marital discord and family psychopathology.[56] Patient 7.5 illustrates several of these problems.

Patient 7.5

Following the birth of his son, a 30-year-old man became depressed. The son was colicky, keeping the parents awake much of the night. The father became depressed, unable to sleep even when he went to another room in his house. He lost his appetite and substantial weight. He became uncertain and was unable to make decisions at work or in daily chores. He ruminated about angry fleeting thoughts that his discomfort was due to his son keeping him awake. He became fearful that he would hurt the infant and avoided him, angering his wife who chided him for not helping with the infant's care. He concluded that he was a bad husband and father, became apprehensive, agitated, tearful, and inconsolable. His wife insisted that if he had a more positive and mature attitude they would weather their difficulties. When he hinted that life was no longer worthwhile, his mother contacted a psychiatrist who insisted that the man get immediate psychiatric care and that hospitalization might be needed. The man's wife refused hospitalization, seeing it as abandonment. She wanted him home, but refused to remove a gun from their house, despite the absence of a realistic threat in the neighborhood. When the man's parents agreed to have him stay in their home and watch him, the man's wife insisted that he be taken to her parent's home where he remained for the next two weeks while being treated with an antidepressant. The depression gradually resolved and he eventually returned home, by which time the gun had been removed.

Failure to hospitalize or involuntarily commit

Clinicians are often reluctant to insist on psychiatric hospitalization, and most patients only agree to this dramatic intervention after much urging. The assistance of family members in the effort is invaluable. Involuntary commitment is even more difficult to accomplish as physicians are apprehensive about the prospects of court appearances to justify their action and their fears of legal reprisal by the patient or family. Hospital counsels and defense attorneys, however, prefer to defend a physician with a living patient rather than a physician with a dead patient. When involuntary hospitalization is needed and the clinical concerns appropriately documented, a malpractice action for wrongful commitment is rare, particularly when the family is engaged early in the process, educated to the need for hospital care, and apprised of the risks in not hospitalizing the patient.[57] Patient 7.6 illustrates the consequences of not insisting on hospitalization.

Patient 7.6

A Euro-American man in his mid-40s became depressed while proceeding with a legal separation from his wife. Difficulties at work developed and a physician prescribed an antidepressant. As the patient's depression deepened, his alcohol intake increased. The patient wrote a letter to his father stating that he wanted to kill himself and that he had purchased a shotgun for that purpose. His father did not reveal the contents of the letter to anyone. Because of overt suicidal statements, increasing alcohol use, and worsening mood, the man was hospitalized. Additional medication was prescribed and after two weeks he was discharged with a follow-up appointment in two weeks' time. At home, his wife saw him as more depressed than before hospitalization and insisted that he seek help sooner than his scheduled appointment. He did so, but she declined to accompany him.

He was seen by a mental health worker in an outpatient "urgent care" psychiatric clinic. He was agitated and severely depressed, but denied suicidal thoughts. Rehospitalization was discussed and refused. The mental health worker and a supervising psychiatrist (who did not see the patient) agreed that forced admission to the hospital would destroy any future "therapeutic alliance." They allowed him to leave the clinic when the patient agreed to a follow-up appointment in a week's time. The patient went directly to his office and shot and killed himself.

Failure to administer ECT

Sixty percent of persons who kill themselves do so in the year after a depressive episode. The two weeks following discharge from a psychiatric unit and the first three months post-depression are the most dangerous periods.[58] This striking and disturbing fact has been attributed to progressively shorter hospital stays leading to premature discharge. The patient, still depressed, now has more energy and drive, and is able to act on a suicidal impulse. The recent trend of psychiatrists to accept improvement rather than remission also contributes to this mortality.

Not prescribing ECT is another factor. Successful suicide following hospital discharge after receiving ECT is extremely rare.[59] The studies that document the efficacy of ECT in reducing suicide intent are described in Chapter 8.

Suicide risk assessment

Medical student training does not adequately prepare physicians to assess suicide risk. American training in psychiatry typically provides about 24 classroom hours in the preclinical years and 4–6 weeks of clinical exposure after that. Curriculum time is at a premium, but given that about 25% of the American population (as an illustration of developed countries) will receive a psychiatric diagnosis during their lifetime, and that depressive mood disorder is one of the top five worldwide health-related economic and social burdens, these training experiences are insufficient and inequitable. In many countries, psychiatric training is substantially less than that in the USA, although depressive illness is as common. The rudimentary training of medical students about mood disorders and suicide prevention, combined with an apparent worldwide negative attitude of medical students toward the specialty of psychiatry and the psychiatrically ill, suggests continued low levels of skills in suicide assessment.[60]

The content of medical student training is also problematic because it stresses facts needed to pass external national licensing examinations.[61] US students are taught that suicide risk is higher for protestants, persons from mountain states, urbanites, and the unemployed and the non-pregnant than it is for Catholics, persons from the Midwest, and pregnant women.[62] What is a clinician, taught these arcane facts, to do when faced with a patient who is financially secure, pregnant, Catholic, from rural Indiana, and melancholic? Suicides are more likely to occur during the late fall and on Sundays in the USA[63] but apparently increase with the amount of daylight hours in Australia, peaking in the spring and summer.[64] What should be done for the melancholic patient who expresses the desire to go to sleep and not wake up on a sunny Wednesday in July?[65] Clinically meaningful risk factors are discussed below and summarized in Table 7.2.

Table 7.2. Factors important in suicide risk assessment

Melancholia with anxiety, agitation, or psychosis
Melancholia in manic-depressive illness
Male > 50 years old
Co-occurring heavy alcohol use or abuse
Co-occurring chronic pain from general medical and neurologic illness
Abnormal dexamethasone suppression test or high 4 p.m. control blood level

Melancholia with agitation, anxiety, or psychosis

The more severe the depressive episode, the greater the suicide risk.[66] Profound hopelessness, hypochondriacal ruminations or delusions, and recurring thoughts of death or self-harm accompany suicide.[67] The risk is greater in patients with psychotic depression.[68] The suicide rates among patients with psychotic depression are at least twice that of non-psychotic depressed patients.[69] Over a 25-year period in one facility, delusional depressed patients were five times more likely to kill themselves than were non-delusional depressed patients.[70] This increased risk is not due to delusional content or numbers of symptoms,[71] but because the patients are less likely to receive adequate treatment[72] and are more likely to use more violent suicide methods.[73] Discrepancies in assessments relate polarity of the mood disorder to overall severity, with the more severely ill and bradykinetic patients unable to act upon their self-destructive impulses.[74]

Despite an absence of risk factors, an anxious and agitated melancholic patient is in a life-threatening state and is best treated in a hospital where 24-h protection can be maintained.[75] Of suicide victims clinically assessed seven days before their death, 79% were rated as severely anxious and agitated.[76] A follow-up of melancholic patients reported that those with less psychomotor retardation during their first episode were at greater long-term suicide risk.[77] A patient who is so despondent to have devised and voiced a plan is at high risk and is best treated in the hospital.[78]

A family history of depressive illness or of suicide increases suicide risk. Suicide runs in families.[79] Rates are twice as high in families of persons who killed themselves,[80] with rates particularly high among siblings.[81] Twin and adoption studies support a genetic interpretation accounting for part of this familial aggregation.[82] An estimate based on twin data concluded that genetic factors account for about 45% of the determinants of suicide.[83] The search for "suicide" genes, however, has not been fruitful.[84]

Such family histories also increase the likelihood that the patient being assessed is depressed and is in a state of illness that carries increased risk.[85] In an Amish community, almost three-quarters of suicides clustered in only four families, all of whom also had heavy loadings for mood disorder.[86] In a study of suicide in twins, the familial aggregation of suicide was related to co-occurring psychiatric disorder with suicide rather than for suicide alone.[87] Even after controlling for psychiatric illness, however, familial transmission of suicide remains high.[88] Impulsive aggressive temperament traits, themselves highly heritable, increase the risk of suicide.[89] Sexual and physical abuse during childhood is associated with suicide risk in families with mood disorder.[90]

Other personality traits affect a person's response to suicidal feelings and risk.[91] A characteristic of openness in discussing private matters and feelings correlates with the likelihood of expressing suicidal intent. Tendencies not to talk about one's feelings add to the difficulty in assessment.[92] Identifying premorbid personality traits is useful when evaluating a patient's suicide risk. The more impulsive, the more harm-avoidant, the less open the patient, the greater is the risk.[93]

Suicide in manic-depressive illness

Persons who are depressed and exhibit a manic-depressive course are at risk for suicide. The patients experiencing hypomania alone are at particular risk.[94] About half of persons with manic and depressive phases in their illness make a suicide attempt.[95] Their risk may be as high as or higher than that of patients who only experience recurrent depressions.[96] Of 100 consecutive suicide victims, 46% were diagnosed as having bipolar II disorder and 53% recurrent depression. Only 1% of this sample had experienced both mania and depression.[97] Although 59% had medical contact during the depressive episode that ended in the suicide, many were undiagnosed, untreated, or undertreated. Averaged across studies, the suicide rate for persons with recurrent depressive illness is 12%, while for all forms of manic-depressive illness it is about 19%.[98]

Men over age 50

Men over age 50, *when depressed,* are at greatest risk of suicide. In a psychological autopsy study of 18 suicide victims 50–92 years of age (15 men), somatic preoccupation, sleep disturbance, anergia, and anhedonia were the most prevalent symptoms. Almost half the men abused alcohol. Many had seen a physician shortly before killing themselves.[99]

Mild to moderate cognitive impairment increases suicide risk, whereas severe impairment makes deliberate planning less likely while not affecting impulsive attempts.[100] Studies finding abnormal executive functions in suicidal but not in non-suicidal depressed patients are consistent with this understanding.[101] Importantly, these observations are independent of Hamilton Rating Scale scores and other indicators of depression severity, suggesting cognitive function as an independent, clinically practical measure in assessing suicide risk. Supporting this idea is the greater suicide risk in persons with first depressive episodes later in life, and in those with brain vascular disease[102] and cytoarchitectural brain abnormalities.[103] When assessing suicide risk in a depressed person over age 65, it is helpful to evaluate the patient's attention and executive function. This can be done quickly using tests of working memory (e.g., digit span, letter cancellation), verbal fluency (e.g., animal-naming), and set-shifting (e.g., trails B).[104]

The most important factor in suicide risk in depressed men is access to firearms. The connection between guns and suicide is worldwide.[105] When a firearm is not available, men are still more likely than women to use more lethal means like hanging or jumping from heights.[106] An example follows.

Patient 7.7

A 70-year-old man with several prior depressive episodes had been asymptomatic for many years while taking phenelzine. Recently diagnosed with a form of leukemia, he was advised (incorrectly) that his antidepressant might adversely interact with chemotherapy, and he reduced the dose from 90 to 15 mg daily. Melancholia quickly emerged. He was anxious and agitated and required constant reassurance. He believed the leukemia was untreatable, although he had been told he had a treatment-responsive form. He was unable to sleep and ate little, constantly paced, and was unable to participate in any vacation activities while on holiday. He was flown home under the supervision of an acquaintance. His wife was warned that her husband was depressed and advised that he needed hospital care. She took him home. Upon arrival, she went into the kitchen to prepare a meal. He walked directly to the back of the house and hanged himself.

Alcohol use

Alcohol is found in the blood of many suicide victims and attempters.[107] Suicidal thoughts correlate with an increase in alcohol use.[108] Nearly half of suicide victims are intoxicated at the time of death. Non-alcohol illicit substance abuse is also associated with suicide attempts.[109] Cocaine use imparts the greatest risk.[110]

In addition to using alcohol to "gain the courage," alcoholic depressed persons are more likely than are non-alcoholic depressed persons to respond with a suicide attempt to the stresses of a recent loss or withdrawal of social support.[111] Depressed patients who drink alcohol even moderately are better off abstinent to avoid the co-occurrence of depression during a holiday period when greater alcohol use is socially accepted. Alcohol abusers who successfully cease alcohol use and then kill themselves tend to be older men with depressive illness or younger men with a psychotic disorder.[112]

General medical and neurologic Illness

A general medical illness without an associated depressive illness is not correlated with suicide risk.[113] Fewer than 3% of patients treated in general medical settings express suicidal thoughts.[114] Among persons over age 65 who kill themselves, however, one-third are in ill health.[115] When a patient in a general medical setting is depressed, other risk factors still pertain.[116] In a study of patients who killed themselves following discharge after general medical care, depressive mood and illicit substance abuse were the leading risk factors. The rate of suicide among patients discharged from general medical services is about three times the suicide rate of the general population.[117] Rates are higher among patients with neurologic disease, particularly those with cognitive impairment, including among those under age 60 and who have a history of mood disorder.[118] The highest risk combination of these factors is a chronic and painful illness in a melancholic man over age 60.[119]

Laboratory measures

Efforts to find laboratory indicators of suicide risk focus on biologic correlates at the time of a suicide attempt or completion. Neurochemical studies are complicated by sample heterogeneity, problems linking postmortem findings to complex retrospective clinical data, the lack of multifactorial analyses, and the conflicting findings across studies.[120]

Low serotonin function in brain measures is a persistent finding among suicide victims.[121] Suicide is associated with impulsivity and aggression, with these behaviors in turn correlated with low levels of measured brain serotonergic activity.[122] While the study of serotonin activity may eventually reveal something about the neurobiology of suicide in depressed persons, it provides no help in suicide assessment.[123]

Reduced frontal circuitry metabolism, abnormal findings on computerized EEG, abnormal hormone responsiveness, and rapid eye movement (REM) sleep disturbances have all been associated with suicide risk. Only sleep and hormone findings, however, offer practical clinical guides to suicide prevention.[124]

Severe sleep disturbance in depressed patients is associated with suicidal behavior.[125] Reduced REM latency and increased REM density are reported findings. Sleep studies are available at many clinical facilities, and continued abnormalities at hospital discharge correlate with rapid relapse.[126] Medications that are pharmacologically activating as selective serotonin reuptake inhibitors (SSRI) exacerbate these abnormalities, another indication of why they are not first-line agents for melancholia.[127]

The *dexamethasone suppression test* (DST) is a measure of the severity of depressive illness.[128] The connection to suicide, however, is unclear. Patients with abnormal DST findings are more likely to have made a recent suicide attempt[129] and are more likely to make another attempt.[130] But some studies have not found the DST helpful in predicting suicide attempts.[131] In a meta-analysis of this literature, cortisol non-suppression was consistently associated with subsequent completed suicide but there was no consistent association with prior attempts.[132] A retrospective study of 310 hospital admissions in which the dexamethasone/corticotropin-releasing hormone test was administered within 10 days of admission found no differences in test responses between the patients with and those without recent suicide attempts.[133]

The rates of abnormal DST, however, are higher in depressed patients who subsequently killed themselves.[134] A 13-year follow-up of hospitalized depressed patients whose DST was recorded within a week of admission reported that those with abnormal responses had a 14-fold increase in the likelihood of a serious suicide attempt in the follow-up period.[135] The results are biased by the lesser likelihood that psychotic and manic patients are assessed with a DST.

The many factors that affect the likelihood of a melancholic patient making a suicide attempt are not incorporated into the analyses of DST studies. Depressed persons with co-occurring personality disorder are reported to have low pre- and post-DST cortisol levels, and personality disorder has not been accounted for in most studies of the relationship between the DST and suicide.[136] Studies that do not find an association between non-suppression and suicide nevertheless often find that suicide risk is associated with elevated 4 p.m. cortisol levels, a time when levels should be low.[137] Thus, a 4 p.m. cortisol level and a follow-up complete DST assessment add important suicide prediction power once the patient is identified as melancholic.

The effect of specific treatments on suicide rates

For the acute prevention of suicide in melancholic patients, ECT is superior to all other treatments. It elicits the most rapid response and the highest remission rate. It is the treatment of choice for the suicidal melancholic patient.[138]

Lithium treatment and suicide

Lithium has the strongest supporting evidence among medications for reducing suicide rates. Many authors consider lithium to reduce suicide risk independent of mood stabilization.[139] The greater the long-term compliance with lithium therapy, the greater is its effect on lowering rates.[140] In a follow-up of patients with manic-depressive illness, no patient who had made a suicide attempt before entering the study made an attempt while lithium was prescribed.[141] A similar experience is reported with 11% of patients not receiving lithium making a suicide attempt, compared to no attempts in patients who received lithium therapy.[142] In 378 patients randomized to different medications in a two and a half-year period, no suicides or attempted suicides occurred in the lithium group.[143] A review of 28 studies published between 1976 and 1996 found that the risk of suicide or attempted suicide in the lithium-treated group was 0.37 per 100 patient-years compared with a risk of 3.2 for patients not receiving lithium – an almost nine-fold difference.[144] When patients with mood disorders fully comply with lithium treatment, their suicide rates may be no different from that of the general population.[145] A review of 34 studies published between 1970 and 2002 that included over 16 000 patients receiving on average 3.5 years of lithium treatment reported a 14-fold reduction in the number of suicides compared to similar patients receiving other medications.[146] As patients meeting bipolar II criteria have the highest suicide rates, lithium therapy is their best long-term treatment.

No other chemical agent defined as a mood stabilizer has been shown to diminish suicide rates. In a retrospective cohort study of over 20 000 persons in two large health plans, patients receiving lithium had one-third the suicide rate of those receiving valproic acid. Lithium-treated patients had 2.5-fold fewer hospitalizations for a serious attempt.[147]

Antidepressant drug treatment and suicide

The effect of antidepressant medication treatment on suicide rates is unclear. The clinical trials assessing the efficacy of antidepressant drugs usually exclude suicidal patients.[148] In a sample of 10-to-19-year-old patients, a small drop in suicide rates with usage of antidepressants was reported.[149] An assessment of prescriptions for SSRIs and tricyclic antidepressants (TCAs) reported a decreased suicide rate with SSRI prescription in over 500 different US regions identified by zipcodes. No other relevant clinical data were gathered.[150] In a National Institute of Mental Health-sponsored collaborative study of depression, fluoxetine was found to have a modest effect on reducing suicide rates compared to placebo.[151] Paroxetine (and one assumes similar drugs) is also cited to lower suicide rates but the evidence is conflicted.[152]

No effect for fluoxetine in reducing or increasing suicide rates was reported in one study.[153] In a later report, flupenthixol, an antipsychotic used in Europe, was claimed to be the "only treatment that has been found to lower suicide attempt rates," and psychotherapy "significantly" increased rates.[154] The use of maprotiline and amitriptyline was also claimed to increase rates of attempted suicide. The claim that the rate of attempted suicide was higher during follow-up with psychotherapy than with standard follow-up treatment for depressive illness is not surprising since no clinical trial has found psychotherapy alone to be effective in preventing serious depression or in reducing suicide risk.[155] These authors also report more suicide attempts among patients receiving amitriptyline than the comparison drug mianserin. But, there was no control for the preselection of patients with greater suicide risk in the amitriptyline group.[156]

In contrast, a naturalistic study of 2776 patients treated in an emergency room for deliberate self-harm reported the self-harm rates to be highest for those on SSRIs and lowest for those taking TCAs. Fluoxetine use was associated with the highest rate and amitriptyline with the lowest rate. Hospital length of stay, however, suggested that if an overdose with medication did occur, the consequences were more severe for a TCA overdose.[157] In a UK study comparing thousands of patients receiving mianserin or amitriptyline, suicide attempt rates were similar.[158]

In a meta-analysis of this literature, no benefit for antidepressant drugs over placebo in reducing suicide rates was found in persons with serious depressive illness.[159] In a further review of US Food and Drug Administration reports of controlled clinical trials for 15 approved antidepressant drugs of several different classes given to over 48 000 depressed patients, the authors again could find no effect on suicide rates for any antidepressant medication.[160] Another review of short-term randomized placebo-controlled trials also could find no evidence that antidepressant drugs reduce suicide rates or suicide attempts in depressed patients.[161] A survey of Australian government databases from 1991 to 2000 also showed no change in overall suicide rates in relation to antidepressant drug prescriptions.[162]

A consistent finding, however, is the association of inadequate prescription of antidepressant medication treatment in patients who kill themselves. The implication is that with adequate treatment, depressive episodes will resolve, will recur less frequently, and suicides will be fewer. This assumption may be valid. In some countries the suicide rates are lower when rates of treatment are higher.[163] A lack of treatment is associated with increased suicide rates, as is discontinuation of antidepressant medication during maintenance treatment.[164] Whether this effect is due to the medications or more attention paid to the patients receiving pharmacotherapy is unknown. The incidence of side-effects does not increase suicide rates in depressed patients taking antidepressant medicines.[165] While it appears reasonable that antidepressant medications reduce suicide risk in adults with depressive illness, the evidence of such effect is poor.[166]

Of concern, however, are reports that suicide rates increase in children and adolescents with the use of SSRI antidepressants. British drug regulators have warned against the use of paroxetine, sertraline, citalopram, venlafaxine, and fluvoxamine in children and adolescents in response to findings of increased suicide risk in this age group with these drugs. The U.S. Food and Drug Administration has issued a less definitive warning than its British counterparts.[167] A single multicenter, industry-independent, 12-week randomized controlled trial with 439 adolescent outpatient volunteers, ages 12–17 years old diagnosed as having major depression found that participants receiving combined fluoxetine (10–40 mg daily) and cognitive-behavior therapy had a lower suicide attempt rate than those receiving either treatment alone or placebo.[168] The forms of depressive illness were not defined, however, but those with psychosis, severe suicide risk, and a manic-depressive illness course were excluded.[169]

The investigators in a UK case-control study of over 159 000 users of four antidepressant drugs (amitriptyline, fluoxetine, paroxetine, and dothiepin) concluded that the risks of suicidal behavior after starting any one of the antidepressant drugs were statistically similar in patients 10–19 years of age.[170] Inspection of the data, however, shows the risk lowest for amitriptyline and highest for paroxetine, a pattern identified in the Donovan *et al.* (2000) study. Any increased risk of suicide in young patients is ascribed to a hypothecated activating effect of SSRIs in the face of their weak antidepressant effect for melancholia.

A caveat to these assessments is offered by a review of the prescriptions of antidepressants in the past 15 years in the UK. The number of prescriptions has more than doubled while population suicide rates have fallen. The decline in suicide rates, however, has been at a much lower rate than the increase in numbers of prescriptions.[171] Gunnell and Ashby conclude that if the risks of suicide behaviors seen in children prescribed SSRIs were to apply to suicides in adults, the number of "antidepressant-induced" suicides would be too small to detect and would be masked by ongoing favorable suicide trends. They interpret their findings as not supporting an increased risk of suicide with the prescription of SSRI antidepressants in young persons. A critique of this assessment considers that the increased rate of prescription may not reflect an increased number of patients undergoing treatment but may be due to the accumulation of long-term users of SSRIs.[172] A second commentator critiqued the assessment on the basis that the rates of suicide are estimated when the proper assessment would require actual numbers of suicides.[173] Such a direct assessment has found that "deliberate self-harm (suicidal behavior) is increased in the first one to nine days after starting an antidepressant but without major differences between individual antidepressants."[174]

In a US examination of the national suicide rate and the prescription of antidepressant medications, unemployment, and use of alcoholic beverages for 1985–1999, the suicide rate was found to have declined by 13.5% with a greater decline among women. During this same period, the prescription rates for SSRIs and other second-generation antidepressants were inversely associated with suicide risk.[175] Assessing suicide rates, antidepressant prescriptions, unemployment, and alcohol consumption for 1985–1999 these authors reported a decrease in suicide rates (with a greater decline among women) with a fourfold increase in antidepressant prescriptions of non-TCA agents.[176] They associated the reduction in suicide rate with medication prescription and suggest that the relationship is causal.[177] More patients receiving treatment, rather than the class of antidepressant drug prescribed, is the more likely explanation of this finding.

If SSRI medications alter suicide risk, the effect is indirect and complex. Their association with an increased risk of suicide in young patients can be attributed to their modest and delayed antidepressant effect combined with their activating properties eliciting agitation in impulsive, depressed persons. There is no evidence that they pharmacologically elicit suicidal thoughts. The increased numbers of prescriptions during a period of declining suicide rates indirectly suggests that effectively treating and preventing depressive illness will reduce suicide rates because most suicides occur during an episode of depression. The number of prescriptions, however, does not define compliance.[178] There is no evidence that SSRIs pharmacologically resolve suicide thoughts, but may be effective over time in reducing suicide rates by preventing recurrences of depressive illness.[179]

Lethality of the overdose from different antidepressants

SSRIs in overdose are much less likely to be fatal than are TCAs or MAOIs in overdose.[180] TCA overdose is associated with cardiotoxicity and encephalopathy with seizures.[181] Monoamine oxidase inhibitor overdose is associated with the serotonin/malignant catatonia syndrome.[182] Pure SSRIs, however, are not first-choice drugs for melancholia, limiting clinical options. In addition, venlafaxine is reported to induce seizures and serotonin toxicity in overdose.[183] Mirtazepine overdose is considered more benign and may be the compromise choice.[184] Both these agents are sedating (the latter more so) and are less likely to increase agitation.

Yet, secondary amine TCAs offer a more effective choice for the treatment of melancholia (see Chapters 10 and 11). As the lethal dose is about 15–20 mg/kg, however, a week's supply or less is prescribed. Optimally, such prescription is made when an adult companion accepts the responsibility to sequester and administer medication.[185] The greater risk of TCAs, however, must be weighed against the therapeutic advantage they have over other antidepressants in treating melancholic patients.[186] A medicine with less overdose lethality that is ineffective is not a "safe" choice if the depressive illness is not resolved.

Management of the suicidal melancholic patient

If caring for a suicidal melancholic patient and preventing suicide were easy, suicide rates would have plummeted long ago. Even if all the concerns cited above are resolved, the task of suicide risk assessment and reduction is daunting. The most difficult decision is whether to hospitalize the patient. Although the American Psychiatric Association offers guidelines for the management of suicidal patients, no studies quantify the severity or number of features that warrant hospitalization.[187] From experience, the unambiguous presence of any item cited in Table 7.3 warrants hospitalization. If any one of the obviously more severe criteria are present (e.g. psychosis, catatonia, suicide plan), hospitalization is mandatory.

Table 7.3. Indications for hospitalization of a potentially suicidal melancholic patient

Severe agitation and anxiety
Immobilized by indecision or ruminations
Psychosis (especially somatic or guilty delusions)
Stupor or catatonia
Physiologically compromised by not eating or drinking
Failure to sleep
Does not immediately and forcefully reject suicide intent
A suicide attempt within the present episode
Voicing a suicide plan
Co-occurring alcohol or illicit substance abuse
Does not meet safety criteria for outpatient care

Inpatient care of the suicidal melancholic patient

Hospitalization is an active treatment for suicide prevention. Nevertheless, suicide is the leading cause of death in psychiatric hospitals.[188] Hospitalization does not guarantee safety. Special efforts are needed to insure that the hospitalized suicidal patient will not commit suicide.[189] Supervision needs to be continuous, and the patient's room and bathroom need to be safe. Seclusion or restraints may be needed.

Examples of suicidal behavior while hospitalized include a patient who repeatedly ran full-tilt across the room, smashing his head into the opposite wall; a patient who climbed on top of an armoire and dove off, sustaining a traumatic brain injury; and a patient who climbed on to the hall wall railing and jumped headfirst to the floor. Completed suicides while hospitalized include a patient who partially kicked open the window of his room, squeezing through and falling to his death; and a patient who used his bedclothes to make a noose that he attached to his bathroom sink, hanging himself.

In a study of 76 patients who committed suicide while hospitalized or immediately after discharge, 49% had a prior suicide attempt and 25% were admitted with concerns about suicide. Seventy-eight percent denied intent before suicide. Twenty-five percent were "on pass" from the hospital, prematurely discharged, or had absconded from the unit. Depressive mood with anxiety and agitation was the best predictor of suicidality.[190]

To hospitalize a melancholic patient because of high suicide risk and prescribe a medication trial that requires 4–6 weeks to be effective but then discharge the patient from hospital care within a week or two is not an adequate course of treatment. For hospitalized, suicidal melancholic patients, ECT is the treatment of choice. It offers a sharp reduction in suicide intent within two weeks. If a patient receives ECT beginning within the first five days, hospitalization costs are less and length of stay is shorter than with medication.[191]

Patients should be encouraged, but not forced, to participate in unit and group activities. Group activities should be directive and goal-oriented. Introspective psychotherapy is not helpful. Daily observations of the patient's sleeping and eating, and weighing the patient every other day are semiquantitative measures of change in clinical status.

Because many different staff members observe the patient, the reliability and responsibility of reporting the patient's clinical features are often unclear. Regular assessment using a single depression-rating scale by the patient's primary nurse or assigned aide provides the most consistent charting of the course of change. Questioning about suicide intent and feelings is best done daily. Most units describe "levels of suicide precaution." All members of the staff interacting with the patient should fully understand the limits of each criterion. The patient and family also need to understand the restrictions. Suicidal patients are often terrified by their self-destructive feelings and gain comfort from knowing that they will be closely supervised.

Ideally, discharge from hospital care should not occur until the patient is in remission. If ECT is the treatment used, this is typically achieved within 3 weeks. With medication, remission requires a longer treatment course. If previous cognitive testing or a DST were abnormal, these assessments should be repeated and the patient not discharged until the abnormal findings are normalized. Continued abnormalities may forewarn of an early relapse. Discharge is best to a safe, supervised, gun-free environment. If there is turmoil in the household, relapse is likely.

Outpatient care of the potentially suicidal melancholic patient

When a patient does not meet criteria for hospital care, but also does not meet criteria for outpatient care, hospitalizing the patient is the prudent course. If a patient impulsively decides to commit suicide, the attempt will likely occur but the frequency and lethality of these attempts can be minimized.

Supervision

Around-the-clock supervision for the first week is vital. A responsible spouse, family member, roommate, or friend must directly express the willingness to assume responsibility and to fulfill the prescribed restrictions. The patient must also understand and agree to the restrictions, and accept that the treating clinician will be speaking frequently with the supervising person. The patient should not leave the outpatient setting until such a person is present. Melancholia is a severe, often fatal illness, and the usual privacy standards of care for mildly depressed outpatients do not apply.

Removal of lethal means

A melancholic patient cannot be permitted to return to a home with firearms. Arrangements for their removal are necessary, or for the patient to agree to go to another location *before* the patient is permitted to leave the outpatient setting. The patient must also be willing to surrender all previous medications from all sources and the supervising person at home should check the usual household locations for keeping medication (e.g., medicine and kitchen cabinets, bedstand drawers).

Frequent contact

Daily phone rounds and, at least, weekly office visits provide the opportunity to monitor treatment. Empathic listening and restrained reassurance calm patients. The belief that "contracts for safety" prevent suicide is unproven and has no legal standing.[192] Nor does intensive psychotherapy reduce suicide risk. Probing interactions often make patients worse.[193] Patient 7.8 illustrates this effect of psychotherapy.

Patient 7.8

A 21-year-old woman had just been discharged from a hospital following treatment for depression and a suicide attempt by medication overdose. Before leaving the hospital, she agreed to a video-taped interview for teaching purposes.

She was still depressed, but in substantially less distress than on admission. She recalled that her father had died of a heart attack while attending her 12th birthday party. Rather than a simple empathic response and then moving on, the psychiatrist probed the possible psychodynamic consequences of this event. The patient became increasingly agitated. Following the interview, she went home, but ruminated about her father's death and how it might have been her fault. She ingested a substantial overdose of medications and had to be rehospitalized.

Rapid relief of symptoms

Rapid improvement is the best evidence that a patient can receive that the situation and illness are not hopeless and that remission is possible. Reducing anxiety and improving sleep are practical initial goals. These are facilitated by prescribing pharmacodynamic broad-spectrum, sedating antidepressant medication, minimizing the need for an additional hypnotic or anxiolytic agents. For some patients, outpatient ECT is a useful consideration.

NOTES

1 Martha Manning's *Undercurrents, A Life Beneath the Surface* (San Francisco: Harper, 1994) is an excellent diary of her struggle with depression and her ultimate recovery with electroconvulsive therapy (ECT). For additional descriptions of suicidal ideation in depression relieved by ECT, see: Endler, N. S. (1982, p. 167); Rosenberg, L. E. (2002); and Nuland, S. B. (2003).
2 Barraclough *et al.* (1974); Conwell *et al.* (1996); Dhossche *et al.* (2001); Conwell *et al.* (2002).
3 Kessing (2004a).
4 Westrin *et al.* (2003); Kunugi *et al.* (2004); Pfennig *et al.* (2005).
5 Bradvik (2003).
6 Grunebaum *et al.* (2004b).
7 Guze and Robins (1970); Goodwin and Jamison (1990).
8 Inskip *et al.* (1998); Bostwick and Pankratz (2000); O'Leary *et al.* (2001).
9 Suicide is reported to be the leading cause of death for Chinese people aged 15–34 (*New York Times*, September 21, 2004, p. A4).
10 Reza *et al.* (2001).
11 Szanto *et al.* (2001).
12 Hemenway and Miller (2000, 2002).
13 Maris (2002).
14 McQuillan and Rodriguez (2000). Accident and homicide rates at 36% and 17%, respectively, top the list of causes of death in teenage adults.
15 Bukstein *et al.* (1993); Beautrais (2003).
16 Kessler *et al.* (2005).
17 McClure (2001).
18 Cantor *et al.* (1999).
19 Lambert *et al.* (2003).
20 Maris (2002).
21 Blair-West *et al.* (1999); Oquendo *et al.* (2001).
22 Lewinsohn *et al.* (2001b).
23 Isacsson *et al.* (1994); Luoma *et al.* (2002).
24 Shneidman (1981); Conwell *et al.* (1991, 2000); Brent *et al.* (1993); Suominen *et al.* (2002); Cavanagh *et al.* (2003). A remarkable book detailing the lives of 134 persons before their suicides is *The Final Months* by Eli Robins (New York: Oxford University Press, 1981).
25 Keller *et al.* (1982, 1986b, 1995); Kocsis *et al.* (1988).
26 Osvath and Fekete (2001).
27 Conwell *et al.* (1991).
28 Suominen *et al.* (1998).
29 Uncapher and Arean (2000).
30 Faber (2003).
31 Triavil is a combination of an antidepressant (amitriptyline) and an antipsychotic (perphenazine) that is formulated so that both are given in subtherapeutic doses; otherwise, when the dose of the antidepressant is therapeutic, it will result in an unnecessary large dose of the antipsychotic. Patient 7.1's long period of remission could likely have been achieved with low to moderate doses of amitriptyline alone.
32 For the role of ECT in delirium, see Kramp and Bolwig (1981), Strömgren (1997), Fink (1999b, 2000b), and Malur *et al.* (2000).

33 Kessler (1997).
34 Slimmer *et al.* (2001).
35 Matussek *et al.* (1981).
36 Isometsa *et al.* (1994c, d).
37 Kessler (1997).
38 Karam *et al.* (1998).
39 Devanand (2002).
40 Oquendo *et al.* (2004).
41 Kessler and Magee (1993).
42 Hammen (1991).
43 Kendler (1998).
44 Pokorny (1993); Maris (2002).
45 Zimmerman *et al.* (1995).
46 Isometsa *et al.* (1994c).
47 Runeson *et al.* (1996).
48 Kovacs *et al.* (1976); Litman (1982); Radke (1999). One of the most poignant responses to the question, "Would others be better off if you were dead?" came from a melancholic man in his late 30s who had been depressed for the previous 18 months without relief. He said "Yes. Everyone would be better off if I were dead. I'm like a mole on someone's face. They should just cut me off."
49 Keller *et al.* (1982, 1986b, 1995); Isometsa *et al.* (1994a, b); Young *et al.* (2001).
50 Suominen *et al.* (1998).
51 Isometsa *et al.* (1994b).
52 Maris (2002).
53 Oquendo *et al.* (1999).
54 Oquendo *et al.* (2002).
55 Excluding family members from the care of a depressed patient because of concerns about privacy is a conceptual holdover from the psychoanalytic model of psychiatry. When first meeting the patient it is common practice also to meet family members accompanying the patient and invite them to join the evaluation after the patient's private assessment. Prior to the family joining the process the patient is given the opportunity to request what should and should not be mentioned to others. Some patients are so apprehensive that they want their family members present during the evaluation. This situation requires tactful balancing of questions and comments among the family, but can be very helpful in getting all members to understand the patient's condition and agree to the treatment plan. "Family meetings" during the acute phase of treatment is a useful practice.
56 Brent *et al.* (2000).
57 Reeves *et al.* (1998); Stone-Harris (2000).
58 Guze and Robins (1970); Malone *et al.* (1995); Gladstone *et al.* (2001).
59 Isometsa *et al.* (1996).
60 Ney *et al.* (1990); Block (1994); Zulkifli and Rogayah (1997); Oyebola and Adewoye (1998); Bilikiewicz (1999); Feifel *et al.* (1999); Baxter *et al.* (2001).
61 One of us has extensively taught in the preclinical and clinical medical student courses at several universities, and has often been the prime teacher in these courses. The examinations students must pass are the national Step I, II, and III. Course material is often separated into "this is what you need to know for the examinations" and "this is what you need to know to take care of patients."

62 Moscicki (1997); Murphy (2000); Qin *et al.* (2003).
63 Bradvik (2002).
64 Lambert *et al.* (2003).
65 Some clinically unimportant suicide statistics may have theoretical interest. For example, seasonal patterns of suicide in Australia have been linked to amounts of daylight hours (Lambert *et al.* 2003). This finding is consistent with the observed abnormalities in circadian rhythms in depressed patients and may reflect a fundamental aspect of the pathophysiology of depression.
66 Roose *et al.* (1983); Fawcett *et al.* (1987); Coryell *et al.* (1992); Brown *et al.* (2000); Kessing 2003, 2004a); Coryell and Young, (2005).
67 Schneider *et al.* (2001b).
68 Grunebaum *et al.* (2001); Lykouras *et al.* (2002); Kessing (2003).
69 Miller and Chabrier (1988); Hori *et al.* (1993); Vythilingam *et al.* (2003).
70 Roose *et al.* (1983).
71 Grunebaum *et al.* (2001).
72 Mulsant *et al.* (1997).
73 Isometsa *et al.* (1994b).
74 Black *et al.* (1987b, 1988); Chen and Dilsaver (1996); Sharma (1999); Oquendo *et al.* (2000); Grunebaum *et al.* (2001); Lee *et al.* (2003). The assessment of suicide intent was similar among patients in the two multisite studies of ECT in patients with recurrent depressive illness. In the three-hospital study, the mean rating of the HAMD item 3 (suicide intent) was 1.8, reducing to 0.07 among the ECT responders (and 1.6, reducing to 0.9 among the non-responders) (Prudic and Sackeim, 1999). In the four-hospital study the mean score on item 3 for the total sample was 1.7 (Kellner *et al.*, 2005). The intake and exclusion criteria in the two studies were identical.
75 Not all reports find that the highest mortality rates are in the melancholic form of depression (Buchholtz-Hansen *et al.*, 1993). These authors reported a higher mortality rate in non-melancholic women. In selecting patients for follow-up over a 3-year period, however, they *excluded* from study "severely suicidal patients with retarded depression requiring ECT, patients with serious somatic disease, chronic drug or alcohol abuse or paranoid psychosis." These, of course, are the depressed patients repeatedly shown to have the highest risks.
76 Busch *et al.* (2003).
77 Bradvik (2003).
78 Nemeroff *et al.* (2001a).
79 Maris (1981); Murphy and Wetzel (1982); Egeland and Sussex (1985); Mann *et al.* (2001a).
80 Runeson and Asberg (2003).
81 Brent *et al.* (2003).
82 Schulsinger *et al.* (1979); Roy *et al.* (1991).
83 Statham *et al.* (1998).
84 Zalsman *et al.* (2002). Also see recent report of an association between suicide and the S-HTTLPR polymorphism (Correa *et al.*, 2004).
85 Statham *et al.* (1998).
86 Egeland and Sussex (1985).
87 Roy *et al.* (1991).
88 Brent *et al.* (1996); Cheng *et al.* (2000).
89 Pfeffer *et al.* (1994); Brent *et al.* (1996); Johnson *et al.* (1998).

90 Brodsky *et al.* (2001); Brent *et al.* (2002); McHolm *et al.* (2003).
91 Brent *et al.* (1996); Turecki (2001); Fu *et al.* (2002a).
92 Duberstein (2001).
93 High harm avoidance would seem at first contrary to increased self-harm; however, persons high on this personality dimension try to avoid stressful or anxiety-provoking situations, and thus the depressive situation (see Taylor (1999, Chapter 6).
94 Such patients are identified as bipolar II in DSM-IV.
95 Goodwin and Jamison (1990); Jamison (2000); Rihmer and Kiss (2002).
96 Although there is no evidence that the different variations of manic-depressive illness are distinct conditions, they have been given specific labels and different treatment algorithms. Bipolar I refers to an illness course in which the patient experiences episodes of both mania and depression. Bipolar II refers to an illness course in which the patient has episodes of depression that require treatment and occasionally hospitalization, but who only experiences hypomania or other mild versions of mania. Bipolar III is a chronic, low-grade mood disorder that mimics personality disorder. These patients experience periods of mood swings of varying intensity and duration, but not discrete episodes. While it is important to recognize the full spectrum of manic-depressive illness, the fractionation of treatment algorithms needlessly complicates patient care.
97 Rihmer *et al.* (1990a).
98 Rihmer and Pestality (1999).
99 Conwell *et al.* (1991).
100 King *et al.* (2000).
101 King *et al.* (2000); Keilp *et al.* (2001).
102 Ahearn *et al.* (2001).
103 Rubio *et al.* (2001).
104 Test results consistent with mildly impaired cognition would be a digit span of 3–4 digits backwards (5–6 is the norm), 2–3 errors on letter cancellation (0 is the norm), naming only about 8 animals in a minute (15–18 is the norm) and performing the trails B test with one or two corrections needed but taking more than 90 s to complete the task. Drawing a clock face from memory with the hands indicating 10 of 2 is another easy assessment task. Persons with poor executive function have great difficulty with this task. For a detailed discussion of bedside cognitive testing, see Taylor (1999), Chapter 4.
105 Hemenway and Miller (2000, 2002).
106 Polewka, *et al.* (2002).
107 Cooper-Patrick *et al.* (1994); Preuss *et al.* (2003).
108 Waern *et al.* (2002b).
109 Aharónovich *et al.* (2002).
110 Cornelius *et al.* (2001).
111 Barraclough *et al.* (1974); Murphy *et al.* (1992).
112 Conner *et al.* (2000).
113 Conwell *et al.* (2002).
114 Cooper-Patrick *et al.* (1994).
115 Snowdon and Baume (2002).
116 Cooper-Patrick *et al.* (1994).
117 Dhossche *et al.* (2001).
118 Arciniegas and Anderson (2002).
119 Dorpat *et al.* (1968); Harris and Barraclough (1994); Fishbain (1999); Waern *et al.* (2002a).

120 Gross-Isseroff *et al.* (1998).
121 Stockmeier (1997); Mann *et al.* (1999).
122 Kamali *et al.* (2001); Mann *et al.* (2001a); Nemeroff *et al.* (2001a); Spreux-Varoquaux *et al.* (2001).
123 Prefrontal cortex and related subcortical structures (Allard and Norlen 2001; Arango *et al.*, 2002; Austin *et al.*, 2002; Oquendo *et al.*, 2003), midbrain dorsal raphe nucleus activity (Bligh-Glover *et al.*, 2000), serotonin receptor genes (Bondy *et al.*, 2000), and serum cholesterol and tryptophan levels (Almeida-Montes *et al.*, 2000) have received research attention, but have produced limited conclusions. A serotonin transporter gene polymorphism on chromosome 17 linked to response to selective serotonin reuptake inhibitor drugs has also been linked to suicide (Lin and Tsai 2004).
124 A reduction in ventromedial prefrontal cortex metabolism is reported in depressed patients who made high-lethality suicide attempts (Oquendo *et al.*, 2003).

Female adolescents who made a recent suicide attempt are reported not to have the expected greater alpha activity over the right when compared to the left hemisphere on computerized EEG (Graae *et al.*, 1996). Studies of cortical evoked potentials in severely depressed suicidal patients find reduced efficiency of information processing that may reflect altered arousal (Ashton *et al.*, 1994; Fountoulakis *et al.*, 2004). These findings may represent the bradyphrenia of depression that is readily observable clinically.

Insulin sensitivity (Golomb *et al.*, 2002), a diminished thyroid-stimulating hormone response to thyroid-releasing hormone (Loosen 1985), and a blunted growth hormone response to catecholaminergic challenge (Pichot *et al.*, 2003) have also been suggested as markers of suicidality. The validity of these measures is unknown.

125 Agargun *et al.* (1997).
126 Goetz *et al.* (1991); Singareddy and Balon (2001).
127 Armitage (2000).
128 The DST is considered a state marker, not a trait measure (Chapter 4).
129 Targum *et al.* (1983); Banki *et al.* (1984); Lopez-Ibor *et al.* (1985); Pfeffer *et al.* (1991); Yerevanian *et al.* (2004a).
130 Targum *et al.* (1983); Coryell (1990).
131 Brown *et al.* (1986); Secunda *et al.* (1986); Ayuso-Gutierrez *et al.* (1987); Schmidtke *et al.* (1989); Norman *et al.* (1990); Roy (1992); Black *et al.* (2002).
132 Lester (1992).
133 Pfennig *et al.* (2005).
134 Carroll *et al.* (1980b); Coryell and Schlesser (1981, 2001); Yerevanian *et al.* (2004a).
135 Coryell and Schlesser (2001).
136 Westrin *et al.* (2003).
137 Norman *et al.* (1990); Roy (1992); Mathew *et al.* (2003).
138 Prudic and Sackeim (1999); Kellner *et al.* (2005).
139 Modestin and Schwartzenbach (1992); Müller-Oerlinghausen *et al.* (1992); Tondo *et al.* (1998).
140 Kallner *et al.* (2000); Baldessarini *et al.* (2001).
141 Rucci *et al.* (2002).
142 Modestin and Schwartzenbach (1992).
143 Thies-Flechtner *et al.* (1996).
144 Tondo *et al.* (1998).
145 Tondo and Baldessarini (2000); Tondo *et al.* (2001).

146 Baldessarini *et al.* (2001).
147 Baldessarini and Tondo (2003); Goodwin *et al.* (2003).
148 Malone (1997).
149 Olfson *et al.* (2003).
150 Olfson *et al.* (2003).
151 Leon *et al.* (1999).
152 Verkes *et al.* (1998).
153 Montgomery *et al.* (1994).
154 Montgomery, (1997).
155 Moller (1992).
156 Montgomery *et al.* (1978).
157 Donovan *et al.* (2000).
158 Inman (1988).
159 Khan *et al.* (2000).
160 Khan *et al.* (2003b).
161 Baldessarini (2001).
162 Hall *et al.* (2003b).
163 Rihmer *et al.* (1990b); Rutz *et al.* (1992); Isometsa *et al.* (1994a); Isacsson *et al.* (1996, 1999).
164 Isacsson *et al.* (1994; 1996, 1999, 2005); Yerevanian *et al.* (2004b).
165 Tollefson *et al.* (1994b).
166 Kessler *et al.* (2005) find that the trends in suicide ideation and attempts in the USA between 1990–1992 and 2001–2003 did not change despite a dramatic increase in antidepressant treatments.
167 *New York Times*, December 16, 2003, section D pp. 1 and 6; *New York Times*, February 3, 2004, section A p. 12; *New York Times*, March 23, 2004, section A pp. 1 and 18; *New York Times*, April 9, 2004, section A p. 16
168 March *et al.* (2004). The study is defined as TADS.
169 The hazards and efficacy of the newer agents in adolescents and adults are poorly known since the majority of studies in the past two decades have been multisite collaborative efforts organized and funded by industry contracts with consortia of drug assessors. The contracts contain protective clauses that prevent the publication of information from these studies unless approved by the funding companies. Since the funding sources have an economic interest in the published outcome, more than half the studies are not reported in the public literature (Angell, 2004; Healy, 2004).
170 Jick *et al.* (2004).
171 Gunnell and Ashby (2004).
172 Aldred and Healy (2004).
173 Mitchell (2004).
174 Jick *et al.* (2004).
175 Grunebaum *et al.* (2004a).
176 Grunebaum *et al.* (2004b).
177 The authors' conclusion is, of course, subject to the limitations of association as an assessment of causality. The argument of Aldred and Healy (2004) is as applicable to the assessment by Grunebaum *et al.* (2004a) as it is to that of Gunnell and Ashby (2004).
178 Mitchell (2004).
179 Cipriani *et al.* (2005).

180 Kapur *et al.* (1992); Henry (1997).
181 Molcho and Stanley (1992).
182 Henry (1997). The characteristics of the toxic serotonin syndrome are so like those of the neuroleptic malignant syndrome that both have been considered examples of malignant catatonia (Fink and Taylor 2003).
183 Whyte *et al.* (2003).
184 Velazquez *et al.* (2001).
185 The average American woman weighs about 50 kg and the average man 65 kg. Using the most conservative lethal dosing of 15 mg/kg, the lethal doses for women and men are 759 mg and 975 mg, respectively (Henry 1997). A starting dose of nortriptyline might be 50 mg daily at bedtime. The 7-day supply of 350 mg is well within the safety margin. For most patients, however, that dose will need to be increased. A week's supply of 75 mg daily or 525 mg weekly is also within the limit. Blood level monitoring permits careful titration, and for women blood levels will on average be 20% higher for the same dosing. Because failure to achieve full remission is a substantial risk factor in suicide, the drugs most likely to obtain a remission may be the safest in the long run.
186 Chapter 10.
187 APA (2000).
188 Maris (2002).
189 Goh *et al.* (1989).
190 Busch *et al.* (2003).
191 Olfson *et al.* (1998).
192 Miller *et al.* (1998); Simon (1999); Gunderson and Ridolfi (2001).
193 Moller (1992); Montgomery (1997).

8

Electroconvulsive therapy for melancholia

Diseases desperate grown
By desperate appliance are relieved,
Or not at all.

Shakespeare[1]

Among the more remarkable medical discoveries of the twentieth century, convulsive therapy is an unheralded success. At a time when the only effective treatment for a major psychiatric disorder was fever therapy for neurosyphilis, the reports that the induction of seizures relieved the psychosis of dementia praecox were rapidly and widely accepted. Seizures were first induced by intramuscular injections of camphor by Ladislas Meduna, a Hungarian neuropsychiatrist. Within a year, he described the benefits of intravenous pentylenetetrazol, known commercially as Cardiozol and Metrazol.[2] The benefit of convulsive therapy in patients with mood disorders was quickly recognized, but nowhere is its efficacy more striking than in the relief of melancholia. When and how was this association made?

The first detailed reports on the effects in manic-depressive disorders appeared in 1938: "The facility with which so many diverse reactions were influenced by cardiozol fits led me . . . to experiment with emotional and conduct disorders of non-schizophrenic type."[3] Cook described four manic patients whose excitement and psychosis were quickly relieved. An agitated psychotic depressed patient recovered; of three depressed patients with severe psychomotor retardation, two recovered; and a postpartum depressed patient became hypomanic and left the hospital much improved. Simultaneous reports were made by Bennett, who reported relief within two weeks in 21 seriously depressed patients treated with Metrazol-induced seizures and by Küppers (1939), who described the augmentation of insulin coma by Metrazol seizures.[4]

The antidepressant benefits of Metrazol seizures were quickly confirmed.[5] Of 27 patients with manic-depressive psychosis in the manic phase, seven recovered but 20 did not. The duration of illness in the non-responders was, on average, double that of responders (21.5 versus 10.5 months). Of 13 patients in the depressed phase, five recovered, and of two in a mixed-mood episode, both recovered. Two patients with the then recognized diagnosis of "involutional depression" recovered. The success in the latter two patients was particularly impressive considering that the mortality among patients with the diagnosis of involutional melancholia was the highest rate among the "functional" psychoses, being twice the rate for manic-depressive illness, and four times that of dementia praecox.[6] The excess death rate was 6.2 times that of the general population.[7]

Relapse rates were high with the premature cessation of treatment. One writer hypothesized: " A possible explanation of these events is that the production of some essential biochemical substance, lacking in the maladjusted organism, or the removal of an abnormal noxious substance, is affected by the stimulus of the convulsions" – a view that is consistent with the present image of the mechanism of convulsive therapy.[8]

A high incidence of incomplete and missed seizures complicated these reports. Induction of a seizure with intravenous Metrazol was difficult and successful inductions varied from 30% to 90% of the injections. Thus, the use of electricity to induce seizures, described in 1938, rapidly replaced Metrazol for efficacy of induction, ease of use, and lesser expense. The experience with Metrazol attests to the conclusion that the therapeutic benefit resides in the seizure and not in the induction method.[9]

Compelling data supporting the use of convulsive therapy in mood disorders came from the studies by Ziskind *et al.* (1942, 1945). In their first report, they compared the immediate and long-term effects of Metrazol seizures and electroconvulsive therapy in 38 patients who accepted treatment with 47 who did not. In the treated group, remission occurred in 82% (92% if partial remissions are added), with one death, compared to 38% remission (72% if partial remission is included) and five deaths. The suicide death in a convulsion-treated patient occurred 9 months after the last treatment and full remission.

Updating their experience in 1945, Ziskind and colleagues described full remission in 78%, improvement in 18%, and failure of improvement in 4% in 88 patients with seizures induced over 3–6weeks. In 109 patients who refused ECT, nine died in suicide and four from exhaustion, compared to a single death by suicide in the treated patients. The investigators cited two salient factors that limited the benefit of convulsion therapy – missed or partial seizures (subconvulsive doses) and a foreshortened course of therapy.

Confirmation of these effects quickly followed.[10] Myerson (1944), a leader in the psychoanalytic movement, described four patients with grief reaction successfully treated with ECT after extensive trials of psychotherapy, sedatives, hormones, amphetamines, vitamins, and institutional care had failed. The severe depression in each of the four patients resolved rapidly with ECT.

In a study from the Brooklyn State Hospital, 59% of 87 involutional patients and 77% of 134 manic-depressive patients left the hospital at a time when discharge rates for these illnesses treated by other means was extremely low.[11] Among depressive disorders in mid-life, the melancholic form showed more favorable results, with 76% leaving the hospital, compared to those with prominent persecutory delusions, among whom 45% left the hospital.

In the early experience at the Henry Phipps Psychiatric Clinic of Johns Hopkins Hospital insulin coma therapy was given to 59 patients, Metrazol seizures to 16, and combined insulin and Metrazol to 29 patients.[12] Immediate favorable responses were reported in 75% of the 92 manic-depressive patients and in 46% of the 58 patients with schizophrenia. Of 12 schizophrenic patients with affective features, all responded well. Convulsive treatment decreased the duration of manic-depressive attacks, with better results in illnesses of shorter duration, better in mood disorders than in schizophrenia, and shortened periods of hospitalization.[13]

In an experience with 1500 patients, Kalinowsky (1943) reported that, of 60 depressed patients with manic-depressive psychosis, 52 (87%) recovered. Of 32 manic patients, 27 (84%) recovered or were much improved. Of 76 with the involutional melancholia diagnosis, 66 (87%) recovered, and, of 32 with the diagnosis of "involutional paranoia," 14 (44%) were so rated.

The first text on somatic therapies noted:

> Metrazol convulsive treatment was originally proposed as a therapy for schizophrenia, but, during the years following its institution, it became increasingly evident that the main field of its effectiveness was not schizophrenia but the affective disorders . . . The results in depressive psychoses are often striking . . . Convulsive therapy is indicated if the depression lasts longer than is expected, if the patient becomes exhausted from excitement or agitation, if repeated suicidal attempts endanger the patient's life or if his suffering becomes unbearable."[14]

The spate of convulsive therapy texts that appeared during and at the end of the Second World War clearly endorsed induced seizures for patients with manic-depressive illness and "involutional depression."[15]

ECT in melancholia

Attempts to define melancholia as a clinical entity have a complex history (Chapter 1). The assumption that different depressive illnesses are to be treated alike makes assessment of the efficacy of ECT for melancholia difficult. The best approximation in diagnosis in the older studies is to focus on patients identified as having "manic depression (depressed)", "involutional psychosis" (especially when the sample is divided into "melancholic" and "paranoid" forms), and "endogenous depression." These groups probably contained the highest concentration of patients that we now recognize as melancholic.

The compelling case for a life-saving benefit of convulsive therapy in patients with the then-accepted diagnosis of involutional depression is presented by Ziskind *et al.* (1942, 1945), cited earlier.[16] Huston and Locher (1948) retrospectively compared the effects of ECT in 61 depressed patients treated between 1941 and 1943 with 93 patients treated with psychotherapy and other means between 1930 and 1939. In the non-ECT comparison group, 46% recovered after an average of 49 months' hospitalization, 18% remained ill, 13% died by suicide and 18% died from other causes. In the ECT-treated group, 77% recovered within an average of six months. Melancholic patients had better outcomes than those with the paranoid form.[17]

The rapid introduction of antidepressant and antipsychotic medications in the 1950s changed the focus of interest. Whether the antidepressant medicines were as effective as ECT became a dominant question.

Three random assignment studies compared the effects of ECT with antidepressant drugs in depressive illnesses.[18] In each study, ECT elicited greater benefits than did the medications. The participants, however, were mixed groups of depressive patients so these findings are not clearly transferable to the issue of melancholia. For example, Greenblatt *et al.* (1964) included patients identified as manic-depressive depressed, involutional psychotic, psychoneurotic depressed, and a large group categorized as "other."

Other comparisons of ECT and antidepressant drugs reported a quicker onset of action and, decreased chronicity, morbidity, and mortality for those treated with ECT.[19] The antidepressants were mainly tricyclic antidepressants and, to a much lesser extent, monoamine oxidase inhibitors. The one comparison of ECT and a selective serotonin reuptake inhibitor, found ECT markedly superior in short-term benefit compared with paroxetine in patients who had failed multiple medication trials.[20]

Many meta-analyses of the reports of ECT and medications have been published. In a review of 18 studies, an average response rate for ECT was 20% higher than that for TCA and 45% higher than that of MAOI.[21] A similar examination a few years later concluded that ECT was superior to the medicines but cautioned that the dosages of the medicines were low, and that the studies did not meet standards of good evidence.[22] The most recent detailed analysis is that of the UK ECT Review Group (2003). After reviewing the available randomized controlled trials of ECT and pharmacotherapy and of different forms of ECT for patients with depressive illness the authors concluded: " Real ECT was significantly more effective than simulated ECT (six trials, 256 patients). Treatment with ECT was significantly more effective than pharmacotherapy (18 trials, 1144 participants). Bilateral ECT was more effective than unipolar ECT (22 trials, 1408 participants)."[23] Other reviews and two official governmental efforts come to the same conclusion.[24] An extensive ethical analysis of the use of ECT focused on the effects of the treatment on memory concluded that ECT is an effective treatment for major depression and mania.[25]

Although ECT is more effective than antidepressant drugs in the relief of mood disorders, the ease of use, lesser cost, and intensive marketing of the medications assure their widespread use. A major contribution to the failure to use ECT, even when it is clearly indicated and superior to medication, is its persistent stigmatization.[26]

In treating patients with mood disorders, ECT is usually reserved for those who have not responded to psychotherapy and medications. For such patients, ECT still effectively relieves their mood disorder. Two recent National Institute of Mental Health supported multisite studies examined the effects of ECT in patients with recurrent unipolar depression.[27] At the time of referral the patients averaged 27–52 weeks of illness in their present episode, had experienced 2.4 prior episodes and 1.7 prior hospitalizations for depressive illness. A 55% remission rate was reported in one study and 87% in the second, the difference best interpreted as resulting from the choice of ECT parameters. The efficacy of ECT in non-psychotic melancholia is seen in patient 8.1.

Patient 8.1

?tlsb=-.01w?>A 66-year-old woman with recurrent psychiatric illnesses since age 26 was hospitalized with depressed mood, slow speech, suicidal thoughts, rigidity, posturing, and severe motor retardation. She had lost 5% of her body weight and complained of poor sleep for many weeks. The $HAMD_{21}$ was scored as 28. Serum cortisol levels at 0800 and 1600h were elevated and failed to suppress with 1 mg dexamethasone. Despite treatment with both SSRI and TCA medications, augmentation with atypical antipsychotics and high doses of lorazepam, her illness progressed. By the fifth week, she became mute and required intensive nursing care. As medications failed to relieve her condition, bilateral ECT was begun.

After two treatments, she answered questions, walked with assistance, ate, and went to the bathroom by herself. After the third treatment, she spoke spontaneously, walked unaided, but slowly. After five treatments, she became more interactive, cared for herself, and could not recall why she was in the hospital. After seven treatments, she was smiling, no longer depressed, and had slept and eaten well. The $HAMD_{21}$ was seven. Serum cortisol levels were normal at all times except 1600h, and this suppressed with dexamethasone. Continuation ECT was offered but refused and nortriptyline was prescribed. Examination at 1, 4 and 12 months later found her caring for herself without signs of depressive illness.

ECT for psychotic depression

The benefits of ECT in patients with psychotic depression are well established. The efficacy is so great that ECT is recommended as a primary treatment, without the necessity of prior trials of medication.[28]

In hospitalized non-psychotic depressed patients, TCA medications elicit improvement in the majority of those treated with an 82% response rate to amitriptyline and 54% to imipramine in depressed patients.[29] The response rate in deluded patients, however, was less than 20%. None of the 17 imipramine-treated and only 4 of the 10 amitriptyline-treated delusional patients improved.

A landmark study described 10/13 patients with delusional depression who had failed to respond to imipramine even when treated with high dosages and monitored serum levels. When the non- responders were treated with ECT, 9/10 sustained improvement.[30]

The 1964 Italian study by de Carolis and co-workers offers the best evidence of the efficacy of ECT in patients with psychotic depression.[31] A sample of 437 hospitalized depressed patients was treated with imipramine for a minimum of 25 days at dosages of 200–350 mg/day. Patients with endogenous depression constituted the largest subgroup (282); of these, 172 (61%) responded to imipramine. In a second subgroup of 181 delusional depressed patients, 72 (40%) had responded to imipramine treatment. Of the 109 imipramine non-responders who went on to ECT, 91 (83%) responded. This study convincingly demonstrated that delusional depressed patients, as a class, are less responsive to imipramine, but are responsive to ECT, even after a poor response to imipramine.

The poor response of delusional depressed patients to antidepressant drugs and superior response to ECT is a consistent finding in numerous studies[32] and reviews.[33] In one review, 17 investigations met acceptable research criteria and reported the results of medications and ECT in psychotic depressed patients.[34] The improvement rate was 34% in those treated with a TCA alone, 51% with an antipsychotic drug alone, 77% with combined TCA and antipsychotic medications, and 82% for ECT. The other reviews found similar differences in response rates.

The most recent meta-analysis considers the results reported in 15 selected ECT studies published since 1978.[35] Considering the variables of age, duration of illness, prior medication, "medication resistance," and psychosis, they find the greatest impact on outcome for psychosis. Its presence yielded the greatest effect size and the authors conclude that "Overall this meta-analysis has found evidence . . . that ECT is more efficacious in the treatment of depression with psychosis than without psychosis."[36]

Two new studies offer more evidence of the efficacy of ECT in delusional depressed patients. In the Consortium on Research in ECT (CORE) study, 67 patients (31%) were both psychotic and depressed. At baseline, the mean $HAMD_{24}$ scores of the psychotic patients were greater than the scores of the non-psychotic (37.8 versus 33.8). The overall remission rate for the sample was 87% (189/217), with 96% (64/67) of the psychotic depressed and 83% (125/153) of the non-psychotic patients remitting.[37] Interestingly, the psychotic patients responded faster and with greater reductions in $HAMD_{24}$ scores at all time points than the non-psychotic depressed. The difference was evident after 5 ECT, and was sustained throughout the study.[38]

In another report the remission rates for psychotic patients were better than for the non-psychotic depressed.[39] Of 55 depressed patients, 26 met criteria for psychotic depression. Using a 50% reduction in HAMD as criterion, 92% of the psychotic depressed and 55% of the non-psychotic depressed improved. Using a more rigorous criterion of remission (HAMD < 7), 57% of the psychotic depressed and only 24% of the non-psychotic depressed remitted.

It is difficult to identify delusions in severely depressed patients, and many such patients are inadequately treated. In the three-hospital collaborative study an elaborate rating scale was used to assess the adequacy of prior medication trials.[40] Only 2 of 52 patients with psychotic depression had been adequately treated before referral for ECT.[41] In the CORE study, using the same scale assessing treatment adequacy, 51% of the referrals for ECT had been adequately treated with medications. Of the psychotic depressed patients, however, only 6.5% were adequately treated.[42] The seven institutions that participated in these studies were academic training medical centers where treatment standards are expected to be superior to general practice.

The painfulness of the experience of psychotic depression is described by patient 8.2.

Patient 8.2[43]

"From my late thirties until my early forties, I underwent a period of depression that gradually deepened into an intensity that I finally required admission to a mental hospital, where I stayed for more than a year. Neither medication, psychotherapy, the determined efforts of friends nor the devotion of the few people whose love never deserted me had even the most minimal beneficial effect on my worsening state of mind. Finally, faced with my resistance to all forms of treatment till then attempted, the senior psychiatrists at the institution in which I was confined recommended the draconian measure of lobotomy.

I was, in fact, completely disabled by pathological preoccupations and fears. Obsessions with coincidences; fixations on recurrent numbers; feelings of worthlessness and physical or sexual inadequacy; religious anxieties of guilt and concerns about God's will; ritualistic thinking and behavior – they crowded in on one another so forcefully as to occupy every lacuna of my mind. I cowered before them, not only emotionally but physically, too – my hunched-over posture reflected my decline into helplessness.

I was saved from the drastic intervention of lobotomy by the refusal of a twenty-seven-year-old resident psychiatrist assigned to my case to agree with his teachers. At his insistence, a course of electroshock therapy was reluctantly embarked upon. I would learn later that virtually everyone familiar with my case despaired of the possibility of recovery.

At first, the newly instituted treatment made not a whit of difference. The number of electroshock treatments mounted, but still no improvement took place. The total would eventually reach twenty. Somewhere around the middle of the course, a glimmer of change made itself evident, which encouraged the skeptical staff to continue a series of treatments they had begun only to mollify a promising young man in training. I recovered so well, in fact, that in the four remaining months of hospitalization, I lost all but the dimmest memory of the obsessions and saw my depression disappear entirely.

For seventeen years, I was free of any hint of depression. But in the past decade, I have had a few recurrences, though none remotely approaching the catastrophe of thirty years ago, and none accompanied by more than a whiff of obsessional thinking. When the old pain begins to make its presence known, I return to the wisdom – and the presence – of the former psychiatric resident who saved my life and my sanity."

ECT and suicide risk

Suicide risk is high in patients with melancholia.[44] The impact of medications on suicide risk is not well defined. Compared to ECT, the efficacy of medication is less favorable.[45] Comparisons of ECT and TCA across different treatment eras find the frequency of suicides decreased in the ECT era.[46] In a study of the post-depression psychiatric status of 519 patients six months after discharge from hospital treatment found 0.8% of the ECT-treated patients had made a subsequent suicide attempt compared to 4.2% for those rated as receiving adequate and 7% of those receiving inadequate courses of antidepressant drugs.[47] At the 6-month follow-up no suicides were reported in 34 women treated with ECT, but two suicides occurred in the 84 patients treated with antidepressants (2.4%). Antidepressant drugs proved to be no more effective than placebo in reducing suicide rates in another study of seriously ill depressed patients.[48]

Following hospital discharge after a course of ECT, the incidence of suicide is rare.[49] In an examination of 1397 completed suicides in Finland within a 12-month period, only 2 patients had received ECT. In both, the quality of ECT was questionable, and suicide occurred during a depressive relapse.

The same benefits for ECT are reported in a literature review of suicide risk in patients treated with ECT.[50] These authors also examined the expressed suicide intent (changes in item 3 of the HAMD rating scale) in 148 patients treated with ECT. At baseline, the overall average score on item 3 was 1.8. It was reduced to 0.1 in 72 responders and to 0.9 in 76 non-responders to ECT. For the total sample, there was a greater decrease in the suicide item scores than in the overall HAMD scores.

A similar question was addressed in the CORE study.[51] Expressed suicide intent in item 3 of the $HAMD_{24}$ is scored as 0 = absent; 1 = feels life is empty or not worth living; 2 = recurrent thoughts or wishes of death of self; 3 = active suicidal thoughts, threats, gestures; and 4 = serious suicide attempt. Of 444 patients referred for ECT, 118 (26.6%) received a score of 3 as having active suicidal thoughts, actions, or gestures, and 13 (2.9%) received a score of 4, reporting a suicide event during the current episode. The baseline means (± SD) for the item 3 ratings were 1.70 (± 1.2) for the full sample, 1.64 (± 1.2) for 355 patients who completed the full treatment course, and 1.92 (± 1.0) for 89 dropouts.

Of the 131 patients in the high expressed suicide intent group, the ratings in 106 (80.9%) dropped to zero with treatment, occurring in 15.3% (20/131) after one ECT; in 38.2% (50/131) after three ECT (1 week); in 61.1% (80/131) after six ECT (2 weeks); and in 76.3% (100/131) after nine ECT (3 weeks). Among patients in the high expressed suicide intent group who completed the acute course of ECT, the scores of 87.3% (89/102) dropped to zero by the end of the treatment course, with approximately 64% reaching resolution after 6 ECT (within 2 weeks). For the 13 patients with a maximum rating of 4 (suicide attempt) at baseline, all dropped to zero by the end of their treatment.[52]

The data demonstrating the acute reduction in suicide intent with ECT are all the more remarkable because suicide risk is highest in depressed patients in the several weeks following discharge from a psychiatric hospital.[53] This dangerous period is illustrated by the deaths of two patients in the CORE study.[54]

The reduction of suicide risk is an often-cited justification for the use of ECT.[55] Each assessment acknowledges that ECT is a primary consideration when the risk is high.

Patient 8.3[56]

A former dean of Yale University Medical School, Leon Rosenberg, M.D., "went public" describing a recurrent depressive illness and suicide attempt that was relieved with ECT. After retiring from his position at age 65, he suffered weeks of feeling numb, nothing seeming important, and insomnia that led to irritability, loss of concentration, hypophonia, and despondency. He was treated with various antidepressants to little avail. He signed into a local hotel, sat on the bed washing down one antidepressant pill after another with vodka, and went to sleep anticipating dying. Awakening 12 hours later, he called his wife who had been frantically looking for him. Admitted to the psychiatric ward of a local hospital and interviewed by his psychiatrist and an accompanying medical student put a mirror to his condition, that he was ill enough to be discussed with medical students, and this led him to weep. Offered ECT, he registered surprise, thinking that the treatment had been abandoned years before. His negative image of the treatment, developed by images from the 1950s and from movies, had been reinforced by his experiences at Yale, then a center of psychoanalytic practice and theory.

"After the fourth ECT, I was noticeably less depressed. My appetite returned, as did my ability to sleep. After eight treatments, my mood was fully restored. I experienced no confusion, memory loss, headache or any other symptom sometimes attributed to ECT." He returned to work and six weeks after the suicide attempt, he took a train to Washington DC and presented a report of the Institute of Medicine to the leaders at NIH [National Institute of Health]. "My comments were well received, and the committee's report to NIH . . . was well received . . . I am quite certain that none of the people I addressed that day knew that I had recently lost and then retrieved my mind."[57]

ECT for catatonia and depressive stupor

The motor syndrome of catatonia is a frequent feature of depressive mood disorders.[58] Classic signs are negativism, mutism, staring, and posturing. The more severe form appears as stupor. An excited form termed delirious mania is also described. Antidepressant medication alone is unsuccessful in relieving accompanying catatonia. The effective algorithm is the use of a benzodiazepine or barbiturate, initially given as an intravenous challenge. If the challenge relieves the catatonic features, treatment with the sedative agent continues. If this medication trial is unsuccessful, ECT becomes the treatment. With ECT, the depressive features also resolve.

The syndrome of catatonia was recognized in the latter half of the nineteenth century.[59] The syndrome was quickly incorporated within the concept of dementia praecox and thus its presence still elicits the prescription of antipsychotic drugs. But catatonia occurs more commonly in patients with major depression, manic-depressive illness, general medical illnesses (including malignant catatonia or neuroleptic malignant syndrome), and as a toxic response.[60]

Convulsive therapy was conceived from the belief of an antagonism between psychosis and seizures. In the first few years, Metrazol-induced seizures were mainly applied to patients with the catatonic form of schizophrenia. The response was excellent.[61] Later, when electricity was introduced as the seizure-inducing agent, the first patient was suffering from delirious mania with catatonia. An early exposition of the favorable effects of ECT was in patients with lupus erythematosus exhibiting catatonia.[62]

The efficacy of ECT in catatonia became clearest in reports of its use in malignant (lethal) catatonia (MC), a syndrome of acute onset and high mortality. In an experience with 34 patients with MC, 18 patients were treated within three days of the onset of the episode and 15 survived. Of the 16 patients treated on day five or later, only one survived, despite the use of daily ECT.[63] Surveys of the experience with MC report that mortality rates of up to 100% were sharply reduced with ECT. When treated with ECT, 40/41 patients (98%) recovered.[64] The efficacy of ECT in MC was confirmed in both a literature review and from the experience at the Mayo Clinic.[65]

A neuroleptic malignant syndrome (NMS) is indistinguishable from MC with the identifiable precipitant of an antipsychotic medication. The syndrome was described soon after the introduction of chlorpromazine and was first thought to be an idiosyncratic response to the dopaminergic actions of the drugs. When the features of NMS were identified as identical to MC, the treatment of MC was applied and was quickly shown to be effective.[66] A review of the published experience in 46 published reports found ECT to be effective in 40 of 55 patients with NMS (73%). ECT also relieved the underlying psychosis in 10 patients (18%).[67] The evidence is strong that NMS is identical to MC and that the treatment for MC needs to be applied within the first five days of the illness when it is severe.[68] A study of an adolescent patient with MC showed ECT to be successful in this age group as well.[69]

While the retarded form of catatonia, dominated by mutism, withdrawal, posturing, negativism, and stupor, is the commonest presentation, a hyperactive form is recognized (delirious mania, excited catatonia). This form is also responsive to ECT.[70]

The first patients in whom seizures were induced exhibited the catatonic form of schizophrenia.[71] While in modern clinical practice it is customary to treat schizophrenic patients preferentially with antipsychotic drugs, ECT still has a role. When the antipsychotic drugs were introduced, comparisons with ECT showed the two treatments to have equivalent benefits. The ease of use of medication and the presumed greater safety led to a marked reduction in the use of ECT.[72] For psychotic patients with catatonia, when medications are not successful, ECT is still a useful choice.[73]

The requirement for individual consent before administering ECT is a restrictive impediment to its use. Obtaining a valid consent is often difficult in catatonic patients where negativism, mutism, delirium, and excitement interfere. Temporary cogent responses in a catatonic patient were achieved by the administration of lorazepam.[74] A detailed discussion of competency and consent is to be found in the monograph by Ottosson and Fink on ethical considerations in prescribing and administering ECT (2004).

The following vignette describes the range of behaviors in recurrent melancholia with prominent symptoms of retardation, depression, pseudo-dementia, and catatonia.

Patient 8.4[75]

A 58-year-old married woman was referred to a university geriatric service for confirmation of the diagnosis of Alzheimer's disease. Nine years earlier, she had been depressed, sleepless, withdrawn, and had refused to eat. After being treated with amitriptyline (150 mg/day), she showed an "immediate response." Two weeks later, she became confused, wandered aimlessly, and withdrew from contact with family and friends. A computed X-ray tomographic study (CT) revealed cortical atrophy, and a consulting neurologist, having made a diagnosis of Alzheimer's disease, advised the family that further intervention was useless.

For 9 years, she was cared for at home by her husband and her daughters. Her weight dropped to 75 lb (pound) (34 kg), and she became incontinent of both bladder and bowel. Her husband retired from work to devote himself to her care and received support from his daughters and friends.

On examination, she was thin and pale, stared aimlessly, kept her arms wrapped around herself or moved an arm and a leg in rhythmic masturbatory motions, appearing like a mechanical doll, oblivious of others. As the examination progressed, her perplexity and anxiety increased. She touched paintings on the wall, and picked up magazines to glance at them momentarily. Her speech was slow and halting, but she knew her name, although she said the year was 1976 instead of 1985. She had experienced previous episodes of depression. When she was 42 she had been withdrawn and non-communicative, had lost weight, and had failed to care for herself or her family. ECT combined with an unspecified antipsychotic medication brought improvement. Five years later, she was again withdrawn and unable to care for herself or her family. She received a second course of ECT and once more recovered. At age 49, she again became ill and was hospitalized. These experiences suggested that the dementia was depressive in origin, not the consequence of a degenerative brain lesion.

She was admitted to an inpatient psychiatric unit. Admission laboratory evaluations and a CT of the head were normal. Nortriptyline (75 mg/day) was prescribed, her appetite improved, and she engaged in brief conversations. When she appeared to respond to internal auditory stimuli, haloperidol was added, and she received the combined treatment for three weeks. Her appetite improved; she became continent and minimally verbal. She remained depressed, however, and ECT was recommended. Consent was obtained from her husband and oldest daughter.

After the fifth treatment, she was alert and communicative. After 13 treatments, she was fully oriented, achieved 30/30 on the MiniMental State Examination, and was able to take care of her daily needs. She was discharged with both ECT and nortriptyline as continuation treatments.

Over the next four months, she received ECT on average once every six days. Between treatments, she cared for herself, cooked for the family, and enjoyed her grandchildren. She traveled with her husband and attended softball games, keeping score and cheering for her favorite team.

In succeeding years, her symptoms returned periodically. On each occasion she became hesitant about decisions and progressively less able to work or cook. She would stand still for many minutes, staring into space; she answered questions with "I don't know," and no longer dressed herself or cared for her home. This sequence occurred over 2–5 days. When she was seen at these times, she was withdrawn and perplexed, and she performed poorly on cognitive and memory tests. For 10 years, she received 10–16 ambulatory ECT each year. Lithium therapy with serum levels between 0.7 and 0.9 mmol/l replaced nortriptyline in the second year. The formal consent for ECT was renewed annually. In 1995, the anticonvulsant sedative lorazepam, in daily doses of 0.5 mg three times a day, was added to her other medications. For 2 years, she remained well and required no further ECT.

ECT in pregnancy and postpartum depression

The physiologic and psychologic stresses of pregnancy increase the risk of both intrapartum and postpartum exacerbation of melancholia. During pregnancy, especially during the first trimester, antidepressant and antipsychotic drugs are reluctantly prescribed as these medications pass from the mother through the placenta and enter the blood circulation of the fetus. At critical stages of development, especially the first trimester, congenital abnormalities have been described.[76] What of ECT?

Two aspects of ECT are considered: (1) the impact of the seizure on the fetus and the risk of miscarriage; and (2) the impact on fetal development by the sedatives, muscle relaxants, oxygen, and anticholinergic agents used in ECT.

ECT is used safely in all stages of pregnancy without affecting fetal development.[77] We lack direct comparative studies of medicines and ECT so that all obstetricians and psychiatrists are obliged to apply their experience to the individual patient. Some psychoactive agents prescribed during pregnancy carry a teratogenetic potential, encouraging the use of ECT. In an extensive literature very few reports associate ECT with miscarriage or congenital anomalies. Indeed, the risks are sufficiently small as to encourage the preferential use of ECT over medications in psychotic pregnant women, especially in the first trimester.

Monitoring of fetal activity during ECT finds no alterations in fetal heart rate, fetal movement, or uterine tone.[78] Some authors perform ECT under endotracheal intubation during pregnancy, but such defensive intervention is unnecessary and adds risks.[79] For women with psychiatric illness during the first trimester of pregnancy, ECT is considered a safe treatment.[80]

Whether antidepressant drugs administered in the second or third trimesters of pregnancy adversely affect the fetus is unclear. Most practitioners rely on medications, but ECT remains a first-line treatment for depression in a hospitalized pregnant woman at any time during pregnancy,[81] ECT is also recommended when medications fail to control the illness or when the patient has had a good result with ECT in an earlier episode.

In the postpartum period, ECT is an effective treatment and no special considerations apply. As medications may appear in the breast milk of nursing mothers, the preferential use of ECT may be justified.

A particularly sad tale of an inadequately treated postpartum depression is described in the widely reported story of a Texas mother who carried out her psychotic thoughts to murder her children.[82]

Patient 8.5

A 29-year-old married Texas woman developed a postpartum depression with psychotic features after the birth of her first child in 1994. She responded to antidepressant medications. She had three more pregnancies and, in 1999, after the birth of her fourth child, she again became despondent, mute, withdrawn, and incapable of caring for her children. She was guilt-ridden with feelings of worthlessness; twice she attempted suicide by medication overdose. She was hospitalized; treatment with sertraline gave minimal relief but insurance limitations led to her discharge. She attempted suicide again by cutting her throat. She described visual images of knives and thoughts of harming herself and her children. ECT was recommended but refused by the patient and her husband. Haloperidol was added to venlafaxine and bupropion and the combination rapidly ameliorated the psychotic depression, but she never fully recovered.

In March 2001 her depression worsened and she expressed guilt over the death of her father. She was hospitalized; ECT was again considered but rejected. She was again treated with haloperidol but her delusions persisted. She was allowed to return home despite the persistence of her illness. In May, 2001 she serially drowned and killed each of her five children and called her husband at his work and urged him to come home immediately as the children had come to harm. He returned to find the children dead.

In the prison hospital, Mrs. Yates described visions of men, children, and horses on the jail walls. She had killed her children because they were "not righteous," were "doomed to perish in the fires of hell," and "to save them from Satan." She was placed on suicidal precautions and for a month she was mute, unresponsive, staring, and posturing. The court found her guilty of murder and not to be insane, and ordered her to be imprisoned for life.

ECT in children and adolescents

The role of ECT in adolescents and children is perplexing. The reasonable questions, whether ECT is effective, for whom it is indicated, and whether it is safe, are overshadowed by legislative proscriptions. Although no persistent egregious effect of ECT has been reported, its use is restricted in at least four American states. Californian legislation enacted in 1974 prohibits its use in children under the age of 12. It is banned in persons less than 16 years of age in Colorado and Texas. A 1976 Tennessee law banned ECT in minors less than 14 years of age. Such legislation implies that this medical treatment is so dangerous as to warrant citizen protection by the police powers of the state. Indeed, only euthanasia and assisted suicide receive the same legislative interdiction.[83] The restrictions are based on political, not medical, rationales.

ECT in adolescents and children is both safe and effective. The prevalence of depression in these age groups is increasingly recognized. The morbidity and mortality are substantial despite the intensive application of psychotherapy and medicines, and as a consequence, the pediatric use of ECT is increasing. A workshop titled Using ECT in Adolescents: The Cutting Edge was presented at the 1998 meetings of the American Academy of Child and Adolescent Psychiatry, and a practitioner review of ECT was subsequently published in a journal dedicated to pediatric mental health.[84] Proper experimental studies of ECT in adolescents and children are lacking, so an evaluation must be based on individual clinical experiences.

In a review of 60 reports of ECT in 396 adolescents and children, improvement rates of 63% for depressive disorders, 80% for mania, 80% for catatonia, and 42% for schizophrenia are reported.[85] These rates were experienced despite the fact that ECT was used as a last resort in 92% of the applications, after the patients had failed extensive courses of psychotherapy and many psychoactive medications.

At a 1993 annual meeting of the Child and Adolescent Consortium, clinicians from five academic centers reviewed their experience with 68 adolescent patients who had received ECT. A report from one university treatment center cited an experience with eight adolescent patients (5 bipolar, 3 unipolar) with ECT. Each patient had failed multiple trials of medications or had exhibited signs of NMS. The baseline HAMD scores of 32–59 dropped uniformly to between 5 and 10 at the end of the treatment course. Treatments were given three times a week, with the numbers of treatments ranging from 6 to 18. On follow-up, three patients sustained their recovery and went on to schooling and careers, three relapsed in the second year after treatment, one relapsed within a few weeks, and one was lost to follow-up.[86]

The Mayo Clinic experience with 20 adolescent patients reported a reduction or elimination of depressive and psychotic symptoms.[87] No adverse effects were reported, even in patients with co-occurring general medical illness. In a university-based inpatient service between 1983 and 1993, 12 adolescents (10 male and 2 female) received ECT.[88] Each patient was hospitalized for at least three weeks and had failed treatment trials of at least two psychotropic drugs. Ten of the 12 patients improved with remission of all target symptoms. Each patient had symptoms of mood disorder, six also had signs of catatonia, and nine presented with psychosis. Those with both mood and catatonic symptoms benefited most. Improvements were seen in the patients with psychotic depression, manic-depressive illness, and psychosis. The two non-responders were diagnosed as ill with schizophrenia. Although their psychosis persisted after 18 and 20 ECT, respectively, their affective symptoms and their suicidal tendencies remitted. While they did not return to their premorbid state, both were well enough to be discharged to a day hospital.

A Canadian experience offered ECT to 20 adolescents with manic-depressive illness (ages 16–22 years) who had not responded to medication trials, or who were severely suicidal requiring continuous observation, or in whom the side-effects of medications limited adequate clinical trials. Six subjects refused ECT, leaving 14 (8 male, 6 female) in the study. ECT was given twice weekly, with bilateral ECT in 87% of the treatments. The average number of seizures in a course was 10.4. Scores on the Brief Psychotic Rating Scale (BPRS) were reduced to 10% of the baseline at discharge. While the same general reduction in BPRS scores was achieved in the "ECT- refusers," the number of hospital days after ECT was recommended was 75 days for those treated with ECT, and 170 days for the "ECT-refusers."[89]

A review of the experience at the University of Michigan reported ECT to be effective in female adolescents with major depression (4), manic-depressive illness (2), and mood disorder secondary to intracranial tumor (1). Four patients had a history of childhood abuse and six exhibited self-injury.[90] A more recent case described a near-tragic course of a 17-year-old woman in a delirious manic state who was treated with antipsychotic drugs and developed NMS.[91] After multiple hospital transfers and delayed treatment over more than six weeks, she finally received ECT and recovered.

In the Australian experience with ECT between 1990 and 1996, 42 adolescents underwent 49 courses of ECT comprising 450 treatments. The treatment in adolescents represented 1% of the ECT given to all persons.[92] Symptoms resolved or markedly improved in half the patients who completed their ECT course. Patients with mood disorders derived the most benefit. Side-effects were transient, with easily terminable prolonged seizures observed in two of 450 treatments. The authors concluded that ECT is an effective treatment with few side-effects and that the indications, response, and unwanted effects of ECT in adolescents are similar to those observed in adults. They decry that it is seldom used.

A French group reviewed their experience with 21 adolescents. All 10 psychotic depressed patients, three of four manic patients, and three of seven schizophrenic patients improved with ECT.[93] The relapse rates were high, however, with four of the 10 depressed patients relapsing at one year. None of the patients were continued on ECT after the index course of treatment. A follow-up report found no persistent adverse effects, although 2% of the seizures had been prolonged.[94] While we lack proper experimental studies of ECT in adolescents, the combined clinical experience compels the conclusion that adolescents respond to ECT in much the same way as adults.

A retrospective analysis of the results of ECT in adolescent and adult patients found that 61% of the adolescents had improved with treatment and 53% were not rehospitalized in the subsequent year.[95] The findings were considered comparable to the effects of ECT in adults.

The experience with ECT in prepubescent children is limited to case reports. An 11-year-old depressed boy with suicidal intent and severe head-banging received 12 unilateral ECT with remarkable improvement of his depressive symptoms.[96] A 12-year-old girl with mania responded similarly.[97] In four pediatric cases treated with ECT, a prepubescent boy responded well to ECT.[98] Another prepubescent boy with depressive stupor, who exhibited changes in the dexamethasone suppression test which paralleled similar observations in adults, was successfully treated with ECT.[99] More recently, the successful treatment of an 8 1/2-year-old girl with major depression and catatonic symptoms was described. She returned to school and had no observable deleterious side-effects.[100]

The reason offered for the failure to use ECT in pediatric populations is a fear of an impact of seizures on the maturating brain. An examination of cognitive and personality measures in 16 children who received ECT found no impact on intellectual efficiency.[101] Performance was reduced immediately after ECT but in the follow-up examinations, all the subjects had recovered. Simple cognitive and perceptual tests were unimpaired within 48 h of the end of an ECT series. In another study, the follow-up after a mean of 3.4 years of 10 adolescent patients who received courses of ECT found no persistent memory or learning defects.[102] The authors used controls matched for age, psychiatric illness, and social functioning before ECT.

The more difficult hurdle to the use of ECT in pediatric populations is consent. The guidelines for informed voluntary consent for ECT call for the physician to provide adequate information to a patient capable of understanding and acting intelligently upon such information, and to do so without coercion.[103] Such prior consent contrasts with patient acquiescence that is considered sufficient to allow medicines to be prescribed and psychotherapy to continue. In some states, special procedures are mandated for consent for ECT and these are particularly onerous for children. For patients too young to consent knowingly to treatment, or who are deemed incompetent, treatment is given with guardian consent or following a court proceeding.

In 1990 and again in 2001, the American Psychiatric Association Task Force on ECT recommended the concurrence in the diagnosis and treatment by an independent consultant, preferably a psychiatrist qualified in child and adolescent psychiatry. For adolescent patients referred for ECT they recommended one consultation; for children, they recommended two. But the number of child psychiatrists with experience with ECT is so few that sophisticated consultations are almost impossible to obtain. Such a recommendation places an undue burden on the use of effective treatments in adolescents and children.[104]

Individual case reports (patients 8.6, 8.7, and 8.8) reflect the experience in adolescents and children.[105]

Patient 8.6

A 16-year-old boy with a 2-year history of depressed mood, feelings of worthlessness and incompetence, self-isolation and withdrawal from school was hospitalized. One year earlier a suicide attempt by overdose with aspirin and acetaminophen had also led to hospitalization. After discharge he was admitted to a residential school, continued psychotherapy, and received various antidepressant drugs. His thoughts of depression and suicide persisted, and he was referred for evaluation for ECT.

Lean and well-groomed, he was alert, oriented, and responsive. He reported a weight loss of 40 lb (18 kg) over the previous four months. He was obsessed by thoughts of helplessness, dying, and inability to maintain his coursework in school. Speech was circumstantial. There was no evidence of psychosis. He was aware that he was ill, wanted help, and was concerned that if ECT was the last effort, what would he do if it failed? On the inpatient unit, he slept late, missed meals, remained in his room, and did not participate in activities.

Examination revealed a $HAMD_{17}$ of 18, Beck Depression Inventory of at least 36, and he performed at the "superior" level on the WISC-III IQ test. Thinking was circumstantial, mood depressed, and ideation obsessional.

A course of ECT was recommended and accepted by the patient and his parents. Seven ECT given three times a week elicited a euphoric-denial response in which the patient denied prior illness and felt relieved of mood symptoms.[106] He was discharged home for continuation ECT. Treatment continued twice weekly. When schooling was reinstated, he again became depressed. Treatment frequency was increased and his feeling of well-being returned. Four months after his first ECT, and after a full course of 25 treatments, he was euthymic, sustained on lithium and phenelzine continuation treatment, in weekly psychotherapy, and able to continue his schooling.

Patient 8.7

A 17-year old boy with a two-month history of persecutory delusional ideas, insomnia, and manic behavior periodically requiring restraints was hospitalized. He was hyperactive, spoke incessantly, and was grandiose. Treatment with haloperidol resulted in rigidity, fever, altered consciousness, hypertension, tachycardia, and elevated serum creatinine phosphokinase (CPK). This episode of NMS was treated symptomatically with the administration of dantrolene in an intensive care facility. NMS resolved but he was left in a psychotic and manic state that warranted transfer to another hospital.

On admission he was agitated and confused, with waxing and waning periods of lucidity. Speech was slurred, monotonous, and disorganized. He was anxious, delusional, and suspicious. At times, he was mute and failed to answer questions, staring past the interviewer. He was oriented to time, place, and person, but unable to recall three items over 5 min. His ability to do calculations was impaired and he was unaware of current events. Temperature, heart rate, blood pressure, and CPK were normal. On admission, he was under treatment with clonazepam, chlorpromazine, lithium, and lorazepam. All except lithium were discontinued.

His behavior required periodic restraint and injections of droperidol or lorazepam were used to control excitement. Sedatives resulted in periods of cooperation, but he remained delusional and delirious, with poor self-care.

Because various treatments for more than two months had not relieved the syndrome of manic delirium, ECT was recommended and consent obtained from the patient and his parents. Immediately after the first seizure, he was more rational, no longer overactive nor delusional, and no longer required restraint. After the fourth treatment his thoughts and mood were appropriate; delusional ideas had disappeared; and self-care was normal. After the sixth treatment he was discharged for continuation treatment with lithium maintained at approximately 0.8 mg/L. Four additional ECT were given, and at the time of his last visit he was in remission. Lithium therapy was sustained for four months, at which time he was discharged from the clinic.

Patient 8.8[107]

An 8 1/2 -year-old girl experienced persistent low mood, tearfulness, self-deprecatory comments, social withdrawal, indecisiveness, decrease in appetite, and initial insomnia of 1 month's duration. She had frequently commented to her parents, "I don't feel like myself." They had observed a new obsessive preoccupation about "good versus bad behavior," in her and in others. She had to think about her behavior constantly for fear that she would do something bad. There was no report of suicidal ideas or psychotic symptoms. Her condition had developed acutely after a week-long summer camp. Past psychiatric history was unremarkable, as were her birth and development. She was an excellent student, described as "moody" and creative.

Diagnosed with major depression, she was prescribed paroxetine, 20 mg/day, and weekly individual psychotherapy. One week later, appetite and communication decreased, and she began hitting herself with her fists. She became mute, refused to eat, and was admitted to a child psychiatry inpatient unit.

She spoke in a whisper, and only with prompting. She would not eat unless assisted. Her psychomotor retardation worsened. Paroxetine was continued. Her refusal to eat necessitated nasogastric tube placement. She became mute, communicating by gestures or writing, but that soon ceased as well. She was bedridden with board-like rigidity, and was enuretic. On other occasions she was briefly combative.

Laboratory examinations found no pathology. Paroxetine was discontinued and a brief trial of haloperidol begun, but was discontinued at the parents' request. Other medications failed to alter her condition.

ECT was begun, and she received 19 treatments. After the first several treatments, she had increased awareness of her surroundings. After the eighth treatment, she blinked in response to verbal commands, cooperating with activities of daily living, bearing weight, and attending to a video game. Haloperidol, 5 mg/day, was added. After the 11th treatment, she was taking adequate fluids and food orally and the nasogastric tube was removed. She improved dramatically with each treatment. The skills she had lost during the deteriorating phase of her illness gradually returned, in approximately the reverse order in which they had been lost. She tolerated the treatments well, but was mildly disinhibited and had some anterograde memory loss for the period encompassing the last three or four treatments. Once the ECT course ended, haloperidol was discontinued and she began a regimen of fluoxetine, 20 mg/day.

She quickly reintegrated into her previous public school setting and was discharged home to her family 3 weeks after the completion of the ECT course. Re-examinations over 6 months found her well, receiving fluoxetine and regular psychotherapy, without recurrence of depression.

ECT in the elderly

The record of ECT in the elderly is highly favorable; indeed, elderly patients have better responses in depression scale scores to ECT than do younger adults.[108] They tolerate ECT well despite co-occurring general medical illnesses.[109] For many years, a long list of absolute contraindications to ECT were commonly described in ECT texts, but during the 1970s and 1980s, practitioners challenged each contraindication and developed procedures to manage the risks safely. With modern ECT procedures, there are no *absolute* contraindications, although some patients with co-occurring general medical illness warrant special attention.[110] Neurologic disorders, whether a stroke, parkinsonism, multiple sclerosis, or seizure disorder, do not preclude the use of ECT.[111] Specific aspects of the role of ECT in patients with general medical illnesses in the elderly have been detailed.[112]

Greatest attention has been paid to cardiovascular disease. During seizures the heart rate and blood pressure rise. These effects were anticipated to incur additional risks for the elderly but ECT under modern anesthesia guidelines is remarkably benign.[113] The principal requirement is that the efficacy of each seizure needs to be assured by proper physiologic monitoring. Patients 8.9 and 8.10 are illustrative.

Patient 8.9

Following a second surgical repair of an aortic aneurysm, a 76-year-old retired physician became increasingly concerned with dying. He forced the sale of his home and he and his wife moved to an apartment in a retirement community. He obsessed that he should not have made the sale. His sleep and appetite deteriorated and he lost weight. Psychomotor retardation became severe. He was withdrawn. Seeking reassurance with a therapist, he insisted on taking sertraline and when that was ineffective, fluoxetine.

Over the next two weeks he became helpless and hopeless, seeing suicide as a solution. He refused ECT. Ruminations of death left him housebound. When his wife found a stash of antidepressant pills in the house, she insisted on a course of ECT.

After an independent re-examination of his cardiac status, outpatient ECT was begun. No special precautions were needed. After two treatments, his appetite returned. After six ECT, his sleep improved and he was able to leave his home. In the third week, ruminations were much less and when asked about suicide, he said "that was foolish, wasn't it?" Weekly treatments for 5 weeks were followed by resolution of his depression. Seen at a dinner by a colleague, he joked about the illness and politics, and was optimistic about the future.

Patient 8.10

A 68-year-old retired man with Parkinson disease rigidity of four years' duration was treated with a wide range of dopamine agonists, each with transient relief. Rigidity progressed so that he was bed-ridden much of the time, unable to dress or feed himself. When *l*-dopa dosages were increased to levels that allowed movement, he became fearful and anxious, occasionally excited and psychotic, and the dosages had to be reduced. He became increasingly depressed, lost weight, slept poorly, and did not respond to antidepressant medications. ECT was recommended and, after much consideration, he and his wife consented.

After the third treatment, rigidity decreased and he was able to clothe and feed himself and to walk slowly with assistance. After the fifth treatment, he walked unaided, and was no longer depressed. Treatments continued once weekly and over the next two months he was sustained at home, able to care for himself. For the next year, he returned for ECT on a self-demand schedule, varying from every two weeks to monthly. This schedule allowed the patient to care for himself and take part in an active social life.

ECT and characterological conditions

"Neurotic" traits

In the experience of ECT in patients with severe mood disorders, patients suffering from "neurotic depression" have less robust responses than those with melancholic or psychotic depression. In predictor scales designed to identify patients for whom ECT would be useful, the presence of overt anxiety, hypochondriasis, and emotional lability was identified as predictors of poor outcome with ECT.[114]

A report from the CORE ECT study is consistent with these experiences.[115] Two-hundred and fifty-three patients with recurrent depressive illness received an index course of bilateral ECT. From the $HAMD_{24}$, baseline psychic anxiety, somatic anxiety, and hypochondriasis were determined. Among less severely depressed patients, high baseline somatic anxiety and hypochondriasis predicted a low likelihood of a sustained remission with ECT. Among patients with more severe depression at baseline, these traits did not preclude sustained remission. This finding indicates that milder depressions associated with abnormal personality traits are not melancholic, while severe depression is likely to be melancholic and responsive to ECT regardless of co-occurring personality disorder. The investigators confirmed the clinical experience that patients with traits defined in past classifications as *neuroses* are not responsive to ECT.[116]

Patient 8.11

A middle-aged woman developed dental pain which persisted despite extensive orthodontic care. She "fell into a deep depression" and lost her appetite, with a 20% loss in weight. She began a course of psychotherapy and when she continued to ruminate about her mouth and gums, and that she had become ugly, she was admitted to a psychiatric hospital. A 9-week stay was uneventful but left her no better. "I am on a rest cure with do-it-yourself treatment." Under the care of the Chief of Psychiatry, she wrote to her parents that "He does not understand my case." On another occasion she wrote: "After being turned into a monster by the orthodontist, I must adjust to life as a damned ugly woman."

A course of ECT was recommended and, after 8 ECT, she wrote: "I felt just fine, perfectly relaxed and comfortable and also very hungry, as if I were making up for lost time." Although she had been playing bridge throughout the hospital course, she now felt that she could no longer recall the cards. She returned home and described "a déjà-vu experience." She said that her memory was altered: "I was puzzled – but only vaguely. I really felt too vague to care. Nothing really bothered me . . . I felt physically very well . . . and calm. I didn't have enough memory to think, or even worry . . . . Work was just something that drifted across my mind from time to time. It didn't interest me. I was too comfortable doing nothing."

After a month at home, she returned to work. Although her associates and her work appeared familiar, and she remembered some of their names, she found the terms of her work unfamiliar and she returned home in panic. "I was terrified. I've never been a crying person, but all my beloved knowledge, everything I had learned in my field during 20 years or more, was gone. I'd lost the body of knowledge that constituted my professional skill. I'd lost everything that professionals take for granted."

The preoccupation with dental pain and feelings of ugliness were now gone, replaced by a persistent preoccupation with her memory. She retired on medical disability. "I mean, I mustn't give the impression that my experience with electric shock was a total disaster. There have been some beneficial results. For one thing, my physical health has improved. I am beginning to eat again, my digestion is much improved, and I have no trouble with sleep. I also feel emotionally relaxed. And I've lost a lot of bothersome inhibitions." She went on to a public career as a critic of psychiatry.[117]

Personality disorder

The presence of comorbid personality disorder in depressed patients is another predictor of poor outcome with ECT. A comparison of outcomes for 76 depressed patients with comorbid personality disorder with 152 patients without such a disorder found those with personality disorder to have a younger age of onset, multiple prior hospitalizations, and to have reported more suicidal thoughts and attempts.[118] They were more symptomatic on discharge and eight times more likely to be rehospitalized than those without the disorder.[119] Others report similar higher relapse and poorer response rates.[120] The diagnosis of dissociative identity disorder is associated with poor outcomes,[121] as is that of borderline personality disorder.[122]

The more severe the character pathology, the less effective is ECT in remitting depressive illness and the more likely that the patient will have complaints of persistent memory deficits and bodily complaints. Such patients often challenge their treatment and allege malpractice, citing persistent and severe memory defects and failure to warn of the consequences of ECT.[123]

ECT in unipolar and bipolar depression

Cross-sectional signs and symptoms do not distinguish recurrent major depression from bipolar disorder. The distinction is made by the history of a manic or hypomanic episode.[124] The belief that the administration of antidepressant treatment may elicit a manic episode in one and not the other condition separates samples in research projects. Two NIMH-supported studies of ECT were required to omit patients who met the Structured Clinical Interivew for DSM-IV-TR (SCID) criteria for bipolar disorder.[125] The data assessing the treatment response differences between such patients, therefore, are limited and based on older reports.

The appearance of hypomanic symptoms during the course of ECT is a basis for the concern that ECT is mania-inducing. Such responses, however, are not uncommon and do not warrant a change in treatment.[126]

Convulsive therapy relieves the manic as well as the depressive phases of manic-depressive illness.[127] During the treatment of depressed mood, patients often pass through a hypomanic or manic phase. The first signs of relief of severely retarded, mute, and stuporous patients are often a surprise and are looked upon as a switch to mania.

The association of manic episodes in patients with melancholia was recognized repeatedly in the descriptions of psychopathology in the eighteenth and nineteenth centuries.[128] Of patients with major depressive disorders, 40–50% develop mania or hypomania during the course of their illness.[129] It is in this environment that "switching" from depression to mania became an issue in psychopharmacology, one that is highly commercialized. In a retrospective review of 1057 hospital admissions over 60 years, a switch to mania of 12% in patients with "endogenous depression" and 10% in psychotic recurrent depressive illness was reported.[130] Of the non-psychotic patients treated with medication, 3.6% switched to mania. In psychotic manic-depressive patients the switch rates were 30% for ECT and 32% for medications.[131] Switches in presenting mood occur spontaneously, most often for reasons that are obscure. They also occur during the course of treatment and the relation of spontaneous and treatment-induced switches has not been resolved. There is little justification to see the switch as more than a change in the phase of the illness. For patients undergoing ECT, the treatment continues since ECT is as effective in mania as it is in depression.[132]

ECT is effective in relieving both manic and depressive mood disorders and as continuation treatment.

Patient 8.12[133]

A 53-year-old woman with a history of bipolar-I disorder since the age of 22 had repeated hospital admissions. In the 10-year period from 1991 to 2001, she spent 41% of the time (1499 days) in hospital despite multiple medication treatment regimens of antidepressants, antipsychotics, and mood stabilizers. As lamotrigine, reboxetine, and haloperidol were tapered, a course of ECT was begun. After six weeks of right unilateral ECT on a twice-a-week schedule the mixed manic state remitted. Continuation ECT at weekly intervals sustained the patient for a month. When the schedule was changed to one treatment every two weeks, signs of relapse appeared and the weekly schedule was reinstated.

Over the next 17 months she was sustained with weekly and then bi-weekly treatments. Treatment intervals increased to every three and then every four weeks. She remained clinically stable and after 37 months and 85 treatments, maintenance ECT was discontinued and valproate was prescribed.

Three months after the last treatment session, she was readmitted in a manic relapse. RUL ECT was reinstated and after four weeks she was discharged from hospital, with mild depressive symptoms. Weekly continuation ECT was started on schedule and she remained well at the 4-month follow-up.

At the age of 22, the patient had a WAIS-IQ score of 115. Prior to her first ECT at age 51 years, the IQ was 63. The Hasegawa Dementia Screening Scale (HDSS) showed "pre-dementia, probably secondary to the multiple episodes of the disease." Six months later, at the end of the continuation phase of the ECT -treatment, testing showed an IQ of 96 with minimal deficits in short-term memory functions and no retrograde amnesia on semantic/autobiographical tests. HDSS was normal. Eleven months later, when treatments were given once every 4–5 weeks, the WAIS-III-IQ was 94 (verbal IQ 98 – performance IQ 90). Signs of mental deterioration had decreased, and cognitive flexibility had increased.

Conclusion

The merits of ECT in relieving melancholia are undisputed. The issues in clinical practice are the identification of patients with melancholia, the early administration of adequate treatments, and assuring continuation of treatments until all signs of the illness have been extinguished. But treatment trials of depressive disorders rarely use "melancholia" as a diagnostic term. Nevertheless, patients suffering from manic-depressive, involutional, psychotic (delusional), agitated, endogenous, and vital forms of depression typically have melancholic features and meet the criteria for melancholia. The outcome with ECT is excellent in patients with these descriptors. The efficacy of ECT is not limited by gender, age, pregnancy, severity of illness, or prior courses of treatments. Throughout the 70 years of experience with convulsive therapy, all comparisons with alternative treatments – medications and psychotherapy for the most part – clearly demonstrate the superiority of induced seizures as effective therapy.

The principal impediments to the successful use of ECT are its stigma and restrictions in its use, the special requirements for consent, and other non-clinical aspects that restrict its use. An equally limiting factor is the failure to assure adequate treatments once the treatment course is adopted. Assuring treatment adequacy is a principal feature of effective ECT practice.

NOTES

1 *Hamlet*, act IV, scene 3, line 9.
2 Meduna (1935, 1937a, b, 1985). Pentylenetetrazol is a central nervous stimulant. Intravenous boluses elicit seizures.
3 Cook (1938).
4 Bennett (1938, 1939, 1972); Küppers (1939).

5 Read *et al.* (1939).
6 Malzberg (1937).
7 Metrazol treatments were not without risk (Read, 1940). Vertebral and other fractures occurred in 51/320 patients and the acute exacerbation of tuberculosis (8% versus 3% in non-seizure-treated patients) was another severe risk. Myocardial damage was assessed in a "relatively small number of patients" and "Defects of memory were not obvious enough to be reported upon."

Another assessment of risks in convulsive therapy found no deaths in 144 patients treated (Wyllie, 1940). Summarizing the risks from prior published reports, 12 deaths were reported in 2875 patients treated. Of these, one was associated with cerebral hemorrhage and two with prolonged seizures.

Prolonged seizures occur in a small number of patients with electroconvulsive therapy. The occurrence is minimized by proper use of anesthetic agents (Bailine *et al.*, 2003) and successfully treated by the intravenous administration of a rapid-acting benzodiazepine such as diazepam, lorazepam, or midazolam. A unique risk of Metrazol injections is the occurrence of tardive seizures – spontaneous seizures later in the day of a treatment. Tardive seizures are extremely rare with ECT (American Psychiatric Association, 1978, 1990).
8 Wyllie (1940). While many hypotheses have been offered to explain the mechanism of convulsive therapy, the neuroendocrine is most consistent with the clinical data (Fink, 1979, 1999a, 2000a).
9 Fink (1979, 2000a).
10 Kalinowsky (1943), Rennie (1943), Bianchi and Chiarello (1944), Myerson (1944), and Tillotson and Sulzbach (1944), among many others.
11 Bianchi and Chiarello (1944).
12 Rennie (1943).
13 Reports from Europe by Mader (1938), Kronfeld (1939), and Lapipe and Rondepierre (1942), among many others, additionally described the benefits of convulsion therapy in the affective disorders.
14 Jessner and Ryan (1941), p. 73.
15 Lapipe and Rondepierre (1942); Delmas-Marsalet (1943); Delay (1946); Kalinowsky and Hoch (1946); Roubicek (1946); Sargant and Slater (1946); von Braunmühl (1947); von Baeyer (1951).
16 Today, these patients would most likely be identified as suffering from major depression with melancholic features. Their middle age and female gender would not be considered relevant to the diagnosis of depression.
17 Huston and Locher (1948) define their sample:

> Involutional psychosis is a psychosis occurring in middle life and the following years, without evidence of either "organic" intellectual defects or previous affective disorder. The subtype melancholia is characterized mainly by agitation and depression, with a mental content of self-condemnation, hopelessness and a tendency toward hypochondriasis. The paranoid subtype shows delusions of persecution or grandiosity, suspiciousness and misinterpretation. The mixed subtype shows a combination of these two types, with the addition of strong somatic delusions in some cases.

18 Greenblatt *et al.* (1964); Medical Research Council (1965); Gangadhar *et al.* (1982).
19 The literature supporting the use of ECT in depression is extensive but considered controversial in that few studies assigned patients to the treatments randomly, the dosages of medication and even ECT were not optimal, and the assessments were not independent

(Abrams, 1982; Rifkin, 1988). The better recent additional reviews are by American Psychiatric Association (2001), McCall (2001), Abrams (2002a), Salzman *et al.* (2002), Fink and Taylor (2003), and Ottosson and Fink (2004), among many others. For the older literature, see Fink (1979).

20 Folkerts *et al.* (1997).

21 Janicak *et al.* (1985). Using the Mantel-Haenszel statistic to estimate the overall difference between treatments, Janicak *et al.* (1985) reported the advantage of ECT over tricyclic antidepressants at $P = 4.8 \times 10^{-7}$; for the advantage over MAOI as 1.1×10^{-18}; and ECT compared to placebo as 1×10^{-15}.

22 Rifkin (1988).

23 The authors conclude (p. 799):

> ECT is an effective short-term treatment for depression, and is probably more effective than drug therapy. Bilateral ECT is moderately more effective than unilateral ECT, and high dose ECT is more effective than low dose.

24 Agence d'Evaluation des Technologies et des modes d'Intervention en Sante', (2002); National Institute for Clinical Excellence, (2003); Pagnin *et al.* (2004).

25 Reisner (2003). The study concludes: "Scientific study of ECT spanning many decades suggests that it is an effective treatment for, at minimum, major depression and mania." Considering the venue and the author's search for evidence of brain damage, his conclusion is of interest (p. 216):

> Its effects on memory, and particularly the mechanisms by which these effects come about, have been an ongoing source of controversy. There is a possibility that a very small percentage of ECT patients may sustain debilitating cognitive effects, although the most recent studies suggest that with the use of high-intensity unilateral treatment and with the use of brief pulse current, fewer and less serious cognitive deficits are produced by ECT.

Another ethical analysis of ECT concludes that modern psychiatric practice meets the ethical principles of beneficence, non-maleficence, and autonomy, but not that of justice (Ottosson and Fink, 2004). Also see Nuttall *et al.* (2004) for a review of the morbidity and mortality in the use of ECT, further documenting its safety.

26 The stigmatization of ECT as an intrusive, mind-altering, brain-damaging intervention further discourages its use. In the past decade, despite the acknowledged weakness of modern antidepressant medicines, some psychopharmacologists actively disparage its use (Fink, 1991; Ottosson and Fink, 2004; Shorter and Healy, in preparation).

27 The three-hospital study used right unilateral electrode placement with energies set at 2.5 × calibrated seizure threshold; the four-hospital study used bitemporal placement with energies at 1.5 × calibrated seizure threshold. Chapter 9 discusses the relative efficacies of unilateral and bilateral ECT.

28 Fink (1999a); American Psychiatric Association, (2001); Abrams (2002a).

29 Hordern *et al.* (1963).

30 Glassman *et al.* (1975).

31 The study was translated and published by Avery and Lubrano (1979).

32 Hickie *et al.* (1986); Buchan *et al.* (1992); Parker *et al.* (1992b).

33 Kroessler (1985); Vega *et al.* (2000); Kho *et al.* (2003).

34 Kroessler (1985).

35 Kho *et al.* (2003).

36 The authors found 15 studies published between 1978 and 2001 that met their strict inclusion criteria. The findings of the two more recent reports, those of Petrides *et al.* (2001) and Birkenhäger *et al.* (2003), were not included. The positive findings of these latest studies would reinforce the significance of psychosis as a predictor of good effect for ECT in depressive illness.
37 Petrides *et al.* (2001).
38 Husain *et al.* (2004).
39 Birkenhäger *et al.* (2003).
40 Prudic *et al.* (1990, 1996).
41 Mulsant *et al.* (1997).
42 Evidence-based medical standards dictate that psychotic depressed patients should not be labeled as having "treatment-resistant depression" until they have had a full course of bilateral ECT (Fink 1987a, 1993, 1997, 1999a; American Psychiatric Association, 1990).
43 Yale Professor of Surgery Sherwin Nuland (2003).
44 Chapter 7.
45 Prudic and Sackeim (1999); Maris (2002); Kellner *et al.* (2005).
46 Tanney (1986).
47 Avery and Winokur, 1977.
48 Khan *et al.* (2000).
49 Isometsa *et al.* (1996).
50 Prudic and Sackeim (1999).
51 Kellner *et al.* (2005).
52 Among the 25 patients in the high expressed suicide intent group whose ratings did not resolve to zero, 48% (12/25) discontinued their treatment before receiving an adequate course. Of the remainder, 46% (6/13) had a rating of 1 at the end of the acute course. Over half (7/13) rated zero during the treatment course but did not retain it at the final rating. Patients whose expressed suicide intent ratings did not resolve were younger than those whose ratings resolved ($P = 0.02$), but were not different with respect to percentage psychotic or baseline severity of illness.
53 Chapter 7.
54 Two Euro-American men, 76 and 80 years of age, who were depressed without psychosis died by suicide in the course of the study, one each at different sites. At the outset, one patient had an $HAMD_{24}$ of 29 with an expressed intent that was scored one on item 3. He received seven ECT and ended the course with a $HAMD_{24}$ of eight and a score of zero on item 3. He was in the 1-week interim phase awaiting randomization, and on day six after the last ECT, he died by gunshot. The second patient had a baseline $HAMD_{24}$ of 22 and expressed no suicide intent, scoring zero on item 3. After 10 ECT, his $HAMD_{24}$ score was 8 and one week later he was randomized to continuation ECT. Two weeks later, after the second continuation ECT ($HAMD_{24}$ of 16 and item 3 score of 2), he overdosed with medications.
55 NIH-NIMH Consensus Conference on ECT (Consensus Conference, 1985). Also cited by commissions of national associations in the UK and the USA. (American Psychiatric Association, 1978, 1990, 2001; Freeman 1995), and in the most recent assessments by the Canadian Agence d'Evaluation des Technologies et des modes d'Intervention en Sante'(AETMIS) Commission (2002) and the British National Institute for Clinical Excellence (NICE) Commission (2003).
56 Rosenberg (2002).

57 This episode was the fourth that Dr. Rosenberg recalled, the others occurring in 1959, 1965, and 1980, each at a time when he changed his academic position.
58 Fink and Taylor (2003).
59 Kahlbaum (1874).
60 Fink and Taylor (2003).
61 Meduna (1937b, 1985).
62 Guze (1967).
63 Arnold and Stepan (1952).
64 Mann *et al.* (1986, 1990, 2001b).
65 Philbrick and Rummans (1994).
66 Greenberg and Gujavarty (1985); Pearlman (1986).
67 Troller and Sachdev (1999).
68 Fink and Taylor (2003).
69 Ghaziuddin *et al.* (2002b).
70 Alexander *et al.* (1988); Fink (1999b); Fink and Taylor (2003).
71 Meduna (1937b, 1985); Accornero (1988).
72 Fink and Sackeim (1996).
73 Fink and Taylor (2003); Suzuki *et al.* (2003).
74 Bostwick and Chozinski (2002).
75 Abstracted from Fink (1999a) (p. 40–2).
76 Chapter 12.
77 Ferrell *et al.* (1992); Miller (1994); Walker and Swartz (1994); Altshuler *et al.* (1996); Echevarria *et al.* (1998); Moreno *et al.* (1998).
78 Repke and Berger (1984); Wise *et al.* (1984). Fetal heart rate monitoring was performed in pregnant woman undergoing ECT. Remarkably, although the mother's heart rate increased during the seizure, the fetal heart rate was unaffected. The finding was replicated in six patients, leading to the discontinuation of routine fetal monitoring during ECT (Fink, personal experience, 1995–6).
79 Wise *et al.* (1984); Folk *et al.* (2000).
80 American Psychiatric Association, (1990, 2001); Abrams (2002a).
81 During the late stages of pregnancy, ECT is given with the patient in a lateral position, to move the fetus and uterine contents away from the diaphragm, to allow better ventilation.
82 O'Malley (2004). The patient's history is abstracted in Ottosson and Fink (2004), pp. 116–17, as an example of the influence of legal restrictions on ECT and public stigmatization leading to a tragic murder of five children by their mother while she was in a psychotic episode.
83 Ottosson and Fink (2004).
84 Walter *et al.* (1999).
85 Rey and Walter (1997).
86 Strober *et al.* (1998).
87 Schneekloth *et al.* (1993).
88 Moise and Petrides (1996).
89 Kutcher and Robertson (1995).
90 Ghaziuddin (1998).
91 Ghaziuddin *et al.* (2002b).
92 Walter and Rey (1997).
93 Cohen *et al.* (1997).

94 Cohen *et al.* (2000a, b); Taieb *et al.* (2002).
95 Stein *et al.* (2004).
96 Black *et al.* (1985).
97 Carr *et al.* (1983).
98 Guttmacher and Cretella (1988).
99 Powell *et al.* (1988).
100 Cizadlo and Wheaton (1995).
101 Gurevitz and Helme (1954).
102 Cohen *et al.* (2000b).
103 American Psychiatric Association (1990, 2001); Abrams (2002a); Ottosson and Fink (2004).
104 Ottosson and Fink (2004).
105 Additional patient vignettes of adolescents treated with ECT can be found in Fink (1999a), Fink and Taylor (2003), and Ottosson and Fink (2004). They include examples of psychotic depression occurring in persons with mental retardation and manic delirium.
106 Fink and Kahn (1961).
107 Cizadlo and Wheaton (1995).
108 O'Connor *et al.* (2001).
109 Abrams (1989, 2002a); American Psychiatric Association, (2001).
110 The general medical conditions offered as "conditions associated with substantial risk" are severe cardiovascular conditions, aneurysm or vascular malformations, increased intracranial pressure, "recent" cerebral infarction, pulmonary conditions (chronic obstructive pulmonary disease), and patient status rated by an anesthesiologist as ASA (American Society of Anesthesiologists) 4 or 5 (American Psychiatric Association, 2001). The "recent" cited in the text is not defined, leaving the patient in the limbo between the recommendation for treatment by the psychiatrist and the opinions of internists and neurologists with little to no competence or experience with ECT. The reality of modern ECT practice is similar to surgical practice. The risk–benefit analysis of the general medical conditions and the psychiatric illness must give strong consideration of the experience of the treating ECT team.
111 Abrams (1989, 2002a).
112 Hay (1989); Alexopoulos *et al.* (1989).
113 Abrams (1989, 2002a); Kalayam and Alexopoulos (1989); Tancer and Evans (1989); Welch and Drop (1989); American Psychiatric Association, (1990, 2001).
114 Hobson (1953), Carney *et al.* (1965), and Mendels (1967).
115 Rasmussen *et al.* (2004).
116 An interesting report of the effects of ECT in a patient with obsessive thoughts of ugliness and persistent dental pain is related in the series "Annals of Medicine" by B. Roueché in *The New Yorker*, 1974. pp. 84–100.
117 Although not mentioned by name in the article, the patient described by Roueché was later identified as Mrs. Marilyn Rice, founder of the anti-ECT advocacy group Committee for Truth in Psychiatry. She attended open meetings of psychiatrists and complained that ECT had been administered without prior explanation that the price would have been a loss of her memory. She read and critiqued the ECT literature thoroughly. At a meeting dedicated to reports on progress in ECT research in 1982, Mrs. Rice debated the literature with ECT experts, citing articles correctly. She was a gadfly that did much to stigmatize ECT.

118 Black *et al.* (1988).
119 Zimmerman *et al.* (1986b).
120 Kramer (1982); Pfohl *et al.* (1984); Stein (1992); Sareen *et al.* (2000); Feske *et al.* (2004).
121 DeBattista *et al.* (1998).
122 DeBattista and Mueller (2001).
123 Abrams (2002a).
124 Chapter 2.
125 The three-hospital study of continuation treatment (placebo, nortriptyline, or lithium–nortriptyline combination after ECT (Sackeim *et al.*, 2001a) and the four-hospital study known as CORE (O'Connor *et al.*, 2001; Petrides *et al.*, 2001; Husain *et al.*, 2004) limited their sample of depressed patients to those who met SCID criteria for unipolar depression. Patients with a history of mania or hypomania were excluded.
126 Chapter 2.
127 Fink (1979); Abrams (2002a); Small *et al.* (1988).
128 Chapter 1.
129 Benazzi (2004).
130 Angst *et al.* (1992).
131 The study was retrospective. The patients referred for ECT were clearly more severely ill since the use of this treatment was reserved for patients who had failed extensive other trials.
132 Treatment-induced switches from depression to mania (and from mania to depression) are a significant problem in treating patients with manic-depressive illness with anticonvulsant and antidepressant medications. The switch to depression in a manic patient calls for judgment as to whether the anticonvulsant medication or lithium should be continued or augmented. The literature of this difficulty with medication is extensive. See Sarwer-Foner (1988) and Goodwin and Jamison (1990). Also see Mukherjee *et al.* (1994) for a review of the efficacy of ECT in mania.
133 Courtesy of Pascal Sienaert and Jozef Peuskens, University Center Sint-Jozef, Catholic University of Leuven, Kortenberg (Belgium).

9

Achieving effective ECT

Practice makes perfect.[1]

Remission of melancholia is achieved in 80–95% of patients treated with electroconvulsive therapy (ECT).[2] Lesser remission rates, however, are commonly reported.[3] What accounts for the differences in clinical outcome?

The technical practice of ECT is complex and not all treatment courses are optimized to assure the maximum therapeutic benefit. Inappropriate frequency and inadequate numbers of treatments, energies too low to assure an effective seizure, elevated seizure thresholds, inefficient electrode placements, and missed or incomplete seizures result in courses of treatment with limited benefit.

Patient selection

Convulsive therapy relieves depressive mood disorders, yet the benefits are best established in those with melancholia.[4] The relief of severe disorders in mood was discovered early in ECT history.[5] In patients with both the depressed and manic phases of "manic-depressive insanity" and "involutional depression," the introduction of ECT was quickly identified as a life-saving treatment. To assure proper selection of patients, an intensive search for predictors of good response examined identifiable symptoms and syndromes, demographic features, severity of illness, and duration of illness. An excellent and rapid clinical response found in melancholia of recent onset with severe vegetative signs, suicide intent, and delusional thinking occurred in older rather than younger patients. A poor outcome was associated with chronic illness, limited impairment that allowed sustained employment, comorbid personality disorder, "neurotic symptoms" (pervasive anxiety, dysthymia, hypochondriasis), and substance abuse.[6] Specific behavior-rating scales designed as predictors were developed.[7] But these were no better predictors of treatment outcome than traditional clinical evaluation that carefully defined patients with melancholia.[8] Laboratory tests were evaluated as predictors of outcome.[9] The methacholine (Mecholyl) test,[10] the sedation threshold,[11] personality variables,[12] and the dexamethasone suppression test (DST)[13] were studied. Except for the DST, none was found useful.[14]

Table 9.1. Clinical characteristics associated with good outcome with electroconvulsive therapy (ECT)

Episode < 1 year[a]
Age over 50 years
Psychosis (delusions) prominent
Anorexia severe and > 10% weight loss
Insomnia severe
Stupor, motor retardation, agitation prominent
Suicidal thoughts or acts requiring 24-h observation
Catatonia
Delirium (related to a depression or mania)
Previous good response to ECT

[a] Although patients whose episodes are less than 12 months in duration may have the best remission rates, most patients who receive ECT have been ill much longer without responding to multiple medication trials. They still respond well to ECT.

Outcome is still best defined by clinical criteria. The more severe episodes of mood disorder, the presence of vegetative signs, suicidal and delusional thoughts, and catatonic signs are associated with rapid clinical response (Table 9.1). Considering the remarkable efficacy of ECT, the proper diagnosis of melancholia is sufficient to support and encourage its use. On balance, the efficacy rate for melancholia with psychosis is better than that of melancholia without psychosis, arguing that the presence of psychosis in an episodic illness should encourage the use of ECT.[15]

Older patients (age > 65 years) have higher remission rates than younger patients (< 45 years), an argument for an earlier consideration in the elderly.[16] Severe vegetative signs, motor retardation and agitation, or suicidal preoccupation in the elderly compel consideration of ECT rather than repeated medication or psychotherapy trials. Indeed, ECT is favored as the main treatment in such patients by the ECT Task Forces of the American Psychiatric Association: "As a major treatment in psychiatry with well-defined indications, ECT should not be reserved for use only as a 'last resort'."[17] After citing the speed of response and efficacy of ECT in patients at high risk of suicide and with co-occurring general medical illness, the task force concludes: "Severe major depression with psychotic features, mania with psychotic features, and catatonia are conditions for which there is a clear consensus favoring early reliance on ECT."[18]

The clinical characteristics associated with a poor outcome in ECT are cited in Table 9.2.

While the disorder in mood and suicide intent may be relieved in patients with comorbid character pathology or severe "neurotic" symptoms, the adjustment to a normal life is not improved. A persistence of pretreatment difficulties is then

Table 9.2. Clinical characteristics associated with poor outcome with electroconvulsive therapy

Defined personality disorder
Indefinite onset; prolonged illness
"Neurotic signs" of anxiety, somatization
Comorbid alcoholism, substance abuse

ascribed to the treatment, a development that closely follows the history of other somatoform disorders.[19] Poor responders to ECT who overly complain about the treatment's side-effects, despite an absence of objective signs of disability, are often persons under age 50 with C traits described in psychiatric classifications as histrionic, antisocial, and high novelty-seeking.[20] Co-occurring substance abuse and a history of non-compliance with treatment recommendations also compromise outcomes.

Technical considerations

Convulsive therapy is akin to a surgical treatment. It requires anesthesia and the full paraphernalia of anesthesiology, nursing, intravenous line, and loss of consciousness. The technical procedures to assure effective treatment are undergoing continuing reassessment. Variations in the form of the electrical current, placement of the electrodes, frequency of treatments, and augmentation with chemicals affect efficacy. Clinically effective seizures are defined by motor, electroencephalogram (EEG), and cardiovascular characteristics.[21] Our present techniques seek to minimize risks and patient discomfort by anesthesia and muscle relaxation but these do not increase treatment efficacy.[22]

Panic and fear of treatment, missed seizures, and secondary (tardive) seizures that developed later in the treatment day were risks that were peculiar to the chemical induction of seizures. When chemical inductions were replaced by electrical stimulation, panic and fear of the treatments and the occurrence of tardive seizures were much allayed, and are no longer impediments to treatment. Missed seizures, however, remained a hurdle to effective practice.

Fractures of the dorsal vertebrae, less often of a shoulder, hip, or jaw during the motor convulsion, were risks. Many muscle paralytic agents were tested and, by 1952, succinylcholine was shown to be an effective, rapid, and safe method to paralyze muscles.[23] The incidence of fractures was sharply reduced. But succinylcholine paralyzed not only the skeletal muscles but it also inhibited respiration. Patients strongly objected to the momentary feelings of suffocation. To minimize this awareness, an intravenous barbiturate (or other anesthetic such as etomidate, propofol, or ketamine) was accepted as standard practice.[24]

Both the seizure and the anesthetic impair orientation and memory. On awakening, the patient is disoriented, often severely enough to be characterized as delirious.[25] By ventilating patients with pure oxygen rather than room air, however, the severity and duration of the delirium are reduced.[26] Oxygenation, barbiturate sedation, and muscle paralysis are accepted procedures in effective and safe "modified" ECT.

The first electric currents used to induce a seizure were the alternating current forms readily available from the mains. The energy dose was often more than was needed to elicit an effective seizure and the high doses exaggerated the immediate effects on cognition and memory. Different current forms were tested and square-wave pulse currents were shown to have lesser effects on memory than the alternating currents.[27] This current form is in standard use today.

Electrode placement

In ECT, two electrodes are placed on the head to allow passage of the current to stimulate a seizure. Bilateral (bitemporal) placement (BL-ECT) was the first widely used application. To reduce the immediate cognitive effects of seizures and anesthesia, electrode locations on different parts on the head were tested. By the mid-1970s, a unilateral positioning on the non-dominant hemisphere, characterized as the d'Elia placement, came to common use. In this configuration, one electrode is placed on the temple, and the second near the vertex about one in. (2.5 cm) to one side of the midline. To minimize the direct effects of the currents on the brain's memory centers, the practice focused on the non-dominant hemisphere.[28] This alignment is described as right unilateral electrode placement and the seizures so induced are labeled RUL-ECT.[29]

At first, RUL-ECT was believed to be as effective as BL-ECT, with lesser immediate effects on cognition and memory. It was widely favored for the minimal psychological effects. But clinicians soon reported that RUL-ECT was clinically less effective than BL-ECT.[30] An explanation for the lesser efficacy of RUL-ECT comes from an examination of current path and characteristics of the induced seizure. The lesser efficacy is explained by the path of the electric currents not impacting on the brain regions believed essential to the behavioral response.[31] RUL-ECT has other disadvantages. Because the seizure threshold must be significantly exceeded to achieve clinical efficacy, the threshold must be calibrated, assuring that the first session has no clinical efficacy.[32] RUL-ECT is also hampered by the need to deliver high energies beyond the device's capacity to induce effective seizures in some patients, especially the elderly.[33]

The experience of 70 years has so reduced the risks of ECT that the list of contraindications to its use has virtually disappeared. Many general medical conditions that were once thought to limit the use of ECT can now be managed, so that no *absolute* contraindications to ECT are cited.[34] The decision when to use ECT is based on medical algorithms that balance risks and benefits. The death rate with ECT is so remarkably low that the balance tilts favorably toward ECT.[35]

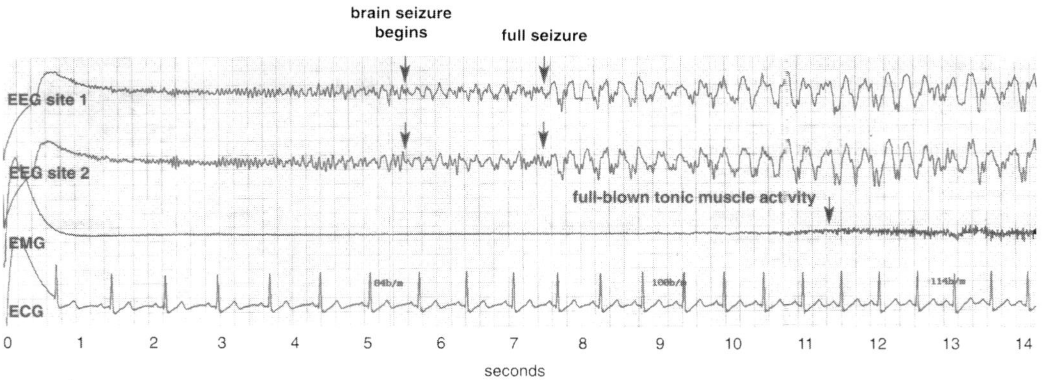

Figure 9.1 Recording of induced seizure with two electroencephalogram (EEG) derivations, electromyogram (EMG), and electrocardiogram (ECG). This record shows the seizure onset with build-up of EEG slow-wave and spike activity.

Optimizing seizures

The efficacy of convulsive therapy resides in the quality of the induced seizures.[36] An "effective seizure" is characterized by measurable motor, EEG, cardiovascular, and hormonal changes. Modern ECT devices include EEG, electromyogram (EMG), and heart rate recorders, making seizure monitoring available to all clinicians.

An effective seizure is defined by the tonic and clonic motor effects. A motor duration of 25 s or longer is one sign of effective treatment.[37] This minimal duration is accompanied by tachycardia and a longer EEG seizure.[38]

After the stimulus, the ictal EEG changes rapidly, with a build-up of amplitudes and the expression of high-voltage bursts of slow waves (delta) that include "spikes" (they look like the spires on top of church steeples; Figure 9.1). The record changes to strings of symmetric and rhythmic slow waves, followed by a period of waxing and waning of slow waves, and an abrupt (sharp) endpoint to the rhythms, leading to a period of electrical quiescence (Figure 9.2). EEG seizures with durations between 30 and 120 s are considered effective. Longer seizures are not associated with better clinical results so present practice is to abort longer seizures by intravenous benzodiazepines.

For effective courses of ECT, it is necessary to achieve seizures that meet criteria for an adequate ictal EEG. Interest is now centered on seizure duration, the development of distinct phases of high-voltage slowing with spike activity, rhythmic high-voltage slowing, and a precise endpoint.[39] Considering the safety of the induction procedure, failure to induce an adequate seizure warrants immediate re-stimulation while the patient remains paralyzed and under anesthesia.[40]

The changes in the interictal EEG have also been correlated with clinical outcome. With increasing numbers of seizures the interictal EEG recordings made 24 h after a seizure show progressive slowing of frequencies and increased amplitudes. As the number and frequency of seizure inductions increase, the characteristics of the interictal EEG change.[41]

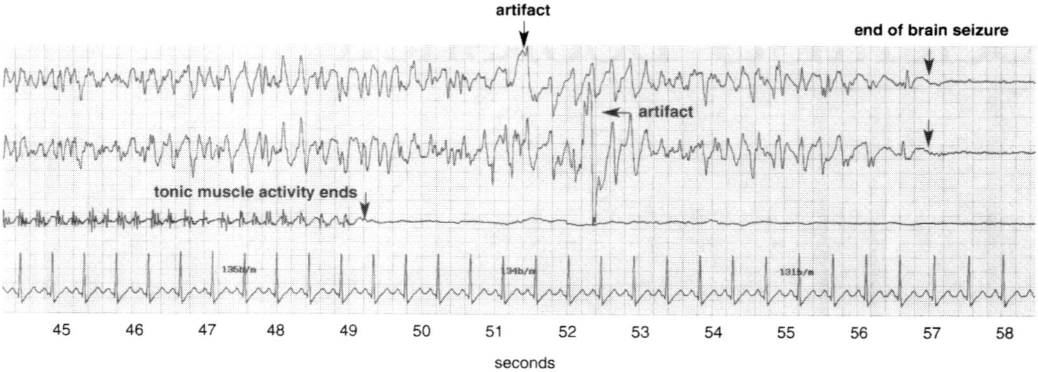

Figure 9.2 The last phase of the seizure exhibiting rhythmic slow-wave activity terminating abruptly in electrical silence.

The symmetry and degree of EEG changes vary with electrode placement. The changes with bitemporal electrodes are symmetrical and generally of higher voltages and slower frequencies than seizures induced through unilateral electrodes.[42] The rapid development of high degrees of symmetric bilateral EEG slowing is associated with a good behavioral outcome.[43] Failure to develop interictal slowing is associated with failed treatment courses.

If the physiologic indices of EEG, heart rate, and EMG are difficult to interpret, an alternate index is the measurement of the release of hypothalamic hormones. While many brain hormones may be measured in the blood after a seizure, the most frequent index is serum prolactin.[44] The peak release is 20–30 min after a seizure.[45] An increase in serum prolactin of two to four times the reference value is evidence of an effective seizure.[46]

Electrode selection and energy dosing

Selective energy dosing is critical to achieve maximum efficacy with unilateral electrode placement (RUL), but is less critical in bilateral (BL) electrode placements such as bitemporal (BT) or bifrontal (BF).[47] The practical and effective choice in ECT is to treat melancholic patients through BL electrodes. Energy levels are selected as 50% above the titrated seizure threshold, or, more practically, by applying the experience that seizure thresholds rise with increasing age.[48] A simple assessment for BT energy selection is the half-age formula.[49] If the stimulus does not elicit the EEG and motor duration that meet minimal criteria, and the ictal EEG does not express the typical patterns of an effective treatment, stimulation is repeated immediately with 50% more energy under the same anesthesia.

Treatment frequency

Frequency is determined by severity of the illness. Treatments are given more frequently, even initially on a daily basis, for the more malignant conditions, especially those characterized by severe psychomotor retardation, agitation, delirium, suicide risk, psychosis, or in those patients who have had substantial weight loss.[50] For most depressed patients, treatments are induced two or three times weekly. Clinical improvement appears earlier with more frequent treatments, but so too do the immediate cognitive effects. Twice-weekly treatments minimize anterograde confusion in older patients.[51]

As patients improve, the time between treatments is lengthened, so that a typical course may be three treatments the first week, two treatments for the next 2–3 weeks, and then one treatment a week until the illness has ameliorated and remission has been achieved.

An effective course

The benefits of induced seizures are additive, typically requiring from four to nine seizures to achieve remission in melancholia.[52] After two to three treatments, appetite and sleep return, followed by decreased suicidal thoughts, heightened affect, and increased interest and energy. Psychotic thoughts and guilt are the last signs to disappear.

The immediate relief is often so great that some patients decline further treatment. Premature conclusion of a treatment course, however, is a common cause for relapse. Every effort should be made to assure that the patient continues treatments until full relief is obtained. A useful analogy is the course of antibiotic therapy. Symptom resolution of an infection occurs within a few days, but therapy needs to proceed for longer periods to avoid relapse and complications.[53]

The benefits of ECT may be seen immediately but for sustained relief, the changes in body physiology require stabilization. Using percentage reductions in rating-scale scores to assess the endpoint of the course of ECT is a poor method. It allows the illness to be incompletely resolved at the time that the treatment course is ended.[54] It is usually necessary to stabilize the recovery with continuation treatment, either continuation ECT or establishing an effective medication schedule. For many patients, however, the signs of the mood disorder are still present and re-emerge despite antidepressant medication treatment. Continuation ECT is an effective method to sustain the benefits. Evidence-derived criteria are lacking, however, for how many treatments should be given and at what frequency once melancholia has remitted. Remission is best sustained by offering additional continuation treatments at weekly and then bi-weekly intervals until all signs of illness are dissipated.[55] Once a patient has accepted the risks and stigma of ECT, it is unreasonable to offer a limited treatment course with a high likelihood of relapse.[56]

Although these and similar guidelines have been the basis for ECT practice for decades, reports of ineffective treatment and high relapse rates are frequent. Guidelines are poorly followed. A survey of practice patterns in ECT facilities in the greater New York City metropolitan area in early 1997 found a diversity in electrode placements, the continued use of sine-wave stimulating currents, multiple treatments in one session, haphazard dosing strategies, and a wide range of medication and ECT continuation practices.[57]

A naturalistic prospective study of 347 patients at seven metropolitan hospitals found the sites to differ markedly in the selection of patients and in ECT techniques. The remission rates were 30.3–46.7%, in marked contrast to those reported in research studies. Among remitters, the relapse rate during follow-up was 64.3%. Patient selection included many who did not meet criteria for successful ECT and episode durations were longer than those usually reported for the patients who respond best to ECT. Clinicians frequently ended the ECT course prematurely, believing that the patients had benefited fully, yet formal assessments showed the persistence of residual symptoms.[58]

Concurrent medications

The same antidepressant medications that did not relieve the depressive illness are often prescribed during the treatment course. We have little evidence that any of the established antidepressant medications alter either the seizure threshold or the seizure quality. Nor do they augment the acute antidepressant response of ECT. Their continuation is a matter of clinical choice.[59]

Medications that are known to affect the seizure, such as benzodiazepines, lidocaine, high-dose beta-blockers, and anticonvulsant drugs, are usually discontinued. Theophylline is associated with prolonged seizures and its administration is modified so that seizure durations do not become prolonged. The hypoglycemic effects of insulin may be augmented during the seizure, driving serum glucose levels lower than expected.[60] Monitoring of glucose levels before and after a treatment are useful guides to changes in insulin dosages.

Lithium use in ECT warrants special attention. Cerebrospinal fluid levels of lithium rise with seizures and a transient confusional syndrome immediately after a seizure has been described in patients with high serum lithium levels. It is customary to withhold lithium dosing on the evening before and the morning of a treatment and this sufficiently reduces serum lithium levels so as not to be a hazard.[61]

Some synergistic benefits have been associated with the concurrent use of antipsychotic medications. When these have been a feature of the pre-ECT treatment schedule, their continuation has been encouraged.[62]

Continuation tactics – ECT versus medications

The effects of each seizure and the series of seizures are transient, as the body's homeostatic processes rapidly restore the altered physiology.[63] Changes in cognitive functions and EEG, for example, resolve within 2–6 weeks, often sooner after the last ECT. Changes in mood and thought are also transient unless treatment is continued.

How to sustain the acute benefit of ECT is a challenge. In treating melancholic patients with medication, patients are urged to continue the prescription for up to a year or more after the symptoms resolve.[64] For patients with recurrent melancholia, antidepressant medication is usually prescribed indefinitely. When the antidepressant medicines were previously unsuccessful and ECT was administered, the prescription of the same medicines has small benefit, with unacceptable relapse rates. In one study, after a course of ECT, a 30% relapse rate was reported with continuation with imipramine, 10% with paroxetine, and 65% with placebo.[65] In another, the relapse rate after the course of ECT (with monitored blood levels) was 39% with the combination of lithium and nortriptyline, 60% with nortriptyline alone, and 84% with placebo.[66] The rate of relapse with lithium and nortriptyline was confirmed in an independent study.[67]

Continuation ECT is difficult to achieve. Each ECT treatment requires an accompanying adult to be present for much of the morning. Starting the intravenous line for anesthesia and post-ECT confusion can be discomforting. Some patients are fearful of anesthesia and the treatments. Treatments are expensive. Every effort is made to achieve benefits with the least number of seizures.

In the first decades of ECT use, treatments were repeated as soon as any signs of illness recurred. Practitioners would ask patients to come for return visits prepared for treatment, and when the examination showed signs of recurrence, treatment was induced that day.[68] Such individual management was abandoned in the belief that continuation antidepressant medication would suffice. Two decades later, with recognition that the relapse rates were unacceptably high, tentative trials with ECT as a continuation tactic were undertaken.[69] In one study of continuation ECT once or twice weekly for two months after remission was achieved found better patient acceptance for the schedule of once every two weeks than once weekly.[70] Of 19 patients assigned to the study and who completed a 1-year re-examination, eight received ECT once a week and 11 received ECT once every two weeks. Three of eight patients treated once a week and nine of 11 patients treated once every two weeks completed the schedule. Compared to depressed patients who were continued on various antidepressant medications, one of 13 (8%) relapsed by six months, compared to 10/25 (40%) on medication alone.

Based on these experiences, two large 6-month continuation trials were undertaken, a three-hospital study assessing continuation medications and a four-hospital study comparing medication to continuation ECT. The 6-month relapse rate for continuation ECT was 37% compared with a 32% rate for continuation lithium and nortriptyline combination.[71]

In experimental studies, such as the CORE study, after remission with ECT the patients receive treatments once a week for four weeks, once every two weeks for two months and then monthly until remission has been sustained for 6 months. Another schedule prescribes weekly treatment for six weeks, then every two weeks for up to six months. An alternative is to offer continuation treatments on demand at the first sign of relapse, offering two to three treatments in the week after signs of relapse.[72] These methods are reported to be successful, with the demand method most easily accepted by patients and their families.

Lithium therapy prophylaxis is an effective tactic.[73] After reviewing the sparse literature on continuation medication, the combination of lithium and nortriptyline was assessed as probably the most effective.[74] This combination has the advantages that serum blood level criteria are available to monitor dosing for both drugs, and it sustained remission more effectively than nortriptyline alone in the three-hospital continuation medication study (39% for the combination compared to 60% for nortriptyline alone). This combination sustained ECT remission for six months at the same rate as a rigorously prescribed continuation ECT schedule.[75]

Conclusions

ECT at three times a week, using BF or BT electrode placement, standardized regimens of anesthesia, ventilation with oxygen, and muscle relaxation, minimizes risks and elicits remission rates in more than 80% of melancholic patients. Physiologic monitoring offers guides to effective treatments. Rating each treatment by the quality of the ictal EEG and seizure duration, restimulating if a seizure is deemed ineffective, maximizes response rates. Continuation treatment until remission is achieved is essential to prevent relapse. While the majority of continuation efforts are with medication, there are no clear guidelines on the efficacy of different medication regimens. The experimental literature favors the combination of lithium and a tricyclic antidepressant. Clinicians have come increasingly to depend on continuation ECT to minimize relapse rates, and the present guideline calls for continuation ECT for 6 months or as long as symptoms persist.

NOTES

1 Proverb.
2 Chapter 9. Also Fink (1979); American Psychiatric Association, (1990, 2001); Abrams (2002a).
3 Petrides *et al.* (2001) reported a 95% remission rate for patients with psychotic depression and 84% for those with non-psychotic depression. Birkenhäger *et al.* (2003) reported a 55% remission rate in psychotic depressed and 24% in non-psychotic depressed. A variation in remission rates in clinical practice of 30–47% in a survey of metropolitan New York clinical practice is described by Prudic *et al.* (2004). The UK ECT Review Group (2003) meta-analyses cite variations in efficacy rates according to electrode placement and energy dosing. The variations with the form of electricity (alternating current versus brief pulse) and electrode placement are described by Weiner (1988) and Sackeim *et al.* (1987, 1993, 2001a). The variations are cited in texts (Abrams 2002a; American Psychiatric Association, 2001).
4 The benefits of ECT in catatonia and delirious mania are also excellent (Fink, 1999b; Fink and Taylor, 2003).
5 Chapters 1 and 8.
6 Kalinowsky and Hoch (1946); Sargent and Slater (1946); Fink (1979); Hamilton M (1982); Abrams (2002a).
7 Hobson (1953); Weinstein and Kahn (1955); Mendels (1965); Carney *et al.* (1965).
8 Abrams (2002a).
9 Chapter 4.
10 Funkenstein *et al.* (1952); Blumberg *et al.* (1956).
11 Shagass (1954, 1957). Chapter 14.
12 Weinstein and Kahn (1955); Kahn and Fink (1960); Kahn *et al.* (1960a, b).
13 Fink (1986a). The dexamethasone suppression test is discussed in Chapter 4.

14 Chapter 4.

15 Petrides *et al.* (2001); Birkenhäger *et al.* (2003); Kho *et al.* (2003). Patients 8.2 and 9.9 are illustrative examples.

16 O'Connor *et al.* (2001). The elderly have marked reductions in neuroendocrine functions even in the absence of a mood disorder. With a mood disorder, these abnormalities increase. During seizures, the hypothalamic neuroendocrine centers are stimulated, and physiologic functions are restored (Fink, 2000a, b).

17 American Psychiatric Association, 2001.

18 American Psychiatric Association, 2001, pp. 6–7. Also patients 3.2 and 8.5.

19 Trimble (2004) describes syndromes labeled hysteria that became the central feature of the war neuroses in each of the major world wars. He presents an instructive vignette in the Camelford water pollution episode in the UK. After a brownish discoloration of the water when chemicals were inadvertently released into the water supply, some citizens with pre-existing somatic complaints associated new symptoms with the event and sought compensation. Trimble's analysis finds that a somatoform disorder follows an acute traumatic experience in persons with characterological difficulties, expectation of somatic consequences, assertion of such an association by professional opinion, opportunity for compensation, and the absence of any evidence of a systemic biological defect to explain the symptoms.

The same course may be the basis for the persistence of complaints of memory loss that interferes with daily functioning reported by some patients after ECT. ECT is pictured as a traumatic experience with memory loss as an immediate aftermath of each seizure. Authorities repeatedly assert that memory loss is a consequence of seizures and this assertion is codified in the written consent form that is read and signed by patients. Yet, detailed examinations of the brain and brain functions (including extensive cognitive tests) fail to find evidence of the self-reported cognitive deficit. Relief from work on the basis of medical illness and financial compensation is sought. The number of such complaints is few yet their voices and the voices of their supporters are loud. The best predictor of post-ECT somatization is diagnosable character pathology.

20 DSM-IV (American Psychiatric Association, 1994).

21 Fink (1979); Kellner *et al.* (1997); Beyer *et al.* (1998); Abrams (2002a).

22 Anesthesia is an integral part of modern ECT practice. Anesthesiologists are active partners in the treatment and the practical aspects are well described in recent reviews (Folk *et al.*, 2000; Ding and White, 2002). No aspect of anesthesia is essential to therapeutic efficacy as the benefits can clearly be achieved without anesthesia or muscle relaxation. The modifications are meant to reduce the fear and anxiety of patients and the risks of fracture. Unmodified ECT is still widely practiced in societies where the cost of anesthetic agents and the charges of specialists limit the use of ECT (Ottosson and Fink, 2004).

23 Holmberg and Thesleff (1952).

24 Any rapid and short-acting anesthetic may be used. The barbiturates methohexital and Pentothal have a rapid onset and short duration of action. Intramuscular ketamine is an effective anesthetic that is particularly effective in excited manic patients. Propofol and etomidate are alternatives. Propofol raises seizure thresholds sufficiently to find a defined use in the treatment of adolescents in whom seizure durations may be prolonged.

25 Estimates vary, with the incidence highest for bilateral ECT using alternating current (AC) currents, less with unilateral ECT and brief-pulse currents (Fink, 1979; Weiner, 1980; Abrams, 2002a).

26 Holmberg (1953a, b).

27 Weiner (1979, 1988).

28 Careful attention was paid to handedness and all patients were assessed with tests of eye, hand, and foot dominance. As the normal population has an imbalance of right-handedness (90% of the population), and when the assessments after seizures were induced with electrodes on the dominant hemisphere did not show any sustained memory effects, all patients were routinely treated with electrodes over the right hemisphere. On occasion, such placement elicits a transient delirium. When testing for handedness finds the patient to be left-handed, the electrodes for subsequent treatments are placed over the left hemisphere.

29 American Psychiatric Association, (1978); Fink (1979); Abrams (2002a).

30 Abrams *et al.* (1970, 1972); d'Elia and Raotma (1975); Fink (1979).

31 Electric currents are most concentrated in the brain regions between the electrodes. In RUL-ECT the energy density is greatest over the motor strip, eliciting motor seizures with lesser energies (i.e., seizure thresholds are low). In BL-ECT and bifrontal ECT, the energies bypass the motor strip and are densest in the diencephalon (Sackeim *et al.*, 1987, 1993, 2000, 2001a; McCall *et al.*, 2000; Little *et al.*, 2003.)

The path of current influences the physiologic effects of the seizures. RUL-ECT-induced seizures are associated with asymmetric and poorly organized electroencephalogram patterns and the expression of lower amounts of hypothalamic hormones (Abrams *et al.*, 1972; Volavka *et al.*, 1972; Fink, 2000a, b).

For RUL-ECT, the remission rates reported with induction currents at 1.5 and 2.5 times the calibrated seizure threshold are inferior to the remission rates achieved with BL-ECT (30–55% compared to 80–95%). It is only when energies are at least six times the calibrated seizure threshold that the RUL-ECT remission rates approximate those of BL-ECT (Sackeim *et al.*, 1987, 1993, 2000). At the energy dosages needed to achieve clinical efficacy, the saving in immediate cognitive effects is lost (McCall *et al.*, 2000).

32 Administering an anticholinergic agent is essential when assessing seizure thresholds by titration. In the procedure the minimal energy to induce a seizure, selected by age and gender characteristics, is applied to an anesthetized patient. If no seizure occurs, the energy is raised by 50%, and another attempt is made. This procedure is repeated until a seizure is elicited. For bitemporal (and bifrontal) electrode placement, subsequent treatments are given at energies calculated at 50% above the energy that induced the seizure (the seizure threshold).

Missed seizures risk cardiac asystole, so titration must be done with the administration of an effective anticholinergic agent. Further, the titration treatment is admittedly clinically ineffective and is a "wasted" induction, adding to the number of anesthetic inductions and the cost of an effective course of treatment.

33 Governmental regulations limit the energies that can be delivered by ECT devices sold in the USA, making it difficult to deliver effective energies to many patients, especially the elderly late in the course of their treatment. This limitation results from the experience that individual seizure thresholds rise with age (American Psychiatric Association 2001; Abrams 2002a, b). US approved ECT devices deliver a maximum of 576 millicoulombs (mC) of energy. During the course of treatment, seizure thresholds rise, so that about mid-course, the elicited seizure is poorly generalized and loses the characteristics of an effective treatment. (Devices sold in other parts of the world are calibrated to deliver twice that amount of energy, approximately 1000 mC.)

Inducing two seizures rapidly is an approximate way around this hurdle (Swartz and Mehta, 1986).

34 Abrams (1989, 2002a); APA (2001). Texts still list "relative contraindications" to the use of ECT, such as unstable cardiovascular conditions, aneurysm or vascular malformation, increased intracranial pressure, recent cerebral infarction, chronic obstructive pulmonary disease, or high anesthesia risk rates.

An alternative tactic is to use the full-age method (Abrams, 2002a). In this method, the percent energy is selected by approximating the patient's age for the initial treatment energy. The quality of the seizure is assessed and energies for subsequent treatments adjusted accordingly. Modern technical advances make it possible to treat almost all patients in whom ECT is indicated (Abrams, 1989, 2002a; American Psychiatric Association, 2001).

35 The mortality rate with ECT is estimated as two deaths per 100 000 treatments (Kramer, 1985, 1999). It has remained constant for more than 20 years, placing ECT at the low end of the risk range for anesthesia induction alone and about 10 times safer than childbirth. Approximately six times as many deaths are caused by lightning than by ECT in the USA annually (Abrams, 1997).

36 Technical aspects of ECT practice are well documented. The details offered here are to answer specific queries that arise in the treatment of melancholic patients. Texts include Abrams (2002a), American Psychiatric Association Task Force reports (1990, 2001), the handbooks by Kellner *et al.* (1997) and Beyer *et al.* (1998), and a simplified text for patients and their families (Fink, 1999a).

37 Fink and Johnson (1982). Seizure durations vary with age. Adolescents and young adults have very long seizures, the elderly much shorter ones. At times, we are unable to achieve seizures of 25 s in the elderly, and the characteristics do not meet optimal standards, especially in the mid-course of treatment. Changing the anesthesia agent and minimizing soporific medications are useful.

38 Greenberg (1985); Sackeim and Mukherjee (1986); Sackeim *et al.* (1987, 1991); Swartz and Larson, (1989); Swartz (2000); Benbow *et al.* (2003).

39 We lack experimental studies that define the optimal EEG characteristics for effective treatment. Suggestions are to be found in Kellner *et al.* (1997) and Beyer *et al.* (1998). The latest versions of ECT devices record EEG, electrocardiogram, and electromyogram. The devices offer analytic algorithms that measure EEG seizure duration, EEG energy index, and a postictal suppression index (Abrams 2002a). Their merits as predictors of seizure adequacy are under study.

40 In ECT we convert abnormal brain electrical rhythms just as cardiologists convert abnormal heart rhythms in cardioversion. We assume that the brain in a melancholic patient is in a state in which a seizure affects its rhythms much as electricity affects cardiac rhythms. Interestingly, in cardioversion, 200–400 J are delivered in a split second. In ECT from one-tenth to one-third of this amount of energy is used. Sadly, the electrical stimulation of the brain is stigmatized while that of the heart is hailed (Ottosson and Fink, 2004).

41 Fink and Kahn (1957); Fink (1979).

42 Abrams *et al.* (1970, 1972, 1973); Volavka *et al.* (1972).

43 Fink and Kahn (1957); Sackeim *et al.* (1996).

44 Trimble (1978); Swartz and Abrams (1984); Abrams and Swartz (1985a, 1985b); Fink (1986a).

45 Swartz (1984, 1985).

46 When doubts arise as to the efficacy of a treatment, the serum prolactin taken in the 20–30 min post-seizure is compared to a value ascertained the next morning at a comparable time, since serum prolactin levels have a diurnal variation, with peaks in the morning and troughs during the night.

47 Bifrontal electrode placement is described as having equivalent efficacy to BT with fewer effects on cognition and memory (Lawson *et al.*, 1990; Letemendia *et al.*, 1993; Bailine *et al.*, 2000; Delva *et al.*, 2000). These reports encouraged a National Institutes of Mental Health (NIMH)-supported study of the random assignment of depressed patients to BT and BF (at 1.5× calibrated seizure threshold) and RUL (at 6× calibrated seizure threshold.) The results of this ongoing CORE study are expected in 2007.

A retrospective study by Little *et al.* (2004) favors the BT placement for its reduction of the rehospitalization rate. But the patients were not randomly assigned to the electrode placements, not excluding the possibility that a selection bias may have affected the results.

48 Kellner and Fink (1996); Abrams (2002a); Fink (2002b).

49 Petrides and Fink (1996). For modern ECT devices that can maximally deliver approximately 500–600 mC energy, half the patient's age converted to percentage energy for the stimulus yields effective seizures in 80% of inductions. For example, in an 80-year-old patient the starting dose would be 40% of the device's maximum output.

50 When patients are severely bradykinetic, rigid, with signs of catatonia, daily ECT for three to four treatments is necessary (Fink and Taylor, 2003). Also see patients 8.7 and 8.9.

51 Lerer *et al.* (1995). Cognitive effects are related to seizure frequency. Daily ECT has more immediate effects than less frequent seizures. The optimal rate is a balance between need for speed of response (as in suicidal patients) and the unpleasantness of seizure-associated deliria.

52 But many courses are much longer, and prescribing a fixed number of treatments at the onset is poor practice, leading to incomplete remissions and high relapse rates (Ottosson and Fink, 2004).

53 In the recently completed CORE collaborative study of ECT, 530 patients with recurrent major depressive illness with pretreatment $HAMD_{24}$ scores averaging 35.3 (±7.3) were treated three times a week until they had scores less than 10 for one week. In the week before randomization to either continuation ECT or continuation pharmacotherapy, 70 remitted patients developed increased symptoms with $HAMD_{24}$ scores over 10. They were evaluated as relapsed.

Of the 341 remitters, 10 had protocol violations severe enough to terminate their participation; 38 refused further participation (feeling well enough not to want further treatment), seven developed an adverse effect, 12 exited for other reasons, and 204 were eligible for randomization. Three refused and 201 were randomized to the continuation treatments.

The 70 "relapsers" are partly the result of a strict definition of relapse, defined as any score above 10. Thus, if a patient started with a score of 35, reduced to 7 the day after the last treatment, and then returned a week later for randomization with a score of 11, he was rated as relapsed and no longer in the study. Many patients came back for the interim assessment clearly much better than before ECT but slightly higher than a 10 and were identified as relapsers (Kellner *et al.*, submitted).

54 In ECT studies comparing RUL-ECT and BL-ECT, the BL-ECT-treated patients had better post-6-ECT outcomes than the RUL-ECT patients as assessed on the $HAMD_{17}$ rating scale. A concurrent 4-point overall rating of illness persistence showed many patients with apparently resolved HAMD scores of illness who still rated as modestly ill on the overall rating scale. Their mood or animation was still not fully improved (Abrams *et al.*, 1983).

55 The DST is a useful index of relapse. The reappearance of an abnormal DST after normalization with treatment is a harbinger of relapse. The evidence is anecdotal, however, and warrants further evaluation. Chapter 4.
56 Ottosson and Fink (2004).
57 Prudic *et al.* (2001).
58 Prudic *et al.* (2004).
59 American Psychiatric Association, (1990, 2001); Kellner (1991); Abrams (2002a).
60 No clear practice recommendations have evolved. For diabetic patients who require careful dosing of insulin, serum drug studies before and after a seizure may be done to assess the impact of the seizure on serum glucose. Dosing of insulin is adjusted to avoid symptomatic hypoglycemia.
61 Serum lithium levels warrant monitoring if patients become delirious after the first treatments.
62 Chapter 11. For a review of the synergistic effects of antipsychotic agents and ECT, see Braga and Petrides (2005).
63 Fears of "brain damage" resulting from the electric currents or the induced seizures have been the basis of much research. Cellular pathology, neuropsychology, brain imaging, and brain chemistry methods have been applied and no consistent findings have been demonstrated. Indeed, the evidence is compelling that the changes in these measures are transient, making it remarkable that the changes in mood, thought, and motor behavior persist.

Two models of medical intervention come to mind, that of an acute infection or a deficiency disorder. In acute infection, treatments resolve the illness fully and health is restored. In hormone deficiencies, such as diabetes or hypothyroidism, continuing replacement is necessary.

64 Chapters 11 and 12.
65 Lauritzen *et al.* (1996).
66 Sackeim *et al.* (2001a).
67 Kellner *et al.* (submitted).
68 Karliner and Wehrheim (1965); Fink *et al.* (1996).
69 Fink *et al.* (1996).
70 Petrides *et al.* (1994).
71 Kellner *et al.* (submitted). As the early exit rates were 17% for continuation ECT and 22% for lithium–nortriptyline combination, the overall non-relapse rates were 46%.
72 The clinical experience with continuation ECT appears in case reports and small studies that support the view that continuation ECT is safe, even as to cognitive effects (Aronson, 1987; Fink *et al.*, 1996; Rabheru and Persad, 1997; Fox, 2001).
73 Bourgon and Kellner (2000).
74 Sackeim (1994).
75 Kellner *et al.* (submitted).

10

The validity of the pharmacotherapy literature in melancholia

... my few hours of sleep were usually terminated at three or four in the morning, when I stared up into yawning darkness, wondering and writhing at the devastation taking place in my mind and awaiting the dawn, which usually permitted me a feverish, dreamless nap[1]

Melancholia is a severely debilitating illness with a high death rate and high potential for suicide. Its consequences were so dire that the introduction of even so intrusive a treatment as induced seizures was hailed as a remarkable advance.[2] Over the past half-century, medications effective in ameliorating melancholia were developed and the fears that melancholia engendered in earlier centuries lessened.

Our present therapeutic ideal is to select treatments based on scientific study, defined as evidence-based medicine. Randomized controlled clinical trials form the foundation of evidence-based medicine, and the literature assessing the benefits of antidepressant and mood-stabilizing drugs is widely accepted. Reviews of this evidence conclude that all antidepressant medications have equal efficacy for major depression, differing only in side-effects.[3] These conclusions influence clinical guidelines.[4]

Present teaching, as expressed by an expert National Institutes of Mental Health (NIMH) panel states that: "The SSRIs [selective serotonin reuptake inhibitors] are clearly the drug treatment of choice for all forms of depression in the United States . . . These drugs are approximately equivalent to each other and to TCAs [tricyclic antidepressants] in efficacy . . . The SSRIs have a much more benign side effect profile than TCAs and, largely for this reason, have replaced TCAs as first line therapy."[5] The report cites many studies, but many are severely flawed and the conclusions poorly and selectively presented. For example, a meta-analysis of 105 randomized trials looking at pharmacodynamic differences among antidepressant drugs failed to find a difference in outcome between a pure SSRI or one with broader pharmacologic activity.[6]

Because the tertiary amine TCAs have prominent anticholinergic properties and elicit orthostasis and weight gain, and a lethal dose can be amassed by patients who wish to kill themselves, TCAs are said to be neither safe nor well tolerated.[7] SSRIs are reputed to have few anticholinergic properties and to be better tolerated. It is also more difficult for most patients to amass a lethal dose with these agents, leading to the recommendation that SSRIs are preferred for reasons of safety. This viewpoint encourages more patients to receive SSRIs than the older antidepressants.[8]

Over the past decade, however, the evidence that supports this consensus has been questioned. Industry presented only favorable studies to the public, a practice that has led governments to question the safety and efficacy of antidepressant medications. The methodology of the reports has raised further concern that industry statisticians and authors manipulated the data to present biased conclusions.[9] As a consequence, clinicians are faced with unclear choices.

Case reports and open clinical trials with small samples further muddy the picture. Single samples are reported multiple times, giving the false sense of extensive studies.[10] Individual double-blind, placebo-controlled studies can be misleading, particularly when findings among studies conflict.[11] Focusing on the analyses of pooled data, and whenever possible, data collected under state-of-the-art methodology may minimize the distortions inherent in small trials and single studies, but even meta-analytic investigations do not provide clear conclusions.[12] A meta-analysis of published medication studies in major depression from 1980 to 2002 identified 100 other meta-analytic reviews of randomized controlled antidepressant trials. Many analyses were rejected for critical inadequacies in design, biased subject selection, and ill-defined outcome measures. Using a guideline measure of quality of each study, the average quality score for the 32 remaining publications was calculated to be about 50%, or "barely acceptable." The investigators concluded that the data were too flawed to provide clear recommendations.[13]

Any review of the experimental antidepressant literature is best tempered by clinical experience. From this perspective, the claims advancing the "latest" antidepressant drugs are overstated. For uncomplicated melancholia, pure SSRI medications (e.g., fluoxetine, citalopram) are not optimal. They are only weakly effective in relieving melancholia. They "energize" patients, many of whom are already agitated, disrupt sleep, and inhibit sexual activity. These properties commonly call for the concurrent prescription of anxiolytic and hypnotic medications, raising concerns for the increased risk of suicide.[14]

Secondary amine TCAs (e.g., nortriptyline, desipramine, clomipramine) and other antidepressants with broad pharmacodynamic properties (e.g., venlafaxine, mirtazepine) appear to be preferable. They may achieve better remission rates (60–70% compared to 25–40%) and are well tolerated when matched to the patient's side-effect risk (e.g., the absence of glaucoma or substantial heart disease). What is the evidence for the efficacy of these recommendations in the treatment of melancholia?

Industry influence undermines conclusions about newer agents

Recent studies to assess the activity of psychoactive drugs are commonly designed and funded by a pharmaceutical company in multisite collaborative studies. In one review of 500 randomly selected clinical trials published in "influential" journals between 1981 and 2000, almost two-thirds were identified as industry-connected.[15] These studies are designed to develop the minimal definition of a compound's efficacy, safety, and tolerability to meet government licensing requirements.[16]

The study design, medication dosages, evaluation points, duration of the study, and rating instruments are determined by the sponsor. Scoring of the recorded clinical assessments is often done by the sponsor and not by the investigators, whose roles are often limited to the selection of subjects and the entry assessments.[17] The role of the sponsor, so critical to the design and the assessment, is rarely described in the method section in the published reports. In one survey, only eight of 100 studies identified the role of the industry sponsors.[18] Despite efforts to insure better editor oversight of the reports and implementation of strict guidelines to limit conflict of interest, the results are unclear.[19]

The more severely ill depressed patients, those with suicidal risk, and those in hospital are rarely included in clinical trials of antidepressant drugs. Most participants are outpatients or have been recruited for study by advertisements offering free care under research auspices and they comprise the bulk of the data in the industry-supported studies that are the basis for applications for licensing for marketing.

The more quickly subjects can be recruited and the larger their numbers, the greater is the likelihood the clinical site will continue in the project and maintain its financial support from the sponsor. Standards for subjects to meet criteria for "illness" are minimized to allow the largest number of participants. The volunteers who are elderly or adolescent, have general medical illnesses, or are too severely depressed to be likely to complete an outpatient trial are rejected. Suicidal, psychotic, manic-depressive, stuporous, or catatonic depressed patients are excluded. Depressed patients with alcoholism, drug abuse, and anxiety disorder are typically excluded. Melancholic patients are often too ill for a drug trial or are excluded when placebo is a design feature because they are known to have low placebo response rates. The selection criteria assure that the subjects in most therapeutic drug trials are minimally ill and do not represent the bulk of patients with depressive illness seen in clinical practice. In one survey of 346 outpatients with major depression, only 14% would have been eligible for the typical treatment trial study.[20]

It is now common for the sponsor to maintain and analyze the data from these studies, often with little or no investigator input. When results do not meet expectations, and are deemed unsuitable for a government filing, the data are "sealed" and are not published or available for scrutiny.[21] Data favorable to the sponsor's drug, however, are described in reports, many of which are "ghost-written" by professional writers with the acquiescence of academic investigators as the lead authors. The reports are published in journals receiving substantial advertising support from the company.

Such practices account, in part, for the pattern that drug trials from the USA tend to favor SSRIs while drug trials from other countries tend to favor TCAs.[22] As examples, reports published in 2001 from both print and electronic issues of the *New England Journal of Medicine* and the *Journal of the American Medical Association* were analyzed for author conflict of interest and for industry sponsorship. Almost 40% of authors of drug treatment trials were identified as industry consultants, encouraging an association between the acknowledged consulting relationships and positive reports of the efficacy of the medication marketed by the sponsor.[23] In an assessment of 332 randomized trials from eight "leading" surgical journals and five medical journals, industry funding was also associated with pro-industry findings.[24] An examination of all published articles reporting the "cost-effectiveness" of antidepressant drugs applied contingency table analysis and found that studies of SSRIs sponsored by the manufacturer favored their drug over TCAs more than non-industry-sponsored studies.[25] More disturbing is the finding that, among the authors of highly influential clinical practice guidelines published by psychiatric associations, 81% have industry ties, including research funding and direct compensation as consultants or employees. Such a conflict-of-interest relationship is prohibited for government employees.[26] The global Cochrane Collaboration, a major independent data bank of biomedical research, has also had to address concerns about industry sponsorship of its activities.[27]

The standard of treatment efficacy of a 50% reduction in rating-scale scores rather than remission is a weakened and clinically inadequate endpoint, favoring drugs with only modest efficacy and leaving many subjects who are identified as "responders" still significantly ill.[28] In his review of randomized controlled clinical trials of antidepressants and the data filed with the US Food and Drug Administration to license antidepressant drugs, Parker (2004) found their effects to differ marginally from placebo.[29] Kirsch *et al.* (2002) concluded that the "pharmacologic effects of antidepressants are clinically negligible."

Industry influence on much of the data and the acceptance of marginal efficacy is exacerbated by biased study designs and methods. In one industry-sponsored study of the use of an SSRI in 601 primary care patients, 62% were assessed as receiving adequate treatment, yet only 23% achieved remission and 46% were non-responders.[30] Reviews of clinical trial literature conclude that the lesser standards of response contribute to lingering illness and frequent relapse Remission must be the gold standard to judge efficacy.[31]

Head-to-head comparisons are biased to favor newer drugs

Most head-to-head comparison studies of antidepressants are between newly designed agents and tertiary, not secondary amine TCAs. Compared to secondary amine TCAs, tertiary amines (e.g., imipramine, amitriptyline) have greater muscarinic, histaminic (H_1), and alpha$_1$-adrenergic receptor affinity. They elicit weight gain, sedation, and orthostatic effects. The differences in degree of these side-effects and the numbers of patients affected are clinically meaningful.[32] A more appropriate judgment would be between an SSRI and a secondary amine TCA (e.g., desipramine, nortriptyline).

In a meta-analysis of 115 suitable studies comparing SSRIs and TCAs, however, only one study compared an SSRI to nortriptyline and only six to desipramine.[33] Inspection of the relative risks for dropout from side-effects in these studies shows that the rate from the secondary amines is half or less than that of the tertiary amines, but the conclusion reached is a blanket one for all TCAs as a single drug class.

The Freemantle *et al.* (2000) study is instructive. The authors conclude that their analysis "does not provide evidence that antidepressants acting at more than one pharmacological site differ in efficacy from drugs selective for serotonin reuptake in the treatment of 'major' depression." Their meta-analysis included 105 randomized comparison trials. No study of nortriptyline was included, while there were 12 studies of clomipramine, usually at doses below 100 mg daily. In the nine studies with venlafaxine as the comparison drug, only two prescribed venlafaxine doses of 200 mg or greater, with the remainder at 150 mg or less (often 75 mg). The comparison drug doses in head-to-head studies are typically inadequate for melancholic patients.[34] Sample sizes are also typically too small to show real differences and do not allow analyses of efficacy for the varieties of the depressive illnesses.

Another meta-analysis of comparison studies in elderly depressed patients that met rigorous quality standards defined by the authors concluded that "all antidepressants were equally effective."[35] In the five studies where amitriptyline was the comparison TCA, however, its daily dose is reported as 75, 75, 50–150, 50–100, and 75 mg. One could easily conclude that low-dose amitriptyline has equivalent efficacy to SSRIs. The use of inadequate dosing (e.g., imipramine 75–100 mg daily) in recent studies comparing TCAs to other agents or to placebo is the rule rather than the exception.[36]

The low doses of amitriptyline and other TCAs in these comparison studies is critical. A review of 186 randomized control trials found that amitriptyline had a better recovery rate than any of the alternative drugs, although it was less well tolerated.[37]

Methodology issues

Maintaining "blindness" to avoid observer bias is problematic in head-to-head studies when the comparison is between drugs with either strong or weak anticholinergic effects. Anticholinergic effects are frequent with TCA tertiary amines and are easily detected. An analysis of all clinical trials for depressive disorders reported in the *American Journal of Psychiatry* and in the *Archives of General Psychiatry* between 1996 and 2000 found few studies that adequately documented the number of raters, rater training, assessment of interrater reliability, and rater drift. Of 22 multicenter studies where such methodological concerns are critical, only two reports documented rater training and only three reported interrater reliability, despite the use of up to 20 different raters. Without reliability assessments, the validity of observation is unknowable.[38]

The placebo effect inflates response rates

Another substantive problem is the variability of placebo response rates across studies. Low placebo response rates are associated with neurovegetative features, psychomotor retardation, rapid eye movement (REM) sleep disturbances, thyroid-stimulating hormone blunting to thyroid-releasing hormone, plasma cortisol non-suppression to dexamethasone, and an insidious onset of the depression over three months or longer. These are classic characteristics of melancholia.[39] Placebo responders do not exhibit melancholic features. They often exhibit mood reactivity and a comorbid personality disorder.[40] Response rates are likely to be inflated when such placebo responders are included in medication trials. Further, most head-to-head comparisons do not include a placebo group, so the placebo and drug response rates are unknown. Because severely depressed patients are typically excluded from trials, melancholic patients are less likely to be studied, further blurring differences between the new drugs and TCAs.

The magnitude of the placebo response in a medication trial correlates with the magnitude of effect of a medication. Studies with a large placebo effect show a larger medication effect than do studies with a small placebo effect.[41] Industry-sponsored trials favor "positive" studies so overrating occurs, increasing both the medication effect and the placebo response. To provide a fair assessment of the new agent while at the same time not overinflating its efficacy, a placebo group is essential in any trial. Because patients who respond to placebo are similar to patients who respond to SSRI agents like fluoxetine, the response rates of SSRIs are inflated with placebo responders.[42] This effect becomes particularly important when moderate scores or even low scores on depression-rating scales are accepted for patient selection and samples are recruited in response to advertisements. This practice leads to the inclusion of subjects who are not clinically ill. In one study of persons identified as "depressed" by the Beck Depression Inventory, only 35% of persons with scores 16 or below were identified as depressed by cluster analysis, whereas 86% with scores of 21 or greater were defined as depressed.[43] Some patients with low depression-rating scale scores will report improvement regardless of to which study group they are assigned.

Using a 50% reduction in symptom scores as a criterion of efficacy, rather than remission, and the increasing use of mild to moderately ill subjects to test efficacy decrease the value of recent studies even further. The rates of both placebo and drug responders have increased annually over the past decade.[44] As more and more placebo responders are included in clinical trials, and as the quality of responses is diluted, more study subjects are called "responders" and differences among classes of antidepressants are increasingly masked.

Antidepressant drug efficacy: TCA versus pure SSRI[45]

Meta-analyses of head-to-head studies conclude that the antidepressant efficacy is about equal between SSRIs and TCAs *if the measure is mean reduction in symptom scores.* But one meta-analysis which reached the conclusion of equivalence was only able to assess 11 of 130 studies, rejecting 112 (91.5%) because they were commercially funded, reported small samples, or had critical methodological flaws. Seven other studies were rejected because publications reported the same data twice.[46] The majority of the studies examined for efficacy (7 of 10) found a small advantage for TCAs, but this pattern was not statistically significant. Rather than concluding that the two classes of antidepressants have similar efficacy, however, one could equally conclude that the samples reported were not homogeneous and that efficacy depends on the form of depressive illness under study. Navarro *et al.* (2001), for example, found nortriptyline treatment monitored by plasma levels to be superior to citalopram in a sample of elderly patients with endogenous or psychotic depression. Another meta-analysis of 108 antidepressant drug trials also found the quality uneven and cautioned against generalizing the findings to clinical practice.[47]

Using pooled data for meta-analysis assumes that the subject samples are reasonably homogeneous, but samples of depressed patients gathered for various purposes are regularly shown to be heterogeneous. There is little effort to separate patients by patterns of clinical features, such as melancholia or psychosis. Studies assume subject homogeneity when they report mean changes in symptom severity. There is, however, great likelihood that patient heterogeneity masks heterogeneity of response. As an example, Miller and Freilicher (1995) conducted a retrospective chart review of patients over age 65 hospitalized for major depression, and concluded "SSRIs are equal to TCAs in the treatment of major depression in hospitalized geriatric patients." Fluoxetine and sertraline were compared with desipramine and nortriptyline by calculating dosing equivalents. The SSRI group received (on average) 27 mg fluoxetine while the TCA group received (on average) 145 mg desipramine. Forty-one percent and 39% of each group were considered responders, defined as improvement of at least 20 points in a Global Assessment of Function (GAF) score and an absolute total score above 50 out of 100, indicating adequate self-care or better. One TCA-and two SSRI-treated patients dropped out of the study, each for unacceptable side-effects. However, 35% of the TCA but only 7% of the SSRI groups were psychotic. The investigators dropped these patients from further analysis, and reported equivalent responsiveness between the remaining patients. They dismissed the issue of psychosis by stating that all the psychotic patients were receiving an antipsychotic medication, implying treatment adequacy when none was demonstrated.

Using an alternative naturalistic strategy, Parker *et al.* (1999c) asked 27 Australian psychiatrists to assess the records of 341 non-psychotic depressed patients for the effectiveness of their previous treatments. Electroconvulsive therapy (ECT) was judged highly effective for melancholic and non-melancholic depression. TCAs and monoamine oxidase inhibitors (MAOIs) were rated more effective than SSRIs, venlafaxine, mianserin, and moclobemide for melancholia. Such estimates of efficacy favoring TCAs reflect that the goal of the clinician is to achieve remission, not just to demonstrate that the agent is better than placebo. A similar survey of Australian psychiatrists by Hickie *et al.* (1999) found a consensus that antidepressant drugs are not clinically equivalent. Venlafaxine and high-dose TCAs received the highest ratings for antidepressant efficacy. MAOIs were also considered effective. Venlafaxine was rated the most useful because of its speed of onset, antidepressant effect, and low side-effect burden.

In a review of the literature, an advantage was reported for TCAs over other antidepressants when remission is used as the outcome criterion.[48] Preskorn and associates (Preskorn and Fast, 1991; Preskorn and Burke, 1992) observed that when remission rates rather than percentage change in Hamilton Depression Rating Scale scores are considered, 40–55% of depressed patients remit on SSRIs while 60–70% remit with TCAs, especially when treatment is guided by plasma level monitoring.[49] A number of randomized controlled studies have found this advantage most prominent in melancholic and more severely depressed patients.[50]

In a meta-analysis of controlled trials comparing amitriptyline with other TCAs, heterocyclic antidepressants, and an SSRI, overall efficacy significantly favored amitriptyline.[51] Dropout rates were similar for the groups, but the TCA group had 13% more reported side-effects than the SSRI group. A meta-analysis also found efficacy to favor TCAs dramatically for hospitalized depressed patients, but not for other groups.[52] Hospitalized depressed patients are also more likely to be melancholic.[53] Desipramine was reported to be superior to fluoxetine in the treatment of patients with severe depression.[54] Another report found TCAs superior to SSRIs for melancholic patients.[55] These studies are supported by a meta-analysis that found TCAs more effective than SSRIs in severely depressed and elderly patients[56] A recent comparison of nortriptyline 150 mg daily versus fluoxetine 60 mg daily in a double-blind 6-week trial in moderate to severe depression found the TCA superior. Dropout rates were similar and there were no significant cardiovascular problems with nortriptyline.[57] Three Danish double-blind randomized controlled antidepressant drug trials that included 292 inpatients, most of whom, with melancholia, report clomipramine to be superior to the comparison drug (citalopram, paroxetine, or moclobemide).[58]

In contrast, industry-sponsored studies report SSRIs and TCAs to be equally effective for severe melancholia.[59] A multicenter industry-sponsored study reported nortriptyline and paroxetine to be equally effective in treating depressed outpatients with cardiovascular disease.[60] Higher SSRI doses than typically prescribed may, however, be necessary to treat melancholic patients effectively.[61] The need for additional medication to encourage sleep is also more likely when an SSRI is used rather than a TCA, as SSRIs worsen the sleep of depressed patients.[62] Benzodiazepine use has become routine for patients receiving SSRIs, despite warnings of the dangers of dependence and abuse.[63]

Repetitive reviews by industry-sponsored authors that report no differences in efficacy among classes of antidepressants cloud understanding of the literature unless the reader is prepared to forgo reviews and instead analyze original reports. A review by Burke discussing "selected" randomized double-blind placebo-controlled trials of outpatients with recurrent depressive illness accepts the conclusion of no meaningful difference in efficacy between TCAs and SSRIs.[64] The reviewed studies selected volunteers with modest depressions and reported high placebo rates, low TCA dosing, and reductions in HAMD scores to compare drugs rather than remission rates. Burke also discusses the Geddes *et al.* (2000) Cochrane analysis of head-to-head TCA and SSRI studies and dismisses the clear TCA advantage for hospitalized patients as due "merely to chance." The Danish University Antidepressant Group's finding that clomipramine was superior to paroxetine and citalopram for inpatients is often cited.[65] Most of the patients were identified as having endogenous depression, and clomipramine's greater benefit is ascribed to its sedating properties and not to its antidepressant effects. Burke also challenges the idea that venlafaxine as representative of a "dual-action" neurotransmitter reuptake inhibitor is more effective as an antidepressant than pure SSRIs. The same literature flaws ignored in the TCA versus SSRI studies are used to reject studies that report advantages for venlafaxine, while studies that report no efficacy differences between venlafaxine and an SSRI are accepted despite venlafaxine often being prescribed in minimally effective dosages.

Table 10.1. Tricyclic antidepressant-responsive depressed patients

Neurovegetative signs present (anorexia, weight loss, amenorrhea, poor sleep quality with loss of deep sleep)
Diurnal mood variation (worse in the morning)
Unremitting, apprehensive mood with ruminations, often expressed as self-blame
Psychomotor retardation
Agitation
Insidious onset (weeks to a month or two)

The choice of antidepressant in persons whose mood disorder is complicated by a general medical or neurologic condition is discussed in Chapter 12. Although SSRIs are proffered as the treatments of choice, some studies report TCAs to be more effective than SSRIs in the treatment of patients with complicated conditions.[66] Nortriptyline is reported to be superior to fluoxetine in treating melancholic elderly patients with cardiovascular disease, precisely the patients who are said not to tolerate a TCA but who are thought to respond best to an SSRI.[67]

Another report finds nortriptyline up to 100 mg daily to be superior to fluoxetine up to 40 mg daily in the treatment of depression in post-stroke patients.[68] Success rates measured by the fall in Hamilton Rating Scale scores were 77% for nortriptyline, 14% for fluoxetine, and 31% for placebo. Fluoxetine was accompanied by unwanted and substantial weight loss (average 8% of body weight). Average age for these patients was in their mid-60s, but, contrary to accepted ideas about tolerance, the dropout rate in the fluoxetine group was three times that of the nortriptyline group.[69] The characteristics of depressed patients who are particularly responsive to TCAs are cited in Table 10.1. Melancholic patients with a premorbid personality disorder or who have a psychotic depression are less likely to respond to TCAs.[70]

Antidepressant drug efficacy: pure SSRIs compared to non-TCA agents

Non-TCA antidepressant medications are not equal in efficacy. The literature assessing these drugs against placebo and head-to-head, however, is plagued by the same problems detailed above. Most are industry-sponsored multisite studies. Careful reading finds that the broader the pharmacodynamic effects of the agent, the more effective it is for melancholia. The magnitude of this effect is not clear, however, because placebo groups are rarely included and, when they are, placebo improvement rates are high. Nevertheless, in a randomized, double-blind comparison of fluoxetine (20–40 mg daily) and sertraline (100–150 mg daily) in 286 outpatients, sertraline elicited substantially better outcomes among patients with melancholic features and psychomotor retardation, and was better for the more severely ill patients with lower anxiety. It was also superior to fluoxetine in inducing sleep, minimizing weight loss, and improving cognition.[71]

In a 6-week random assignment study in depressed inpatients and outpatients, mirtazepine was as effective and as well tolerated as fluoxetine.[72] A meta-analysis concluded that mirtazepine may elicit some benefit in severely ill patients, both in and out of hospital.[73]

Venlafaxine has been reported to be useful in relieving major depression.[74] The efficacy is not greater than high-dose fluoxetine.[75] The same efficacy may be true for nefazodone.[76] The overall evidence, however, favors venlafaxine over more specific SSRIs in head-to-head studies and in patients unresponsive to SSRIs.[77] In a literature review of multisite studies, venlafaxine achieved as high remission rates as comparison medications.[78] Another review reported venlafaxine equivalent to TCAs in reducing symptom scores.[79] A meta-analysis of studies including over 2000 patients 18–83 years old reported venlafaxine to be superior to pure SSRIs (50% versus 35% 8-week remission rates) and to be faster in therapeutic onset. Men and women improved equally well with venlafaxine, and it was well tolerated.[80] Another meta-analysis is consistent with these findings.[81] A pooled analysis of 1454 outpatients from five double-blind randomized studies found the 6-week efficacy of venlafaxine and fluoxetine to be superior to placebo in reducing depression, with the onset of the effects of venlafaxine earlier than that of fluoxetine.[82] The authors report a reduction in anxiety scores of venlafaxine as a major influence on outcome and suggest that its benefits in anxiety may explain its superiority over fluoxetine. Another meta-analysis of randomized trials found venlafaxine to be superior to pure SSRIs (20 studies), but not to TCAs (seven studies) in achieving remission.[83] Venlafaxine is also reported to prevent relapse in the 12 months following remission for depression.[84]

Venlafaxine is well tolerated in elderly patients, with the added advantage of being only a weak inhibitor of cytochrome P450 liver enzyme systems and therefore less likely to induce drug–drug interactions in this age group, who are often exposed to multiple medications. Hypertension was uncommon (about 1.5% of patients) and only occurred at doses above 150 mg daily.[85] A meta-analysis of venlafaxine's effects on blood pressure in 3744 patients concluded that the effect was dose-dependent above 300 mg daily and "should not deter first-line use of this effective antidepressant."[86]

Side-effects

No medicine is without side-effects. Matching the likely side-effects to the patient's tolerance is standard practice. A hypertensive patient with a moderate to severe melancholia and likely to require high-dose treatment might not be a candidate for venlafaxine. Medications with pronounced anticholinergic properties should be avoided in patients with narrow-angle glaucoma or Alzheimer's disease, so paroxetine and TCAs would not be suitable choices for these patients.[87]

Sleep is typically disturbed in depressed patients. Sleep electroencephalogram (EEG) abnormalities, particularly elevated REM density, are sensitive indicators of depression.[88] Poor sleep in a depressed person is a predictor of self-harm.[89] TCAs are potent REM sleep suppressors, prolonging REM latency and decreasing total amount of REM sleep time, enhancing sleep efficiency. MAOIs also suppress REM sleep in depressed patients. Fluoxetine and other SSRIs increase REM latency but have minimal effect

Table 10.2. Co-occurring conditions affecting antidepressant choice

Condition	Considerations
Risk of bleeding	SSRIs deplete platelet serotonin, increasing risk of gastrointestinal bleeding three- to fourfold[a]
Dehydration, risk of hyponatremia	SSRIs induce hyponatremia, increasing the risk of delirium, catatonia, and psychosis, leading to the mistaken prescription of antipsychotics[b]
Basal ganglia disease	SSRIs elicit dystonia and may worsen Parkinson's disease[c]
Insulin-dependent diabetes	TCAs interfere with insulin utilization and blood glucose control. They worsen glaucoma
Alzheimer's disease	Early treatment tries to enhance cholinergic brain function. Using any drug with anticholinergic properties is counterproductive
Cardiovascular disease	Anticholinergic properties of TCAs interfere with vagal tone, reducing heart rate variability and increasing the risk for adverse cardiac events in patients with pre-existing heart disease. SSRIs increase vagal tone and may be protective in such patients. They reduce platelet agglutination.[d]

Notes:

[a] In a Danish study of over 26 000 adults taking antidepressants, the use of pure SSRIs increased the risk of a gastrointestinal bleed 3.6 times. Concomitant use of a nonsteroidal anti-inflammatory agent increased the risk 12.2 times. Antidepressants like venlafaxine and mirtazepine increased the risk 2.3 times. Drugs without the serotonin transporter action showed no increased risk (Dalton *et al.*, 2003).

[b] *Psychiatry Drug Alerts*, August 2002, p. 59.

[c] Richard and Kurlan (1997); *Psychiatry Drug Alerts*, August 2002, p. 61.

[d] Chapter 12 provides references and a discussion.

on total REM time. They also increase stage 1 (light) sleep and increase awakenings. Sleep efficiency is significantly decreased.[90] Trazodone and nefazodone increase sleep efficiency.[91] Thus, it is now common practice to combine SSRI treatment with a hypnotic in hopes of avoiding their adverse effects on sleep architecture.[92]

Table 10.2 lists the more important concerns as to side-effects. General medical and neurologic co-occurring conditions also put patients at increased side-effect risk from certain antidepressants.[93]

Conclusions

For patients with uncomplicated melancholia, the evidence for efficacy indicates that TCAs, not SSRIs, are the first-choice agents. SSRIs are weak antimelancholic agents and rarely achieve remission. Their energizing effects increase agitation and anxiety in melancholia and degrade sleep. Additional medications are commonly needed to counter their activating and sleep-disrupting properties.[94] Secondary amine TCAs, specifically nortriptyline and desipramine, have modest side-effects and are more effective in melancholia, particularly when dosing is guided by plasma monitoring.[95] Venlafaxine and mirtazepine may have minimal advantages in efficacy and safety over pure SSRI drugs. Paroxetine and sertraline in high doses may be useful choices in patients with cardiovascular disease.

NOTES

1 Styron (1990) p. 449.
2 Chapter 9 presents the history of the impact of convulsive therapies on the death rates for melancholia.
3 Anderson and Tomenson (1994); Perry *et al.* (1997); Tollefson and Rosenbaum (1998).
4 Depression Guideline Panel (1993).
5 Tamminga *et al.* (2002).
6 Freemantle *et al.* (2000).
7 We use the well-recognized acronym *TCA*, tricyclic antidepressant, as a categorical term for the older antidepressant agents such as imipramine, amitriptyline, and nortriptyline.
8 Sclar *et al.* (1998).
9 Healy (1997, 2004); Gelman (1999); Angell (2004); Medawar and Hardon (2004).
10 Melander *et al.* (2003).
11 Many studies detailed here and in Chapters 11 and 12 illustrate the limitations of randomized controlled trials.
12 Casacalenda *et al.* (2002); Jainer and Chawala (2003); Rifkin (2003).
13 Hemels *et al.* (2004).
14 One industry study reported no advantage for using a "sedating" antidepressant rather than the company's antidepressant (Tollefson *et al.* 1994a).
15 Buchkowsky and Jewesson (2004).
16 Reports of the flaws in present drug evaluation were prominent in the news in 2003 and 2004. See Healy (1997, 2004); Angell (2004); Medawar and Hardon (2004).
17 Safer (2002).
18 Gross *et al.* (2003).
19 Vanderbroucke (2002). Contract payment for the work is based on the submission of the completed schedule forms for each patient visit. Bonuses are paid for completion of all the patient's scheduled records.
20 Zimmerman *et al.* (2002).
21 In a randomized controlled trial sponsored by Pfizer of hospitalized depressed patients assigned to sertraline, imipramine, or placebo, the data were sealed and the investigators were not given access to the code defining which patients in their site had received which medication (Fink, 2002a). The ostensible reason given was that the records were incomplete, but the investigators remained concerned that the company's decision was because the company's agent, sertraline, was not distinguishable from placebo, or that the imipramine was found superior.
22 Bech *et al.* (2000).

23 Friedman and Richter (2004).
24 Bhandari *et al.* (2004).
25 Baker *et al.* (2003).
26 Choudhry *et al.* (2002).
27 Moynihan (2003).
28 Melander *et al.* (2003).
29 Hickie (2004) criticized Parker's review and suggests that real-world clinical experience supports the efficacy of the newer antidepressants.
30 Corey-Lisle *et al.* (2004).
31 Keller (2004).
32 Potter *et al.* (1991); Preskorn and Burke (1992).
33 Anderson (2000).
34 To achieve maximum benefit, antidepressant drugs often need to be prescribed at the higher end of their dose range. In the treatment of melancholic patients, clomipramine typically needs to be prescribed in doses of 200 mg daily while 300–400 mg of venlafaxine is required.
35 Menting *et al.* (1996).
36 In a recent meta-analysis, Furukawa *et al.* (2002) examined 41 studies and found low-dose TCAs to be better than placebo. They were unable, however, to determine the minimal effective dose or to establish a dose–response curve.
37 Barbui and Hotopf (2001).
38 Mulsant *et al.* (2002).
39 Nelson *et al.* (1990).
40 Rabkin *et al.* (1987); Elkin *et al.* (1989).
41 Khan *et al.* (2003a) examined the literature from 1985 through 1998 as well as Food and Drug Administration-reviewed but unpublished studies. Over 9000 patients were included in the treatment trials assessed. Among placebo patients there was a 30% drop in Hamilton Rating Scale scores, compared to 42% drops for the new antidepressant drug being studied and the competitors.
42 Ackerman *et al.* (1997).
43 Cox *et al.* (2001).
44 Walsh *et al.* (2002).
45 The discussion that follows applies to the treatment of adult patients. In treatment trials of preteen children with depression, TCAs are reported to be ineffective (Maneeton and Srisurapanont, 2000). Chapter 12 discusses the antidepressant literature in young persons.
46 MacGillivray *et al.* (2003).
47 Anderson (2001).
48 Thase (2003).
49 Preskorn and Fast (1991); Preskorn and Burke (1992). Remission rates for other pharmacodynamically narrow agents are also low, e.g., buproprion 47% (Thase *et al.*, 2005); duloxetine 44% (Mallinckrodt *et al.*, 2005).
50 Danish University Antidepressant Group (1986, 1990, 1993); Vestergaard *et al.* (1993); Roose *et al.* (1994); Perry (1996); Nobler and Roose (1998); Bagby *et al.* (2002).
51 Barbui and Hotopf (2001).
52 Anderson (2000).
53 Danish University Antidepressant Group (1999).
54 Schatzberg (1998).

55 Perry (1996).
56 Anderson and Tomenson (1994).
57 Akhondzadeh *et al.* (2003).
58 Hildebrandt *et al.* (2003).
59 Pande and Sayler (1993); Hirschfeld (1999).
60 Nelson *et al.* (1999).
61 Dunner and Dunbar (1992).
62 Armitage (2000); Clark and Alexander (2000). The Armitage review found that TCAs generally suppress REM sleep and prolong REM latency. Clomipramine, however, acts more like an SSRI. SSRIs increase wakefulness and decrease sleep efficiency. MAOIs may also decrease sleep efficiency while suppressing REM.
63 Uhlenhuth *et al.* (1999).
64 Burke (2004), discussing the report by Walsh *et al.* (2002). Burke is on the board of directors of Forest Laboratories, Pfizer, and Cyberonics and receives support from Forest, Lilly, GlaxoSmithKline, Merck, and Cyberonics. His review derives from a symposium supported by Forest Laboratories.
65 Danish University Antidepressant Group (1986).
66 Tamminga *et al.* (2002).
67 Roose *et al.* (1994).
68 Robinson *et al.* (2000).
69 Andersen *et al.* (1994) found citalopram, a pure SSRI, to be more effective than placebo for patients who develop depressive features immediately post-stroke but not for depressive illnesses that developed after seven weeks post-stroke.
70 Nelson *et al.* (1994).
71 Flament *et al.* (1999).
72 Wheatley *et al.* (1998).
73 Kasper (1995); see also Carpenter *et al.* (2002).
74 Guelfi *et al.* (1995).
75 Clerc *et al.* (1994); Costa e Silva (1998).
76 Baldwin *et al.* (1996).
77 Nierenberg *et al.* (1994); de Montigny *et al.* (1995); Dierick *et al.* (1996); Poirier and Boyer (1999); Thase *et al.* (2001a); Kaplan (2002); Mbaya (2002). Saiz-Ruiz *et al.* (2002) Shelton (2004).
78 Rudolph (2002).
79 Wong and Bymaster (2002).
80 Entsuah *et al.* (2001).
81 Stahl *et al.* (2002).
82 Davidson *et al.* (2002).
83 Smith *et al.* (2002a).
84 Montgomery *et al.* (2004).
85 Staab and Evans (2000).
86 Thase (1998).
87 A full discussion of psychopharmacology is beyond the scope of this book. For details of side-effects and risks, see Stahl (2000).
88 Benca *et al.* (1992); Brunello *et al.* (2000).
89 Wolfersdorf *et al.* (1990).
90 Keck *et al.* (1991); Armitage *et al.* (1997a, b).

91 Brunello *et al.* (2000).
92 Lian (1997).
93 Chapter 12 discusses the use of antidepressants in patients with co-occurring general medical or neurologic disease.
94 A report that SSRIs induce melancholia has not been replicated (Swartz and Guadagno, 1998). Reports that pure SSRIs are associated with an increased risk of suicide await systematic study (Vorstman *et al.*, 2001; King *et al.*, 1991; Mann and Kapur, 1991). The association is discussed in Chapter 7.
95 Preskorn and Fast (1991). More patients complain about the sexual side-effects of SSRIs than they do about the anticholinergic side-effects of TCAs. The therapeutics of using a TCA when the patient is a suicide risk is discussed in Chapter 7.

11

Basic pharmacotherapy for melancholic patients

I, who have always seen him so serene, so completely the master of his wonderful emotional instrument . . . so sensitive to human contacts and yet so secure from them; I could hardly believe it was the same James who cried out to me his fear, his despair, his craving for the "cessation of consciousness," and all his unspeakable loneliness and need of comfort, and inability to be comforted! "Not to wake – not to wake –" that was his refrain; "and then one does wake, and one looks again into the blackness of life, and everything ministers to it."[1]

Among the interventions for the relief of melancholia, electroconvulsive therapy (ECT) is the most effective and should be considered in the treatment of every melancholic patient.[2] Although superior to medications in the treatment of depressive illness, ECT is intrusive, not widely available, and most psychiatrists are not trained to prescribe or administer it.[3] ECT has been so stigmatized that it is widely considered the treatment of last resort. The cost per treatment is substantial.[4] The efficacy and optimal use of ECT are discussed in Chapters 8 and 9.

Melancholia is an illness that requires *acute treatment* to resolve the episode of depression, *continuation treatment* to preserve the remission and prevent relapse, and *long-term treatment* to reduce the risk of recurrence.

The basic pharmacotherapy for adult melancholic patients in uncomplicated circumstances warrants simplified algorithms. Seeking to evaluate the efficacy of various treatments for melancholia is difficult, however, as melancholia has not been recognized in the principal classifications in use during the introduction of the newer antidepressant agents. Because melancholic patients are frequently hospitalized for recurrent episodes of illness, the recommendations that follow stress the value of medication found most effective in depressed patients characterized as "severely ill" or in a hospital setting. The efficacy of newer agents has been primarily examined in outpatients or in volunteers.

Secondary amine tricyclic antidepressants (TCAs, such as desipramine, nortriptyline, and protriptyline) are first choices for melancholic patients. Tertiary amine TCAs (amitriptyline, imipramine) benefit patients equally, but their prescription is limited by greater anticholinergic effects and toxicity of overdose. Among newer agents, the evidence is sparse but venlafaxine and, perhaps, mirtazepine may be alternatives for melancholia. Augmenting these medications with lithium and the concurrent use of monoamine oxidase inhibitors (MAOIs) are other useful options.

Table 11.1. Treatment setting: inpatient or outpatient?

Factor	Implication
Suicide risk	Err on the side of safety. Persons with expressed risk require hospitalization. If the risk is deemed moderate or less, hospitalization may be avoided if around-the-clock home supervision is available
Level of functioning	Stupor, catatonia, severe bradykinesia and bradyphrenia, psychosis, or cognitive impairment that disables the patient from meeting responsibilities or providing adequate self-care is the basis for hospitalization
Polypharmacy	Many depressed patients receive multiple medications that may do more harm than good. Hospitalization offers the opportunity to detoxify such patients, especially the elderly
Treatment needs	ECT is usually begun when the patient is hospitalized
Health risks	Serious general medical problems worsen when a person is depressed. Hospitalization allows stabilization of the co-occurring illnesses and treatment of the mood disorder

Acute treatment

The goal is remission

The successful treatment of melancholic patients requires optimistic and aggressive therapeutics. Treatment choice is based on the balance between the likely benefit and the probability of severe side-effects. Selecting treatments primarily for their favorable side-effect profiles rather than strong efficacy is overly defensive.[5] The most effective treatments should be considered first, and from among these, the safest and most practical chosen. Because the goal of acute treatment is remission, the efficacy of any approach is defined by remission rates and not by lesser standards.[6] Patients who obtain only a partial response and remain dysfunctional are prone to relapse.[7]

The first decision in the care of the melancholic patient is to offer continuous protection in the hospital or at home. The factors determining the venue for treatment are summarized in Table 11.1.

Rapid response is the goal

The broad array of available antidepressant and mood-stabilizing drugs that are slow in effective onset encourages multiple single-drug trials and combination trials, resulting in a prolonged "acute" treatment course, often without remission. The therapeutic yield, however, maximal with the first medication, progressively diminishes with successive trials. The longer patients remain ill, the greater the social and economic losses, the more depressive episodes they are likely to suffer, the more "treatment-resistant" they are likely to become, and the more neurotoxic will be the effect of their illness. Rapid treatment that results in remission shortens the duration

Table 11.2. Planning acute treatment for a melancholic patient

Factor	Some treatment implications
Type of depression	Melancholia responds to pharmacodynamically broad-spectrum antidepressants and to ECT
Polarity of the depression	Depressed manic-depressive patients may require a mood stabilizer combined with an antidepressant agent, or require ECT
Severity of the depression	Psychosis, stupor, catatonia, dehydration, or suicide risk requires hospitalization
Co-occurring conditions	Alcohol and illicit drug abuse are the basis for non-compliance. Some general medical (e.g., insulin-dependent diabetes) and some neurologic (e.g., basal ganglia disease) conditions may be exacerbated by antidepressants (TCAs affect insulin utilization; sertraline elicits dystonia). Some general medical conditions interfere with responsiveness (e.g., hypothyroidism) or the drug's pharmacokinetics (e.g., liver disease)
Demographics	Age and gender impact drug pharmacokinetics and pharmacodynamics
Personality traits	Personality traits affect compliance (e.g., impulsive persons do not tolerate even modest side-effects and require rapid relief of symptoms to be compliant)
Environment	Depressed outpatients should be in a weapon-free environment with friend or family support. Patients must be able to afford their medication to be compliant
Point in illness course	Number of previous episodes and pattern of episodes (e.g., stable or increasing frequency) determine the need for long-term treatment. The tolerability and efficacy of previous treatments influence treatment choices for the present episode

of the next episode when it occurs.[8] If the first antidepressant medication is effective, the response is seen within two weeks and remission is achieved within eight weeks.[9] After two unsuccessful drug treatment trials, however, any additional yield drops precipitously and ECT becomes the treatment of choice for the melancholic patient, even if the severity of the melancholia does not in itself warrant hospitalization.[10] Depressed patients who fail two medication trials are frequently labeled as "treatment-resistant." Yet among these patients, 50% or more remit with ECT within 2–3 weeks.[11] Among psychotic depressed patients, the remission rates are higher and occur earlier.[12]

The success of acute treatment also depends on the thoroughness of the evaluation. Table 11.2 summarizes factors affecting management choices.

The first weeks of treatment are critical. If the first-choice medication is not quickly effective, the likelihood of eventual remission with that medication is reduced. In assessing pooled data, patients who fail to have a 20% or more deduction in symptoms within four weeks have only a 4% chance of substantial further improvement.[13] Switching to a different antidepressant or augmenting with a second agent provides modest benefit for patients who did not respond to the first medication. In a review of 24 analyzable investigations from 1986 to 2001 assessing augmenting an antidepressant medication with additional agents, 62% of non-psychotic patients ultimately responded.[14] This rate is not substantially different from those achieved with a single original TCA at maximum dose for a sufficient length of time.

Switching from one drug class to another is reported to be beneficial in up to 30% of patients who did not respond within 12 weeks of either moderately dosed imipramine (150 mg) or sertraline (50 mg).[15] When the second agent was prescribed, the dose was maximized. This study presents no evidence, however, that similar results could not have been achieved by simply increasing the dose of the initial medication. Other authors conclude that augmenting a first choice or switching to a second choice are equivalent in therapeutic yield and that if one approach does not work there is little merit in trying the other.[16] The practice of switching to yet a third medication or adding more agents has even less support.

If the first-choice medication is chosen with care, improvement in sleep usually occurs within 10 days. Appetite also improves. Because unpleasant side-effects may occur as doses are increased, the first weeks are critical for compliance, and every effort must be made to insure the patient's cooperation. Frequent telephone contacts (*phone rounds*) during the early weeks of treatment are helpful.[17] During these calls, symptoms and side-effects are reviewed and dosing changes initiated. Suicide thoughts are assessed, and patient and family concerns are addressed. Feelings of isolation and "going it alone" are minimized. When customary side-effects occur (e.g., dry mouth with TCAs), the patient and family are assured that these effects are expected and are "good signs," indicating the medication is beginning to "do its job." If side-effects are substantial or suicide risk is increased, proper decisions can be made.[18]

Dosing of many newer antidepressants is usually started at the lower end of their therapeutic dosing range. Some clinicians incorrectly assume that these lower doses are sufficient. Melancholic patients who respond to antidepressants do so at the higher end of their therapeutic range. In 285 depressed subjects treated in the National Institutes of Mental Health (NIMH) collaborative depression study, re-examined over 20 years, and who had at least one additional episode of depression during the follow-up, those who initially received higher antidepressant doses were more likely to remit and not to relapse. Those who received lower initial doses were no more likely to recover than those who received no somatic treatment.[19]

Limiting augmentation and switching drug trials

Augmenting the first-choice antidepressant is justified if the patient remains clinically ill. Using a rating scale to quantify severity, more than a 33% but less than a 75% decrease from the pretreatment score suggests augmentation is needed if the patient has received 3 weeks of maximum dosing (often 8–12 weeks into the treatment trial) and the patient's rating-scale score remains in the illness range (typically above 8 for the HAMD).

Switching to a different class of antidepressant medication is justified if there is no meaningful improvement with the first-choice medication at maximum dose for several weeks (e.g., a depression-scale score dropping less than a third from baseline).[20] If meaningful improvement has not occurred with the first-choice medication, the yield is low with the second. There is also an increased risk of relapse with only a partial response.[21] Thus, offering ECT at this point is preferable but not always available.[22]

When switching to another antidepressant agent, broader pharmacodynamic spectrum agents (e.g., TCAs, venlafaxine, mirtazepine) are still preferable as the data favor these medications in the treatment of melancholia. If augmentation of the first-choice antidepressant is considered, the data and clinical experience favor lithium.

Augmentation with lithium

Results from double-blind, placebo-controlled studies are mixed.[23] Lithium in adequate doses has modest to moderate antidepressant effects when added to an antidepressant medication.[24] Melancholic patients benefit most from lithium augmentation, 57% of patients responding compared to 25% of non-melancholic patients.[25] One study found that patients with a "hypersensitive" adrenal response as measured by dexamethasone and corticotropin-releasing hormone challenge were less likely to respond to lithium augmentation.[26] The response was interpreted as reflecting chronicity.

Melancholic patients who suffer recurrent depressions or who have both manic and depressive episodes have similar response rates. Doses that achieve lithium blood levels of 0.5–0.7 mg/L are adequate, with levels above 0.7 mg/L rarely providing additional symptom relief.[27]

Improvement is typically seen within several weeks and, if no response is obtained, continued lithium augmentation is unlikely to be of benefit. If lithium augmentation is effective, some authors recommend that treatment should be continued for at least one year.[28] Maintenance lithium therapy has long-term benefit in preventing future depressive episodes, even in patients without a history of mania or hypomania.[29]

Augmenting antidepressant medication with lithium, however, may be no better than maximizing the dose of the first-choice antidepressant. In a study of partial responders to various antidepressants, 33% improved further when lithium was added while 50% improved further by maximizing the dose of the original antidepressant alone. Among non-responders, about 20% benefited from the addition of lithium while 35% responded to maximizing the antidepressant dose. Dropout rates were similar for all groups.[30]

In studies that report a benefit in lithium augmentation, the therapeutic yield is modest. In one study in which lithium was added to desipramine, 65% responded to desipramine alone while 75% responded to the combination.[31] In all, 11 double-blind controlled trials of lithium augmentation are reported with an additional 50% of patients responding to augmentation.

While most augmentation trials have added lithium to a TCA, several trials have added lithium to a selective serotonin reuptake inhibitor (SSRI), and case reports describe the results of its addition to an MAOI. Although treatment advantages differ in the selection of the first-choice medication, no therapeutic advantage is gained to which agent lithium is added. Adverse effects from lithium–TCA combinations do not differ from those that occur when the two classes of medications are used alone. Weight gain and tremor are the most common troubling side-effects. Adverse effects with a lithium–MAOI combination are also no different from those that occur when the two agents are used alone. Combining lithium with an SSRI increases the risk for a toxic serotonin syndrome.[32] When lithium augmentation is anticipated for the melancholic patient, it is better to select a non-SSRI antidepressant as the first-choice medication.

Other augmentation options

Although several other agents are reported to enhance the effect of the first-choice antidepressant, the data supporting these options are weak. The benefit of adding thyroid or pindolol is unproven. They may accelerate the response rather than augment a partial response. Adding stimulants is limited to patients with apathetic syndromes misidentified as depressive mood disorder. Adding an MAOI to a TCA may increase the benefit, but other antidepressant medication combinations are no better than maximizing a first-choice agent. The addition of an antipsychotic in the treatment of a non-psychotic melancholic patient has few supporting data, but adds the risk for the acute and long-term adverse effects of antipsychotic agents. Thus, if lithium augmentation is not helpful or its use is contraindicated, additional augmentation trials provide little benefit but will probably prolong illness. ECT is a better option. If not available, switching to a different class of antidepressant medication would be the next step.

Triiodothyronine (T_3) (25–37.5 μg daily) affects thyroid functions more rapidly than does thyroxine (T_4).[33] For some patients T_3 may correct subclinical hypothyroidism.[34] T_3 has been added to TCAs, MAOIs, and SSRIs without adverse reactions. Meta-analyses indicate a clinically meaningful effect only in women: T_3 accelerates the antidepressant response rather than providing a better therapeutic yield.[35] The effect, however, is clinically no more meaningful than lithium augmentation.[36] A positive effect is reported to occur within 2–3 weeks. When improvement is seen, dosing is continued until maximum benefit is achieved or two months have elapsed. T_3 at that point is slowly tapered and then stopped. T_3 is not recommended for elderly patients with cardiac insufficiency.[37]

Pindolol, a beta-blocker with 5-HT_{1A} autoreceptor antagonistic properties, has been tested in the enhancement of the effects of SSRIs in double-blind, placebo-controlled studies. No efficacy is demonstrated.[38]

Stimulants (e.g., methylphenidate 10–40 mg daily; dextroamphetamine 5–20 mg daily) *and related agents* (bromocriptine) added to an antidepressant have minimal benefit for melancholic patients.[39] No proper experimental studies support the use of stimulants as augmenting agents. Two double-blind studies report that bromocriptine has an equivalent antidepressant effect as imipramine and amitriptyline.[40] This claim is unlikely and any effect is due to relief of symptoms of apathy not depression.

Two antidepressants given simultaneously is a strategy that began in the early 1960s as MAOIs were added to a TCA. The MAOI is introduced after the TCA dosage has been maximized and a partial response achieved. Reversing the sequence and adding a TCA to a MAOI is not done because that sequence may precipitate a hypertensive crisis. Patients with anxiety disorder and depressed mood, depressive illness comorbid with somatization disorders and cluster B personality traits, or atypical depressive features are reported to have some benefit from this combination.[41]

Recent claims that other antidepressant combinations are better than one antidepressant alone have weak support and most studies are industry-sponsored. A 15-year Medline review identified 27 studies with adequate methodology that examined 667 patients. No combination was clearly best and the overall response to any combination was 62% in patients who had previously not recovered with the first medication.[42] A life-threatening toxic serotonin syndrome has also been reported with SSRI combinations.[43] Delirium and grand mal seizures have been reported with several combinations.[44] Thus, the risks outweigh the benefits of combining antidepressants, with the possible exception of adding an MAOI to a TCA.

Antipsychotic medications added to an antidepressant are claimed to benefit both psychotic and non-psychotic patients.[45] In a multicenter, industry-supported, outpatient study, low-dose olanzapine (10 mg or less daily) and risperidone (2 mg daily) were reported to be effective adjuncts to antidepressants and mood stabilizers, with response beginning rapidly and full remission seen in some patients.[46] The sedating properties of olanzapine that may encourage sleep and reduce anxiety may explain its claimed antidepressant effect. An open multicenter clinical trial involving 560 depressed outpatients who received an olanzapine–fluoxetine combination for 76 weeks reported a mean decrease in the MADRS scores of about two-thirds, with 56% of patients remitting.[47] No placebo or comparison treatment group was included, and the initial one-third drop in mean scores by one week suggests that the benefit was in the relief of insomnia and anxiety rather than of depressed mood. Half the patients remitted after about 18 months, which is the natural course for melancholia.

A reduction of depressive features in schizophrenic patients provides the primary support for the use of risperidone in depressed patients.[48] An unlikely 70% remission rate was reported in an open trial of a risperidone–fluvoxamine combination in outpatients.[49] Combinations of SSRIs and antipsychotic drugs, however, increase the risks for delirium and severe movement disorders.[50] The evidence is weak that antipsychotic agents provide enough benefit for non- psychotic depressed patients to outweigh their risks.[51]

Switching antidepressants

Switching from one antidepressant agent to another is considered if the first-choice medication has had no effect. Augmentation with a second agent is only useful if the first agent has had a measurable benefit. The half-lives of the two agents and the liver enzyme systems that metabolize them shape the merits and speed of the switch.[52] Before switching, discontinuation of MAOIs and a washout period are required before the second agent is introduced. For other classes of antidepressant agents, switching within the class is usually done in a direct substitution, medication A being stopped abruptly and medication B beginning immediately in its usual starting dose.

Many authors recommend that a switch should be to an agent with a different pharmacodynamic profile.[53] Up to 65% of patients unresponsive to the first antidepressant are reported to respond subsequently to the second antidepressant.[54] As these studies rarely consider the type of depressive mood disorder and do not take melancholia into account, there is little evidence that switching resolves the illness of patients with moderate to severe melancholia who have failed an adequate trial with a TCA.

Combining drugs and psychotherapy

It is a daunting task to assess the efficacy of the psychotherapies in relieving mood disorders. So many different therapeutic maneuvers are offered as individual treatments and as concurrent interventions. The multiplicity of disorders in which psychotherapy has been proffered makes the literature difficult to assess. The prevailing belief is that combining psychotherapy and medication is more effective than either treatment alone.[55] Yet, some authors assess the claims for efficacy, even for depressive disorders of modest severity, as overstated and that psychotherapy should not be applied indiscriminately to what is a clinically heterogeneous condition.[56] About 50% of patients with mild to moderate non-melancholic depression with features of anxiety disorder or anxious-fearful personality traits are reported to benefit from *cognitive-behavior therapy* or *interpersonal therapy*.[57] These patients are similar to those in drug trials who respond to "placebo."[58] A benefit was reported for psychotherapy in women with depressive mood during pregnancy in an open, uncontrolled trial.[59]

One review found no advantage for any psychotherapy approach, although the evidence for efficacy was weakest for brief dynamic therapy.[60] A large 6-month randomized trial of psychodynamic supportive therapy and antidepressants found no objective benefit for the addition of verbal therapy, although patients perceived a benefit.[61]

The addition of psychotherapy to pharmacotherapy is thought to benefit patients who have had *only a partial response* to medication.[62] It may improve social adjustment in older depressed patients.[63] This effect, however, is not seen in persons *who have remitted*.[64] An assessment of interpersonal therapy during maintenance treatment in outpatients reported that once-monthly psychotherapy sessions in addition to adequate doses of imipramine lengthened the times between episodes and improved overall survival time.[65] The intervention probably reinforced medication compliance.[66] In a 2-year follow-up of 83 depressed women receiving interpersonal psychotherapy, some benefit in their responses to stress is reported, although severity of depression was modest and the form of depression is not reported.[67]

Although supportive reassuring comments, counseling, education, and empathic listening are helpful during the acute treatment of a melancholic patient, probing and intense psychotherapy makes these patients more anxious and ruminative, and is inappropriate. Melancholic patients who feel worthless or guilty respond to comments about their maladaptive thinking as proof of their self-doubt, adding to their misery, rather than relieving depression. The more severe the depression, the less likely the patient will respond to formal psychotherapy.[68] In assuring compliance in the treatment of patients with bipolar depression, a form of "psychoeducation" has been formulated.[69] Psychotherapy serves primarily to enhance compliance and partially insulates the patients from the normal stresses of daily living in the treatment of melancholia.

Continuation and maintenance treatment

The goal of continuation treatment is to prevent relapse once remission is achieved. Up to one-half of depressed patients who improve with medication relapse within 9 months if treatment is not continued. The rates for patients with psychotic depression are particularly high.[70] Younger patients, those with co-occurring conditions that interfere with treatment, patients taking multiple medications (particularly an additional benzodiazepine), and patients with several previous episodes have high relapse rates.[71] The persistence of hypothalamic–pituitary axis hyperactivity identified in the course of treatment by an abnormal dexamethasone suppression test (DST) is associated with relapse and signals the need for further treatment.[72] If the first episode of depressive illness is severe, the risk of relapse and subsequent suicide is high, warranting extended treatment.[73] Patients who are not treated to remission or who do not fully comply with continuation treatment are most likely to relapse.

Continuation treatment reduces relapse rates.[74] Clarity of instructions to the patient about dose and length of continuation treatment, phone rounds, and three or more visits during the continuation period enhances compliance.[75] Unfortunately, even in university settings antidepressant continuation treatment is often inadequate, despite the continued risk for suicide.[76]

The evidence for efficacy of continuation medication treatment is similar to that for acute treatment.[77] The medicines that resolved the depressive episode are likely to be superior to placebo in maintaining the response.[78]

When medications are discontinued after a year of remission, 60% of patients with two episodes or more will have a recurrence within the next year. Among patients at risk for recurrence who continue treatment in the maintenance phase, 10–30% will have a depressive illness in the next year.[79]

In 380 successfully treated depressed patients re-examined up to 15 years, about 55% had a recurrence within eight years. Women, the never married, persons with a prolonged index depressive episode, and persons with more previous episodes were most likely to relapse. For every previous depressive episode the risk of recurrence increased 18%.[80] In a 10-year follow-up of 318 patients, the risk of recurrence increased with each episode.[81] In a 27-year follow-up of 186 patients with recurrent depressive illness and mean age in the late 40s, and 220 patients with manic-depressive illness with mean age in their 20s, 55% had died, with 17% of the deaths by suicide.[82] Chronic depressive features occurred in 11% of the sample. Lifetime treatment is often needed, especially when the initial depressive illness is not fully resolved.

Studies of long-term antidepressant treatment most often assessing relapse rates following medication withdrawal after a maintenance period of 3–5 years find that all classes of antidepressants impart some prophylactic effect. Yet, following withdrawal of medication treatment, even after 5 years, many patients develop a recurrence of a depressive mood disorder.[83]

Social factors appear less important in influencing recurrence among melancholic patients.[84] High recurrence rates are most likely to be observed in patients who have had an episode lasting longer than a year, two or more episodes of melancholia, or episodes of depression with mania or hypomania. In one report, over the 15 years following a unipolar depressive illness, close to 90% of patients experienced a recurrence.[85]

Non-compliance because of dissatisfaction with side-effects is also a factor in relapse.[86] Melancholic patients with more frequent episodes, incomplete acute response, and those with complicated clinical situations are most likely to have recurrences when treatment is discontinued.[87] Patients who are partial responders or who have abnormal hypothalamic–pituitary–adrenal neuroendocrine responses before treatment that fail to convert to a normal pattern are more likely to relapse during treatment.[88] They are also more likely to have recurrences following discontinuation of treatment, no matter how long the treatment has been maintained.[89]

Recurrence rates are also high after a first episode after age 50, even in patients who have remitted. These patients require continuing treatment for several years to a lifetime to minimize the risk of new episodes. New episodes, however, do occur despite adequate dosing of medication and careful follow-up.[90] Yet, when treatment sustains remission of the mood disorder for several years or more, mortality rates, including suicide, are reduced.[91]

Pharmacotherapy for melancholia

Acute treatment

Patients with uncomplicated melancholia respond quickly and fully to treatment. The prescription of the antidepressant with the most favorable risk–benefit ratio at optimal dosing typically elicits a favorable response within two weeks. A substantial improvement is usually present by the fourth week. Most patients will have a full remission within eight weeks. Table 11.3 summarizes guidelines for adequate treatment.

Lithium is the first-choice augmenting agent. Lithium augmentation differs from lithium treatment for acute mania. Dosing is lower (600–900 mg daily) and the treatment trial is shorter (several weeks). If improvement is not seen within several weeks of the addition of lithium, the likelihood is low that further combined treatment will be effective. ECT is the best option. Adding an MAOI to a TCA is a long-standing practice, but there is little experimental evidence to support it. There is no advantage in endless augmentation trials, and there is no evidence that switching is better than augmentation.[92]

Table 11.3. Acute treatment guidelines for melancholia

The goal is remission
Secondary amine TCA or ECT are first-line treatments
Antidepressant doses are maximized as rapidly as possible
Switching to a different class of antidepressant when there is no reduction in symptoms to the first-choice medication at maximum dose for several weeks
Augmentation with lithium if the first-choice medication at maximum dose for several weeks has elicited improvement but not a remission
Medication trials should not be prolonged; if remission is not achieved after two medication trials, ECT is the best option

With no reduction in symptoms *at all* to the first-choice medication within several weeks at the maximal tolerated dose, switching to a different class of antidepressant is considered. Failure to respond fully to the second agent within six weeks or so compels consideration of ECT. If there is a partial response to the second agent, an augmentation trial with lithium is again the first choice. If augmentation following a switch in medications is not effective, ECT is considered, because the duration of the acute treatment trial is now four months or more.

Additional evidence for the utility of lithium comes from two reports of lithium and nortriptyline combination in continuation treatment after successful ECT in patients with major depression. In a three-hospital collaborative trial, ECT referrals treated to remission were randomly assigned to placebo, nortriptyline alone, or the combination of lithium and nortriptyline.[93] In the 6-month follow-up, 80% of those treated with placebo, 60% of those treated with nortriptyline, and 39% of those treated with the combination relapsed. In the four-hospital collaborative study, a similar population was treated to remission with ECT and continuation treatment was either scheduled ECT or the same lithium–nortriptyline combination. The relapse rates at 6 months were 37% for ECT and 32% for the medication combination among the patients who completed the treatment.[94]

Refusal of ECT after two periods of adequate but unsuccessful medication treatment requires the reassessment of the diagnosis, suicide risk, health risk factors, and the capacity to make treatment choices. Involvement of the family or significant others is essential to effective care. An independent opinion from a clinician experienced in pharmacotherapy and ECT reassures the patient and family that ECT is the best option. The alternatives are a change of physician, or seeking alternative legal routes for ECT.[95] Table 11.4 summarizes these decision points and options.

Long-term treatment

Treatment needs to be continued for long periods for every melancholic patient who has successfully remitted. After a maximum response has been obtained, treatment is continued until the maximum response has been sustained for 9–12 months, or

Table 11.4. Acute treatment strategy for patients with melancholia

Treatment stage	Weeks into treatment	options and considerations
First-choice antidepressant	4–8	Secondary amine TCAs provide the best risk–benefit ratio. Venlafaxine and mirtazepine are compromise agents when TCAs are contraindicated. If full response, continue treatment for at least 9 months. If no response at maximum tolerated dose for 3 weeks (< 33% symptom reduction), switch. If partial response at maximum tolerated dose (33–75% symptom reduction), augment
First switch from first-choice to different-class second choice	9–16	If full response, continue treatment. If no further response, offer ECT
First augmentation of first-choice agent with lithium	9–12	If full response, continue treatment. If inadequate response, offer ECT

longer. Many patients with a history of one or two episodes who are in remission have their medication tapered and slowly discontinued. Patients who have had three episodes or more or who have never achieved remission warrant indefinite treatment.

Treatment of severe melancholia

Of the principal forms of melancholia, special consideration in treatment is given to patients with psychotic depression, catatonic and stuporous depression, and manic-depressive illness.

Melancholia with psychosis (psychotic depression)

About 20% of persons with recurrent depressive illness have psychotic features.[96] Older patients are at particular risk.[97] Feelings of worthlessness or guilt are harbingers of psychosis.[98] The mortality rate within the 15 years after an episode among psychotic depressed patients is higher than among other depressed patients (41% versus 20%).[99] The increased mortality is associated with incapacitating agitation or psychomotor retardation leading to exhaustion, cognitive impairment reducing self-care to dangerous levels, and higher suicide rates. Patients cease eating and drinking or taking medications. Hallucinations command suicide and self-injury. Delusions lead to dangerous decisions (patient 11.1).

Patient 11.1

A middle-aged, depressed, diabetic man believed there was a plot to kill him and that the prescribed insulin had been poisoned. He refused doses of insulin and developed ketosis with blood glucose levels > 300 mg%. Admitted to a medical service, his metabolism was stabilized and he was transferred against his will to a locked psychiatric unit. Once the psychosis was treated, he agreed to continue insulin therapy.

Suicide rates are twice that of non-psychotic depressed patients,[100] although not all studies report this.[101] In one facility over a 25-year period, delusional depressed patients were five times more likely to kill themselves than were non-delusional depressed patients.[102] This increased risk is not due to delusional content or severity of illness alone,[103] but because the patients use more violent suicide methods.[104]

ECT

The treatment of choice for psychotic depression is ECT. Remission rates are between 80% and 95%.[105] Most impressive data come from an ongoing multicenter study of continuation and maintenance ECT.[106] Seventy-seven unipolar depressed patients with psychosis were treated with bilateral ECT on a 3 × /weekly schedule. The *remission* rate was 95%. Consistent with this finding is a meta-analysis of 44 studies of psychotic depressives that found bilateral ECT to be superior to unilateral ECT and both superior to the more widely used antidepressant–antipsychotic combination.[107] The drug combination was only slightly better than either class of medication alone.

Antidepressant–antipsychotic combinations

Combining an antidepressant and an antipsychotic is the commonest strategy for treating psychotic depression. Early studies report the combination to be better than either class of agent alone and that about 70% of patients improve substantially. The remission rate for psychotically depressed patients with TCA agents alone was approximately 35%.[108] Dependable studies of SSRI agents are lacking. A single double-blind study of olanzapine plus fluoxetine was reported to have a better response rate than placebo (55% versus 29%).[109] The remaining evidence for an antipsychotic agent combined with fluoxetine,[110] paroxetine,[111] fluvoxamine,[112] venlafaxine,[113] or sertraline[114] is limited to small-sample open case studies. In treating psychotic depressed patients, the literature supports the use of TCA and typical antipsychotic agents.[115]

Prolonged use of typical antipsychotics, however, elicits extrapyramidal uncontrolled movements, falls, and tardive dyskinesia.[116] Atypical antipsychotics are in vogue, but are not better tolerated than low-dose typical agents.[117] Case reports and open trials claim efficacy for all the atypical agents added to an antidepressant.[118]

Caution, however, is needed in prescribing an antipsychotic for a patient, particularly an older patient.[119] Clozapine, with its substantial anticholinergic properties and need for repeated blood testing, is not a first choice.[120] Olanzapine used alone has been reported effective but is marketed as a mood stabilizer.[121] Olanzapine also has substantial anticholinergic properties and weight gain is a problematic side-effect.

Both clozapine and olanzapine elevate blood sugars and elicit diabetes within 6 months of exposure.[122] Despite claims that risperidone has antidepressant properties beyond its antipsychotic effect, the evidence is weak, and its use offers no advantage, even in low doses in the elderly.[123] Further, in a double-blind parallel-group multicenter trial, risperidone alone was less effective than an amitriptyline and haloperidol combination.[124] Adequate studies of quetiapine, ziprasidone, or aripiprazol are lacking. Considering their low antipsychotic efficacy, it is unlikely that these agents have a place in the treatment of psychotic depression.

The need to use a combination of an antipsychotic and antidepressant to treat psychotic depression has been questioned. Some authors find efficacy of antidepressant agents alone. Nefazodone[125] and venlafaxine[126] alone are proffered for psychotic depression, providing relief equivalent to moderate-dose amitriptyline plus low-dose haloperidol. A study of elderly patients with psychotic depression found that, after four weeks of treatment, 50% of those treated with nortriptyline plus perphenazine responded, while 44% receiving nortriptyline alone responded[127] – not a compelling advantage for the combination. Earlier studies report that about 40% of patients with psychotic depression responded to a TCA alone, although nearly 80% were reported to respond to the combination.[128] Using blood level monitoring, however, imipramine alone achieved an almost 70% response rate in psychotic depression.[129] Thus, for some patients with psychotic depression, an antidepressant alone may be sufficient. An antipsychotic may be added when the response is poor.

Adding to concerns about immediately prescribing an antipsychotic agent in patients with psychotic depression is a survey of over 50 000 women in the New Jersey Medicare and Medicare supplemental medication program and mandatory cancer registry.[130] Patients prescribed antipsychotic or antiemetic dopamine blockers that chronically increased prolactin levels were more likely to develop breast cancer. The increased risk appeared dose-related.

Conclusion

Applying evidence-based decision-making to the treatment of patients with psychotic depression dictates that ECT should be immediately offered. Its use as a primary indication for psychotic depression is widely accepted. If refused, a broad pharmacodynamic spectrum antidepressant medication trial is warranted, with the best evidence for the classical TCAs amitriptyline and imipramine. If this response is only partial and ECT is still refused, the addition of a classical antipsychotic agent is the best documented choice. If the patient is not fully recovered within 4 weeks, ECT should again be offered, and if refused, alternative routes sought to provide the treatment.

Catatonia and depressive stupor

Some melancholic patients have profound psychomotor retardation and are listless, anergic, and unresponsive. They are said to be in stupor. Stuporous melancholic patients also have more specific catatonic features. They are often dehydrated and have lost large amounts of weight. They are at substantial risk for neuroleptic malignant syndrome/malignant catatonia, and exposure to an antipsychotic increases this risk.[131] Intravenous lorazepam relieves stupor, mutism, and other signs of catatonia, and permits further evaluation to confirm the diagnosis of melancholia. If the patient responds to a challenge of intravenous lorazepam, a trial of oral or intramuscular lorazepam (doses starting at 1–2 mg TID and increasing if needed to 4–8 mg TID) resolves catatonia. The definitive treatment is bilateral ECT which resolves stupor, the other signs of catatonia, and the underlying melancholia.[132]

Manic-depressive illness

Effective treatment for the depressed phase of patients with a history of both manic and depressive episodes is controversial.[133] US guidelines limit the use of antidepressants on the basis that they are ineffective and may induce mania and hypomania. TCAs are antidepressants that are most often indicted.[134] SSRIs are generally recommended.[135] Bupropion is considered on the basis of anecdotal reports in a small handful of subjects in whom the risk of a switch into mania appeared small.[136] Similarly, the recommendations for lamotrigine and olanzapine are questioned as they are based on industry-sponsored multisite studies.[137] European authorities challenge these recommendations.[138]

Risk of switch

Estimating the risk of a treatment-induced switch into mania must be compared with the natural rate of switching within a depressive phase of illness. In the scant literature, among persons with an initial depressive illness, 10–15% will experience manic or hypomanic episodes in their next decade.[139] The patients with the greatest experience are those with onsets of illness early in life or where the initial episodes exhibit psychosis or vegetative signs.[140] Cross-sectional clinical features do not distinguish an initial unipolar from an initial bipolar illness.[141] The patients with a bipolar expression may be associated with more agitation and racing thoughts.[142]

The frequency of depressed switches to mania among patients who first had a depressive episode is similar in the period before the introduction of modern antidepressant agents, as in the recent decades.[143] The concept that antidepressant medications induce mania in treated hospitalized patients is challenged, although the recognition of switching is somewhat greater in recent decades.[144] The US guidelines are supported by recent reviews.[145] These authors later reported observations of 41 patients who had a 48% switch rate and cautioned the use of antidepressants.[146] Another report of 258 patients, however, observed a 9% switch rate, mostly in the first 16 weeks of treatment, and reported that patients under treatment with antidepressants had fewer depression relapses.[147] One study found that patients receiving antidepressants were four times *less* likely to develop mania or hypomania.[148]

Distinguishing patients who have experienced flagrant manic episodes from those who experienced hypomania alone reconciles conflicting findings. A switch rate of 3% is reported among bipolar II patients (depression and hypomania) receiving imipramine, a rate similar to that among patients with recurrent depression.[149] Another review could cite no compelling data to preclude the use of antidepressants in depressed persons with a history of hypomania alone.[150] A different review concludes that the risk is higher for depressed patients with a history of mania.[151] While lithium might ameliorate this risk, it was unclear whether the anticonvulsants could do so. Increased switch rates among depressed patients with a history of mania has also been reported by others.[152] One study calculated a 10% switch rate with TCAs compared with 0–7% for placebo, 0% for lithium, and 4–5% for lamotrigine, suggesting that TCAs induced mania in only some manic-depressive subjects, and that anticonvulsants might reduce the risk of switching.[153] Given the weak evidence, the risk of a switch from depression to mania in depressed patients, while taking an antidepressant medication alone is probably not elevated in those with a history of hypomania and only slightly elevated in patients who experience mania.

Antidepressant drug class and risk

Claims that antidepressant agents can be differentiated by the switch rates are weakly supported. In an open study of mood shifts in depressed patients and a review of 113 medication trials (37 with bupropion), the investigators found no switch advantage for any medication. While 16% of patients receiving SSRIs switched into a maniform episode, 28% of patients receiving bupropion also switched.[154] Others also could not find an advantage for bupropion over sertraline or venlafaxine in reducing the rate of switching.[155] These switch rates are similar to those reported for TCAs.[156]

Few studies compare different classes of agents. A reanalysis of the data presented by Cohn *et al.* (1989) reported a 7% switch rate for both fluoxetine and imipramine.[157] In a later report, the same authors concluded there were no differences in clinical response or in switch rates among classes of antidepressants despite finding the highest switch rate with SSRIs (22%) and the lowest rate with TCAs (13%).[158] Twenty percent of the bupropion patients switched. Others found a 7% switch rate for imipramine, but observed no switches with paroxetine.[159] Another found an 11% rate with TCAs but only a 4% rate with SSRIs.[160]

Some depressed patients become manic when treated.[161] For those with a mild to moderate depressive illness, particularly those who only experience hypomania, antidepressant monotherapy is effective treatment without the expectation of precipitating a manic state. For depressed patients, regardless of severity, who also experience mania, an antidepressant alone is not recommended.

Antidepressants in manic-depressive patients

A recent retrospective study reported that depressed manic-depressive patients receiving SSRIs, bupropion, venlafaxine, mirtazepine, or a MAOI did no better than those patients who did not get medication.[162] Retrospective examination of the records of over 2000 depressed patients find equivalent responses to antidepressants (mostly TCAs and MAOIs) between those with only recurrent depressions compared to those with both manic and depressive episodes.[163] Similar findings are reported from small open clinical trials.[164]

A randomized trial comparing the reversible MAO-A inhibitor, moclobemide with imipramine as monotherapy or as additions to ongoing mood stabilizer treatment reported that both antidepressants offered equal benefit for depressed manic-depressive patients.[165] Two studies report that paroxetine combined with a mood stabilizer has antidepressant efficacy in depressed manic-depressive patients.[166] The benefit of imipramine is reported, although among patients with adequate lithium serum levels no additional benefit was offered.[167] Another study found different classes of antidepressants to have equally poor cost/benefit in treating depressed manic-depressive patients.[168] Thus, the antidepressant benefit of an antidepressant agent when offered alone for the depressed manic-depressive patient is at best modest.

Mood stabilizers

Monotherapy with an anticonvulsant mood stabilizer is recommended when the severity of the depression is mild to moderate.[169] Mood stabilizers alone are claimed to be as effective as antidepressants under these circumstances and with little risk of precipitating a mania, but the evidence for this claim is weak.[170]

Lithium is the best treatment for manic-depressive illness.[171] Its usage has declined, however, as the anticonvulsant agents have been heavily marketed.[172] Lithium requires more careful monitoring and has a narrower therapeutic window. Nevertheless, lithium is a first choice because its effective therapeutic dose can be reached more quickly than with the anticonvulsant mood stabilizers. It is a better antidepressant. An extensive experience of lithium combined with antidepressants attests to the safety of the combination. It is inexpensive compared to the other choices.[173]

The evidence supporting lithium monotherapy for depressive mood disorders shows that patients with melancholic depression respond best.[174] Small, open trials report lithium to be equally effective as TCAs in depressed manic-depressive patients. The largest double-blind study, however, found imipramine to be superior to lithium.[175] Response rates vary widely (44–100%) but about 80% of manic-depressed patients with mild to moderate depression eventually respond over a several-month trial.[176]

Lithium prevents recurrent episodes, and it has a substantial effect in reducing suicide rates.[177] In a 10-year follow-up study of 100 patients, suicide attempts were 24 times higher when not taking lithium than when taking it.[178] In a Danish naturalistic study in which unselected patients who were prescribed lithium and re-examined over 16 years, the mortality from suicide was high, mostly in the first two years of continuation treatment and associated with non-compliance.[179]

Lithium can be safely used in all age groups, as long as specific side-effect and toxicity risk factors are avoided (Table 11.5).

Elderly patients tolerate lithium well. They experience higher brain to blood level concentrations than are usually seen in younger patients, so blood levels around 0.5 mg/L are often clinically effective.[180] In a study of 50 elderly patients recovering from depression, lithium or placebo was added to an antidepressant. After six months, 17% of the placebo group but none of the lithium group had relapsed. After two years 33% of the placebo group and only 4% of the lithium group had

Table 11.5. Side-effect and toxicity risk factors in lithium therapy[a]

Factor	Potential Consequences
Renal disease	Poor lithium clearance results in high levels and toxicity
Cardiac conduction disorder	Heart block, potentially fatal
Thyroid or parathyroid disease	Lithium-induced hypothyroidism and hypoparathyroidism without prior disease, the latter causing fatigue, concentration problems, loss of interest, and other depression-like features[b]
Previous major stroke	Lithium may elicit features of an old stroke without causing further stroke
Pregnancy	Lithium is associated with deadly fetal cardiac anomalies during the first trimester, and floppy-baby syndrome in late pregnancy
Concurrent use of non-steroidal anti-inflammatory agents	These agents affect renal clearance of lithium, resulting in higher blood levels than predicted from the dose[c]

[a] In rare instances, lithium induces thyrotoxicosis which may be mistaken for a breakthrough mania, so all patients taking lithium who are rehospitalized for mania should have serum T_4 and T_3 serum levels measured (Barclay *et al.*, 1994).
[b] Aspirin and over-the-counter doses of naproxen and acetaminophen have little effect on lithium plasma levels and can be used safely with lithium (Levin *et al.*, 1998).
[c] Niethammer *et al.* (2000); Fahy and Lawlor (2001).

relapsed.[181] Despite lithium's effect on the parathyroid glands, no apparent risk for osteoporosis is reported.[182] Men and women of all ages have similar response rates for acute depressive or mixed depressive and manic episodes of 60–80%.[183] Relapse rates are 30–70% lower than among patients receiving placebo.[184] Neither the menstrual cycle nor oral contraceptives affect serum lithium levels.[185] Lithium therapy is particularly useful in premenopausal women since valproic acid and perhaps other anticonvulsant mood stabilizers affect ovarian functioning, thereby interfering with fertility.[186]

The necessity for long-term maintenance treatment is a consideration in the choice of an acute treatment. A Cochrane pooled data review concluded that the prophylactic benefits of valproic acid compared with placebo were unclear and that the present shift to valproic acid over lithium is not supported by the evidence. The review encourages a preference for lithium over valproic acid.[187] Lithium's long-term administration also has the advantage of reducing suicide rates, an effect not demonstrated for other mood stabilizers.[188] Thus, if the depressed manic-depressive is likely to need long-term treatment, lithium is the best choice.

Anticonvulsant mood stabilizers are strongly advertised to moderate the manic features in patients who are mild to moderately depressed. These agents are offered when a depressive illness is closely linked with a period of mania or hypomania, during rapid cycling, when lithium is contraindicated or is ineffective, and when the course of illness suggests limbic sensitization is developing.[189]

Experience is greatest with *valproic acid* and *carbamazepine*. Fewer than 50% of depressed manic-depressive patients respond to carbamazepine.[190] Other studies fail to find greater benefit than with placebo.[191] Similar disappointing improvement rates are reported for valproic acid.[192] The evidence for an antidepressant effect of valproic acid is weak, although in an open trial of 33 patients, two-thirds were reported to benefit.[193]

Lamotrigine is the most recent anticonvulsant recommended to reduce manic episodes.[194] It is marketed as safe and easy to use without inducing increased liver enzyme activity.[195] It is well tolerated.[196] Although lamotrigine is reported to have better efficacy as a mood stabilizer than other new anticonvulsants (gabapentin, topiramate, oxcarbazepine, zonisamide, and tiagabine), the evidence favoring lamotrigine is minimal and industry-generated.[197] The evidence comes from anecdotal open trials with few patients in each report.[198] In a double-blind, placebo-controlled industry-sponsored study of patients characterized as moderately depressed, lamotrigine at 50 mg ($n = 64$) and 200 mg ($n = 63$) were both statistically better than placebo ($n = 65$) between 4–7 weeks of treatment. Mean 17-item Hamilton Rating Scale scores dropped by 13 points for both lamotrigine groups and by 9 points for the placebo group. Mean 21-item Hamilton Depression Rating Scale scores fell 19 points for the lamotrigine groups and 15 points for the placebo group. Few clinicians would consider the difference of four points sufficient reason to prescribe lamotrigine alone. In a comparison of lamotrigine to lithium in a double-blind, placebo-controlled study over 76 weeks of maintenance following an open-labeled successful acute clinical trial, lithium was slightly better at preventing recurrences of mania while lamotrigine was reported to be slightly better at preventing recurrences of depression.[199]

The manufacturer identified 202 manic-depressive patients who received lamotrigine alone in placebo-controlled trials. After 10 weeks of treatment, lamotrigine was no better than placebo, and 7% of the lamotrigine patients switched to mania.[200] A review of the evidence concluded: "When efficacy, adverse effects, and cost are considered, lamotrigine should be reserved as a second-line agent for bipolar depression." [201]

Further, because the introduction of lamotrigine typically takes weeks to reach therapeutic levels, it is not suitable when there is need for a rapid antidepressant effect.[202] The slow dose build-up is for concerns of a lamotrigine-induced rash that occurs in about 10% of patients within the first 2 weeks of treatment.[203] Lamotrigine is, at best, an add-on in manic-depressive illness and, at worst, a poor adequate antidepressant therapy.

Optimizing treatments for manic-depressive illness

Mild to moderate melancholia

If the depressed manic-depressive patient is not suicidal, psychotic, or stuporous, and is able to meet daily responsibilities, there is no anticipated need for hospitalization (a 17-item HAMD score < 20), and the patient has only experienced hypomania that has not disrupted functioning, antidepressant monotherapy is offered. Antidepressant drug choice should be based on remission rates and not on fears of inducing a switch into mania. Broad pharmacodynamic spectrum antidepressants (TCAs) are the first choices. Lithium is the best augmentation.

When a mood stabilizer alone is to be prescribed, lithium has the best antidepressant efficacy. If lithium alone does not achieve remission, adding a broad pharmacodynamic spectrum antidepressant would be the next step. If that does not fully resolve the mood disorder, ECT should be offered. The efficacy rate of ECT for manic-depressive depression is about 80% and would be superior to adding a second anticonvulsant mood stabilizer.[204]

If ECT is declined, a second trial with a different mood stabilizer combined with an antidepressant is suggested. If the second combination trial does not work, there is no evidence that continued switching or adding medications has any substantial benefit, and ECT becomes the treatment of choice.

Severe melancholia

If the depressed manic-depressive patient is moderately to severely ill (a 17-item HAMD score of 21 or higher), an antidepressant and a mood stabilizer or ECT alone are the first choice. When hospitalization is needed, ECT is the treatment of choice. In two prospective and seven retrospective studies, ECT achieved remission rates of 43–100%.[205]

Combining an antidepressant and a mood stabilizer is standard practice, and lithium again is the mood stabilizer of choice. The choice of mood stabilizer depends on side-effect and pharmacokinetic considerations (e.g., liver and kidney functioning). If resistant to the initial combination, ECT should be offered again, rather than multiple trials of medication combinations. The simultaneous use of two mood stabilizers rather than a mood stabilizer and an antidepressant has no greater benefit, but does lead to higher dropout rates from increased side-effects.[206] Combining an antidepressant with a mood stabilizer lowers the risk of a breakthrough mania in patients with a history of mania.[207] Venlafaxine and paroxetine are also reported to be effective for depressions when added to a mood stabilizer, with only a few patients switching into mania.[208] In contrast, a recent double-blind, placebo-controlled trial of paroxetine or imipramine added to a mood stabilizer could find little benefit for adding either agent, and there were substantial dropouts with imipramine.[209]

In depressed patients who are also psychotic, catatonic, or in stupor, or the patient's condition requires hospitalization, ECT is the treatment of choice.[210]

Comparing these recommendations with those of authoritative sources in published treatment algorithms is instructive. In an "expert consensus" series, the algorithm of a mood stabilizer alone for mild to moderate depression and ECT or a medication combination for more severe episodes is presented.[211] Lithium is the first-choice mood stabilizer followed by valproic acid and then lamotrigine. The choice of, however, focuses on non-TCA drugs. Common ground would be venlafaxine or mirtazepine. The recommendation that bupropion is the antidepressant of choice is not supportable.[212]

Lithium and lamotrigine are given equal prominence as mood stabilizers. Thus, the conflicting focus remains the choice of antidepressant – TCAs, bupropion, or broad pharmacodynamic spectrum newer agents (venlafaxine, mirtazepine, paroxetine) or antidepressants with a narrower pharmacodynamic profile.

NOTES

1 A description of Henry James in the depths of one of his melancholic depressions is described by his friend Edith Wharton; cited in Lewis (1991), p. 580.
2 UK ECT Review Group (2003).
3 The evidence for the usefulness of psychotherapies in the relief of melancholia is weak. A small benefit is reported in encouraging compliance.
4 Although hospital care is not always required for ECT, it is preferable to treat elderly patients and those who have co-occurring illnesses in the hospital. Outpatient treatments take most of the morning and the patient must be accompanied by a responsible person, a requirement for every patient receiving a general anesthesia in an outpatient procedure. Anterograde memory problems during the acute treatment course may interfere with work or the meeting of other responsibilities.

   In one setting, ECT is administered in a postanesthesia recovery unit by an attending psychiatrist and two nurse anesthetists and a resident physician. An anesthesiologist circulates into the room regularly, and a recovery room nurse cares for the patient after treatment. Total billing can be $2000 per treatment. For a detailed discussion of the bias against the use of ECT, see Ottosson and Fink (2004).
5 Tranter *et al.* (2002); Bakish (2001).
6 Thase (2003).
7 Antidepressant medications are approved for marketing on the basis of a 50% reduction in rating-scale scores in two or more studies of large samples. Such a standard leaves many patients ill despite meeting this arbitrary standard (Healy, 1997, 2004; Angell, 2004; Medawar and Hardon, 2004). That symptom reduction alone is not adequate for patients with melancholia is a concern because the risks of relapse and suicide are substantial during the year following an episode.
8 Kupfer *et al.* (1989).
9 Posternak and Zimmerman (2005).
10 Fink (1987a, 1990, 1997, 2001).
11 Petrides *et al.* (2001); Husain *et al.* (2004).
12 Petrides *et al.* (2001); Birkenhäger *et al.* (2003).
13 Boyer and Feighner (1994); Faltermaier-Temizel *et al.* (1997).
14 Lam *et al.* (2002). Also see Diego *et al.* (2004).
15 Thase *et al.* (2002).
16 Marangell (2001).
17 Gilbody *et al.* (2003).
18 Side-effects are the necessary consequences of a compound's pharmacodynamic properties. Some, but not all, unpleasant effects can be avoided by matching the side-effect profile

of the medication with the patient's likely risks (e.g., avoiding a strongly anticholinergic drug such as clozapine in an elderly man with prostatic hypertrophy). Adverse effects are rare and unpredictable from the medication's basic pharmacodynamics (e.g., agranulocytosis from carbamazepine). Side-effects can also be used therapeutically. For example, using an antidepressant with sedating properties in a bedtime dose encourages sleep, giving some early relief to the patient, and lessening the need for a second medication for sleep.

19 Leon *et al.* (2003).

20 Hirschfeld *et al.* (2002a, b).

21 Flint and Rifat (2001).

22 That ECT is not available at many psychiatric hospitals, and that fewer than 10% of US psychiatrists are sufficiently experienced in the treatment to use it, is a sad consequence of the stigmatization of this treatment (Ottosson and Fink, 2004).

23 Nine double-blind placebo-controlled studies of lithium augmentation were reported between 1983 and 1995. The two largest samples comprise 33 and 60 subjects; five were small samples. Six studies found a benefit in adding lithium, three did not. Among the "positive" studies, response rates were 50–63% (Angst *et al.*, 1969; Price *et al.*, 2001).

24 Bauer and Dopfmer (1999); Fava (2001).

25 Alvarez *et al.* (1997).

26 Bschor *et al.* (2003).

27 Lithium augmentation of an antidepressant medication does not require the same dosing that is needed in the treatment of acute mania. Daily doses of 600–800 mg offer adequate augmentation benefit.

28 Bauer *et al.* (2000); Bschor *et al.* (2002).

29 Baethge *et al.* (2003c).

30 Fava *et al.* (2002a).

31 Block *et al.* (1977).

32 The toxic serotonin syndrome looks like the neuroleptic malignant syndrome (NMS) with additional gastrointestinal symptoms of cramps and diarrhea (Schweitzer and Tuckwell, 1998). We have argued that both NMS and the serotonin syndrome are variants of malignant catatonia and are best treated as catatonic syndromes initially with a course of high-dose benzodiazepine, and if the response is not rapid, ECT (Fink and Taylor, 2003). Lithium affects the serotonergic system, increasing presynaptic synthesis and turnover and postsynaptic binding (Price and Heninger, 1994). For patients who may have pre-existing basal ganglia sensitivity, even small doses of an SSRI may precipitate the syndrome (Voirol *et al.*, 2000).

33 The mechanism of action of supplementary thyroid products in depressed patients with normal thyroid function is unknown, but is hypothesized to impact the noradrenergic system (Whybrow and Prange, 1981) or dampen the relative increase in thyroid hormone levels observed in some melancholic patients (Joffe *et al.*, 1984).

34 Gold *et al.* (1981).

35 Aronson *et al.* (1996); Altshuler *et al.* (2001a; 2003); Appelhof *et al.* (2004).

36 Joffe *et al.* (1993).

37 Schweitzer and Tuckwell (1998).

38 Charney (1996); Berman *et al.* (1997); Rabiner *et al.* (2001); Perry *et al.* (2004).

39 Fava (2001).

40 Sitland-Marken *et al.* (1990); Inoue *et al.* (1996).

41 Davidson *et al.* (1989); McGrath *et al.* (1992); Quitkin *et al.* (1993); Stewart *et al.* (1997); Sotsky and Simmens (1999).
42 Lam *et al.* (2002).
43 Fink and Taylor (2003); Houlihan (2004).
44 Hansten and Horn (2002); Solai *et al.* (2002).
45 Thase (2002); Tohen *et al.* (2004).
46 Corya *et al.* (2003).
47 Corya *et al.* (2003).
48 Myers and Thase (2001).
49 Hirose and Ashby (2002).
50 Lambert *et al.* (1998); Bozikas *et al.* (2001). One of us saw a 42-year-old depressed woman who was resistant to various antidepressant treatment trials. On one occasion, she was given olanzapine, 10 mg daily, and quickly developed oculogyric crisis with total body dystonia, eyes rolled up and her back extended in spasm, difficulty breathing, and spatial disorientation. She required emergency room care and benztropine and diphenhydramine were administered over a 4-h period to resolve the crisis.
51 One study of clonazepam (3 mg daily for 4 weeks) as an augmenting agent reports a reduction in HAMD scores of 80% in patients with recurrent depressive illness, but only 10% in manic-depressive patients and patients identified as treatment resistant (Morishita and Aoki, 2002).
52 Marangell (2001).
53 Hirschfeld *et al.* (2002b).
54 Stern *et al.* (1983); Othmer *et al.* (1988); Preskorn and Burke (1992); Joffe *et al.* (1996); Zarate *et al.* (1996) (2002).
55 Segal *et al.* (2002).
56 Parker *et al.* (2003).
57 Ablon and Jones (2002); Casacalenda *et al.* (2002); Garland and Scott (2002); Harkness *et al.* (2002); Scott (1995a).
58 Markowitz (1996). The term "placebo responder" is misunderstood to mean that the placebo condition is inactive and that patients who improve are not ill. Recent studies, however, demonstrate that the placebo condition is "active" for some patients. In controlled clinical trials blood pressures may be lower in the placebo condition (Queneau *et al.*, 2002). Patients with Parkinson's disease also respond to placebo, a phenomenon that is explained to be due to dopamine release in the striatum secondary to the placebo's effect on reward systems (de la Fuente-Fernandez and Stoessl, 2002). Unipolar depressed patients who improve with placebo have brain glucose metabolism changes similar in pattern and degree to patients responding to fluoxetine (Mayberg *et al.*, 2002), and depressed placebo responders also have quantitative electroencephalogram changes in prefrontal regions, but these are different in pattern from drug responders, suggesting there is an effect, but that it is different from that of the medication (Leuchter *et al.*, 2002). Because 30% or more of patients in recent antidepressant drug trials are placebo responders and patients with melancholia may be less likely to respond to placebo than patients with other forms of depressive illness, the placebo group becomes scientifically and ultimately clinically just as important as the group receiving the active medication (Walsh *et al.*, 2002).
59 Spinelli (1997).
60 Arean and Cook (2002).
61 de Jonghe *et al.* (2004).

62 Fava *et al.* (1996); Thase *et al.* (1997b); Paykel *et al.* (1999).
63 Lenze *et al.* (2002).
64 Perlis *et al.* (2002); McPherson *et al.* (2003).
65 Frank and colleagues (1989, 1990).
66 Rush (1998).
67 Harkness *et al.* (2002).
68 Elkin *et al.* (1989); Thase *et al.* (1991b). The Enhancing Recovery in Coronary Heart Disease (ENRICHD) study demonstrates that psychotherapy worsens the condition for some depressed patients. For discussion of psychotherapy within the medical model of psychiatric practice, see Guze and Murphy (1963); Guze (1988).

One analysis of pooled data found cognitive-behavior therapy (CBT) helpful for hospitalized, severely depressed patients (DeRubeis *et al.*, 1999). Most strikingly, CBT was thought equivalent to medications. The analysis was of four comparison studies of an antidepressant versus CBT. However, a significant placebo response in these reports is likely as baseline mean depression-rating scale scores were low to moderate and there were substantial drops in scores early in treatment, a typical placebo pattern (Murphy *et al.*, 1984; Hollon *et al.*, 1992).

69 Psychoeducation is briefly discussed in Chapter 2.
70 Kocsis *et al.* (1996, 2002); Reimherr *et al.* (1998); Paykel (2001b).
71 Claxton *et al.* (2000).
72 O'Toole *et al.* (1997). The DST is discussed in Chapters 4 and 6.
73 Kessing (2004a).
74 Montgomery (1996); Altshuler *et al.* (2001b); Hirschfeld (2001).
75 Katon *et al.* (2001); Bull *et al.* (2002). In a recent study of compliance that used electronic drug exposure monitors, over 70% of 82 patients during SSRI continuation treatment missed at least one day of dosing and about 30% missed two days or more. These are considered serious lapses in treatment (Meijer *et al.*, 2001).
76 Oquendo *et al.* (2002).
77 Entsuah *et al.* (1996); Koran *et al.* (2001); Paykel (2001b); Thase *et al.* (2001b).
78 Keller (1999).
79 Keller, (1999); Hirschfeld (2001); Wilkinson *et al.* (2002).
80 Mueller *et al.* (1999).
81 Solomon *et al.* (2000).
82 Angst and Preisig (1995).
83 Paykel (2001b).
84 Andrew *et al.* (1993); Paykel *et al.* (1996); Hayhurst *et al.* (1997).
85 Keller (1999).
86 Tollefson (1993).
87 Coryell and Winokur (1992); Paykel *et al.* (1995).
88 Hatzinger *et al.* (2002) (Chapter 4).
89 Nemeroff and Evans (1988); Tranter *et al.* (2002).
90 Byrne and Rothschild (1998).
91 Takeshita *et al.* (2002).
92 Posternak and Zimmerman (2001).
93 Sackeim *et al.* (2001a).
94 Kellner *et al.* (submitted). Overall, 46% of both groups survived the 6-month follow-up. Dropouts were 22% for the medication treatment and 17% for ECT.

95 Ottosson and Fink (2004).
96 Johnson *et al.* (1991); Ohayon and Schatzberg (2002); Zaratiegui (2002). The incidence is higher in populations referred for ECT, approximating 30% (Petrides *et al.*, 2001; Sackeim *et al.*, 2001a).
97 Lykouras *et al.* (2002).
98 Ohayon and Schatzberg (2002).
99 Vythilingam *et al.* (2003).
100 Miller and Chabrier (1988); Hori *et al.* (1993).
101 Grunebaum *et al.* (2001); Lykouras *et al.* (2002); Kessing (2003).
102 Roose *et al.* (1983).
103 Grunebaum *et al.* (2001).
104 Isometsa *et al.* (1994b).
105 Kroessler (1985); Flint and Rifat (1998a, b).
106 Petrides *et al.* (2001).
107 Parker *et al.* (1992a, b).
108 Kroessler (1985); Spiker *et al.* (1986); Chan *et al.* (1987); Khan *et al.* (1991); Rothschild (2003a).
109 Dube *et al.* (2002), cited by Rothschild (2003b).
110 Rothschild *et al.* (1993).
111 Wolfersdorf *et al.* (1995).
112 Gatti *et al.* (1996).
113 Zanardi *et al.* (2000).
114 Zanardi *et al.* (1996).
115 Chapters 9 and 10. For a different view, see Wheeler Vega *et al.* (2000).
116 Meyers *et al.* (2001).
117 Geddes *et al.* (2000); Lieberman *et al.* (2005).
118 Sajatovic *et al.* (2002); Rothschild (2003a).
119 The US Food and Drug Administration has recently placed a "black box" warning around atypical antipsychotic drugs for older patients with dementing conditions, finding death rates to be substantially higher than in those patients not prescribed these agents.
120 Hrdlicka (2002) reported that the combination of clozapine and maprotiline was effective. Each agent can induce seizures, however, making this combination high risk.
121 Rothschild *et al.* (1999); Bruijn *et al.* (2001).
122 Koller and Doraiswamy (2002).
123 Myers and Thase (2001).
124 Muller-Siecheneder *et al.* (1998).
125 Grunze *et al.* (2002).
126 Zanardi *et al.* (2000); also see Simpson *et al.* (2003), reporting sertraline alone as effective for patients with psychotic depression.
127 Mulsant *et al.* (2001).
128 Spiker *et al.* (1986).
129 Bruijn *et al.* (2001).
130 Wang *et al.* (2001b).
131 Fink and Taylor (2003).
132 Fink and Taylor (2003).
133 Blanco *et al.* (2002).

134 Prien *et al.* (1984); Peet (1994); Boerlin *et al.* (1998); Nolen and Bloemkolk (2000); American Psychiatric Association (2002a); Hirschfeld *et al.* (2002a); Keck *et al.* (2003b).
135 Silverstone and Silverstone (2004).
136 Sachs *et al.* (1994).
137 McElroy *et al.* (2004).
138 Ghaemi *et al.* (2003).
139 Johnson *et al.* (1991); Akiskal *et al.* (1995); Coryell *et al.* (1995b); DelBello *et al.* (2003).
140 Ghaemi *et al.* (2000).
141 Dorz *et al.* (2003).
142 Benazzi (2003); Maj *et al.* (2003).
143 Lewis and Winokur (1982).
144 Angst (1985).
145 Ghaemi *et al.* (2003).
146 Ghaemi *et al.* (2004a, b).
147 Post *et al.* (2003).
148 DelBello *et al.* (2003).
149 Kupfer *et al.* (1988).
150 Thase and Sachs (2000).
151 Parker and Parker, (2003).
152 Kilzieh and Akiskal (1999).
153 Grunze *et al.* (2002b).
154 Joffe *et al.* (2002); MacQueen *et al.* (2002).
155 Post *et al.* (2001, 2003).
156 Maj *et al.* (1994); Altshuler *et al.*, 1995.
157 Ghaemi *et al.* (2003).
158 Ghaemi *et al.* (2004a, b).
159 Nemeroff *et al.* (2001b).
160 Peet (1994).
161 Wehr and Goodwin (1987).
162 Frankle *et al.* (2002).
163 Moller *et al.* (2001).
164 Baumhackl *et al.* (1989); Cohn *et al.* (1989); Zornberg and Pope (1993).
165 Silverstone (2001).
166 Young *et al.* (2000b); Nemeroff *et al.* (2001b).
167 Nemeroff *et al.* (2001b).
168 Ghaemi *et al.* (2004b).
169 American Psychiatric Association (2002a). Valproic acid is reported to benefit patients with mixed affective states and in those who no longer respond to lithium (Bowden, 2004).
170 Goodwin *et al.* (1972); Post *et al.* (1986).
171 Emilien *et al.* (1995); Pies (2002).
172 In 1992 about half of manic-depressive patients were receiving lithium. By the century's end, this figure had dropped to 30%, largely replaced by valproic acid, which now accounts for 27% of prescriptions for mood stabilizers (Blanco *et al.*, 2002).
173 Grunze (2003); Kleindienst and Greil (2003); Maj (2003).
174 Serretti *et al.* (2000a).

175 Fieve *et al.* (1968).
176 Goodwin and Jamison (1990); Strakowski *et al.* (2000b).
177 Ahrens *et al.* (1995); Bocchetta *et al.* (1998); Goodwin (2002).
178 Rucci *et al.* (2002).
179 Brodersen *et al.* (2000).
180 Price and Heninger (1994); Johnson (1987); Taylor (1999).
181 Wilkinson *et al.* (2002).
182 Cohen *et al.* (1998); Pieri-Balandraud *et al.* (2001).
183 Viguera *et al.* (2001).
184 Price and Heninger (1994).
185 Chamberlain *et al.* (1990).
186 Herzog *et al.* (1986).
187 Macritchie *et al.* (2002).
188 Goodwin *et al.* (2003); Maj (2003).
189 Limbic sensitization is proposed to explain the chronic course observed in 30–50% of manic-depressive patients (Neugebauer *et al.*, 2000). Anticonvulsants that prevent kindling in laboratory animals or restrain kindling once it has started (valproic acid and carbamazepine) were introduced as mood stabilizers based on this model (Berns *et al.*, 2002).
190 Gilmore (2001).
191 Small (1990).
192 Swann *et al.* (1997); Dietrich and Emrich (1998); Winsberg *et al.* (2001).
193 Davis *et al.* (1996).
194 Nolen and Bloemkolk (2000).
195 Meldrum (1994).
196 Bowden *et al.* (2004).
197 Macritchie *et al.* (2002); Evins (2003).
198 Kusumakar and Yatham (1997); Bowden *et al.* (1999); Calabrese *et al.* (1999a); Yatham *et al.* (2002).
199 Calabrese *et al.* (1999b); Bowden *et al.* (2003).
200 Glaxo-SmithKline (1997).
201 Hurley (2002). Also Sporn and Sachs (1997).
202 One guideline for introducing lamotrigine calls for a starting dose of 25 mg daily for two weeks, 50 mg daily for the next two weeks, followed by 50–100 mg increases every two weeks. To achieve an antidepressant dose of 150–200 mg daily takes 8–10 weeks (Guberman *et al.*, 1999).
203 A rash of sufficient severity to discontinue treatment is reported in 12% of treated patients. Instances of the Stevens–Johnson syndrome (immune complex hypersensitivity syndrome) occur in 2% of treated patients (Guberman *et al.*, 1999).
204 Yuen *et al.* (1992).
205 Avery and Winokur (1977); Avery and Lubrano (1979); Homan *et al.* (1982); Black *et al.* (1987a); Srisurapanont *et al.* (1995).
206 Young *et al.* (2000b). Safety concerns limit the use of some combinations (Freeman and Stoll, 1998).
207 Dietrich and Emrich (1998).
208 Vieta *et al.* (2002).

209 Nemeroff *et al.*, 2001b.

210 Many clinicians also resort to combinations of several drugs. The long-term use of olanzapine as an enhancer, the only antipsychotic approved as a mood stabilizer, was no better in preventing future episodes than lithium or valproate alone (Tohen *et al.*, 2004).

211 Sachs *et al.* (2000).

212 Grunze *et al.* (2004) offers World Federation of Societies of Biological Psychiatry guidelines for treating manic-depressive depression that follow the basic algorithm detailed above. They favor bupropion or a pure SSRI followed by an MAOI as antidepressants of choice.

12

Pharmacotherapy for melancholic patients in complicating circumstances

A mood of lassitude and dejection took possession of his spirits. He lost all pleasure in society, would sit for hours at his table, unable to bring himself to work at anything . . . His sleep was troubled by dreams, his waking hours by accusing voices . . . His shaken nerves could muster up no power of resistance . . . Melancholy swelled to obsession, obsessions to delusion . . . Once again he tried to kill himself[1]

Melancholia that is identified early and is treated vigorously by the available methods resolves rapidly. Treatment becomes challenging, however, when the patient has a comorbid general medical or neurologic condition that affects its delivery, or is very young or very old. The presence of psychosis or a history of a manic-depressive course are also complicating circumstances, but acute treatment of a melancholic episode in these circumstances is often straightforward and is discussed in Chapter 11. So-called "treatment-resistant depression" is discussed here.

Melancholia in pregnancy and breast-feeding

From 5 to 10% of women become clinically depressed during pregnancy.[2] A depressive mood disorder is a risk factor for obstetrical difficulties,[3] low infant birth weight,[4] newborn irritability,[5] retarded child development,[6] and neurological deficits.[7] Depressive moods and abnormal vegetative signs during pregnancy anticipate postpartum depression.[8]

Women with mood disorders during the childbearing years and while sexually active need to be educated about the risks for the fetus of the illness and its treatments. They and their partners need a long-range treatment plan.[9]

No psychotropic agent is accepted as fully safe for the fetus as none is in Food and Drug Administration (FDA) "category A" for teratologic risk (stipulating that controlled studies demonstrate no risk to humans). Psychotropic agents and their metabolites cross the placental barrier, usually in concentrations lower than those observed in the mother.[10] Benzodiazepines, often used as adjunct treatment, elicit decreased fetal muscle tone, cleft lip, and when maternal dosing is stopped, withdrawal signs of irritability, tremors, and seizures in the infant. Hypnotics are in FDA "category X" as entailing high risk; their use is contraindicated in pregnancy. Atypical antipsychotic medications are associated with an increased risk of fetal neural tube defects.[11] Any treatment has to be weighed against the risks to the mother, the fetus, and the family of not receiving effective treatment.[12]

Consequences of withholding treatment during pregnancy

Prepartum depression is a high stress response state and the stress response hormones (e.g., glucocorticoids, vasopressin) are elevated. They cross the placenta to the blood stream of the infant.[13] Children who were exposed as fetuses to stress-related intrauterine environments exhibit neuromotor growth delays, neuroendocrine and neurotransmitter abnormalities, and disorganized sleep patterns that alter circadian rhythms.[14] Maternal blood flow to the fetus is reduced in depressed women, leading to low birth weights in the newborn.[15]

Increased rates of premature birth and low birth weight are frequent in women who are depressed during pregnancy.[16] The infants respond less well to stimuli than do comparison infants, are hypoactive, and are less robust and sustained in their movements.[17] They cry excessively and are inconsolable. The more severe the prepartum depression, the more likely the infant will express these behaviors and the more severe they are likely to be.[18] Prepartum depression also increases the risk for pre-eclampsia.[19] It is the most robust risk factor for depressive illness in the offspring because it encompasses a genetic predisposition inherited from the mother with a prolonged adverse environmental impact at a critical phase of neural development. A tragic example of inadequate treatment follows.

Patient 12.1

A 29-year-old émigrée, early in her first trimester, sought treatment for an atypical depressive and psychotic illness. She reported fragmented auditory hallucinations of commenting voices, a delusional mood, and ideas of reference. Her affect was subdued and she was anhedonic. She was slow in movement and speech. Her sleep was disturbed and she had lost weight. Fluoxetine in doses ranging up to 40 mg daily was prescribed with some benefit, but she remained severely ill. Because of her poor functioning, her family concluded that she would be unable to care for a child and convinced her to have an abortion. Ten days after the abortion the psychotic depression exacerbated and she was hospitalized. She made a slow recovery with medication treatment.

Effects of treatment during pregnancy

The effects of psychoactive agents, including selective serotonin reuptake inhibitors (SSRIs), in pregnancy and to the fetus are uncertain.[20]

Malformations

There is little evidence that antidepressant agents are teratologic.[21] Tricyclic antidepressants (TCAs) do not increase the risk of congenital anomalies, although neonatal lethargy and anticholinergic effects have been observed.[22] Nortriptyline and desipramine are least likely to be associated with these effects.[23] Similarly, the SSRI antidepressants are not associated with teratologic risk. One investigation of

226 children exposed prenatally to sertraline, paroxetine, or fluvoxamine could find no increase in rates of major malformations.[24] A prospective study using the Swedish Birth Registry assessed 969 children exposed to citalopram, paroxetine, sertraline, or fluoxetine and found no increase in rates of malformations.[25] The same was true for venlafaxine.[26] In a recent multicenter study in which 150 pregnant women received venlafaxine, there was no increase in rates of infant malformations.[27]

Monoamine oxidase inhibitors (MAOIs) offer limited information. One study of 21 pregnancies found the use of a MAOI to be associated with an increased risk for congenital malformations.[28]

Neonatal problems

SSRI-induced neonatal difficulties are transient *if* the newborn is not further exposed postpartum.[29] SSRI-related neuromotor problems occur and may persist if the nursing mother continues to take the SSRI, and one review cautions that agents with the lowest detectable breast milk levels (nortriptyline, paroxetine, and sertraline) are to be preferred.[30]

Mother–child pairs exposed throughout gestation to a TCA ($n = 46$) or to fluoxetine ($n = 40$) were re-examined in 5–71 months postpartum.[31] Neither TCAs nor fluoxetine adversely affected the child's IQ, language development, or behavior. In contrast, the child's IQ and language development were adversely affected by the length of the mother's mood disorder and the number of episodes of illness following delivery. After screening thousands of persons in a Washington state health plan, 209 children exposed to antidepressant medications during gestation were identified. Compared with similar but not exposed children, the investigators could find no association between TCA or SSRI exposure and either congenital malformations or developmental delay. SSRI exposure, however, was associated with early delivery and thus lower birth weights and Apgar scores.[32] TCAs were not associated with these findings.[33] Another study found that children exposed prenatally to paroxetine were more likely to experience postpartum respiratory distress and to be premature.[34] But in a prospective care survey of 997 Swedish children exposed to antidepressant medications during their third trimester, paroxetine was not singled out, and low birth weight and premature birth were reported to be more likely with TCAs than with SSRIs. TCAs were also associated with an increased risk for neonatal hypoglycemia. Both classes of medication were associated with an increased risk for low Apgar scores, respiratory distress, and neonatal convulsions.[35] These findings, however, were not related to maternal depression factors or treatment response, so whether these adverse events were medication- or disease-related is unknown.

In a prospective study of 20 mothers prescribed an SSRI, an association was found between higher maternal umbilical cord blood levels of the medication, newborn symptoms (e.g., sleep and appetite disturbances, neuromotor problems), and biochemical markers of serotonergic central nervous system abnormality (e.g., 5-hydroxyindoleacetic acid levels).[36] In another prospective study of 17 SSRI-exposed and 17 non-exposed full-birth-weight newborns who had no obvious general medical or neurologic problem matched for maternal age, tobacco use, and socioeconomic status, the SSRI-exposed infants had shorter mean gestational age, were more active and tremulous, were behaviorally subdued, and had more rapid eye movement (REM) sleep and sleep arousals.[37]

Based on this information, secondary amine TCA and SSRI antidepressants appear to carry little teratogenetic or spontaneous abortion risk. Most problems in exposed fetuses are considered transient.[38] SSRI use, however, increases the risk for premature birth and is often prescribed with benzodiazepines, agents that are contraindicated in pregnancy. Thus, for melancholic pregnant women, TCAs offer the best therapeutic effect with the safest profile and the least need for polypharmacy. Electroconvulsive therapy for melancholia in pregnancy is safe and effective; its use is discussed in Chapter 8.

Mood stabilizers are more problematic during pregnancy than are antidepressant agents, making the pregnant woman with a manic-depressive depression most difficult to treat. Lithium is contraindicated because of the risks of Ebstein's anomaly in the infant. This heart malformation consists of a downward displacement of the tricuspid valve into the right ventricle, and redundancy of the valve with variable adherence of the septal and posterior cusps to the right ventricle wall. Open heart surgery is required. Other anomalies are also often present. Re-analyses of the literature, however, indicate that the risks are much lower than previously thought and lithium has again been accepted for use during pregnancy *if* it has been well tolerated and effective in preventing recurrences in the mother.[39] If anomalies do occur, surgical correction is typically performed. Nevertheless, unless the pregnancy is unplanned, it is most prudent to taper quickly and discontinue lithium before conception is attempted.[40] If pregnancy is unplanned and is recognized within the second month of gestation, whatever damage that may occur has already happened. It is probably safer for the mother to continue lithium therapy than to stop it suddenly.

Anticonvulsants have been used extensively during pregnancy to treat epileptic patients. The risk for neural tube defects with valproic acid is well defined. It may be reduced with folic acid supplements, but the remaining risk is higher than the risks to the heart from lithium. Folic acid treatment is also associated with obstetric delayed clotting in both the mother and fetus later in pregnancy. Increased spontaneous abortions are also associated with valproic acid exposure.[41]

In a planned pregnancy it is safer to taper and discontinue an anticonvulsant agent before conception is attempted. If a pregnancy is unplanned and not recognized by the second month of gestation, tapering will take too long to prevent damage to the fetus; abrupt discontinuation elicits withdrawal seizures, non-convulsive status, or recurrence of mania or depression, conditions that are associated with obstetric difficulties. Maintaining the medication prescription with folic acid supplements is considered the better course.

Carbamazepine is associated with dysmorphic facial features, mental retardation, and other malformations and its use follows that of other anticonvulsants.[42] Data about newer mood-stabilizing anticonvulsants are too sparse to assess their risks, but until those risks are known it is reasonable to assume they are similar to other anticonvulsants.

Official guidelines for treating a depressed woman during pregnancy focus on the risks and benefits to the mother, fetus, and family.[43] These guidelines, however, do not separate melancholia from other forms of depression and so recommend psychotherapy as an alternative to medication.[44] The women in these studies were not melancholic or severely ill. All were outpatients, and the treatment effect was weak. One study reports cognitive-behavior therapy to reduce the risk for postpartum depression modestly.[45] Another open trial reports that bright light therapy reduced depression rating-scale scores by about 50% without any adverse effects in 16 pregnant women.[46]

When the prepartum depression is melancholic, however, not to treat with medications or ECT is dangerous to all concerned.[47] The data support the use of nortriptyline or desipramine, with venlafaxine as a possible choice. Multiple medication trials or polypharmacy, never a good practice, are even more problematic in pregnancy. ECT is the best alternative. Discussing the merits and limitations of ECT at the time of planning a treatment course will assure better cooperation from the patient and family if medications fail. On the other hand, the prophylactic use of nortriptyline (and presumably other antidepressants as well) does not prevent recurrence of a postpartum depression.[48] We lack other prophylactic measures.[49]

Postpartum depression

Postpartum depression has adverse consequences to all children in the household. The neonate may be the most vulnerable, showing delayed cognitive and behavioral performance.[50] Maternal parenting is compromised and mother–child interactions disturbed. Depressed mothers are more likely to yell, hit, shake, and neglect children. Infanticide is reported.[51] The severity of such behavior is associated with poor infant cognitive performance at 18 months.[52] Longer-term effects occur when maternal illness lingers.[53] In over half of the households re-examined in one study, both the mother and her partner remained symptomatic 6 months after delivery.[54]

Psychotropic medications are secreted in breast milk and are detected in the breast-feeding infant's blood. With antipsychotic agents infants become lethargic, with long-term effects on the infant's motor functions. Mood stabilizers elicit irritability, drowsiness, abnormal crying, and electroencephalogram seizure rhythms. Sedation, lethargy, irritability, and cyanosis accompany benzodiazepine use. Antidepressants are associated with colic, excessive crying, respiratory distress, and seizures. As the enzymes needed to metabolize these agents develop slowly in newborns, their susceptibility to toxicity is great even when the medication blood levels are low.[55]

As of 2001, there are no controlled studies of the safety of psychotropic use in women who are also breast-feeding their infants.[56] A review of 95 reports of depressed women who were breast-feeding and using 32 agents found no adverse effects for TCAs. Fluoxetine was associated with transient colic and isolated episodes of cyanosis or unresponsiveness as in "a seizure". The effects of other antidepressants were unclear[57]. Later reports of mothers taking sertraline, paroxetine, or fluvoxamine found that serotonin activity in their breast-feeding infants was unchanged.[58] In a study of citalopram, maternal plasma drug levels in 11 mother–infant pairs were higher during pregnancy because of liver enzyme induction and at birth, infant plasma drug levels were two-thirds that of the mother. Concentration in breast milk was two to threefold higher than in maternal plasma, but simultaneously there was only a trace in the infants' blood.[59]

A review of studies in which serum drug levels were obtained from nursing infants concluded that infants older than 10 weeks were at low risk and that "the drugs of choice" were TCAs and sertraline.[60] Another review of 57 research reports and 36 unpublished cases of nursing newborns who had not been exposed prenatally but whose mothers were taking an antidepressant drug postpartum defined an infant drug plasma level of 10% or more above the maternal level as being elevated and potentially harmful.[61] Nortriptyline, paroxetine, and sertraline were associated with undetectable levels. Fluoxetine serum levels were elevated in 22% of infants and citalopram in 17%.

Among women taking benzodiazepines, infant withdrawal symptoms were a concern when the drug was tapered in the mother. Among women taking typical antipsychotic medications, lethargy was reported in infants. Drowsiness, irritability, high-pitched crying, hyperexcitability, and changes in liver function accompanied the maternal use of mood stabilizers.

Although the effects of psychotropic agents in breast milk on the newborn suggest the avoidance of these drugs, that option is not always possible, particularly when the mother's illness is so severe as to require treatment. When medications are used, single daily dosing facilitates the measurement of peak-and-trough maternal blood drug levels.[62] Awareness of the levels permits the pumping of breast milk during troughs so that the newborn is exposed to the lowest possible levels. Because many of the infant reactions to drugs in maternal milk are withdrawal phenomena (e.g., benzodiazepines), the weaning from breast milk needs to be particularly gradual. For mothers with more severe illnesses, ECT is the treatment of choice, with the newborn drinking pumped milk on the day of treatment. Unfortunately, there are no studies assessing these clinical experiences.

Melancholia in childhood and adolescence

Many authors hold that prepubescent depressed children do not improve with TCAs.[63] Although the use of SSRIs in depressed children and adolescents is thought to be effective, such use is restricted by concerns for increased suicide risk. And, among patients who are reported to respond to SSRIs, early relapse rates approach 40% within 6 months.[64]

Small samples of patients and individual case reports examine ECT in the young. Most practitioners have no experience with ECT in children under age 12. One meta-analysis of pooled data from 396 patients (almost all teenagers) found a response rate of 63% for severe depression with the procedure considered safe for young persons.[65]

Psychotherapy for major depression in adults has not been beneficial during the acute phase of treatment and there is no reason to expect better results in children and adolescents.[66] A large controlled comparison of cognitive-behavior therapy, non-directed supportive therapy, and systematic behavior therapy in depressed adolescent outpatients reported that 70% responded to treatment. The mildly ill did best. Non-responders were described as severely depressed and anxious; it is likely that many were melancholic.[67] Cognitive-behavior therapy, although no better than placebo in relieving depression in outpatient volunteers aged 12–17, was reported to enhance the effects of fluoxetine modestly in this age group.[68]

Although melancholia is identified in young children and adolescents, treatment options are limited.[69] Treatment algorithms provide little help because they offer the same unsatisfying multiple medication trials, alone and in combinations, that are offered to adults.[70] The psychopharmacology literature assessing efficacy and safety in children offers little help.

Sample heterogeneity

Epidemiologic studies estimate that 2% of prepubescent children and 5–8% of adolescents suffer depressed moods. Seventy percent have additional episodes and 5–10% of depressed adolescents die by suicide within 15 years of their first depressive illness.[71] The depressed young, however, are no more clinically homogeneous than are other depressed age groups. Further, about 20% of "normal" comparison groups in biologic and treatment studies develop depressive illness.[72] The antidepressant medication literature in the young must be understood within the context of this heterogeneity.

Perhaps a third of depressed children and adolescents are best labeled as manic-depressive, experiencing mania within 5 years of their initial depressive episode.[73] Investigations assessing basal cortisol levels, response to dexamethasone challenge, growth hormone probes, and sleep EEG report highly variable results that are confounded by the clinical heterogeneity of participants.[74] Results vary by the presence of melancholic and psychotic features,[75] prior episodes of depressive illness,[76] and whether the sample is drawn from a hospitalized or an outpatient setting.[77] The presence of co-occurring conduct or oppositional disorders affects results.[78] Such patients, when depressed, are more likely to be placebo responders than depressed children without such diagnoses. Results in adolescents are even more variable, suggesting even greater heterogeneity in the depression category in that age group.

The more severely ill melancholic child, however, is most likely to non-suppress cortisol in response to dexamethasone,[79] exhibit a blunted growth hormone response to clonidine,[80] hypersecrete cortisol,[81] and exhibit elevated nighttime cortisol[82] and have sleep EEG abnormalities seen in depressed adults.[83] Abnormal hypothalamic–pituitary–adrenocortical functions are associated with increased risk of a serious suicide attempt.[84] These identifying laboratory features are not used in selecting patients for inclusion in clinical trials and the proportion of subjects who are melancholic is rarely stated or identified, or their data analyzed separately.

Biologic differences during puberty and the variability in neurodevelopment within and across subsets of normal children and adolescents affect treatment response. Monoamine storage capacity and synthetic processes differ by age, and different neurotransmitter systems mature at different rates.[85] Prefrontal cortex and related circuitry continues to be refined into late adolescence.[86]

Antidepressant treatment trials rarely consider all the study confounds. To dismiss a specific antidepressant treatment for young persons on the basis of poorly designed studies denies potentially useful treatments to these patients.

TCA in the young

Early open clinical trials reported that 60–70% of children with melancholia or endogenous depression responded to TCAs. An abnormal dexamethasone suppression test in these children was associated with responsivity.[87] Symptoms in depressed prepubescent children and adults have many common features of melancholia defined by factor analysis. These features in both age groups predict a favorable response to imipramine.[88]

A double-blind comparison of imipramine and placebo in seven children aged 6–12 years described the patients as withdrawn and having a dysphoric mood associated with feelings of hopelessness and suicidal thought. Imipramine at 5 mg/kg was prescribed and the treatment was monitored with serial electrocardiograms. Results favored imipramine, but are not interpretable because of the small sample.[89]

That early TCA studies reported clinical benefits is instructive for several reasons. The patients were the more seriously depressed children, often identified as endogenously depressed or melancholic. Melancholic patients are most likely to respond to TCAs. Plasma blood levels were used to monitor dosage rather than maintaining a fixed dose by body weight. Dosing by drug blood levels accounts for the pharmacokinetic and pharmacodynamic variability and typically leads to higher response rates. The studies demonstrate that TCAs were well tolerated.[90] In contrast, randomized controlled trials in depressed children report that TCAs are no better than placebo.[91] A meta-analysis of databases from 1966 to 1999 and controlled trials from 1980 to 1999 also reached this conclusion.[92]

Two studies deserve special consideration. In an examination of nortriptyline dosed by a fixed plasma level, 72 outpatients 5–12 years of age were studied.[93] Twelve participants improved during the placebo washout phase, and 50 of the remaining 60 completed the trial. Almost all met Research Diagnostic Criteria for melancholia. Only 30% of the nortriptyline group and 16% of the placebo group were rated as substantially improved. The investigators, however, considered their dosing as too low and that with guidance from blood levels the TCA response rate might have been higher. In a later report, nortriptyline was compared to placebo in 31 adolescents, about 60% of whom were melancholic and all of whom were chronically ill.[94] During the washout period 17 of the 48 participants improved and were not included. Among the 31 participants who completed the study, 8% of the nortriptyline group and 21% of the placebo group were labeled as responders. In both reports, the investigators considered patient chronicity to play a role in non-response.

An explanation for the lack of response is that TCAs are powerful noradrenergic agents and noradrenergic pathways are relatively immature in this age group.[95] While this may be a factor, the controlled studies cannot be considered definitive, and which classes of antidepressant are effective and safe is uncertain. First, placebo response rates in the randomized double-blind studies range from 17% to 92% and average over 50%.[96] Such samples are unlikely to be predominantly melancholic because placebo response rates are low in melancholic samples.[97] Indeed, the high placebo response rates calls into question the diagnoses of major depression.[98] With small heterogeneous samples and high placebo rates, only the most robust therapeutic effect will be recognized. For example, in one study five of 10 adolescents in the amitriptyline group remitted compared with six in the placebo group.[99] Plasma drug level monitoring was not done. Although the two groups did not differ at baseline in clinical rating score means, inspection of individual items finds the amitriptyline group to have more delusional participants. Half the amitriptyline group had made a suicide attempt compared to two in the placebo group. These clinical differences suggest that more members of the amitriptyline group were psychotically depressed, a condition that does not respond well to an antidepressant medication alone.

"Negative" studies are not entirely negative. In a double-blind imipramine and placebo 5-week comparison in 38 prepubertal children, the overall response rates were 56% for imipramine and 68% for placebo.[100] This study is commonly reported as showing a lack of efficacy of TCAs. Yet, over a third of the sample had psychotic features, and 5 of 12 children with psychotic features were considered responders. Among patients identified as endogenous depressed, 50% were responders, while over 80% of children identified as non-endogenous were reported to respond. Another "negative" study compared paroxetine, imipramine, and placebo in mild to moderately depressed 12–18-year-olds and reported paroxetine to be effective, but not imipramine.[101] This study was sponsored by the manufacturer. The responses of a third of patients, identified as having melancholic features, were not separately reported. Among patients completing the study and exhibiting a fall in the Hamilton Depression Rating Scale score greater than 50%, 74% were in the paroxetine group, 65% in the imipramine group, and 57% received placebo.

In a controlled trial of amitriptyline in mild to moderately depressed 12–17-year-olds, amitriptyline was effective on one of two clinical measures.[102] Melancholic patients were not identified.

TCAs are said to be too dangerous to use in depressed children because of a cardiovascular risk.[103] Yet the same agents are widely assessed as safe in children with attention-deficit, anxiety, and sleep disorders.[104] Fears have been heightened by case reports of adverse events. In most of these patients, however, pre-existing heart disease was present.[105] In contrast, the controlled efficacy studies described above that report side-effects consistently find that, while resting pulse rate is increased, the ECG changes are minimal. Studies specifically assessing cardiovascular risk also find the risk of TCAs in children to be no different than in adults, while children tolerate better the anticholinergic side-effects.[106]

Plasma level monitoring of dosing is helpful to good outcomes. An examination of pooled data from 24 studies involving 730 children and adolescents given a TCA and in which the ECG was monitored found increases in heart rate, diastolic blood pressure, and intracardiac conduction interval at high TCA serum concentrations. The authors concluded that cardiovascular changes were "uncertain" and of "probably minor, clinical significance." They recommend baseline ECG and additional recordings after dose increases along with plasma monitoring.[107] Among TCAs, nortriptyline dosing guided by plasma blood level and ECG monitoring offers the best cost–benefit ratio, but this strategy has infrequently been studied in depressed children.[108]

Non-TCA reuptake inhibitors in the young

In contrast to the TCA literature, published randomized controlled studies of fluoxetine, paroxetine, citalopram, sertraline, and their open trials have consistently reported that depressed children respond to SSRIs.[109] These studies, however, are few in number and remission rates are low (30%). Placebo response rates are high, and "positive" studies require careful interpretation.

One study concluded that fluoxetine was effective, although no statistical differences in remission between the medication and placebo were cited for patients who completed the 8-week course. Different clinical instruments also yielded different results.[110]

Another study that defined improvement as an absolute difference in Hamilton Depression Rating Scale scores found no difference between fluoxetine and placebo.[111] A third study reported paroxetine to be better than placebo in an 8-week trial involving 275 depressed adolescents, although the statistical significance was less than commonly accepted levels.[112] Imipramine was not found to be better than placebo. Parent and self-rating measures, however, found the two medications not to differ from placebo. Dosing was not guided by plasma drug level monitoring.

A comparison of paroxetine and clomipramine in an 8-week trial in 121 depressed adolescent outpatients reported the results as equivalent, with around 60% in each group considered responders. Age did not affect results. No placebo group was included for study.[113] Both UK and US oversight groups, however, warn of an increased risk of suicide with paroxetine.[114]

A study of 376 depressed children and adolescents 6–17 years of age from outpatient centers in five countries compared sertraline to placebo.[115] Sertraline elicited significantly reduced mean scores on the Children's Depression Rating Scale-Revised version. The mean score reductions were 22.8 and 20.2 points, respectively, not a dramatic clinical difference. Based on a 40% decrease in adjusted scores, 69% of the sertraline group and 59% of the placebo group were classified as responders. Neither the forms of depression nor the reliability of diagnosticians and raters were specified. These modest changes leave many "responder" children ill, explaining why in such studies parents find the medications no better than placebo.

Using similar methodology, the same group compared citalopram and placebo in the treatment of 174 depressed outpatients 7–17 years old.[116] Response rates were 36% for citalopram and 24% for placebo. Venlafaxine was reported no better than placebo, but dosing and duration of treatment were both inadequate.[117]

The multicenter Treatment of Adolescents with Depression Study (TADS) compared the responses to placebo, fluoxetine, and cognitive-behavior therapy in 439 depressed outpatient adolescents 12–17 years of age.[118] Improvement was 61% in the fluoxetine group, 43% in the cognitive therapy group, 71% in the combined fluoxetine and cognitive therapy groups, and 35% in the placebo group. Suicide attempts were less in combined treatment group compared to placebo. Remission rates are not reported, nor are the forms of depression specified. The results suggest that a third to a half of the patients were still ill at the end of the 12-week trial.

The weak efficacy of published studies of SSRIs for depression in childhood and adolescence was recently reviewed, with the conclusion that their efficacy and safety have not been established for the age group.[119] The published literature is further compromised by unpublished data. A meta-analysis of published and unpublished data of randomized controlled trials that compared the benefits of an SSRI to placebo in 5–18-year-old depressed participants found the risk–benefit to favor only fluoxetine, with weak or equivocal efficacy for paroxetine and sertraline and unacceptable risk–benefit for these agents and for citalopram and venlafaxine.[120] Risk of suicide was the major concern.[121] Unpublished trials were more likely to show no efficacy and substantial risk for the company medication. The omission of these negative trials is unlikely to be by chance as internal documents from one company indicate the withholding of data was advised by pharmacology experts who were paid by the company.[122] The failure to report negative studies to the FDA and the bias in dosing, participant selection, and outcome assessments is widely criticized in recent reports.[123]

MAOI in the young

MAOIs have not been adequately studied in the young. One study reported the combination of phenelzine and chlordiazepoxide to lead to improvement in 78% of depressed children compared to 50% improvement in those receiving phenobarbital.[124] A chart review identified 23 depressed adolescents hospitalized at two university hospitals who received tranylcypromine or phenelzine in a medication switch or add-on. The patients had either not responded or only partially responded to a TCA. The form of the depressive illness is unclear, although two patients were said to have double depression, two atypical depression, three psychotic depression, and two a manic-depressive history. Seventy-four percent were reported to have a "good or fair" response to the MAOI. Six patients failed to follow dietary restrictions, four experienced no effect, one had a headache and a modest rise in blood pressure that resolved, and one experienced myoclonic jerks without a rise in blood pressure or discontinuation of the MAOI. Of the six subjects, three remitted and two partially responded.[125] Nevertheless, concern for hypertensive crisis has limited the use of MAOIs. New MAO-A and MAO-B inhibitors and patch delivery systems that bypass initial liver metabolism and promise fewer dietary limitations and risks for a tyramine reaction need to be assessed in the young.[126]

Conclusion

In planning treatment for a depressed child, the *Diagnostic and Statistical Manual* (DSM) criteria do not identify those with melancholia. The likelihood of manic, psychotic, and melancholic features must be determined. DST and nighttime cortisol levels should be used in the assessment. Patients with melancholic or psychotic clinical characteristics and abnormal laboratory findings are not likely to respond to psychotherapies alone. The use of a secondary amine TCA (e.g., nortriptyline, desipramine) guided by blood level and ECG monitoring is the first choice for the patient who meets criteria for melancholia. This algorithm is particularly compelling because only modest therapeutic effect is attributed to SSRIs.[127] The increased suicide risk for some agents is another deterrent.[128] Rather than an induction of suicidal thoughts and actions, the increased suicide risk reported with SSRIs is more likely due to their weak antidepressant efficacy combined with their ability to induce agitation and to disrupt sleep.[129] Depressed children and adolescents who are anxious or agitated would do best on more sedating antidepressants. Lithium augmentation is recommended with some algorithms.[130] Forty percent of adolescent patients responded to lithium added to a TCA.[131] An MAOI should be considered if switching medications is needed. ECT in young patients is discussed in Chapter 8.

Melancholia in old age

Most depressed persons older than 70 years first seek help from a non-psychiatrist physician and often their care is inadequate. Failure to recognize a depressive mood disorder and failure to treat it properly are the major factors in poor care.[132] Treatment is usually complicated by general medical conditions.

Depressed mood associated with vascular brain changes causes severe dysfunction. Patients stop eating, drinking, and keeping clean.[133] They appear demented and are cognitively impaired.[134] They require hospitalization for nutritional support. Mortality is substantial.[135]

Pharmacologic and methodology factors

Reduced liver metabolism and renal clearance are associated with higher medication blood levels than expected. The half-life of medications is prolonged so that the timing of dose increases needs to be slower than with the same medication given to a younger patient. "Start low and go slow" is a common guide to dosing. Treatment medication trials in the elderly are much longer than trials in younger patients. Older patients are also at risk for drug–drug interactions as they take more prescribed and over-the-counter medications than do the young.[136] As an example, paroxetine autoinhibition of the CPY2D6 liver isoenzyme system is associated with higher than expected blood levels of antiarrhythmic agents, TCAs, typical antipsychotics, risperidone, and several analgesics (e.g., codeine, tramadol).[137] Plasma monitoring is particularly important in guiding treatment in the elderly.

Efficacy studies in the elderly are also plagued by the same problems seen throughout the antidepressant drug literature. Sample sizes are too small to demonstrate potential differences among different classes of agents for different mood disorders, so it is assumed that all classes have similar efficacy.[138] Studies rarely include a placebo group. Tertiary amine TCAs are typically the comparison class. Plasma level monitoring is rarely done so dosing is fixed rather than individually adjusted. Double-blind controlled studies do not identify melancholic patients.[139] Data are scant. A recent review of published and unpublished randomized, placebo-controlled antidepressant treatment trials between 1966 and 2003 in persons over age 55 could identify only 18 studies that permitted analysis.[140]

Therapeutic optimism is needed

Older patients with mood disorder often have co-occurring vascular brain disease and are thought to be less responsive to medication treatment than are younger depressed persons.[141] They are also said to be more prone to chronicity.[142] A recent multicenter drug trial, however, reports a good response rate in patients with moderate to severe late-life depressive illness and "comorbid" vascular disease.[143] Patients randomized under double-blind conditions to sertraline and either fluoxetine or nortriptyline showed equivalent efficacy and rates of adverse events. Rates "much or very much improved" ranged from almost 60% to 90%, making this one of the best antidepressant medication outcomes in the literature. The type of vascular disease did not affect response. Despite the lack of evidence of an advantage for one of the antidepressants, the authors conclude that sertraline is the preferred agent. It was the study sponsor's drug of interest.[144]

Another review of sertraline in persons over age 60 reached similar conclusions.[145] A comparison study reported amitriptyline to be superior to sertraline, but all other studies found sertraline equivalent to other antidepressants and superior on measures of quality of life. Vascular morbidity did not affect response. The side-effects of sertraline were dry mouth, headache, diarrhea, nausea, insomnia, somnolence, constipation, dizziness, and sweating and taste abnormalities.

A study of 156 patients over age 60 with a first-time depressive illness found many patients with cardiovascular risk factors; the degree of risk did not predict remission with nortriptyline, need for additional medication, or recurrence. Maintenance treatment with nortriptyline was associated with reduced recurrence over a 3-year follow-up. The depressed persons over age 80 with vascular brain disease were more likely to have a recurrence than were younger patients.[146] A 6-month follow-up study reported similar response rates between patients with vascular and non-vascular associated depressive disorders in the elderly. The older patients were more likely to have recurrences.[147] A naturalistic 3-year follow-up of patients with "late-life depression" concluded that the condition was chronic. Yet, 62% of the patients "recovered," a rate similar to that of younger patients. In addition, 15% of the patients were underdosed and, even though some were psychotic, none received ECT.[148]

The presence of vascular brain disease or the patient's age over 70 years does not affect acute treatment outcome, although they indicate the need for indefinite maintenance to avoid relapse and recurrence.

TCA in the elderly

Of 12 randomized, placebo-controlled trials of a TCA in the treatment of depressed older patients, two are with nortriptyline while the others are with imipramine. All the studies report the medication to be superior to placebo.[149] Comparison studies of tolerance to antidepressants in the elderly have compared a TCA tertiary amine and SSRIs. Dropout rates for the two classes of drugs are both about 20%, but for different reasons. The elderly are more likely to have orthostasis and falls, renal retention and constipation, and impaired vision with TCAs; while diarrhea, restlessness, anxiety, tremor, sedation, basal ganglia movement disorders, hyponatremia, weight loss, and sexual dysfunction accompany the use of SSRIs.[150] The last, including reduced libido, anorgasmia, delayed ejaculation, and impotence, is common.[151]

It is widely alleged that TCAs adversely affect cognition and that SSRIs do not.[152] However, a study using data from the Baltimore Epidemiologic Catchment Area project identified 65 participants assessed over 11 years with repeated Mini Mental State Examinations (MMSE) and who were also taking a TCA.[153] The patients were compared to over 1400 "non-users." No cognitive differences between the two groups were observed on regression analysis of the data, and the authors concluded that TCAs have no effect on cognition, even among smokers or among different age groups. The MMSE, however, is not a sensitive test battery and does not adequately assess short-term memory, the reported area of dysfunction in older persons receiving TCAs.[154] Nevertheless, this study suggests that TCAs should not automatically be excluded from use because of presumed effects on cognition. Some reports assessing specific acute cognitive effects of TCAs are consistent with this conclusion.[155] Others support the use of SSRIs when cognition is of particular concern.[156] If the patient is melancholic and agitated, however, prescription of an SSRI requires the addition of an anxiolytic and a sedative – classes of drugs that are likely to affect cognition adversely in the elderly, thereby minimizing any SSRI advantage on cognition.

As in the young, the choice of an antidepressant in the elderly is not simple but the same rules apply and the same results are to be expected.[157] Among TCAs, nortriptyline has the most favorable pharmacodynamic profile and minimal effect on the metabolizing liver enzyme system, CYP2D6. It has been used safely and effectively in the elderly and found superior to comparison drugs.[158] A large French study of older depressed persons found TCAs effective and safe, and recommended blood level monitoring to gain maximum benefit and minimize side-effects.[159]

The subjective quality of sleep is improved with nortriptyline as it increases REM sleep phasic activity and reduces sleep apnea.[160] Its moderate anticholinergic side-effects are well tolerated and orthostasis is less than with other TCAs.[161] Therapeutic doses do not affect ventricular function, even in patients with reduced cardiac ejection fractions. In higher doses, however, TCAs have quinidine-like effects slowing cardiac conduction and so should not be used in persons with cardiac bundle-branch block. TCAs may increase the mortality risk in persons with ischemic heart disease and so are usually avoided in persons with ischemic disease.[162] SSRI medications have a lesser effect.[163]

If a TCA is contraindicated, other pharmacodynamically broader-spectrum drugs may be effective. Nortriptyline and paroxetine were reported to have equal efficacy and tolerability in the treatment of depressed persons, including inpatients and melancholic patients.[164] A collaborative study sponsored by the manufacturer of sertraline compared sertraline to nortriptyline in outpatients over age 70, and found sertraline superior to nortriptyline.[165] However, although plasma drug levels were obtained, they were not used to monitor treatment and a substantial proportion of the nortriptyline treated group reported subtherapeutic serum levels (42% at week 6, 29% by week 12). Attrition for side-effects was higher for nortriptyline.

Another manufacturer-supported study concluded that: "sertaline was effective and well tolerated by older adults with major depression." Among patients who completed the 8-week trial, however, the authors reported no meaningful changes in Hamilton Depression Rating Scale scores between patients receiving sertaline or placebo. Melancholic patients in the sample did not benefit substantially from sertraline.[166]

Non-TCA reuptake inhibitors in the elderly

Pure SSRIs exaggerate the anxiety and agitation in melancholia.[167] SSRIs may also be ineffective in this age group when remission is the standard. An industry-organized multisite, 6-week double-blind trial of fluoxetine in 335 depressed outpatients over age 60 reported a remission rate of 32% for fluoxetine compared to 19% for placebo.[168] Remission rates of 35% and 33% for citalopram and placebo were reported in a randomized, placebo-controlled trial in 174 depressed women over age 75 years.[169]

SSRIs are also typically prescribed with a benzodiazepine and a somnifacient. Sedatives and sedating antipsychotics (e.g., quetiapine) are often used, the latter even in non-psychotic patients. These combinations are problematic, however, because SSRIs induce postural instability in the elderly, increasing the risk of falls and fractures.[170] Postural instability is also elicited by benzodiazepines and sedating drugs enhance the instability. Benzodiazepines should be particularly avoided in persons over age 70 because of their adverse effect on cognition.[171] SSRIs alone are not reported to affect cognition adversely.[172] In melancholic patients, venlafaxine is a better choice when hypertension is not an issue. It has no anticholinergic, histaminic or $alpha_1$ properties, and anecdotally is well tolerated and is effective in the elderly.[173] The data for nefazodone, mirtazepine, and bupropion are inadequate in the elderly. Bupropion use is associated with seizures,[174] as illustrated by patient 12.2.

Patient 12.2

A 78-year-old woman living independently and socially active, without a history of seizure disorder, became depressed. Bupropion was prescribed. With increased dosages, she became increasingly unable to care for herself. Alarmed, her daughter brought her to an emergency room where her mother was diagnosed as catatonic and admitted to a neurology service. Catatonia resolved over the time needed to admit the patient. It was then noticed that the patient had periods of "confusion" that occurred when the daughter was in her mother's hospital room. A psychological conversion reaction was diagnosed and the patient transferred to a psychiatry unit.

On that unit the patient was observed to have multiple, sudden, and transient episodes of transcortical sensory aphasia with alterations in responsiveness, interspersed with longer periods of lucidity during which she seemed depressed and very fatigued. She did not recall the brief episodes of "confusion." EEG confirmed that she was in non-convulsive status. Bupropion was discontinued and phenytoin prescribed, resolving the seizures. Her brief catatonia (catalepsy) was believed postictal.

MAOIs in the elderly

We lack carefully controlled, randomized, adequate sample-sized studies of MAOIs in older depressed patients. Orthostasis, weight gain, insomnia, and sexual dysfunction are commonly reported side-effects of non-selective MAOIs in the elderly. Because there is a gradual increase in the medication's steady state, side-effects may take weeks to emerge. MAOIs stimulate minimal anticholinergic effects. A hypertensive crisis induced by ingesting tyramine-rich food or a sympathomimetic drug is the greatest risk of MAOI use. The dietary risks, however, have been overestimated and modern MAOI diets are less restrictive than those of the past.[175] Selective MAOIs (e.g., selegiline) affecting MAO-B in low doses but both A and B in higher doses carry similar risks because of the high dose needed for an antidepressant effect. Moclobemide, a reversible MAOI, avoids many of the therapeutic problems associated with other MAOI agents. One randomized, double-blind multicenter study reports moclobemide (450–750 mg daily) to be about as effective as imipramine (150–250 mg daily) in relieving depressive mood disorders among patients age 65 and under.[176] Placebo-controlled studies are lacking.[177]

Continuation and maintenance treatment for the elderly depressed

Although the elderly respond well to acute and continuation treatment, they are more likely to relapse or have recurrences than are the young.[178] Maintenance treatment is typically needed for an indefinite period.[179] If augmentation is needed during acute treatment, the drug combination may also need to be continued indefinitely as relapse rates increase in the elderly when the enhancing drug is removed.[180] Nortriptyline is reported to prevent relapse and to continue a high level of social adjustment in older patients.[181]

Conclusions

The choices of medications for the elderly melancholic patient are similar to those for younger patients. Short-term prognosis is also no different, although relapse is more likely when treatments are discontinued. TCAs should not be automatically rejected. Other than in the patient with substantial heart disease (see below), TCAs are well tolerated and effective. Non-TCA broad pharmacodynamic spectrum agents may be of equal cost–benefit in this age group, but we lack well-done comparative studies.

Melancholia with co-occurring alcohol or drug abuse

The co-occurrence of depressive illness and substance abuse is common and difficult to manage.[182] Many patients with a primary depressive illness use drugs or alcohol to self-medicate,[183] but some seem to have two independently derived conditions.[184] Severe suicide attempts increase.[185] Alcohol abuse in adults[186] and illicit drug use in teens[187] are risk factors in attempted suicide. Depressed men and women who are heavy alcohol drinkers have increased all-cause mortality rates compared to non-depressed heavy alcohol drinkers.[188] Depressed patients who are active substance abusers or alcoholics are best detoxified while hospitalized, treated for their depressive illness, and then treated for the substance abuse. Resolving the mood disorder increases abstinence rates.[189]

Alcohol

Alcohol abuse and depressive illness co-occur frequently.[190] Manic-depressive patients are most likely to drink heavily during periods of elevated mood.[191] The association is strongest in women, in whom heavy drinking increases after the onset of depressive illness, whereas the drinking patterns in men are independent of depressive illness.[192] Depressive mood disorder is a risk factor for alcohol abuse in women.[193]

Heritable associations are developed for alcoholism and depressive mood disorders, with the genetic risk differing for the two conditions. Although depressive illness carries a risk for alcoholism, the reverse is not true, and drinking patterns do not change the risk for mood disorder.[194] If the depressive illness is successfully treated, alcohol use is substantially reduced, particularly in women.[195] Co-occurring depressive illness also does not confer a poorer prognosis for alcoholism.[196] Unless the mood disorder is directly related to episodes of drinking alcohol, however, discontinuing alcohol use does not in itself reduce recurrence rates other than by increasing compliance.

For the active alcoholic patient, initial detoxification and treatment are best done under hospital care. Both depression and alcoholism need to be treated simultaneously. Naltrexone is reported to reduce craving and consumption and is introduced when the depression begins to resolve.[197] Continuation treatment with naltrexone (50 mg daily) sustains abstinence in patients responding to acute treatment.[198] Cognitive-behavior therapy modestly influences cooperation for naltrexone.[199] Naltrexone use, however, is toxic in persons with liver disease.[200] Serotonin-3 receptor antagonists (e.g., ondansetron) are also reported to reduce alcohol consumption.[201]

In double-blind, placebo-controlled studies, imipramine and desipramine are effective antidepressants for patients who are also alcoholic.[202] Craving was reduced. Fluoxetine,[203] sertaline,[204] and nefazodone[205] reduced depressive moods but did not inhibit craving.[206] No one antidepressant or class of antidepressants, however, has been identified as useful for treating both depressive mood and alcohol craving, and the selection of the antidepressant is based on the choice factors detailed in Chapter 10 rather than on a search for *the* antidepressant for alcoholics.

Illicit drugs

About a third of persons with mood disorder are also illicit substance abusers.[207] Among illicit drugs, *cocaine* is the biggest problem for melancholics.[208] The co-occurrence of depressive illness and cocaine use is associated with poor general functioning.[209] A comorbid personality disorder or manic-depressive illness is frequently diagnosed in cocaine users.

Cocaine withdrawal, the "crash," mimics atypical depression. Patients are often hospitalized for statements of self-harm. Well-designed studies evaluating treatments for the "crash" have not been done, although it is often sufficient to permit the patient to sleep (hypersomnia may last several days) and eat carbohydrates as wanted. In one naturalistic study of 150 patients withdrawing from cocaine, no patient required medications and the dropout rate was 8%. The most common symptoms were craving, insomnia, apprehension, tremor, and agitation. Half the patients were also alcohol abusers.[210] Despite reports that some antidepressants are useful in the long-term treatment of cocaine abuse, a recent review of 18 studies with over 1100 patients could find no evidence supporting their use.[211]

If cocaine usage or withdrawal occurs in association with the signs of a major depression, antidepressant medication is warranted. Cocaine-dependent patients who attempt suicide (as opposed to coming to an emergency room and threatening suicide if not admitted) often have a family history of suicide or mood disorder, as well as a childhood history of abuse or neglect and a more recent history of alcohol abuse and severe depressive illness.[212] No medication, however, is specific for this circumstance, and many are considered useful.[213]

Nicotine

Nicotine, like caffeine, is a widely used addicting drug. Rates of use are doubled among persons with depressive illness.[214] These patients are also at greater risk for relapse of depressive illness after stopping smoking.[215] Depressed patients who smoke are also more likely to abuse alcohol.[216] The hypothesis that the pathophysiology of depression is linked to dysfunction in the brain's hedonistic reward system[217] does not explain the increased rates of smoking in depressed persons.[218] A common genetic predisposition to use nicotine and to experience non-melancholic depression with contributions from shared personality traits has been suggested.[219]

If a patient expresses an interest in ceasing smoking, beginning this process while the patient is under treatment for an acute depressive illness is probably safer than waiting for the depression to resolve and then having the patient enter a smoking cessation program and risk relapse of the depressive illness. A combination of nicotine patch withdrawal and psychotherapy for smoking cessation is considered useful during acute antidepressant treatment.[220] Clonidine has also been tested for cessation of smoking.[221] Although low-dose or sustained doses of bupropion are recommended in smoking cessation,[222] particularly in women,[223] and SSRIs also have some specific effect,[224] there are also negative studies.[225] The choice of the primary antidepressant medication should not be based on its putative effects on smoking, but rather on its efficacy in depressive illness.

Table 12.1. Risk factors for depression poststroke

Left frontal or left basal ganglia lesion
Subcortical atrophy present
Greater impairment of daily activities from the stroke
Personal or family history of mood disorder
Anxious-fearful personality traits (high neuroticism/high harm avoidance)
Younger age at stroke
Poor social support (especially from spouse)
Current additional stressful circumstances

Melancholia with co-occurring neurologic disease

Melancholia does not protect sufferers from other brain diseases and it may be a risk factor for some (e.g., Alzheimer's disease). When neurologic systems that subserve emotional experience and expression are affected by illness, depressive-like syndromes emerge. Co-occurring neurologic disease complicates treatments for melancholia. Some of the more common associations are discussed here.

Stroke

Symptoms of depression (e.g., apathy, anergia, bradykinesia) poststroke are common,[226] and the presence of a depression poststroke increases the risk for stroke-related morbidity and mortality. Peak prevalence of severe depression poststroke is at 3–6 months.[227] Depressive symptoms (e.g., tearfulness, subjective feeling of sadness, pessimism) emerging within days or a few weeks of the stroke are most likely signs of demoralization. However, some features of mood disturbance persist for years poststroke, suggesting that, even if somatic treatment is not initially needed, some interventions will be necessary.[228] Depressions that emerge a year or more poststroke are likely unrelated to the stroke.

The risk for depression increases as the stroke site moves from posterior to anterior and from right to left.[229] This association is disputed.[230] Stroke-related language, movement, and concentration difficulties contribute to chronic dysfunction. Meta-analyses reach different conclusions, but suggest that, while a depressive syndrome emerging within a few weeks of the stroke is associated with left anterior, particularly basal ganglia stroke, depressions occurring several months after the event do not predict location.[231] Patients with "silent" strokes (often subcortical white matter or in the non-dominant hemisphere) who then become depressed respond less well to antidepressant medications.[232] Table 12.1 lists the important risk factors for poststroke depression.[233]

The merit of prophylactic antidepressant treatment immediately poststroke is not adequately tested. One small study found that nortriptyline was superior to placebo in the short run, but that after 6 months it had little preventive effect.[234] Interventions once a depressive illness has emerged are also not adequately tested and one meta-analysis could find no benefit of antidepressant drugs (seven trials) or psychotherapy (two trials). No trials assess ECT in these patients.[235] However, what is effective for melancholia in other circumstances appears reasonably effective when melancholia follows a stroke. One study found nortriptyline superior to fluoxetine and placebo in the treatment of depression poststroke. Weight loss was a problem in the fluoxetine group.[236] Subsequently these investigators found that both nortriptyline and fluoxetine compared to placebo during the first six months poststroke reduced mortality rates in depressed and non-depressed patients.[237]

An open trial of sertraline at either 50 or 100 mg daily reduced depressive symptoms and improved cognition in 20 patients poststroke with nine (45%) becoming symptom-free.[238] A case report associates citalopram with non-convulsive status epilepticus in a stroke patient, but other antidepressants lower the seizure threshold and citalopram cannot be singled out for this effect.[239] In a double-blind, placebo-controlled trial, citalopram was superior to placebo in relieving the depression in poststroke patients.[240] Inspection of those data, however, reveals that, as with other studies evaluating the efficacy of SSRIs in poststroke patients, the dropout rate was high, while the difference between drug and placebo was small. Many of the patients in the placebo group did well – another common theme in this literature. The initial features of depression poststroke may not reflect a depressive mood disorder; waiting several weeks to re-evaluate may better distinguish patients with a mood disorder needing treatment from those who experienced demoralization that spontaneously resolves.

Safety is the principal criterion for selecting treatment among patients who remain depressed. When considered safe, TCAs (the most studied agents) achieved a moderate to marked improvement in 36–75% of patients. About 60% of patients improve with an SSRI. Stimulants achieve improvement rates of 40–80% (suggesting patients with apathetic syndromes rather than depression were included). ECT led to improvement in 95% of patients. Rates of discontinuation because of unacceptable side-effects were 0–45% for TCAs, 4–12% for SSRIs, 0–18% for stimulants, and 0% for ECT.[241] Another study also found ECT to be effective and safe in treating patients with depression poststroke.[242]

Parkinson's disease (PD)

Half or more of patients with PD exhibit features of depression. In non-hospital samples the point prevalence for major depression in patients with PD is about 8% and it is estimated that a third of persons with PD will develop a major depression during the course of their illness.[243] This form of depressive illness is not the result of demoralization. It derives from disruption in frontal lobe basal ganglia circuits. Depressive features may be the first signs of the illness. Persons who develop PD before age 65 and women with PD appear to be at greatest risk for co-occurring depression.[244] The presence of depression in a person with PD is associated with greater decline in motor and cognitive function, but these declines are ameliorated by successful antidepressant treatment.[245]

ECT is a first-line treatment of melancholia in PD patients.[246] Few controlled studies assess the antidepressant drug treatment of major depression in PD and melancholic patients are not specifically identified.[247] In one effort at pooling data for meta-analysis only four articles met selection criteria and these did not use depression-rating scales.[248] TCAs have been helpful. However, the potential added benefit of TCA anticholinergic properties reducing parkinsonian tremor and salivation is offset by the potential for delirium and orthostasis. Nortriptyline or desipramine provides the optimal balance of efficacy and side-effects among TCAs.[249] PD patients are prone to orthostasis because of sympathetic denervation.[250] Prevention with postural change education, wearing support hose, and drinking morning caffeinated beverages or taking a caffeine tablet minimize this concern.

Although SSRIs worsen motor symptoms and elicit dystonia, about half of depressed PD patients are now treated with these agents.[251] In one study, sertraline induced dystonia in 28% of patients with PD and akathisia in 45%.[252] SSRIs interact with selegiline, an irreversible MAO-B inhibitor used to treat parkinsonian patients.[253]

The efficacy of SSRIs in depressed PD patients is unclear. Sertraline was reported to benefit some depressed PD patients, while fluoxetine up to 40 mg daily was not helpful.[254] Citalopram benefited depression in PD and improved bradykinesia without adversely affecting other motor features.[255] One review recommended paroxetine as a first-choice drug among SSRIs.[256] Venlafaxine provides a balance between efficacy and side-effects among the newer antidepressants.[257] Given the inconsistency in efficacy and their motor side-effects, it might be most cost-effective to avoid SSRIs in depressed PD patients.

Selegiline blocks the catabolism of dopamine and is used to treat PD. In low to moderate doses it does not affect gut MAO, so there is minimal need for dietary tyrosine restriction. In daily doses above 20 mg its amphetamine-like metabolites have mild antidepressant properties. Selegiline alleviates depression in PD.[258] In an early double-blind, placebo-controlled small clinical trial selegiline 60 mg daily reduced Hamilton Rating Scale scores by a third in "treatment-resistant" depressed patients.[259] In a double-blind, placebo-controlled study, a 20-mg transdermal selegiline patch applied once daily had a modest antidepressant effect in mild to moderately ill depressed patients without PD.[260] This route of administration would also be useful for treating depression in patients with dementia.

Bromocriptine in daily doses of 85–220 mg moderates the depression in PD,[261] as does amantadine.[262] These benefits, however, more likely result from their energizing properties, relieving apathy and avolition, rather than a true antidepressant effect. In PD patients with melancholia, first-line antidepressant treatment is needed.

Uncommonly, the depression associated with PD is of psychotic severity. Typical antipsychotics are contraindicated because of their extrapyramidal effects. The use of atypical antipsychotics has not been adequately studied, but quetiapine and ziprasidone are reported to be associated with lesser extrapyramidal side-effects.[263]

Huntington's disease (HD)

Depression occurs in about a third of patients with HD, often several years before the motor problems begin.[264] There are no double-blind, placebo-controlled studies of treatment for depression in patients, with HD. However, some cautions are suggested. Because these patients are sensitive to anticholinergic drugs, cognition may be further impaired by TCAs. Motor function may be worsened by pure SSRIs. Venlafaxine has been recommended.[265] MAOIs have also been considered, but the number of patients studied is small.[266] Olanzapine has been reported helpful in low doses in an open trial for treating mood symptoms in HD patients, with the implication that it would also benefit the few patients with HD who become psychotic.[267] However, the anticholinergic effect of olanzapine limits its use in HD patients. When the depression is severe, ECT is an option.[268]

Epilepsy

The reported prevalence of depressive mood disorders among epileptics is 10–20% in community samples and 25–50% in hospital-based studies. Suicide risk is increased.[269] Patients with frontotemporal foci are most likely to develop mood disorders. Male patients and patients with left-sided foci are at most risk.[270] Some anticonvulsant drugs (e.g., valproate) lower folic acid levels, which contributes to the prevalence of depressive features.[271]

When a depressive mood disorder is directly linked to the seizure (either occurring in the prodromal phase or post-seizure), control of seizures is essential to effective antidepressant strategy. Mood-stabilizing anticonvulsants are also effective.[272]

The choice of medications for depressive moods that occur between seizures is made difficult by the propensity of some agents to elicit seizures.[273] The seizure-inducing properties of antidepressants are highly individualized and cross the boundaries of TCAs versus SSRIs. Among TCAs, clomipramine and maprotiline affect seizure threshold most. In a meta-analysis of more than 7000 depressed patients receiving tertiary amine TCAs, the incidence of seizures was zero for imipramine and 0.6% for amitriptyline.[274] This minimal risk has been associated with very high TCA plasma levels.[275] MAOIs also have a low seizure risk. Among non-TCAs, sertraline in high doses may also be a problem, and bupropion should be avoided in the treatment of epileptics. Fluoxetine, fluvoxamine, nefazodone, and paroxetine inhibit isoenzyme systems involved in the metabolism of many anticonvulsants, leading to toxic blood levels of these medications. Venlafaxine and citalopram have minimal effects on these systems, but venlafaxine may induce seizures in some patients.[276]

Anticonvulsants induce isoenzyme systems that metabolize TCAs, leading to lower than expected blood levels.[277] Patients with seizure disorders and depression, however, may respond at lower antidepressant doses, so "start slow and go slow" is a reasonable rule for dosing.[278] ECT has also been used to treat depressive disorders in epileptics; ECT raises the seizure threshold over the course of treatment.[279]

Dementia

Patients with Alzheimer's disease are at increased risk for mood disorder.[280] Depression is most likely when there is a family history, the patient is a woman, and the onset of dementia is before age 70.[281]

Antidepressant treatment trials in Alzheimer's disease are unsatisfactory. Of eight reported placebo-controlled efficacy studies, four are positive and four are negative.[282] Most report a substantial placebo response. Which antidepressant drugs are effective is unclear. Those with anticholinergic properties, however, are best avoided as cholinergic function is compromised in patients with Alzheimer's disease and early treatment intervention includes cholinergic augmentation. TCAs, paroxetine, olanzapine, risperidone, and clozapine are best not prescribed. Bupropion should also be avoided if vascular dementia is present, as bupropion is associated with seizures. High-dose selegiline (20–60 mg daily) is an alternative under study.[283] ECT is anecdotally reported to be effective and safe.[284]

An important consideration in depressed demented patients diagnosed as suffering from Alzheimer's disease is the possibility of pseudodementia, the syndrome that manifests itself as dementia but is causally related to the severity of the depressive mood disorder. This consideration is discussed in Chapter 6.

Traumatic brain injury (TBI)

TBI disables millions of persons worldwide yearly, over one million in the USA alone. At least 25% become severely depressed.[285] Suicide risk is increased.[286] TBI patients, particularly those with frontal lobe damage, commonly experience fatigue, irritability, poor concentration, and avolition that lead to a misdiagnosis of depression.[287] The absence of hopelessness, worthlessness, and anhedonia distinguishes these patients from the depressed TBI patients.[288] Being female is the only reported risk factor for a depressive syndrome post-TBI.[289]

Treatment reports of depression after TBI are mostly anecdotal and none meets present standards for efficacy assessment. No one medication can be said to be "first-choice." SSRIs are commonly used.[290] Also reported to be of some benefit are lithium, carbamazepine, stimulants, and SSRI/norepinephrine reuptake drugs.[291] SSRIs have also been reported to be useful in treating pathological crying secondary to TBI.[292] A few case reports describe ECT as effective in depression post-TBI.[293]

Melancholia co-occurring with general medical conditions

Many general medical conditions are associated with depression, and patients with these co-occurring conditions often require specialized antidepressant treatment.[294] They are also more likely to have greater impairment in overall functioning, reduced job performance, and greater health care costs.[295]

An analysis of antidepressant drug efficacy in patients with co-occurring general medical illness identified 18 suitable studies, half of these employing a TCA. Results in over 800 patients were examined and revealed that there were no significant differences in outcome between depressed patients with co-occurring general medical problems compared to depressed patients without these complicating conditions.[296] This conclusion has been confirmed, indicating that co-occurring general medical disease does not preclude antidepressant drug treatment and does not endorse therapeutic nihilism.[297] Four common situations are reviewed here: (1) heart disease; (2) diabetes; (3) thyroid disease; and (4) drug–drug interactions. General medical diseases that are associated with depressive moods are discussed in Chapter 6 on differential diagnosis.

Heart disease

About 20% of persons with cardiovascular disease have co-occurring depression. Among patients with recent myocardial infarction a third or more have substantial features of depression. About a third of patients in congestive heart failure meet criteria for major depression, particularly younger patients, women, and persons with previous mood disorder.[298]

Depressed patients with acute heart disease have higher mortality rates than do non-depressed persons with similar heart disease.[299] One study reported a fourfold mortality risk within the six months post myocardial infarction increased in depressed patients.[300] In a 50-month follow-up of Dutch adults with heart disease over age 50, those who had a major depression were 60% more likely to die from heart disease than equivalently ill non-depressed persons.[301] Acute cardiac inpatients prescribed benzodiazepines (presumably for anxiety or agitation) who, have a history of mood disorder, are smokers, and cannot stop smoking within six months post myocardial infarction are most likely to have a co-occurring depressive illness.[302]

A depressive mood disorder in patients with heart disease increases the risk for heart failure, particularly in women. This almost twofold increase is thought to result from an imbalance between sympathetic and vagal tone. Tachycardia, the more dangerous arrhythmias, and hypertension ensue.[303] Melancholic patients also experience intrinsic altered heart rates leading to tachycardia.[304] Hospitalized depressed patients have reduced intrinsic heart rate variability, a sign of reduced vagal modulation.[305]

The risk for thrombosis is increased in depression. It is believed to result from aberrations in serotonin-transporter protein function that stimulates platelet activity.[306] Impaired arterial endothelial function, a precursor of coronary heart disease, has also been described in depression.[307] Depressive illness is thus an independent risk factor for heart disease (particularly in women) and successfully treating the depressive illness is a major step in reducing cardiovascular morbidity.[308] Mortality rates, however, are not reduced with antidepressant drug treatment.[309]

Some observers caution the use of TCAs in persons with ischemic heart disease and in patients with bundle-branch block.[310] Nortriptyline, however, has been used successfully to treat depression in patients with heart disease.[311] Bupropion increased blood pressure but not pulse rate in such patients, leading most to discontinue treatment.[312] A comparison of nortriptyline and paroxetine in depressed patients with ischemic heart disease found both to be effective, but nortriptyline to be associated with more adverse cardiac events.[313] In another study, nortriptyline had stronger vagolytic effects on cardiac autonomic functions compared withs paroxetine, the latter claiming some cardioprotective properties.[314] TCAs in low doses, however, offer no greater risk than with SSRIs, but substantially more risks at higher doses.[315]

Thus, for melancholic patients who often require higher doses, TCAs require special care in their prescription.

Venlafaxine in one instance "induced" an acute myocardial infarction in a patient with pre-existing ischemic heart disease,[316] and in rare instances causes reversible conduction disturbances.[317] Citalopram increases Q-T intervals at very high doses.[318] In rare instances it elicits sinus bradycardia, even when prescribed in therapeutic doses.[319] An extensive review of clinical trials between 1978 and 1996, however, concluded that citalopram has no major adverse cardiovascular effects, but does on average reduce resting heart rate about eight beats by min.[320] Fluoxetine was considered safe, but with a weak therapeutic effect for patients with mild to moderate depression.[321] Paroxetine was found safe and also improved depression. It also appeared to return high pretreatment platelet reactivity toward normal and reduced platelet binding.[322] Other SSRIs are also reported to normalize platelet reactivity.[323] On the other hand, SSRIs also block platelet uptake and pulmonary endothelial metabolism of serotonin that may cause vasospastic complications in cardiac patients.[324]

Two multicenter trials report interventions for depression in patients with cardiovascular disease. The Enhancing Recovery in Coronary Heart Disease (ENRICHD) trial includes almost 2500 post acute myocardial infarction depressed patients reexamined over four years.[325] Patients were randomly divided into two groups, one receiving standard post myocardial infarction, care as the "placebo" group, and one receiving the study's "active" treatments of cognitive-behavior therapy or, if severely depressed, sertraline. Several important findings emerged. Severely depressed patients have almost a 40% greater risk for dying than those with mild depressive features. The "active" interventions had no effect on overall survival, nor did they exhibit a specific antidepressant benefit (Hamilton Rating Scale scores dropped about 10 points in the "active" intervention group and 8 points in the "placebo" group). Some reduced mortality, however, is reported among severely depressed patients receiving sertraline. Women and "minority group" patients did substantially worse with "active" treatments, particularly cognitive-behavior therapy.

The Sertraline Antidepressant Heart Attack Randomized Trial (SADHEART) study included 369 depressed patients with acute myocardial infarction or unstable angina.[326] Patients were assigned to treatment with either placebo or sertraline (50–200 mg daily). Sertraline was well tolerated and "severe" adverse cardiac events were less than in the placebo group. The two groups did not differ on changes in scores on the Hamilton Rating Scale, although a global measure of functioning found sertraline to be slightly more effective than placebo. In the most severely depressed patients, however, sertraline was superior to placebo, with response rates of 78% and 45%, respectively. That almost half of all patients in the placebo group improved, including the "severely" depressed, brings into question whether many of the patients in this sample were demoralized rather than clinically depressed. In parallel circumstances, among the bereaved, almost half initially meet DSM criteria for depression despite not thinking of themselves as ill, nor being thought of as ill by researchers applying the criteria.[327] For patients with acute myocardial infarction who appear to be depressed, it may be best to wait several weeks before assigning the diagnosis of a depressive illness. The presence of melancholia after several weeks warrants treatment.

Antidepressant treatment options, however, are limited for the melancholic patient with heart disease. Paroxetine, high-dose sertraline, and low-to moderate-dose citalopram are reported to be safe, but only modestly effective. If anticholinergic effects are a concern, paroxetine and nortriptyline are poor choices. If 6–8 weeks of adequate antidepressant treatment do not produce substantial improvement, ECT should be offered. For severe depression in this patient group, ECT is a first-line treatment.

Diabetes

There is an increased risk for depressive illness among type 1 and type 2 diabetics, with rates for each between 8% and 27%.[328] An association between depression and poor glycemic control is established.[329] Depression and diabetes are both so common that co-occurrence is not surprising. Melancholia often predates the diagnosis of diabetes and its presence is associated with long-term adverse physiologic changes secondary to diabetes.[330] Hyperglycemia alters hypothalamic–pituitary–adrenal activity and other neurophysiologic and neurochemical processes that play a role in melancholia and its treatments.[331]

Antidepressant agents alter blood glucose levels.[332] Chronically elevated glucose levels reduce insulin release and decrease the sensitivity to insulin. Table 12.2 lists the three classes of antidepressant agents studied and their effects on glucose metabolism. Despite the effect of nortriptyline on insulin sensitivity, it was successfully used to treat depression in a double-blind, placebo-controlled trial in diabetics.[333] Results were similar to those in non-diabetic depressed patients. Duration and type of diabetes did not affect outcome. Similar results have been achieved with fluoxetine,[334] sertraline, and other antidepressants.[335]

Table 12.2. Antidepressant drugs and glucose metabolism

Drug	Blood glucose	Consequences
TCA	Raise levels	Decrease insulin levels, decrease sensitivity to insulin, increase carbohydrate craving
SSRI	Lower levels	30% mean reduction in glucose levels associated with anorexia; increase sensitivity to insulin
MAOI	Lower levels	Hydrazine molecule structurally interferes with glucogenesis; increases insulin sensitivity

Neurogenic pain is a complicating factor in diabetes. TCAs are superior to SSRIs in ameliorating this distressing peripheral neuropathy, but their effects on glucose and insulin sensitivity complicate their use.[336] Venlafaxine has been reported to be effective.[337] Its noradrenergic properties, however, caution against its use, as glucose blood levels may be increased.[338] Mood -stabilizing anticonvulsants are believed to be equivalent to amitriptyline in relieving neurogenic pain.[339]

Thyroid disease

A strong relationship between depressive mood and thyroid disease exists. One review finds all patients with severe hypothyroidism to have concurrent depressive illness, reporting hypothyroidism or subclinical hypothyroidism in up to 15% of depressed patients.[340] Others conclude that the depressive signs result from hypothalamic–pituitary–thyroid axis functions and that only a small number of depressed patients have meaningful hypothyroidism that requires intervention.[341] About 10% of depressed patients exhibit elevated thyroxine (T_4) levels, but this does not affect acute treatment outcome.[342]

Low thyroid function (low serum levels of triidothyronine (T_3) and T_4 and elevated thyroid-stimulating hormone) affects treatment response adversely. Whether the depressive illness is secondary to hypothyroidism or hypothyroidism is a co-occurring condition it needs to be corrected before antidepressant drugs can be fully effective.[343] Such treatment may take 2–4 weeks. Once corrected, a maximum response to an antidepressant is more likely.[344] The class of antidepressant medication to be prescribed is determined by the factors discussed in Chapter 10. Thyroid augmentation of antidepressant treatment is also discussed in Chapter 11. There is no compelling evidence that T_3 improves the response in euthyroid depressed patients.[345]

Drug–drug interactions[346]

All antidepressant and antipsychotic drugs, and most mood stabilizers, are metabolized by the liver. Most drugs used to treat general medical conditions are also metabolized by the liver.[347] In older patients the likelihood is substantial for drug–drug interactions, with serious consequences.[348]

Over 30 liver isoenzyme systems have been identified.[349] In selecting psychoactive agents, assessing possible interactions is necessary to assure treatment adequacy and safety. Some agents inhibit and others activate liver enzymes, changing systemic drug concentrations.[350]

Fluoxetine and fluvoxamine will raise blood levels of olanzapine, clozapine, and risperidone. Fluoxetine increases blood levels of many other antidepressants, and using it as an enhancing agent may be no better than increasing the dose of the principal antidepressant. Carbamazepine and phenytoin lower the blood levels of most antipsychotic agents. Valproic acid raises the blood levels of clozapine, olanzapine, chlorpromazine, and thioridazine.[351] Psychoactive agents affect the metabolism of cimetidine, diphenhydramine, and warfarin. Some non-liver-related drug–drug interactions to avoid are listed in Table 12.3.

Melancholia with co-occurring personality disorder

There is no association between premorbid personality and melancholia. Premorbid personality disorder is, however, associated with non-melancholic depression.[352]

Table 12.3. Drug–drug interactions in the treatment of melancholia

Drug combination	Toxic interaction
MAOI and SSRI	Serotonin syndrome/malignant catatonia
MAOI and opiates/opioids	Hypertensive crisis /serotonin syndrome
MAOI and over-the-counter stimulants (e.g., in cold preparations)	Hypertensive crisis
Lithium and potent non-steroidal anti-inflammatory agents	Lithium retention and toxicity if lithium dose not lowered
Lithium and valproic acid	Lithium increases renal excretion of valproic acid, lowering its blood levels[a]
Two SSRI agents	Serotonin syndrome/malignant catatonia
Lithium and bronchodilators	Increased lithium excretion and lower blood levels
Fluoxetine or paroxetine with many systemic agents	Increased blood levels with more severe toxicity for secondary amine TCAs, type 1C antiarrhythmic agents, carbamazepine, phenytoin, and haloperidol

[a] Yoshioka *et al.* (2000); Mula and Monaco (2002).

A study of melancholic and non-melancholic patients using DSM-based personality checklists, however, found equal likelihood of abnormal premorbid personality.[353] Another study assessed 384 currently depressed patients and found 64% to meet DSM criteria for at least one personality disorder and almost 40% met criteria for three or more. After eight weeks of treatment, many no longer met DSM criteria, highlighting the categorical and often state-dependent nature of the DSM axis II system.[354] The validity of checklists to assess personality may not be valid.

Accurately assessing a patient's premorbid personality, however, is best done using structured personality instruments that measure long-standing, habitual patterns of response to specific circumstances, i.e., trait behavior.[355] These behaviors have substantial heritability and are fully matured by early adulthood. These assessments are less affected by the state of depression than DSM-based assessments. Personality traits do not predict response to medication or to ECT in melancholia.[356] Nevertheless, assessing premorbid personality in melancholic patients may predict compliance. The more deviant the patient's personality traits, the more likely the patient will be non-compliant.

Summary recommendations

Treating patients with melancholia under complicating circumstances is summarized in Table 12.4. Each situation, however, is best considered independently but patients, particularly the elderly, often have multiple complicating conditions simultaneously. ECT is the only recommended treatment for melancholia that has progressed

Table 12.4. Recommendations for treating a melancholic patient in complicating circumstances

Clinical situation	Recommendations
With psychosis	ECT is the first choice. Second choice is a broad pharmacodynamic spectrum antidepressant (nortriptyline, desipramine, venlafaxine, and mirtazepine) followed, if needed, by augmentation with an antipsychotic agent
With catatonia or stupor	ECT is the treatment of choice. Antipsychotics should be avoided
High-risk suicide	ECT is the first choice. Second choice is a broad pharmacodynamic spectrum antidepressant and lithium augmentation if needed
Pregnancy/breast-feeding	ECT is the first choice. A secondary amine TCA, venlafaxine, or mirtazepine is an alternative. Mood stabilizers and the prolonged use of benzodiazepines are to be avoided
Children and adolescents	Prepuberty: secondary amine TCAs with plasma drug level and ECG monitoring. Venlafaxine or mirtazepine and MAOIs to be considered. Lithium augmentation as needed Postpuberty: same medication choices and ECT
Elderly	For mild/moderate depression nortriptyline (lower doses may be sufficient). Venlafaxine and mirtazepine are alternatives. ECT for severe depression
Co-occurring alcohol or drug abuse	Antidepressants and ECT indications same as for the elderly. Naltrexone, counseling, and CBT for the alcohol abuse
Depression poststroke	Nortriptyline, venlafaxine, mirtazepine, paroxetine. Avoid pure SSRIs. ECT is also a first-line treatment
Parkinson's disease	For mild/moderate depression nortriptyline, venlafaxine, mirtazepine, selegiline. ECT for severe depression
Huntington's disease	Venlafaxine, mirtazepine, MAOIs
Epilepsy	Tertiary amine TCAs and MAOIs. ECT for severe interictal depressions
Dementia	MAOIs, venlafaxine, mirtazepine
Heart disease	Mirtazepine, paroxetine, citalopram, low-dose nortriptyline, if no bundle-branch block, venlafaxine. ECT for severe depression
Insulin-dependent diabetes	Venlafaxine, mirtazepine, paroxetine, sertraline, MAOI. ECT for severe depression
Thyroid disease	Same as for the elderly

to catatonia or stupor. These are life-threatening conditions and require rapid treatment for the greatest likelihood of success, and ECT meets this need. Further, many medications worsen these conditions.[357] ECT is also recommended as the first-choice treatment of the hospitalized suicidal patient. These patients have likely already failed at least one drug trial, and are not risk-free, even when hospitalized. They also require the most rapid treatment that is most likely to work. ECT and suicide prevention are discussed in other chapters.

Treatment-resistant depression

Treatment-resistant depression (TRD) is identified when the patient has failed to improve with one or two drug treatment trials appraised to be of adequate doses and duration.[358] The label is loosely applied.[359] Two aspects are critical. Adequacy of treatment in dose and time is assumed but rarely tested. And even more rarely has a course of ECT been prescribed. Even when applied, the adequacy of the ECT methods is not assured (chapter 9). To be truly "treatment-resistant" rather than treatment-deprived or labeled a "medication treatment failure," a melancholic patient should also have failed a minimum course of 8–12 bilateral ECT, each producing an adequate seizure.[360]

Using remission rates as the standard, between 30 and 60% of depressed patients are still symptomatic after their first course of drug treatment.[361] Twenty percent are still substantially ill after two years of medication treatment.[362] After five years of multiple drug trials, 10–15% remain ill.[363] The economic, social, general health, and interpersonal costs from prolonged episodes of depression are staggering.[364]

Patients labeled TRD do not have a unique form of depressive illness.[365] The most common causes for continued illness are preventable and well defined.[366] Incorrect diagnosis and improper prescription of treatments, failure to identify concomitant psychosis or catatonia, co-occurring general medical illnesses, inadequate dosing, failure of compliance, and failure to offer ECT in the treatment course are common faults that lead to the application of the TRD label. The best practice in TRD patients is elusive because they represent a heterogeneous population and randomized controlled treatment trials for TRD patients are few and often methodologically limited.[367] Prevention is the best cure.

Incorrect diagnosis

Incorrect diagnosis accounts for a substantial proportion of TRD patients.[368] The patients are not depressed, and a general medical or neurologic illness is not identified. Lumping diverse mood disorders into the major depression category also contributes to incorrect diagnosis.

The patient is not depressed

Among patients considered treatment-resistant and who have failed two adequate medication trials or a medication and an ECT trial, 11% are found not to have a mood disorder. These patients are unlikely to respond to treatments for mood disorder.[369] Failure to identify avolitional or apathetic frontal lobe syndromes leads to needless antidepressant usage.[370] Bereavement, disappointment, or demoralization is accompanied by disturbances that meet DSM criteria for depression.[371] Without a depressive pathophysiology to resolve, antidepressants cannot change the subjective experiences of distress. A substantial proportion of patients hospitalized for depression improve without any treatment, suggesting that their difficulties were misinterpreted as depression.[372]

Melancholia is almost always associated with disturbed sleep, and improvement in sleep is often the first sign that the illness is resolving. Some patients, however, have a sleep disorder that interferes with the response to antidepressant treatment, while others are "pseudo-TRD" because they have a primary sleep disorder, not a depressive illness. Sleep disorders are also associated with anxiety, irritability, fatigue, and loss of interest, psychomotor retardation, and cognitive impairment. Some patients with a sleep disorder say that they have been recently depressed, further linking their depressive features to a seeming mood disorder.[373] In a study of 55 patients with sleep apnea who also had features of depression, continuous positive airway pressure (CPAP) improved their depressive symptoms.[374] In another study, CPAP improved depressive features in 23 patients with sleep apnea.[375] For depressed patients with a specific sleep disorder, correcting the sleep disorder and maintaining good sleep hygiene are essential in preventing relapse and recurrence.

Depression represents an unrecognized underlying general medical illness

Failing to recognize the patient's behavioral condition as an expression of a general medical or neurologic illness denies specific or direct intervention. Cardiac disease, metabolic disorder, and brain diseases are associated with depressive mood and every effort must be made to exclude these causes of a patient's failure to respond to antidepressant treatment. A tragic example of not adequately considering a specific cause of depression follows.

Patient 12.3

A 26-year-old woman with recurrent episodes of depression had been treated with psychotherapy and several different classes of antidepressants since age 13. Early in the course of her illness her episodes occurred once or twice yearly and lasted for a week or so. Psychotherapy with social workers was her only treatment. Her symptoms were moderate in severity and the pattern non-melancholic. Some episodes met DSM criteria for minor depression and later, many met DSM criteria for major depression. As the depressive moods increased in length and severity, medications were added. The depressions always resolved, but for reasons that are unclear she never received continuing medication to prevent recurrence. The patient was in good general medical health and had no obvious neurologic deficits, although a thorough neurologic evaluation was never done. She was presumed to have a primary, treatment-resistant depressive illness.

She was referred for further evaluation. Her most recent episodes were characterized by 3 weeks or so of loss of energy, anhedonia, feeling subdued and tearful, and having reduced interest in usually enjoyable activities, including sex. She had little appetite but did not lose weight. Sleep was not restful. Each episode began with sudden anxiety with mild panic-like features, followed quickly by a "fuzzy-headed" feeling, depersonalization, and feeling "drunk." The depression then unfolded and resolved slowly. Later episodes were associated with a loss of the sense of smell and a need to concentrate on accomplishing simple movements that she took for granted when not depressed.

A seizure disorder with postictal depressions was diagnosed. Brain imaging identified a venous malformation. The malformation, probably originally very small, now involved large aspects of her left frontal lobe with extensions into her left temporal and parietal lobes. It was considered inoperable. Carbamazepine controlled the seizures and for several years she had no further depressive episodes. She was lost to follow-up, but subsequently it was learned that she had died from a massive brain hemorrhage.

Lumping mood disorders under the single label of "major depression"

Despite evidence that different forms of depressive illness (e.g., psychotic, catatonic) respond to different treatments, clinical practice commonly fails to distinguish the different forms of illness and effective regimens are not prescribed.[376] Melancholic patients have a greater responsiveness to TCAs and ECT than to other antidepressant regimens.[377] Patients with atypical depression require alternative antidepressant treatment, usually MAOIs, or ECT.[378]

Applying the melancholia/non-melancholia dichotomy creates a framework for predicting co-occurring conditions, polarity, and responsiveness to treatments. It also immediately and fundamentally shapes acute treatment choices, as illustrated in Table 12.5.

Inadequate treatment

Half or more of TRD patients received inadequate treatment, usually too low a dose.[379] A striking example comes from an analysis of a California Medicaid database from 1987 to 1996.[380] Over 1600 newly depressed patients who received antidepressant medication were identified. Only 17% were given an adequate course of initial therapy, and of these, 8% also inexplicably received an antipsychotic drug. Forty percent of the patients receiving an inadequate dose of an antidepressant were prescribed a second for augmentation. The majority of patients who were prescribed a second antidepressant stopped taking their first antidepressant, thus ending up in a switch in treatment rather than the prescribed augmentation. The second prescribed drugs were often underdosed. With inadequate dosing or poor choice of medication, the illness shows little sign of resolution or side-effects dominate the clinical picture. Non-compliance with the prescription follows.[381]

Co-occurring conditions

Failing to recognize and treat co-occurring conditions that do not cause the depressive illness but do interfere with antidepressant pharmacokinetics and pharmacodynamics limits the efficacy of treatment. Among hospitalized depressed patients, half have co-occurring conditions that influence responsiveness.[382] Among melancholic

Table 12.5. Acute treatment choices and forms of depression

Melancholia	Atypical	Dysthymic/non-melancholic	Secondary to other condition
Broad pharmacodynamic spectrum antidepressants	MAOI	Pure SSRI	Specific treatments whenever possible. Example: hormone stabilization
Augmentation with lithium MAOI or another broad-spectrum agent	Lithium if seasonal	SSRI with noradrenergic properties if comorbid anxiety disorder/OCD	Stimulants for apathetic and avolitional frontal lobe syndromes
Mood stabilizers for manic-depressive patients	Broad pharmacodynamic spectrum agents	Augmentation	Anticonvulsants for ictal-related episodes
ECT	ECT	Psychotherapy	Specific antidepressant depending on causative condition

patients, however, the presence of a co-occurring personality disorder is not associated with a poor response to adequate treatment.[383] Among a less selected group of depressed patients, however, the presence of a personality disorder is associated with a poor response to treatment. Of 92 outpatients characterized as treatment-resistant, 48% without a personality disorder responded to nortriptyline, but only 17% with a personality disorder responded.[384]

Thyroid dysfunction is a common co-occurring condition associated with poor response. About 16% of melancholic patients have abnormal thyroid functioning, but half of TRD patients have evidence of hypothyroidism.[385] Correcting thyroid dysfunction leads to rapid improvement in mood disorder.[386] Prescribing replacement thyroid (T_3), however, is insufficient to insure that the patient is euthyroid, and repeated laboratory testing is needed to monitor treatment. Other implicated conditions in TRD include Cushing's disease, Addison's disease, hyperparathyroidism, PD and other basal ganglia disease, brain tumors, vascular brain disease, pancreatic carcinoma, autoimmune disease (Multiple sclerosis, systemic lupus erythematosus), vitamin deficiencies, viral infections human immunodeficiency (HIV), Epstein–Barr, cytomegalic, influenza), borreliosis (Lyme's disease), lymphoma, paraneoplastic syndromes, and many medications (e.g., beta-blockers, steroids, immunosuppressants, interferon).[387] Stabilizing or normalizing these conditions is necessary before a maximum antidepressant benefit is achieved. The presence of these conditions, however, should not delay the start of antidepressant treatment, but rather heighten the recognition that the duration of the acute treatment phase will be longer than for uncomplicated melancholia.

Failure to offer ECT early in the illness course

Failure to offer ECT early in the course of a depressive mood disorder leads to chronicity, a conclusion that has face validity. The longer a depression goes untreated or is unresponsive because it is undertreated, the more likely that the process will induce chronicity. In one study 40% of the duration of depressive episodes was explained by the time elapsed between onset of symptoms and the start of an adequate therapeutic dose of antidepressant treatment.[388] Most antidepressant trials do not meet standards of adequacy in duration or in dosing. Even if the dosing and duration are adequate, a poor response to the initial medication indicates that for that patient the dose (even the highest possible) was not therapeutic. If a single augmentation trial or switch does not work, that again indicates the treatment was not adequate for that patient. Continued efforts with medication needlessly prolong the episode without substantial benefit, and chronicity results. The second reason to offer ECT sooner rather than later is that ECT is the most effective antidepressant treatment available for melancholia.

The factors leading to TRD are illustrated by a recent study of 92 TRD patients who had not responded to several different antidepressants (95% had received at least one SSRI).[389] About 40% responded to nortriptyline and by the eighth week had a mean Hamilton Rating Scale score of 8. The group's mean nortriptyline blood level was just over 100 ng/ml, suggesting that higher dosing might have achieved an even better response. Thus, even in a defined TRD study, low dosing was a problem. While two-thirds of the sample had experienced two to five drug treatment trials and the sample index episode's mean length was an astounding 96 months (8 years), only 2 patients had received "ECT," with no details of the course provided.

Prevention of TRD

Thorough differential diagnosis is the first step in the prevention of TRD. Recognizing and managing co-occurring conditions is a necessary effort. For the patient with primary recurrent melancholia who does not require hospitalization, a broad pharmacodynamic spectrum antidepressant agent such as nortriptyline, maximizing the dose if necessary, is the first choice. If the patient does not respond, switching to a different class of antidepressant and maximizing that dose is the next step. If the patient has a partial response to the first-choice agent, augmentation follows. Going beyond two augmentation or switch trials or one augmentation and one switch trial is unlikely to benefit and may harm the patient by prolonging the illness. ECT should no longer be delayed. Virtually all patients with primary recurrent melancholia who are in otherwise good general medical and neurologic health will eventually fully respond to this sequence of treatments. Antidepressant treatment failure in melancholia results when the illness is secondary to an underlying general medical or neurologic condition that interferes with treatment or requires specific treatment, exposure to a prolonged series of drug trials elicits chronicity or persistent failure of compliance. For the patient with complicating factors, the recommendations detailed in this chapter offer the best chance of reducing the likelihood of treatment resistance.

NOTES

1 Cecil (1988), pp. 223–5.

2 O'Hara *et al.* (1991); Wisner *et al.* (1993). Estimates of prevalence and lifetime risk for psychiatric illness must be viewed cautiously. For example, in a three-sample assessment of rates of maternal depression in Latin America (Wolf *et al.*, 2002), 35–50% of interviewed women were identified as having experienced a major depression. Such high rates suggest extreme sensitivity but low specificity of the process of diagnosis by symptom scales administered by non-specialists.

3 Kurki *et al.* (2000); Chung *et al.* (2001).

4 Wadhwa *et al.* (1993).

5 Zuckerman *et al.* (1990).

6 Monk (2001).

7 Frontal lobe activity and reactivity are reported (Dawson *et al.*, 1992).

8 Graff *et al.* (1991).

9 This discussion with the patient should also include the possibility of an unplanned pregnancy. About half the pregnancies in the USA are unplanned (Rosenfeld and Everett, 1996; Koren *et al.*, 1998).

10 Hendrick *et al.* (2003).

11 Koren *et al.* (2002).
12 Altshuler *et al.* (2001b, c).
13 Hammen (1990); Glover *et al.* (1998).
14 O'Connor *et al.* (2002); Hulshoff *et al.* (2000); Field *et al.* (2002b); Field (1998).
15 Glover (1997).
16 Copper *et al.* (1996); Hedegaard *et al.* (1996).
17 Field *et al.* (1995); Field (1998); Abrams *et al.* (1995).
18 Zuckerman *et al.* (1990).
19 Kurki *et al.* (2000).
20 Hendrick and Altshuler (2002).
21 Kulin *et al.* (1998); Cohen *et al.* (2000b); Hendrick and Altshuler (2002).
22 McElhatton *et al.* (1996); Ericson *et al.* (1999).
23 McElhatton *et al.* (1996); Hendrick and Altshuler (2002).
24 Kulin *et al.* (1998).
25 Einarson *et al.* (2001).
26 Altshuler *et al.* (1996).
27 Einarson *et al.* (2001).
28 Heinonen *et al.* (1977).
29 Heikkinen *et al.* (2003); Morag *et al.* (2004).
30 Weissman *et al.* (2004).
31 Nulman *et al.* (2002).
32 Apgar (1953, 1962). http://www.childbirth.org/articles/apgar.html.
33 Simon *et al.* (2002).
34 Costei *et al.* (2002).
35 Kallen (2004).
36 Laine *et al.* (2003).
37 Zeskind and Stephens, 2004.
38 Pastuszak *et al.* (1993); Chambers *et al.* (1996).
39 Cohen *et al.* (1994); Schou (1998).
40 One of us saw a manic-depressive woman who had been well controlled on lithium throughout pregnancy She delivered a boy who, in addition to Ebstein's anomaly, had other cardiac defects, making surgical repair impossible, requiring a new heart. No new heart was available and the boy died.
41 Schou (1998).
42 Schou (1998).
43 Wisner *et al.* (2000).
44 Cooper *et al.* (2003); Grote and Frank (2003); Murray *et al.* (2003). Spinelli and Endicott (2003).
45 Chabrol *et al.* (2002a, b).
46 Oren *et al.* (2002). Bright light therapy and other proposed treatments for depressive mood disorders are discussed in Chapter 13.
47 Hendrick and Altshuler (2002).
48 Wisner *et al.* (2001).
49 Lumley and Austin (2001).
50 Sharp *et al.* (1995); Murray *et al.* (1996a, b).
51 Lyons-Ruth *et al.* (2002); Spinelli (2003).
52 Murray *et al.* (1996b); Weinberg and Tronick (1998).

53 Kurstjens and Wolke (2001).
54 Zelkowitz and Milet (2001).
55 Morselli (1980).
56 Hoffbrand *et al.* (2001).
57 Burt *et al.* (2001).
58 Epperson *et al.* (2001); Hendrick *et al.* (2001).
59 Heikkinen *et al.* (2002). The authors invoke the induction of liver isoenzyme CPY2C6 as the explanation.
60 Wisner *et al.* (1996).
61 Weissman *et al.* (2004).
62 Suri *et al.* (2002) report that estimates of antidepressant drug levels in breast milk are highly variable. Thus, although monitoring maternal blood levels is important to determine the troughs, this method does not guarantee that the newborn will in fact receive a low dose of the medication.
63 Findling *et al.* (1999).
64 Martin *et al.* (2000); Heiser and Remschmidt (2002).
65 Rey and Walter (1997).
66 Chapter 11.
67 Birmaher *et al.* (1996a, b).
68 TADS team (2005); March *et al.* (2004).
69 Ryan *et al.* (1987); Birmaher *et al.* (2004).
70 Hughes *et al.* (1999).
71 Kaufman and Charney (2003).
72 Rao *et al.* (1996b).
73 Strober *et al.* (1993); Rao *et al.* (1996b).
74 Rao *et al.* (1996b).
75 Robbins *et al.* (1983); Freeman *et al.* (1985).
76 Klee and Garfinkel (1984).
77 Kaufman and Charney (2003).
78 Hughes *et al.* (1990).
79 Among inpatient depressed children, 50–70% are dexamethasone suppression test (DST) non-suppressors while 40–60% of adolescent samples are non-suppressors. Fifty to 70% of similar adult samples are non-suppressors.
80 Meyer *et al.* (1991).
81 Schildkraut *et al.* (1989).
82 Goodyer *et al.* (1996, 2001).
83 Kaufman and Ryan (1999).
84 Pfeiffer *et al.* (1991).
85 Goldman-Rakic and Brown (1982); Rosenberg and Lewis (1995).
86 Casey *et al.*, 2000; Alexander and Goldman, 1978.
87 Preskorn *et al.* (1982); Weller and Weller (1986).
88 Hughes *et al.* (1988).
89 Petti and Law (1982).
90 Puig-Antich *et al.* (1979); Preskorn *et al.* (1987); Kashani *et al.* (1984).
91 Kraemer and Feiguine (1981); Geller *et al.* (1989, 1990); Kutcher *et al.* (1994).
92 Maneeton and Srisurapanont (2000).
93 Geller *et al.* (1989).

94 Geller *et al.* (1990).
95 Kye and Ryan (1995).
96 Wagner and Ambrosini (2001).
97 Chapter 10.
98 Martin *et al.* (2000). Chapter 10 provides a discussion of placebo response and form of depression.
99 Kraemer and Feiguine (1981).
100 Puig-Antich *et al.* (1987).
101 Keller *et al.* (2001).
102 Kye *et al.* (1996).
103 Werry *et al.* (1995); Gutgesell *et al.* (1999).
104 Wilens *et al.* (1994); Glazener *et al.* (2003).
105 Alderton (1995); Evans *et al.* (1998).
106 Geller *et al.* (1985); Wamboldt *et al.* (1997).
107 Wilens *et al.* (1996).
108 Daly and Wilens (1998).
109 Wagner *et al.* (2004).
110 Emslie *et al.* (1997).
111 Simeon *et al.* (1990).
112 Keller *et al.* (2001).
113 Braconnier *et al.* (2003).
114 Chapter 7.
115 Wagner *et al.* (2003).
116 Wagner *et al.* (2004).
117 Mandkoki *et al.* (1997).
118 TADS team (2005); March *et al.* (2004).
119 Courtney (2004).
120 There is no obvious pharmacodynamic explanation for fluoxetine appearing to have a better risk–benefit ratio than other SSRIs. Longer half-life and thus greater resistance to non-compliance is one consideration. See Valuck *et al.* (2004).
121 Whittington *et al.* (2004). Any increased risk of suicide in young patients receiving SSRIs likely reflects their weak antidepressant effect combined with their adverse affect on sleep and their associated agitation-inducing properties (Armitage *et al.*, 1997a, b).
122 Kondro (2004).
123 Healy (1997, 2004); Healy and Sheehan, 2001; Parker *et al.* (2001, 2002); Angell (2004); Parker (2004).
124 Frommer (1967).
125 Ryan *et al.* (1988a).
126 Robinson (2002).
127 Wagner and Ambrosini (2001).
128 Vitiello and Swedo (2004); Whittington *et al.* (2004).
129 Armitage *et al.* (1997a, b); Vorstman *et al.* (2001); Brent (2004).
130 Ryan (1992); Hughes *et al.* (1999).
131 Ryan *et al.* (1988b).
132 Charlson and Peterson (2002); Unutzer (2002).
133 Forsell *et al.* (1994); Alexopoulos *et al.* (1997).
134 Chapter 6 discusses pseudodementia.

135 Unutzer (2002).
136 Flint (1998).
137 Solai *et al.* (2002).
138 Mittmann *et al.* (1997).
139 Flint (1998); Parker (2004).
140 Taylor and Doraiswamy (2004).
141 Baldwin and Tomenson (1995); O'Brien *et al.* (1998); Simpson *et al.* (1998); Benazzi (1999c); Baldwin (2005).
142 Lavretsky *et al.* (1999); Denihan *et al.* (2000).
143 Krishnan *et al.* (2001).
144 MF participated in a multisite random assignment study of sertraline, imipramine, and placebo sponsored by Pfizer. After the study data had been collected, the randomization of his patients could not be told to him for a concurrent study. The company had "sealed" the files and the data were not submitted to the FDA (Fink 2000c).
145 Muijsers *et al.* (2002).
146 Miller *et al.* (2002b).
147 Krishnan *et al.* (1998).
148 Denihan *et al.* (2000).
149 Taylor and Doraiswamy (2004).
150 Brymer and Winograd (1992).
151 Among the elderly the most significant influence on the frequency of sexual intercourse is partner availability. Among sexually active elderly persons being treated for depression at one clinic the most common unacceptable side-effect of SSRI treatment was loss of libido, and ejaculation and erectile problems (personal communication, N. Vaidya).
152 van Laar *et al.* (1995).
153 Podewils and Lyketsos (2002).
154 Flint (1998).
155 Cole *et al.* (1983); Allain *et al.* (1992); Kuny and Stassen (1995).
156 Settle (1998); Hirschfield (1999); Levkovitz *et al.* (2002).
157 Unutzer (2002).
158 Roose *et al.* (1994); Gareri *et al.* (1998); Robinson *et al.* (2000); Weintraub (2001); Lenze *et al.* (2002).
159 Ballon *et al.* (2001).
160 Buysse *et al.* (1996).
161 Prevention is the best strategy if orthostasis is a concern. Education about gradual position changes and the wearing of support hose help. If not contraindicated, a strong caffeinated beverage on awakening is of benefit.
162 Flint (1998); Hippisley-Cox *et al.* (2001). The increased mortality rate may result from the elderly being more sensitive to the anticholinergic effects of TCAs because vagal tone decreases by 25–50% by age 60 or so. Low vagal tone has been associated with increased cardiac death (Lehofer *et al.*, 1999).
163 Goodnick *et al.* (2002).
164 Mulsant *et al.* (1999).
165 Finkel *et al.* (1999).
166 Schneider *et al.* (2003).
167 Sheehan *et al.* (1992); Tollefson *et al.* (1994a).
168 Tollefson and Rosenbaum (1998).

169 Roose *et al.* (2004).
170 Laghrissi-Thode *et al.* (1995).
171 Wang *et al.* (2001a).
172 Hindmarch *et al.* (1990); Hindmarch and kerr (1994).
173 Flint (1998).
174 Pesola and Avasarala (2002).
175 Gardner *et al.* (1996).
176 Silverstone (2001).
177 Bonnet (2003).
178 Opdyke *et al.* (1997).
179 Reynolds *et al.* (1999).
180 Reynolds *et al.* (1996).
181 Lenze *et al.* (2002).
182 Hasin *et al.* (1996, 2002); Grant and Harford (1995); Grant (1997); Oslin *et al.* (2000).
183 Wang and Patten (2001a, b).
184 Weiss *et al.* (1992); Tsuang *et al.* (2001).
185 Aharónovich *et al.* (2002).
186 Cornelius *et al.* (1995).
187 Kelly *et al.* (2002).
188 Greenfield *et al.* (2002).
189 Hasin *et al.* (2002).
190 Grant and Harford (1995); Kessler *et al.* (1996, 1997).
191 Reich *et al.* (1974); Winokur *et al.* (1998).
192 Wilsnack *et al.* (1986, 1991).
193 Dixit and Crum (2000).
194 Tsuang *et al.* (2001); Wang and Patten (2001a, b). In male alcoholic patients personality traits that lead to high-risk impulsive behavior may be what is inherited. This trait then leads to the use of substances that affect the brain's hedonistic reward system. The initial stimulation of dopamine in this system is a neuropharmacologic theme for substances of abuse, including nicotine and caffeine. The alcoholic may be particularly sensitive to this process, and when combined with the anxiolytic effects of alcohol in social situations, a powerful double reward is produced. Replacing the addicting substance with a socially acceptable dopaminergic agent that does not adversely affect health is one approach to treating alcoholics (Taylor, 1999).
195 Hasin *et al.* (1996); Oslin *et al.* (2000).
196 Davidson and Blackburn (1998). This surprising observation may result from a "ceiling effect." Because the relapse rates for alcoholism are so high, as much as 90%, there is little variance left to be affected by additional disease. In other words, "it can't get much worse."
197 Croop *et al.* (1997); Kranzler and Van Kirk (2001).
198 Anton *et al.* (2001).
199 Anton *et al.* (1999, 2001).
200 Swift (2000).
201 Johnson *et al.* (2000); McBride *et al.* (2004). Abstinence may be monitored with periodic assays of serum carbohydrate-deficient transferrin, a liver enzyme elevated during the metabolism of alcohol, even in non-alcoholics (Bell *et al.*, 1994).
202 Mason *et al.* (1996); McGrath *et al.* (1996).
203 Kranzler *et al.* (1995); Cornelius *et al.* (1997a, b).

204 Deas *et al.* (2000).
205 Roy-Byrne *et al.* (2000).
206 Gorelick and Paredes (1992).
207 Kessler *et al.* (1996).
208 McDowell and Clodfelter (2001).
209 Schmitz *et al.* (2000).
210 Miller *et al.* (1993).
211 Lima *et al.* (2001). Desipramine has been anecdotally associated with anti-craving properties. A recent 8-week randomized trial in 146 patients receiving desipramine, carbamazepine, or placebo, however, could find no acute treatment benefit for either medication (Campbell *et al.*, 2003a).
212 Helmus *et al.* (2001); Roy (2001).
213 Weddington *et al.* (1991); Nunes *et al.* (1995); Petrakis *et al.* (1998); McDowell *et al.* (2000); Schmitz *et al.* (2001). If the patient experiencing cocaine withdrawal was using large amounts of the drug for an extended period of time, sudden withdrawal leaves a suppressed dopaminergic state. If the patient complains of auditory hallucinations or other psychotic features, administering powerful dopamine blockers, i.e., antipsychotic drugs, further compromises dopaminergic function and precipitates a malignant catatonia/neuroleptic malignant syndrome (Fink and Taylor, 2003).
214 Covey *et al.* (1998).
215 Tsoh *et al.* (2000).
216 Hamalainen *et al.* (2001).
217 Chapter 14.
218 Cardenas *et al.* (2002).
219 Dierker *et al.* (2002).
220 Patten *et al.* (1998); Thorsteinsson *et al.* (2001).
221 Glassman *et al.* (1993).
222 Tonstad (2002).
223 Lerman *et al.* (2002).
224 Nia *et al.* (2002).
225 Covey *et al.* (2002).
226 Aben *et al.* (2003); Nilsson and Kessing (2004).
227 Whyte and Mulsant (2002).
228 Dam (2001).
229 Robinson (1998); Vataja *et al.* (2001); Narushima *et al.* (2003).
230 Whyte and Mulsant (2002).
231 Robinson *et al.* (1983); Parikh *et al.* (1987); Morris *et al.* (1996); Carson *et al.* (2000).
232 Yamashita *et al.* (2001).
233 Narushima *et al.* (2003).
234 Narushima *et al.* (2003).
235 Hackett *et al.* (2004).
236 Robinson *et al.* (2000).
237 Jorge *et al.* (2003).
238 Spalletta and Caltagirone (2003).
239 Hagebeuk *et al.* (2002).
240 Andersen *et al.* (1994).
241 Cole *et al.* (2001).

242 Murray *et al.* (1986).
243 Slaughter *et al.* (2001a).
244 Zesiewicz *et al.* (1999); Slaughter *et al.* (2001a).
245 Norman *et al.* (2002).
246 Andersen *et al.* (1987); Faber and Trimble (1991); Aarsland *et al.* (1997); Wengel *et al.* (1998).
247 Zesiewicz *et al.* (1999).
248 Klaassen *et al.* (1995).
249 Richard (2000).
250 Goldstein *et al.* (2002).
251 Slaughter *et al.* (2001a).
252 Leo (1996); Hauser and Zesiewicz (1997).
253 SSRIs affect liver isoenzyme systems (particularly 2D6), influencing the metabolism of many medications used in the elderly. Citalopram is least likely to do this (Slaughter *et al.*, 2001a).
254 Caley and Friedman (1992).
255 Rampello *et al.* (2002).
256 Richard (2000).
257 Slaughter *et al.* (2001a). Case reports suggest that bupropion may relieve the depression and anergia of the parkinsonian syndrome (Leentjens *et al.*, 2003). However, bupropion also elicits delirium in persons with PD.
258 Allain *et al.* (1993); Jansen Steur and Ballering (1999).
259 Sunderland *et al.* (1994).
260 Bodkin and Amsterdam (2002).
261 Jouvent *et al.* (1983).
262 Silver and Yudofsky (1992).
263 Poewe and Seppi (2001).
264 Hayden (1981); Slaughter *et al.* (2001b).
265 Rosenblatt and Leroi (2000).
266 Ford (1986).
267 Squitieri *et al.* (2001).
268 Evans *et al.* (1987); Ranen *et al.* (1994).
269 Arciniegas and Anderson (2002); Martinez Perez *et al.* (2002).
270 Altshuler *et al.* (1990).
271 Harden and Goldstein (2001).
272 Harden *et al.* (2000).
273 Rosenstein *et al.* (1993).
274 Peck *et al.* (1983).
275 Preskorn and Fast (1993).
276 Schlienger *et al.* (2000).
277 Harden (2002).
278 Fromm *et al.* (1972); Legg and Swash (1974); Blumer and Zielinski (1988).
279 Kellner and Bernstein (1993); Regenold *et al.* (1998); Lambert and Robertson (1999).
280 Zubenko *et al.* (2003a, b).
281 Lyketsos *et al.* (1996); Harwood *et al.* (1999).
282 Lyketsos and Olin (2002).
283 Sunderland *et al.* (1994).

284 Rao and Lyketsos (2000).
285 Bowen *et al.* (1998); Holsinger *et al.* (2002).
286 Arciniegas and Anderson (2002).
287 Jorge *et al.* (1993).
288 Kreutzer *et al.* (2001); Seel *et al.* (2003).
289 Levin *et al.* (2001).
290 Newburn *et al.* (1999); Fann *et al.* (2000); Zafonte *et al.* (2002).
291 Persinger (2000); Kanetani *et al.* (2003).
292 Muller *et al.* (1999).
293 Ruedrich *et al.* (1983); Crow *et al.* (1996).
294 Koike *et al.* (2002).
295 Katon (1998).
296 Gill and Hatcher (2000).
297 Krishnan (2003).
298 Freedland *et al.* (2003).
299 Burg and Abrams (2001); Carney and Jaffe (2002).
300 Carney *et al.* (1999).
301 Penninx *et al.* (2001).
302 Strik *et al.* (2001).
303 Shabetai (2002). Increased renin–angiotensin–aldosterone activity also affects blood pressure and increases circulating cytokines and their cachexia-inducing properties.
304 Moser *et al.* (1998).
305 Nahshoni *et al.* (2004). ECT has a variable effect on heart rate variability, but patients with low baseline variability and thus more likely melancholic are reported to recover rapidly with ECT (Karpyak *et al.*, 2004).
306 Whyte *et al.* (2001).
307 Broadley *et al.* (2002).
308 Charlson and Peterson (2002).
309 Carney *et al.* (1999).
310 Shores *et al.* (1998).
311 Hartling *et al.* (1987); Roose *et al.* (1994).
312 Roose *et al.* (1991).
313 Roose *et al.* (1998).
314 Yeragani *et al.* (2002).
315 Ray *et al.* (2004).
316 Reznik *et al.* (1999).
317 Combes *et al.* (2001).
318 Catalano *et al.* (2001).
319 Isbister *et al.* (2001).
320 Rasmussen *et al.* (1999).
321 Strik *et al.* (2000).
322 Sauer *et al.* (2001).
323 Musselman *et al.* (2000).
324 Skop and Brown (1996).
325 ENRICHD investigators (2000, 2001); Glassman (2005); Taylor *et al.* (2005).
326 Glassman *et al.* (2002). This study is sponsored by the maker of sertraline, Pfizer.
327 Clayton (1982).

328 Goodnick (2001).
329 Lustman *et al.* (2000).
330 Lustman and Clouse (2002).
331 Fonagy *et al.* (1989); Bellush and Reid (1994).
332 Goodnick (2001).
333 Lustman *et al.* (1997b).
334 Lustman *et al.* (1997a).
335 Holliday and Plosker (1993); Goodnick (2001).
336 Goodnick (2001).
337 Lithner (2000).
338 Goodnick (2001).
339 Kochar *et al.* (2004).
340 Haggerty and Prange (1995).
341 Fava *et al.* (1995).
342 Styra *et al.* (1991); Joffe and Marriott (2000).
343 Howland (1993); Hickie *et al.* (1996); Rao *et al.* (1996a); Corruble *et al.* (2004).
344 Joffe and Levitt (1992).
345 Lasser and Baldessarini (1997).
346 See www.drug-interactions.com for continued updated literature on drug–drug interactions.
347 Adson *et al.* (1998).
348 Doucet *et al.* (1996).
349 Nemeroff *et al.* (1996); Preskorn (1997); Wang *et al.* (2001a); Mula and Monaco (2002).
350 The prominent liver isoenzyme systems 1A2, 2C19, 2D6, and 3A4 are affected by many pharmaceutical agents (Hansten and Horn, 2002). Commonly prescribed inducers (increasing activity and thus reducing the blood levels of drugs metabolized by those systems) include barbiturates and several anticonvulsants. Nicotine, cannabis, and St. John's Wort also induce these systems. Commonly prescribed inhibitors (decreasing activity and thus increasing the blood levels) include fluoxetine, fluvoxamine, other antidepressents, valproic acid, cimetidine (Tagamet), and omeprazole (Prilosec). Pharmaceuticals whose blood levels can be substantially affected by drug-induced isoenzyme changes include antidepressants, beta-blockers, non-steroidal anti-inflammatory agents, warfarin, anticonvulsants, benzodiazepines, antihistamines, sildenafil (Viagra), tolbutamide (Ornase), and angiotensin II blockers and many others.
351 Mula and Monaco (2002).
352 Maier *et al.* (1992b).
353 Tedlow *et al.* (2002).
354 Fava *et al.* (2002b).
355 Sato *et al.* (2001). Non-melancholic depression is associated with anxious-fearful personality traits that aggregate in the first-degree relatives of patients with non-melancholic depression (Maier *et al.*, 1992b). Many studies report that patients with non-melancholic depression also have comorbid personality disorder (Alpert *et al.*, 1997; Perugi *et al.*, 1998).
356 Tse and Bond (2001); Marijnissen *et al.* (2002).
357 Fink and Taylor (2003).
358 If the first choice medication has been maximized and the response has not been adequate, eight weeks or more are likely to have passed, and so that duration is usually accepted as adequate for a treatment trial of an antidepressant. For augmentation with lithium or T_3,

3–4 weeks are usually enough to determine if this strategy will succeed. If a second antidepressant is used, another eight weeks is needed. Antidepressant drug trials of only a few weeks are inadequate. For ECT the number of treatments, electrode placement, and quality of seizures all affect adequacy (see Chapter 9). Antidepressant drug dose adequacy varies with each drug, but in general, adequacy of dose is the maximum. Thus, if a patient cannot tolerate more than 100 mg daily of sertraline, that is not an adequate trial, even though many patients will respond to that dose.

359 The label "blames the patient." A better label is "medication treatment failure." Such patients are at increased risk of suicide (Oquendo *et al.*, 2001).

360 Fink (1987a, 1989, 1990, 2000, 2003c).

361 Preskorn and Fast (1991); Preskorn and Burke (1992).

362 Winokur *et al.* (1993); Paykel (1994).

363 Winokur *et al.* (1993).

364 McCombs *et al.* (2001).

365 Fagiolini and Kupfer (2003); Fava (2003).

366 Kennedy and Paykel (2004); Nelsen and Dunner (1995); Kornstein and Schneider (2001).

367 Stimpson *et al.* (2002).

368 Keller *et al.* (1986b); MacEwan and Remick (1988); Nelsen and Dunner (1995).

369 MacEwan and Remick (1988).

370 Starkstein and Manes (2000).

371 Clayton (1982).

372 Nelson *et al.* (1978, 1980).

373 Szuba *et al.* (2001).

374 Millman *et al.* (1989).

375 Ramos Platon and Espinar Sierra (1992).

376 Guscott and Grof (1991); Mulsant *et al.* (1997).

377 Nelson *et al.* (1990).

378 Quitkin *et al.* (1991). In the CORE study, the patients with atypical depression responded as well as those with typical depression to ECT.

379 Quitkin (1985); Keller *et al.* (1986b); Nierenberg and Amsterdam (1990); Scott (1995b).

380 McCombs *et al.* (2001).

381 Delgado (2000a).

382 Keitner *et al.* (1991).

383 Petersen *et al.* (2002a, b, 2001).

384 Papakostas *et al.* (2003).

385 Howland (1993); Peteranderl *et al.* (2002).

386 Gold *et al.* (1981).

387 Musselman *et al.* (2001a, b); O'Reardon and Amsterdam (2001).

388 Scott (1992); Scott (1995b).

389 Nierenberg *et al.* (2003). No placebo group was included.

13

Proposed treatments for melancholia

There is a woman in this town who had lost three of four foetuses from epileptic attacks immediately after birth . . . It is clear that those foetuses died from a taint in the blood transmitted to the brain . . . In dealing with her next three children, immediately at birth, we had a fontanelle inserted in the neck and leeches applied behind the ears in order to drain off the impurities from the brain; they completely escaped epilepsy and still do to this day.[1]

It is fair to say that most treatments prescribed today have little evidence to support their efficacy[2]

Novel treatments for depression have been proposed. Some derive from observations of the neurobiology of mood disorders (e.g., light therapy (LT)) while others are opportunistic applications of new technologies (e.g., transcranial magnetic stimulation (TMS)). None has proven efficacy. Commonly promoted alternatives to standard treatments are discussed here.[3]

Light therapy

Evidence for a seasonality in the incidence of mood disorders with higher incidence in the winter months encouraged thoughts that reductions in hours of sunlight affected brain neuroendocrine mechanisms and elicited mood disorders. The description of a *seasonal affective disorder* (SAD) (winter depression) and its inclusion in the psychiatric classification system encouraged extensive studies of LT. LT has also been assessed in patients with non-seasonally related depression.

This intervention presents high-intensity light from light boxes for varying lengths of time to subjects.[4] Exposure time is 30–60 min daily for two weeks or more, typically between 6 and 9 a.m.[5] There are no absolute contraindications to LT and no evidence that it adversely affects the eyes, although patients report "eye strain," headache, and nausea. These symptoms are usually mild and transient.[6]

Few studies assess the efficacy of LT beyond anecdotal evidence or small open treatment trials. The patients studied are characterized as mild to moderately depressed. Few were likely to be melancholic. The investigations do not show a clear benefit. Among the few controlled studies, LT of various strengths, duration of exposure, and delivery time of day are compared to dim red light or negative ionized air.

Exposure to bright light was reported to enhance better antidepressant medication therapy than did dim light, with a mean reduction in Hamilton Rating Scale scores after one week of 27% versus zero change.[7] Another report concluded that the exposure of 400 lux daily added to 40 mg of citalopram elicited greater reductions in depressed mood than did the medication and "ionized air." Response time was faster with the "active" combination.[8] Other reporters did not find any enhancement effect of 5000 lux added to adequate doses of imipramine.[9]

Patients whose depressive moods occurred primarily in the winter months benefited more from morning rather than afternoon delivery, and exposure to bright light (10 000 lux) was better than exposure to ionized air.[10] When patients with SAD in a primary care setting were exposed to bright light, 74% had some improvement compared to 57% of patients who experienced dim red light.[11] This study was criticized, however, for its small effect size and when strict response criteria were used, bright and dim light responses were 30% compared to 33%.[12] Others found no difference between 7000 lux and ionized air among 32 patients with SAD assigned to bright or dim light. In both groups Hamilton Rating Scale scores significantly dropped from baseline, suggesting to the investigators that the "placebo" condition of dim light might in fact have a therapeutic effect.[13] An alternative explanation is that both conditions offer only a placebo effect. In another, larger sample, these investigators also found morning and afternoon exposure to be equivalent. Hamilton Rating Scale scores dropped more than 50% in 61% of patients exposed to morning light, compared to 50% exposed to afternoon light, and 32% exposed to morning ionization. Response onset, however, was not observed until the third week of treatment.[14] While other reports fail to differentiate conditions of light and no light in persons with winter depression. A recent single-blind comparison of bright light (10 000 lux) to high-density and low-density ion flow in 32 mildly depressed volunteers with a first-episode SAD lasting over two years reports remission rates of 50%, 50%, and 0%, respectively.[15] A meta-analysis of selected studies concluded that LT was modestly effective for patients with seasonal or non-seasonal affective disorder.[16] Another meta-analysis reaches a similar conclusion, but cautions that "many reports of the efficacy of light therapy are not based on rigorous study designs."[17]

"Dawn simulation" is a modification of LT in which a dawn effect is imitated for 90 min beginning between 4 and 5 a.m. as light increases in the patient's bedroom from darkness to 250 lux. Compared to dim red light and morning 10000 lux LT, patients in the dawn simulation condition had a higher rate of remission.[18] Overall, any meaningful benefit appears to be with daily morning 10000 lux light.[19]

LT has also been reported to benefit patients with postpartum depression,[20] those with late luteal-phase dysphoria,[21] and pregnant women with mild to moderate depressive mood disorders.[22] In a small randomized trial, however, the authors report LT to have been effective in relieving prepartum depression, but group mean HAMD score changes were not significant.[23] While LT may have a role as an adjunct intervention for persons with mild, non-melancholic depressions, for almost all other circumstances, clearly active treatment needs to be provided.

Transcranial magnetic stimulation

TMS is a method of stimulating the motor cells of the brain in patients who have developed motor paralyses. TMS maintains motor tone in deafferentiated muscles. The availability of the instrumentation and the possibility of directly stimulating brain centers led to trials in patients with psychiatric disorders, particularly those identified as "medication-resistant" depressive mood disorders.[24] The hope that TMS would elicit the benefits of electroconvulsive therapy without effects on cognition and memory was another stimulus.[25] This hope has not been fulfilled and the interest in TMS as a non-seizure-producing method has shifted; it is now being tested as a method of inducing grand mal seizures in direct imitation of ECT (see below).

TMS stimulates the brain by repetitive magnetic stimulation through large coils placed over the scalp.[26] The energy levels are just sufficient to stimulate a motor response in a small muscle bundle (usually the thumb). The electromagnet generates brief pulses (100–300-ms durations) of energies of 1.5–2.0 T. The magnetic energies pass through the skull and depolarize brain cells, a process at the cellular level that is identical to the effects of electric currents. Pulses of energy are delivered at varying frequencies (slow or rapid), at different intensities, for varying durations, at varying weekly frequencies, for varying lengths of application, through electrodes that vary in shape, size, and head location.

Slow or very-low-frequency TMS is reported to reduce the reactivity of the targeted brain region.[27] Higher frequencies increase brain excitability. High-frequency application produces loud clicks requiring the patient to wear protective earplugs. Rarely, inadvertent seizures occur. Because slow TMS appears to reduce brain reactivity it has been used to study disorders of apparent hyperexcitability such as action myoclonus, focal dystonia, and epilepsy. It has also been used in persons with anxiety disorder and obsessive-compulsive disorder as an experimental tool.[28] No efficacy has been established for TMS in these conditions.

Studies comparing TMS and sham TMS in depressed patients find a wide range of effect sizes, none dramatic, and only in patients with mild to moderate anxiety and depression.[29] None of the favorable studies report a mean Hamilton Rating Scale score drop greater than 50% (a common criterion for response in medication studies). Among studies reporting numbers of responders 14%, on average, were considered responders in the TMS groups and 8% in the sham treatment groups. Unlike ECT, the reports supportive of TMS find the better results in younger patients and lesser results in the older patients.[30] TMS, also unlike ECT, is not associated with normalization of hypothalamic–pituitary hyperactivity.[31]

In a study of daily suprathreshold high-frequency left frontal TMS compared to ECT, the outcomes for TMS and ECT were considered equivalent for the non-psychotic depressed. ECT was more effective than TMS for the psychotic depressed.[32] This study was criticized for its small sample size and inadequate ECT methodology.[33] Another study compared substandard 2.5× threshold unilateral-ECT to TMS and found the two treatments equivalent in reducing HAMD scores. The number of ECT administered was substandard.[34] In a second comparison study using the same design, these investigators report left TMS to be equivalent to right unilateral ECT at 2.5× threshold.[35] The use of low-dose unilateral ECT is a critical problem in these comparisons as a recent analysis of the ECT literature reports unilateral ECT to be no better than sham ECT.[36] Another comparison study of TMS and unilateral ECT also reports the two treatments to be equivalent, but suffers from the same problems in the ECT delivered.[37]

TMS has been offered as a continuation treatment strategy.[38] The 6-month relapse rates in a study of TMS as a continuation treatment after successful ECT in samples of 20 and 21 each found relapse rates of 20%. Patients, however, also received continuation medications.[39]

Two double-blind, placebo-controlled studies of TMS versus sham TMS are reported. TMS reduced mean Hamilton Rating Scale scores from 25.8 to 16.6 after one week.[40] By the end of the 2-week daily session trial, however, mean scores had only dropped another few points to 13.7. The investigators concluded that their study demonstrated the efficacy of TMS because the mean scores for the sham TMS group had only dropped from 25.3 to 19.7. Clearly sham TMS was not effective, but the failure of TMS to reduce scores substantially after the first week suggests inflation from a placebo effect. The sham TMS group's standard deviation of 10.3 (large for a mean of 19.7) is consistent with this interpretation, and the effect size was less than 1.0.

A second study employed a double-blind, placebo-controlled cross-over design of TMS versus sham TMS.[41] During the first 10 sessions of sham TMS the Hamilton Rating Scale scores dropped substantially and then only modestly in the TMS condition for the next 20 sessions. These authors concluded that TMS was not an effective treatment for the depressed patients in their study.

No advantage for left or right TMS over sham TMS as an add-on treatment has been reported.[42] In another double-blind randomized 4-week trial of low-frequency right TMS, however, high-frequency left TMS and sham TMS in depressed outpatients in both active treatment conditions significantly reduced some but not all of the clinical scales without inducing cognitive changes.[43] Another study also found no cognitive effects of TMS.[44]

Among studies that conclude that TMS is effective, it is unclear which patients respond best. Less severely ill, non-psychotic, non-melancholic patients are proposed as the likely target group.[45]

Despite the conflicting reports, some writers state: "the majority of controlled trials demonstrated significant antidepressant effects of active rTMS compared with a sham condition."[46] Meta-analyses of TMS studies are less sanguine in their conclusions. One found only a few reports indicating "substantial.. . . clinical response." Among open studies the conclusion was that "relatively few patients in these studies would meet standard criteria for response, let alone remission." Among controlled or sham studies the conclusion was that "the magnitude of the therapeutic effect was of doubtful clinical significance," with the average difference in improvement between active and control conditions of only 16.25%.[47] In another analysis that failed to find evidence of efficacy, the analysts concluded that there is "no strong evidence for benefit from using transcranial magnetic stimulation to treat depression."[48] While the literature lacks evidence of clinical efficacy, a review in the *American Journal of Psychiatry* concludes: "Most data support an antidepressant effect of high-frequency repetitive TMS administered to the left prefrontal cortex . . . TMS shows promise as a novel antidepressant"[49] A parallel analysis in the *British Journal of Psychiatry* that found the 2-week difference between TMS and sham TMS not to be significant concludes: "Current trials are of low quality and provide insufficient evidence to support the use of rTMS in the treatment of depression."[50] A 2005 meta-analysis concludes: "rapid-fire rTMS is no different from sham treatment in major depression, however, the power within these studies to detect a difference was generally low".[51]

Almost all the TMS studies and reviews are directly or indirectly financed by the device manufacturers. An ongoing multicenter trial designed by the manufacturer who also controls all data and data analysis is unlikely to provide additional guidance on the role of TMS as a treatment.[52] Despite the weakness of the evidence for efficacy, TMS methodology is highly touted and in some countries its use in the relief of depression that has failed multiple medication trials has been approved.[53]

Magnetic seizure therapy (MST)

MST is designed to apply the energies of TMS to induce a therapeutic grand mal seizure. MST requires the same monitoring, general anesthesia, and other medications needed for ECT.[54] The feasibility studies in laboratory animals and the early uncontrolled trials in humans demonstrate that grand mal seizures can be elicited. The first reports of the quality of the seizures and their electroencephalogram characteristics show that the seizures are of lesser efficacy than are needed in effective ECT (Chapter 9). The authors emphasize that the induced seizures are associated with lesser effects on cognition.[55]

A single case report of a course of MST in a 66-year-old woman with recurrent depressions offers some suggestion as to the safety of MST.[56] Despite being ill for many years, she had never received ECT. Her index episode is described as a non-psychotic major depression with melancholic features. Her pretreatment 21-item Hamilton Rating Scale score was 33. After 12 MST sessions the score dropped to 6. The patient tolerated the procedures well.

The use of magnetic energies is within the tradition of inducing seizures for therapeutic purposes by alternate means. Intramuscular camphor, intravenous pentylenetetrazol, inhalant flurothyl, and electrical inductions, as well as different electrode placements and different electrical energies, have been studied. Brief-pulse ECT is established as the effective induction method for ease of use, efficacy of induction, and minimal expense. MST is an alternative method of inducing electrical changes in the motor cells of the brain. There is no reason to expect that the clinical effects of MST will be greater than ECT or the effects on cognition less or that it will supplant ECT.[57]

Vagal nerve stimulation (VNS)

VNS has been marketed for the treatment of various forms of intractable epilepsy since the mid-1990s.[58] Under general anesthesia, electrical leads are wrapped around the left vagus nerve in the neck and attached to a pocket-watch-sized generator in the left subclavian chest wall. The device is comparable to cardiac stimulators. The electric current depolarizes afferent sensory fibers in the nerve, which in turn stimulates the locus coeruleus and its noradrenergic projections to the amygdala, thalamus, and hypothalamus. About a third of patients with intractable partial complex seizures are reported to exhibit lower seizure rates. Throat pain and hoarseness are the most common side-effects.[59] An industry-sponsored study reports that patients who tolerate and benefit from the acute phase of treatment improve further over the next 12 months.[60]

Anecdotal reports of reduction in depressed mood and anxiety among epileptic patients responding to VNS suggested its application in psychiatric patients.[61] The mood-stabilizing effects of some anticonvulsants also encouraged trials of VNS in depressed patients. A multicenter industry-supported study describes 60 patients with mild to moderate non-psychotic depression who had previously failed at least two "robust medication trials."[62] Dosing is not detailed. In their initial report, about 40% of the sample had also failed a prior course of ECT, but the details of ECT are not presented. Overall, about 30% of the patients are said to exhibit falls in Hamilton Rating Scale scores of 50% or more. Seventeen percent are said to remit. The average time for improvement onset was about 45 days.The benefits are said to improve with time, with greater benefits later in the year of treatment than at the beginning. Ten "serious" adverse events occurred during the study, listed as headache, neck and other pain, and dysphagia. The study does not report a placebo group or comparisons of periods of time when the generators were on and off. In a naturalistic 3-month follow-up of 30 of these patients, response rate was sustained and remission rate increased to 29%.[63]

Functional brain-imaging studies in depressed patients receiving VNS report inconsistent findings.[64] A study of sleep architecture at baseline and at 10–12 weeks after VNS implantation in a cohort of 7 patients revealed decreased awake time and a normalization of ultradian sleep EEG rhythms.[65] Despite the absence of definitive findings, a Food and Drug Administration review committee has recommended approval for clinical use of VNS in patients with major depression who are considered to be pharmacotherapy treatment failures.[66]

Glucocorticosteroid receptor agonists

Cortisol levels are elevated and hypothalamic–pituitary–adrenal activity is abnormal in melancholic patients.[67] Some antidepressant drugs increase glucocorticoid receptor functioning.[68] Because cortisol derangement is assumed to contribute to dysphoric mood, agonists to this system have been investigated as possible antidepressants. Mifepristone (RU486) is an antiprogesterone agent used in terminating pregnancy. In higher doses (400–800 mg daily) it is an antagonist of glucocorticosteroid action and has been reported to relieve depressed mood and psychosis observed in some patients with Cushing's disease.[69] Small numbers of patients with primary major depression were also reported to respond.[70] More recently, 30 patients with psychotic depression were given mifepristone in daily doses of 50, 600, or 1200 mg for seven days. Eight of 19 patients receiving $>$ 600 mg responded with falls in the Hamilton rating scale scores and 12 of 19 had decreases in psychosis scale scores of 50% or more. Patients receiving low-dose mifepristone did not do as well. Although reported to tolerate the high doses, other studies describe side-effects to include rash (mostly in men), fatigue, nausea, anorexia, and hot flashes.[71] A 6-week, double-blind cross-over study of 20 manic-depressive outpatients with "residual depressive symptoms" (mean of 18 on the 17-item HAMD and 23 on the MADRS) treated with 600 mg mifepristone daily reported improvement in cognitive performance, but no clinically meaningful reduction in depression ratings.[72]

The studies of other glucocorticoid antagonists describe small samples in open-label trials.[73] In one double-blind, placebo-controlled study of 20 patients, ketoconazole (an antiglucocorticoid) was superior to placebo among depressed patients with abnormal cortisol functioning ($n = 8$) but not among those with normal cortisol levels ($n = 12$).[74] An open trial of ketoconazole reports it to be better than placebo in reducing symptoms in another small sample, this one of psychotic patients with depressive features.[75]

Despite the unclear results of glucocorticoid antagonist treatment in depression, they are theoretically interesting interventions toward understanding depressive illness. At present they are experimental treatments. Corticotropin-releasing hormone receptor antagonists to treat depression are also experimental and unproven.[76]

Targeted neurotransmitter system agents[77]

Despite the overwhelming evidence that the different neurotransmitter systems in the brain work in concert and that depressive illness is associated with changes in multiple neurochemical systems, highly specific medications continue to be developed with the aim that individual customized pharmacotherapy will be possible. Among agents being investigated that affect *serotonin receptor subtypes* are postsynaptic 5-HT1A agonists (gepirone, lesopitron, eptapirone) and 5-HT2C agonists (agomelatine). Some *noradrenergic* and *dopaminergic* agents are available in Europe but not in the USA. Moclobemide, a reversible monoamine oxidase inhibitor (MAOI) with reported clinical antidepressant activity, is not yet available in the USA. Brofaromine, another reversible MAOI, is under study.

GABAergic agents do not appear likely candidates as antidepressants; however, glutamate *N*-methyl-D-aspartate (NMDA) and non-NMDA receptor modulators (remacemide, lamotrigine, topiramate) are being developed or have come on line as mood stabilizers.

Hormones

Estrogen

Observations of the association between fluctuations in levels of estrogen during the menstrual cycle and mood encouraged investigations of estrogen as an antidepressant. Increased serotonin 2A receptor binding in the prefrontal cortex after estrogen administration has been reported to enhance cognitive performance.[78] Estrogen replacement therapy for postmenopausal women, however, has no effect on depressive symptoms.[79]

Studies of the efficacy of estrogens in depressed women are few, methodology is variable, and results are modest.[80] Subjects have generally been outpatients with mild to moderate depressive mood disorders. Most of the reported effects on mood symptoms are attributed to the elimination of thermoregulatory dyscontrol and sleep disturbances that are seen in older women with low estrogen blood levels.[81] An early study compared conjugated estrogen to placebo and found the hormone had antidepressant effects but depressed patients did not remit.[82] Another study could find no benefit for estrogen as an add-on to imipramine therapy.[83] A report speculated that fluoxetine seemed to be more effective in older women receiving hormone replacement therapy than in those who were not or who were given placebo.[84] A comparison of an estradiol transdermal patch (100 μg) with placebo in perimenopausal depressed women found estrogen to be superior in ameliorating depressive symptoms. Sixty-eight percent of the sample was reported to remit.[85] Another study of the effects of transdermal estradiol treatment reported 8 of 20 perimenopausal depressed women to have remitted.[86] There were no differences between responders and non-responders in hormonal fluctuations. One report speculated that an estradiol patch might enhance low-dose fluoxetine in perimenopausal women with major depression.[87]

Two double-blind, placebo-controlled studies using estrogen transdermal patches (17-beta estradiol 200 μg daily) found it somewhat better than placebo in improving mood symptoms.[88] Sublingual estrogen relieved mood symptoms in postmenopausal depressed women, those with low serum estradiol levels were the most likely to benefit from this preparation.[89]

In contrast, several studies did not find estrogen superior to placebo in depressive illnesses.[90] Another study could find no benefit for estradiol in preventing relapse in bipolar patients.[91] Given the modest effects even in the positive studies and its potential risks, estrogen treatment for depression is at best an add-on for treatment-resistant perimenopausal women. The American College of Obstetricians and Gynecologists does not recommend estrogen as a primary treatment for women with depressive illness.[92]

Progesterone

The precipitous drop in progesterone levels following delivery is weakly correlated with the emergence of "postpartum blues."[93] Although no causality has been established, this finding has encouraged the evaluation of progesterone as an antidepressant. An early chart review concluded that progesterone was active in the treatment of psychotic depression,[94] while others saw no benefit to progesterone treatment in three patients.[95] In a naturalistic study, women who had previously experienced postpartum sadness of a severity to require medical attention and who were again postpartum were offered progesterone to prevent a recurrence of sadness. The decision to treat was left to the individual's physician. Twelve (7%) of the 181 women who received progesterone had a recurrence, whereas 14 (67%) of 21 women who did not receive progesterone had a recurrence.[96] A double-blind, crossover, placebo-controlled study of a small sample of women, however, could find no benefit for progesterone therapy.[97] Long-acting progesterone administration postpartum increased the risk of depression.[98] The evidence of efficacy for progesterone in relieving depressive mood disorders is weak.

Testosterone

Testosterone has been suggested as a potential antidepressant for older depressed men.[99] Testosterone levels decline in aging men, particularly the bioavailable form of testosterone. This decline is related to reduced hypothalamic–pituitary function, fatigue, reduced muscle and bone mass, sexual dysfunction, and mood changes observed in many elderly men.[100] Depressed elderly men appear to have the lowest levels.[101] In open trials in small samples of patients, testosterone replacement therapy has been reported to have some beneficial effect on mood in elderly, hypogonadal men.[102] One trial reports testosterone (400 mg intramuscularly every 2 weeks) to have enhanced the effect of selective serotonin reuptake inhibitors.[103] Randomized, controlled studies, however, do not find it of benefit in reducing depression rating-scale scores in these patients, although it does improve energy levels.[104] Despite the risks of testosterone therapy – increased blood hematocrit, hypercholesterolemia, cerebrovascular stroke, exacerbation of prostatic cancer – it remains an investigative tool in the study of depression.

Herbal remedies

St. John's wort

Extracts of this plant product have been considered to have antidepressant properties. The extract, hypericum, has an affinity for a variety of brain receptors, particularly serotonin. It also has monoamine oxidase inhibitor properties.[105] A meta-analysis of early clinical trials of over 1700 patients reported a St. John's wort preparation (300–900 mg hypericum daily) to be superior to placebo in relieving depressive symptoms.[106] The methodologies of these studies, however, were criticized.[107]

A double-blind, placebo-controlled, manufacturer-sponsored study compared the antidepressant efficacy of an active extract of hypericum (WS 5570) in 186 patients with 189 patients receiving placebo.[108] Patients were characterized as having "mild to moderate" depressive mood disorder (mean 17-item Hamilton rating-scale scores for both groups were 21.9). The HAMD scores fell in both groups, about 10 points for the extract group and 8 points for the placebo group. Elaborate statistical efforts produced an extract advantage in the last week of the 6-week trial. A two-point mean difference in HAMD scores, however, is clinically meaningless.

In another double-blind, randomized trial, 140 outpatients with "moderate" depression (HAMD-17 scores of 20–24) received 900 mg of hypericum once daily or placebo. After six weeks the HAMD scores of the hypericum group dropped from a mean of 22.8 to 11.8 while the placebo group dropped from 22.6 to 19.2.[109] A multicenter 12-week trial in Germany including 241 patients said to have "moderate depressive disorder" reported hypericum to be equivalent to 50 mg sertraline, with 68% of the hypericum group and 70% of the sertraline group identified as responders.[110] The dose of sertraline, however, is below the therapeutic range for many depressed patients, suggesting the improvement in both groups was a placebo effect. Another German study of 251 patients identified as having "moderate to severe major depression" reported hypericum equivalent to 20 mg paroxetine.[111] The dose of paroxetine is below the therapeutic range for many patients, again suggesting a placebo effect.

A double-blind, placebo-controlled study conducted at 12 academic centers in the USA compared an extract of St. John's wort, sertraline, and placebo.[112] Patients varied in severity from mild to severely ill ($n = 337$). No statistical differences in Hamilton rating-scale score changes were found among the three groups. Patients receiving sertraline, however, were rated as globally better than the other two patient groups. Depressed patients not responding to St. John's wort are reported to respond subsequently to standard antidepressant drug treatment.[113] Thus, early but methodologically suspect studies support the use of St. John's wort, but recent rigorous studies do not. A meta-analysis of 37 double-blind randomized controlled trials concluded that the evidence is "inconsistent and confusing" with placebo comparison studies. It is said to have minimal benefit and head-to-head comparison studies find it similar to SSRI antidepressants.[114]

The use of St. John's wort is not without risk, however, and it should not be used concurrently with an SSRI or MAOI antidepressant as the combinations increase the risks for a serotonin syndrome or hypertensive crisis. St. John's wort is also contraindicated in pregnancy, breast-feeding, strong sunlight exposure, and pheochromocytoma.[115] It may interfere with oral contraceptives, resulting in pregnancy.[116] It should not be used in persons who have received organ transplants as it can interfere with anti-rejection medications.[117]

Omega-3 fatty acids

Omega-3 fatty acids have also been studied for antidepressant properties, used alone or as an enhancing agent for antidepressant medications in medication-resistant patients.[118] Most reports are anecdotal. In one double-blind placebo-controlled study patients who relapsed during continuation treatment with non-TCA antidepressants were given either 2 g of fatty acid or placebo added to their antidepressant. By week three, six of 10 patients improved compared to one of 10 in the placebo group.[119]

Kava

Kava has been used as a food supplement to treat anxiety and insomnia. Its efficacy is unknown; numerous reports of persons developing liver damage caution that such use is best avoided.[120]

NOTES

1 Willis, T. (1667), cited by Williams and Birmingham (2002). William and Birmingham detail that the children who died had brain trauma from being violently shaken and that Willis' "cure" was not his surgery and leeches, but his close monitoring of the mother, preventing her from hurting subsequent children.
2 Williams and Birmingham (2002).
3 Other proposed treatments include partial opioid agonists (Bodkin *et al.*, 1995), synthetic peptides (Feighner *et al.*, 2000), substance P receptor antagonists (van der Hart *et al.*, 2002), enhancement of neural plasticity with *n*-methyl-D-aspartate antagonists, alpha-amino-3-hydroxy-5-methyl-4-isoxazolepropionic acid (AMPA) potentiators, cyclic adenosine monophosphate inhibitors, glucocorticoid receptor agonists, and agents that regulate F growth factor activity and kinase cascades (Manji *et al.*, 2003; Trivedi, 2003).
4 The boxes are about 36–48 in. (90–120 cm) in size. Patients sit at an angle within about 12 in. (30 cm) in front of a box that delivers up to 10 000 lux of light (treatment courses range from 3000 to 10 000 lux) Patients do not look directly at the screen except for brief periods every several minutes.
5 Levitt *et al.* (2002).
6 Lam and Levitt (1999).
7 Loving *et al.* (2002).
8 Benedetti *et al.* (2003a).
9 Prasko *et al.* (2002).
10 Terman *et al.* (1998).
11 Wileman *et al.* (2001).
12 Jainer *et al.* (2001).
13 Eastman *et al.* (1992).
14 Eastman *et al.* (1998).
15 Koorengevel *et al.* (2001); Goel *et al.* (2005).
16 Thompson *et al.* (1999).
17 Golden *et al.* (2005).
18 Avery *et al.* (2001); Golden *et al.* (2005).
19 Of theoretical interest, however, is an open trial reporting that LT enhanced the transient antidepressant effect of sleep deprivation in non-psychotic, depressed manic-depressive patients. Response was linked to a variant in the serotonin transporter gene (Benedetti *et al.*, 2003b).
20 Corral *et al.* (2000).
21 Lam *et al.* (1999).
22 Oren *et al.* (2002).
23 Epperson *et al.* (2004).
24 George and Belmaker (2000).

25 O'Connor *et al.* (2003b); Hausmann *et al.* (2004a).
26 Coil shapes vary depending on the technique used and placement may be guided by functional magnetic resonance imaging.
27 Hoffman and Cavus (2002).
28 Hoffman and Cavus (2002).
29 McNamara *et al.* (2001).
30 Figiel *et al.* (1998); Padberg *et al.* (1999); Januel *et al.* (2004).
31 Zwanzger *et al.* (2003).
32 Grunhaus et al. (2003).
33 Kellner *et al.* (2002). Initially, all ECT patients received right unilateral treatments at 2.5 times their calibrated seizure threshold. Seven of the 20 were switched to bilateral ECT after their sixth treatment because they did not respond. Means and standard deviation figures indicate that no patient received more than 14 ECT. Hamilton Rating Scale scores dropped equally for both groups, but the final mean scores of 13 for each treatment condition indicate that at the end of the trial some patients in each group were still ill. The sample sizes were too small to identify differences (type II statistical error).
34 Janicak *et al.* (2002).
35 Grunhaus *et al.* (2003).
36 Greenhalgh *et al.* (2005).
37 Pridmore *et al.* (2000).
38 A woman with recurrent episodes of depression was successfully treated with ECT and maintained for three years. When ECT was discontinued she relapsed, with a $HAMD_{24}$ score of 18. Acute TMS applied to the right dorsolateral prefrontal cortex on a daily basis for five days elicited a 50% reduction in $HAMD_{24}$. TMS was applied three times a week for three weeks as continuation treatment. She relapsed two days after the last TMS treatment; ECT was administered and she was successfully maintained on continuation ECT (Conca *et al.*, 2004).
39 Dannon *et al.* (2002).
40 Klein *et al.* (1999).
41 Loo *et al.* (1999).
42 Hausmann *et al.* (2004b).
43 Fitzgerald *et al.* (2003).
44 Martis *et al.* (2003).
45 One study also found that responders had less pretreatment blood flow in the left amygdala on single positron emission computed tomography (SPECT) compared to non-responders and that after treatment the responders had less blood flow in orbitofrontal and anterior cingulate cortex (Nadeau *et al.*, 2002). Another study reports that stimulus intensity needs to be above the motor threshold (which can be painful) and that low-intensity TMS is ineffective (Padberg *et al.*, 2002).
46 Padberg and Moller (2003).
47 Burt *et al.* (2002).
48 Martin *et al.* (2002).
49 Gershon *et al.* (2003).
50 Martin *et al.* (2003).
51 Couturier (2005).
52 Neuronetics, in progress. (Personal communication, D. Avery, May 2005).
53 George and Belmaker (2000); Lisanby (2004).

54 Lisanby (2002, 2004).
55 Lisanby *et al.* (2003).
56 Kosel *et al.* (2003).
57 Fink (2004).
58 Mu *et al.* (2004).
59 Handforth *et al.* (1998).
60 DeGiorgio *et al.* (2000).
61 Elger *et al.* (2000); Harden *et al.* (2000).
62 Rush *et al.* (2000); Sackeim *et al.* (2001b).
63 Marangell *et al.* (2002).
64 George *et al.* (2002); Chae *et al.* (2003).
65 Armitage *et al.* (2003). Chapter 14 provides a discussion of sleep abnormalities in depression.
66 FDA Neurological Devices Advisory Panel meeting minutes, June 15, 2004. http://www.fda.gov/ohrms/dockets/ac/04/minutes/4047m1.pdf. The panel minutes note: "Patients should have failed four or more trials of traditional treatment modalities for TRD [treatment-resistant depression] (medications and ECT) before using the VNS device." See also Cyberonics website for press release, February 2, 2005 (www.cyberonics.com). Deep brain stimulation through implanted electrodes in subthalamic and related nuclei is another proposed surgical procedure for chronically ill depressed patients (Mayberg *et al.*, 2005).
67 Chapter 4.
68 Peeters *et al.* (1994); Barden *et al.* (1995).
69 Kling *et al.* (1991); Van der Lely *et al.* (1991); Murphy (1997); Chu *et al.* (2001).
70 Murphy *et al.* (1993), Belanoff *et al.* (2001a).
71 Belanoff *et al.* (2002).
72 Young *et al.* (2004).
73 Wolkowitz and Reus (1999).
74 Wolkowitz *et al.* (1999).
75 Marco *et al.* (2002).
76 Habib *et al.* (2001); Nemeroff (2002a); Künzel *et al.* (2003b).
77 Farvolden *et al.* (2003) and Blier and Ward (2003) offer detailed reviews.
78 Kugaya *et al.* (2003).
79 Hlatky *et al.* (2002).
80 Grigoriadis and Kennedy (2002).
81 American College of Obstetricians and Gynecologists (2004).
82 Klaiber *et al.* (1979).
83 Shapira *et al.* (1985).
84 Schneider *et al.* (1997).
85 Soares *et al.* (2001).
86 Cohen *et al.* (2003).
87 Westlund Tam and Parry (2003).
88 Smith *et al.* (1995b); Gregoire *et al.* (1996).
89 Ahokas *et al.* (1999, 2001).
90 Campbell and Whitehead (1977); Cooper (1981); Pearce *et al.* (1997).
91 Kumar *et al.* (2003).
92 American College of Obstetricians and Gynecologists, (2004).
93 Granger and Underwood (2001).

94 Bower and Altschule (1956).
95 Hatotani *et al.* (1979).
96 Dalton (1989).
97 Van Der Meer *et al.* (1984).
98 Lawrie *et al.* (1998).
99 Pope *et al.* (2003).
100 Sternbach (1998); Seidman (2003).
101 Seidman *et al.* (2002).
102 Margolese (2000).
103 Seidman and Rabkin (1998).
104 Seidman *et al.* (2001).
105 Teufel-Mayer and Gleitz (1997).
106 Linde *et al.* (1996).
107 Volz (1997).
108 Lecrubier *et al.* (2002).
109 Uebelhack *et al.* (2004).
110 Gastpar *et al.* (2005).
111 Szegedi *et al.* (2005).
112 Hypericum Depression Trial Study Group (2002).
113 Gelenberg *et al.* (2004).
114 Linde *et al.* (2005).
115 Gillis (1998).
116 Hall *et al.* (2003a).
117 Beer and Ostermann (2001).
118 Stoll *et al.* (1999); Puri *et al.* (2002).
119 Nemets *et al.* (2002).
120 Walsh (2002).

14

The pathophysiology of melancholia

I am gall, I am heartburn. God's most deep decree
Bitter would have me taste: my taste was me;
Bones built in me, flesh filled, blood brimmed the curse.
Self yeast of spirit a dull dough sours. I see
The lost are like this, and their scourge to be
As I am mine, their sweating selves; but worse[1]

The biological components of depressive mood disorders are the theme of thousands of articles. Despite recognition that mood disorders are clinically and physiologically heterogeneous, few studies assess the biology of different forms of depressive illness. Our knowledge about melancholia is therefore limited, and is based largely on interpolation from hospital samples or patients identified as "severely depressed," the groups most likely to include an abundance of melancholic patients.[2] This chapter examines the neurobiology of melancholia. The association of melancholia with vegetative, psychomotor, and mood disturbances that result from the characteristic hypothalamic–pituitary–adrenal (HPA) axis dysfunction are the basis for the clinical features of melancholia. Their usefulness as diagnostic criteria is discussed in Chapter 4. Biological studies picture a mood disorder as an abnormal physiologic stress response. The neurochemical, electrophysiologic, and cognitive deviations are considered secondary to an abnormal stress response. Melancholic patients also demonstrate abnormal brain metabolism and structure that worsen with increasing numbers of episodes. Most abnormalities, however, resolve with proper treatment. When prolonged, the risk increases for future episodes of the illness.

A genetic predisposition for melancholia has been sought in genomic mapping. While it is unlikely that a single gene error is the basis for melancholia, akin to the error in Huntington's chorea, the influence of genes in affecting the risk for depressive illness appears to be increased with exposure to stressful situations that adversely affect brain function. Of particular interest are the effects of substantial stresses in the intrauterine period, parenting during infancy, and childhood. Temperament and genetically influenced environmental risk factors may further modify the threshold for illness. The genetic–environmental interaction is not understood and little studied.

Why some melancholic patients develop manic episodes is another unanswered question. Is the biology of the two phases of manic-depressive illness a single process with different expressions or is the biology different, as many authors have thought?

Biological studies are highly complex and the methodologies are oversimplified. The samples are heterogeneous. Most studies are compartmentalized, examining a single aspect of the illness. One type of neurotransmitter is studied rather than interactions among neurotransmitters. Brain structure and metabolism are studied but rarely in the same patients. Few compilations seek to bring the literatures together. Many studies utilize laboratory animals and the findings interpreted as relevant to human depressive illnesses, a linkage that has yet to yield clinically relevant conclusions. This chapter summarizes the published studies with the awareness that the literature is far from defining the pathophysiology of depressive illness.

Genetic predisposition

Mood disorders run in families. In the second half of the twentieth Century behavioral geneticists sought to quantify the heritability of mood disorder and to identify specific genotype–phenotype relationships by studying patients and their families. The effort is ongoing with the present conclusion that melancholia and other depressive illnesses are modestly heritable. Several genes appear to be involved, each with small, additive effects. Some genes influence psychopathology. Others affect the response to environmental stressors, particularly the response to severe, chronic stress. The greater the number of affected genes and the greater their penetrance, the greater is the risk for a mood disorder.

Vulnerability genes – the tendency to become depressed

Family studies of depressive mood disorders are methodologically limited. Those that examine child probands rarely include a non-ill comparison group of children, poorly concealing parental diagnoses.[3] Diagnosis of relatives may not be blind to proband diagnosis. Both failures encourage overdiagnosis, particularly among the milder forms of the illness. Most critical, melancholia is usually not separately identified.

Family studies find children of parents with major depressive illness to have an increased risk for mood disorder and relatives of depressed children to have increased risks for depressive illness.[4] The studies find moderate familial aggregation in non-bipolar mood disorders and, along with twin data, suggest a heritability of about 0.40,[5] suggesting a substantial gene–environment interaction in the liability for depression.[6] While the scant adoption data are consistent with genetic transmission, showing an increased risk in the biological but not the rearing relatives of ill adoptees, they do not define the degree of heritability.[7] Linkage studies seek candidate genes hypothesized to be involved in the neuropathology of depression (neuroendocrine and neurotransmitter systems), but provide weak associations between depressed mood and serotonin and dopamine receptor genes, G protein, $CREB_1$ gene, and tyrosine hydroxylase genes in the GABAergic system.[8]

The heritability estimate is predicated upon national institutes of mental health catchment area data that report high population lifetime base rates for all forms of depressive illness (21% for females, 12.7% for males). The clinical training and experience of the interviewers in this multicenter study were minimal, encouraging overcounting cases. Patients with psychotic depression are less forthcoming to these interviewers or they are in hospital and not available, leading to an undercounting of the more severe illnesses, including melancholia.[9] Family studies typically begin with hospital-treated probands, and are likely to have higher proportions of melancholic and psychotically depressed patients than are found in community samples. As only 20–30% of samples in multivariate studies meet criteria for melancholia, the comparison of illness rates in the relatives of these patients against the base rates for all varieties of depression is misleading. Some investigations of depressive mood disorders estimate the population lifetime base rate to be 5–10%, substantially lower than the figures from epidemiologic studies and sufficiently different to change the interpretation of the familial nature of depression.[10] A lower base rate determines a higher estimate of the degree of familial aggregation. Family studies of the more severely ill forms of depressive illness find the adult first-degree relatives of patients with recurrent depression to have a morbid risk for depression of 20–25%. This is four to five times greater than the lower population risk figures.[11]

Clinical factors influence heritability estimates. Levinson *et al.* (2003) confirm the long-held view that persons with a first episode of depressive illness before age 40 have relatives with the highest rates of depressive illness. They point out that heritability estimates can be as high as 0.80, reflecting an extremely high genetic contribution. Some studies conclude that depressive illness is associated with substantial familial aggregation and that this aggregation tends to be specific for different forms of depression.[12] They report twin data with analyses by type of depressive illness. Their "severe typical" group (with a melancholic pattern of psychopathology) has high monozygotic twin concordance. Women with high familial aggregation are more likely to experience postpartum, often melancholic, depressive illness. Children of mothers with early-onset depression, particularly postpartum depression, have a high heritability for mood disorder. These findings are consistent with the reports that melancholia is associated with a substantial genetic risk, as much as a 14-fold increased risk for depressive mood disorder before the age of 13 in children whose mothers had their first illness before age 20.[13] High familial risk is associated with persistent HPA abnormal function.[14] From the National Comorbidity Survey, Kendler and associates (1997) concluded that the diagnosis of "major depression" shows substantial familial aggregation even when examining community samples, that transmission is fairly specific, and that gender has little effect on the transmission pattern. Environment had little effect on parent–child transmission.

The most severely ill patients (often melancholic) have the strongest family aggregation for mood disorder.[15] Yet in the few studies that identify endogenously depressed probands, the results are mixed. Higher rates are reported in the relatives of endogenously depressed probands.[16] High rates of depressed mood are also reported in the relatives of children with endogenous depression.[17] These associations, however, are not supported by others.[18] The differences likely reflect the severity of the probands' illnesses, with the more severely ill having the greater familial aggregation.

In a meta-analysis of pooled data, the first-degree relatives of depressed probands had two to three times the population risk for all forms of depressive illness.[19] The investigators further considered twin data from six studies to indicate a heritability of about 40%, with the remainder of the variance due to non-shared environmental factors. Other analyses of these data indicate that the genetic contribution to depressive illness is about equal to the environmental contribution, and that the genetic transmission is additive, i.e. the degree of a person's risk increases in a linear fashion with the number of affected relatives.[20] Also, the greater the illness is expressed in relatives, the younger the first episode of depressive illness occurs in offspring.[21] This degree of heritability is similar to that for type 2 diabetes, hypertension, asthma, and some forms of cancer.

Lastly, family and twin studies reveal substantial comorbidity in patients with major depression. Overlap has been reported with recurrent depressive illness, alcoholism, anxiety disorder, and substance abuse.[22] Some of the comorbidity with alcohol abuse may be gender-specific, with different explanations of comorbidity for men and for women.[23] Cannabis and alcohol abuse during the teens has been associated with non-melancholic depression later in life.[24]

It is unclear, however, whether the co-occurring disorders should be considered part of a depression phenotype and to which form of depressive mood disorder they best relate. Segregation analyses of families of probands with depressive illness find a major gene effect for alcoholism in the pedigrees and conclude a shared vulnerability between alcohol abuse and recurrent depressive illness.[25] Other analyses also find a shared vulnerability with the abuse of illicit drugs, but conclude it is mostly explained by the presence of antisocial personality disorder in family members.[26]

Some studies report a relationship between recurrent depressive illnesses and manic-depressive illness.[27] And, recurrent depressive disorder is common among the relatives of probands with manic-depressive illness. In a minority of studies the risk for manic-depressive illness is modestly elevated in the relatives of probands with recurrent depressions but not in those with mania or hypomania.[28] In about 20% of monozygotic twin pairs concordant for mood disorder, one twin will exhibit recurrent depressive episodes while the other will express both manic and depressive episodes.[29] One conclusion is that the patients with recurrent manic-depressive illness are those with melancholia or psychotic depression.[30]

Thus, there is a genetic influence on the risk for melancholia, but the pattern and degree of risk do not indicate a major gene effect. Shared and non-shared environmental influences account for the remainder of the variance.[31] The degree of heritability and the relative contributions of shared and non-shared environment have been associated with gender, age of illness onset, and severity of symptoms. Girls with an early onset of illness have particularly severe depressive illnesses, with the highest heritability influenced by both shared and non-shared factors.[32]

Temperament risk factors (a tendency to be "temperamental")

Temperament refers to the behavioral traits that define a person's habitual ways of responding to situations of reward (praise, affection, money, position), non-reward (criticism, anger), and novelty. Fearfulness, impulsivity, and excitability are examples. Temperament is highly heritable (about 50% additive small gene pattern of transmission) and non-shared environmental effects influence individual differences in temperament.[33]

A weak association between personality traits and milder, non-melancholic forms of depression has been reported.[34] Temperament factors in children that have been associated with adult depressed mood states include behavioral inhibition and shyness, low self-esteem, neuroticism (emotional instability, tendency to be anxious and behaviorally inhibited, overresponsive to stress), low sociability, low subjective well-being, and increased expressions of negative emotion.[35] When severe enough to meet criteria for personality disorder, these traits have been associated with chronic depressive mood disorders.[36]

A few genetic studies assess the association between personality and depressed mood. In an analysis of highly heritable temperament traits and depressive symptoms in 201 twin pairs, Ono *et al.* (2002) found novelty-seeking (behavioral activation), harm avoidance (behavioral inhibition), and reward dependence (behavioral persistence) to depend on the same genetic factors as a predisposition for experiencing depressive symptoms or mild depression. A partial overlap between neuroticism and depression is reported.[37] A modest association between a brain-derived neurotrophic factor (BDNF) variant and neuroticism is reported as a risk factor for depressive disorders.[38] These studies do not link specific personality traits to melancholia.

Temperament, however, does modulate response to stress and response to stress is a risk factor for depressive illness. How an environmental situation is perceived determines the degree to which the situation is stressful. Perceptions affect cortisol levels.[39] More socially dominant and self-directed persons have lower cortisol responses to stress.[40] Men with temperament traits of high emotional lability have greater nighttime cortisol fluctuations.[41] Studies that fail to find a relationship between personality and stress response do not focus on the highly heritable temperament traits.[42]

Non-shared environmental experience influences temperament. Both non-shared and shared environment play a role in the predisposition to depression, perhaps interacting with gender. Temperament traits leading toward behavioral inhibition under stress or non-reward may be true risk factors for some forms of mood disorder, but may also be the consequence of experiencing an environment created by parental, particularly maternal, depression (see below). Regardless of origin, deviant temperament traits encourage a child's tendency to select or avoid particular situations (i.e. trying or avoiding unfamiliar experiences). They lead to the child over- or under-responding to caregiver admonition and stressful situations. Thus, these traits lead to experiencing increased stress and an increased risk for depressive illness.

Genetically influenced environmental risk factors (a tendency to create stress)

Parental temperament and cognitive traits alter the home environment and modify the risks for mood disorder in the offspring. For example, monozygotic twins reared apart are more similar to each other in temperament than are dizygotic twins reared apart. Twenty-five percent of the variance in family environment may be genetic in origin.[43] The life events and stressors associated with depressed mood have a genetic contribution, including poor parenting, contributing to family turmoil, and divorce.[44]

Genetically influenced stress response (a tendency to over-react to stress)

Abnormal neuroregulatory mechanisms are a core element of melancholia. Children of mothers who were depressed during pregnancy or during the offspring's infancy are at greater risk for these abnormalities (see below). One study of persons with depressive illness reports that persons carrying two short forms compared to persons carrying two long forms of the 5-HTT gene have two and a half times the risk of becoming depressed after four or more stressful events experienced between ages 21 and 26.[45] This report suggests an interaction between the number or chronicity of stressful experiences and genetic vulnerability. Most data examining the relationship between stress and genotype, however, come from studies of laboratory animals.

Mice bred for either low or high aggressiveness respond differently to chronic social stress.[46] Under stress, the low aggressive mice are more likely to lose body weight and exhibit increased plasma corticosterone levels and mineralocorticoid and glucocorticoid receptor down-regulation in the hippocampus.[47] Mice bred to be deficient in CRH receptor-2 display anxiety-like behavior and are hypersensitive to stress.[48] Stress-susceptible mice under chronic stress have more pronounced variations in monoamine utilization and exhibit fearfulness and motor disturbances.[49] A genetic susceptibility to abnormal dopamine activity has also been observed in mice subjected to the stress of a forced swimming test, with high-response strains becoming maladaptively immobile in association with activation of mesocortical structures and inhibition of the dopamine activity of the mesoaccumbens. Both behavioral and neurochemical abnormalities resolved with chronic clomipramine administration.[50] Antidepressant drugs also promote normalization of glucocorticoid function in such mice.[51] In addition, adult rhesus monkeys have a quantitative trait characterized by excessive fear-related responses in association with increased electroencephlogram activity in right frontal brain regions, increased pituitary–adrenal activity, and increased activity of brain corticotropin-releasing hormone.[52] This pattern is similar to that of infants of depressed mothers (see below). These traits in rhesus monkeys have substantial heritability.[53]

Environmental factors

Environmental factors influence gene expression toward depressive illness and the most consistently observed factors implicate chronic stress. A chronic stress environment affects the fetus in utero when the mother is melancholic; it affects offspring in the home when the mother suffers a postpartum melancholia. A highly stressed home environment is also associated with both maternal and paternal psychopathology, child neglect, and abuse of the children in the home.

Intrauterine

Depressed pregnant women have elevated plasma cortisol, beta-endorphin, and corticotropin-releasing hormone levels.[54] Urinary cortisol and norepinephrine levels are elevated,[55] indicating that these women are in a heightened stress response state during the depressive illness.[56] Maternal cortisol crosses the placenta and accounts for about 50% of the variance in cortisol levels in the fetus.[57] During a maternal depressive illness the fetus is exposed to extraordinary high levels of neuroendocrine hormones. An assessment of 186 women during their second trimester for the degree of anger, depression, and anxiety reported that fetuses of "high-anger" women were more active at birth and more likely to experience neuromotor growth delays.[58] High-anger women had high prenatal levels of serum cortisol and epinephrine and low dopamine and serotonin levels. Similar abnormalities were also observed in their fetuses. The infants of high-anger women showed right frontal EEG activation and low vagal tone. They also had disorganized sleep patterns. Thus, maternal abnormal mood states produce a stress hormone intrauterine environment that affects fetal neurochemical, neuromotor, and behavioral development. Maternal antenatal anxiety and high stress also is associated with behavioral and emotional problems in exposed offspring at age four.[59]

Maternal blood flow to the fetus is reduced when the mother is depressed. In ultrasound studies uterine blood flow is impaired in anxious women.[60] Reduced blood flow is associated with newborn low birth weight. Newborns of women who were depressed during pregnancy have lower birth weights and are hypoactive.[61] Their growth rates lag behind comparison children.[62] Stress during pregnancy is correlated with increased fetal heart rate that is associated with low newborn attention, orientation, and arousal, even in an otherwise uncomplicated pregnancy and delivery.[63]

Depressed pregnant women are less likely to receive adequate prenatal care and are more likely to smoke, eat unhealthy foods, and sleep poorly than are non-depressed pregnant women.[64] These are risk factors for newborn morbidity. Second-trimester exposure to influenza has also been associated with an increased risk for depression in the offspring.[65] Influenza viral infection may be a stressor because it activates the HPA axis and increases cerebral concentrations of norepinephrine.[66]

The increased rates of premature birth and low birth weight in newborns born during a maternal depressive illness are evidence of an abnormal intrauterine environment in such mothers.[67] Such newborns respond less to somatosensory stimuli than do comparison infants (as if they had higher thresholds), are hypoactive and less robust, and less sustained in their movements. They cry excessively and are inconsolable. The more severe the maternal mood disorder during pregnancy, the more likely the infant will express these behaviors, and the more severe they are likely to be.[68]

Maternal care and paternal modulation

Postpartum depression and maternal depressive illness during a child's infancy produce adverse environments. Depressed mothers are more likely to be more self-focused and express more negative thought content and behaviors, leading to others withdrawing from interactions. Depressed mothers are more hostile and angry, more dysfunctional in problem-solving, and more likely to create conflict. Compared to non-depressed psychiatric and normal controls they are more punitive, negative, and retaliatory with their children, and more likely to engage in angry, intrusive, and hostile interactions. Conflict is more common, and they are more likely to alternate between harsh punitive discipline and permissive undercontrol.[69]

Insensitive and unresponsive parenting is associated with infant insecurity (e.g., heightened separation anxiety) and neuroregulatory problems.[70] Children of depressed mothers have lower vagal tone at age 6 months, evidence of delayed development in autonomic regulation.[71] Such children exhibit deviations in neurologic development (e.g., delayed landmarks), show less facial emotional reactivity and spontaneous expression, are less attentive, less able to self-soothe, and have higher cortisol levels than controls. Some have accentuated resting quantitative right frontal and reduced left frontal EEG activation.[72] Neuroregulatory problems at 9 months predict behavioral problems at 3 years.[73] At 4 years of age such children continue to have perceptual and performance problems.[74] At 11 years of age, their IQ scores are lower than age norms.[75]

Behaviorally, children of depressed mothers are more likely to be anxious, less able to sustain attention when tested, over-respond to mild stress, and are less spontaneous in play. They show heightened emotional responsiveness when exposed to mild conflict or distress in others, while at other times they appear emotionally subdued. When older, such children are rated as less popular by teachers without knowledge of the mothers' diagnoses.[76] They develop poor peer relationships in adolescence.[77] They are more self-critical. Substantial depressive symptoms in adolescence (even if not reaching the threshold to meet diagnostic criteria) predict major depression in early adulthood.[78]

Women with early-onset recurrent depressive illness are likely to transmit a genetic vulnerability to their children. If the mother's illness occurs during pregnancy or during the children's formative years, the child's risk for mood disorder increases. A father with recurrent depressive illness appears equally likely to transmit genes of vulnerability.[79] The observation that the fathers of women with depressive illness have a greater likelihood for depressive illness is ascribed to assortative mating.[80]

Although less attention has been paid to the father's effect on child development, the father's illness affects the parental relationship and accounts for some of the variance in the social and emotional functioning of his children.[81] A father's depressive symptoms exacerbate a mother's depressive symptoms,[82] while a healthy father in the home is associated with lower rates of depressive illness in school-aged children.[83] An alcoholic father in the home with a depressed mother adversely affects infant behavior.[84] Healthy fathers rate higher than do depressed mothers on a number of classic mother–infant interactive behaviors (e.g., game-playing, vocalizations, affective state, and expression).[85] Thus, a father in the household has a modest modulating effect on a child's risk for depression.

High-stress childhood environment

Children of depressed mothers are more likely than children of healthy women to experience marital discord and parental social and job-related stress. Children who grow-up in high-stress households have a higher incidence of behavioral problems.[86] If they become depressed their illness is more likely to become chronic than persons with depressive illness without such early experiences.[87] In a community-derived sample of nearly 2000 women, those with a history of childhood sexual or physical abuse, but not rape as adults, had more symptoms of depression and anxiety and were more likely to attempt suicide than women without those experiences.[88] Dysfunctional parenting is considered a specific risk factor for non-melancholic depression.[89]

Persistent stress over many months or several years is critical in the development of psychiatric illness. Repeated parental discord, but not parental death, is associated with childhood behavior problems and severe depression as adults.[90] Melancholic patients are particularly susceptible to physical and sexual abuse and neglect, as these experiences are more common in melancholic patients than in other depressed patients.[91] Other stressors may also increase the risk for a mood disorder by sensitizing the stress response system, resulting in persistent hyperreactivity. Childhood sexual and physical abuse, childhood neglect, and an alternating harsh and neglectful parenting style in depressed mothers have each been associated with depressive illness in the offspring.[92] Women who experience childhood abuse exhibit increased HPA and autonomic responses to stressful events. An increased response is exacerbated by ongoing depressive mood. Early adult traumatic head injury adds to the risk for subsequent depressive illness.[93]

Laboratory animal studies are a model for how early chronic stress in humans elicits adverse brain changes that increase the risk for mood disorder. Early-life chronic stress is associated with long-term alterations in the nucleus accumbens, amygdala, hippocampus, prefrontal cortex (brain circuits that subserve the stress response), with lasting changes in HPA functioning and in norepinephrine systems.[94] Chronic social stress in male rats reduces dendritic arborization in the hippocampus and decreases binding to serotonin transporter sites.[95] Chronic exposure to high levels of stress-response hormones either because of stress or disease elicits hippocampal atrophy in humans and other species.[96] Rhesus monkeys reared without their mothers but with peers have increased cortisol responses to social separation compared to monkeys reared by their mothers, and this response is associated with a preference for alcohol as young adults.[97] Non-human primates reared in social isolation have decreased corpus callosum volumes,[98] a finding reported in chronically abused children.[99]

Hormones

Women are at twice the risk for mood disorders than are men. The greater likelihood of women reporting symptoms and seeking health care does not explain this gender difference.[100] The increased incidence is for a first episode but does not influence the number of episodes.[101] Women have an increased genetic vulnerability lowering the threshold for this first episode.[102]

Estrogen

The increased incidence of mood disorders after menopause is associated with a fall in plasma estrogen concentrations.[103] Changes in estrogen levels are also implicated in postpartum depression[104] and in premenstrual dysphoric disorder.[105] Estrogen modulates serotonin activity, and changes in estrogen levels have been offered as an explanation for some of the abnormalities in serotonergic activity reported in depression.

Women are more sensitive than are males to glucocorticoid negative feedback, and men and women differ in neuroendocrine responses to stress.[106] Estrogen regulates the stress response, and it is hypothesized that diminishing levels of estrogen increase the stress response in women while reducing serotonin activity, contributing to the initiation of a mood disorder in a genetically vulnerable person. The principal support for this hypothesis comes from studies in laboratory animals. In rats estradiol has a dose–response effect on hippocampal glucocorticoid receptors.[107] In female laboratory animals, the ability to condition is partially determined by levels of estrogen in an inverted-U-shaped relationship, the extremes (as in estrus and under stress) contributing to poor performance.[108] An association between estrogen levels, changes in glucocorticoid receptors, and the ability to be conditioned as a model for the increased risk for depression in women, however, remains unproven.

Thyroid

The evidence for efficacy for trüodothyronine (T_3) augmentation of antidepressant treatment is weak[109] and is mostly reported for women.[110] An association between abnormal thyroid function indices and postpartum depression is also reported.[111] Melancholic patients are more likely than non-melancholic depressed patients to have a reduced thyroid-stimulating hormone (TSH) response to thyrotropin-releasing hormone (TRH). This blunted response is a biological marker for the syndrome, particularly in depressed men.

One explanation for a blunted response is chronic hypersecretion of TRH by the hypothalamus that induces down-regulation of TRH receptors. Hypersecretion of TRH parallels the hypersecretion of the hypothalamic corticotropin-releasing factor observed in melancholia.[112] Gender differences in hypothalamic–pituitary–thyroid (HPT) axis functions are independent of mood disorder. Men are more likely than women to have reduced prolactin release when given TRH.[113] While thyroid dysfunction influences the outcome of treatment of depressive mood disorders and is a marker for depression, there is no compelling evidence that it is causally related to primary depressive illness.[114]

Abnormal stress response[115]

An abnormal stress response is a core feature of melancholia and the HPA axis is a central component of the stress response system. It has complex feedback mechanisms that are disrupted in mood disorders.[116] Chronic stress early in life predisposes to this disruption. The studies of the HPA axis have developed a detailed image of the neuroendocrine abnormalities associated with melancholia. The dexamethasone suppression test (DST) and the Dex/corticotropin-releasing hormone (CRH) tests as useful markers of melancholia are detailed in Chapter 4. The broader implications of these studies for our understanding of melancholia are presented here.

The HPA axis, a core component of the stress-response system, has complex feedback mechanisms.[117] Two glucocorticoid receptors (GRS) have been identified: a mineralocorticoid receptor, GR type I with a high affinity for cortisol, and the GR type II receptor with a higher affinity for cortisol, lower sensitivity, but a greater binding capacity. GR type I exerts greatest influence in the morning and is considered a factor in regulating circadian rhythms. In humans, steroid levels peak upon awakening and decline throughout the day.

Glucocorticoids have widespread adaptive effects. They mobilize energy sources and increase cardiovascular tone. They suppress processes unessential in flight/fight situations, including growth, tissue repair, reproduction and sexual behavior, food consumption, sleep, and some immune activity. CRH promotes arousal while simultaneously inhibiting the release of growth and reproductive hormones. [118] CRH, through its effect on the arcuate nucleus, modulates the locus coeruleus in the midpons, and its release of norepinephrine. The HPA axis is also regulated by norepinephrine through projections from the locus coeruleus.[119] CRH neurons in the amygdala subserve classic fear conditioning. CRH receptors in many parts of the brain are involved in regulating flight/fight behaviors. As part of the stress response in humans and in laboratory animals, pulse rate increases and blood pressure rises. The renin–angiotensin system is activated and blood flow is redistributed toward the brain.[120] Stereotyped fear-related and defensive behaviors predominate. In humans, emotional memories of past traumatic events emerge to provide information that may be needed to assess the present situation, influencing the intensity and duration of the stress response. Working memory becomes less accessible and executive functioning is less involved than are procedural memories needed for flight/fight.[121]

Laboratory animals that have experienced repeated stress exhibit chronically high levels of advenocorticotropic hormone (ACTH) despite high levels of glucocorticoids, reflecting an impaired feedback system. A slower, non-rate-dependent feedback mechanism may also be impaired by chronic stress. Persons who have experienced substantial childhood chronic stress are also likely to have abnormal cortisol functioning as adults.[122]

The neuroanatomy subserving the stress response is well delineated in laboratory animals and is relevant to the structural and metabolic abnormalities observed in depressive illness. Recent studies of the thalamus extend its parameters to include the lateral and medial geniculate bodies, and thus its role in visual and auditory information-processing. The thalamus receives input from the reticular activating system and all somatosensory input. The thalamus relays this information to the sensory cortices and the amygdala. The sensory cortices also project to the amygdala. The amygdala involves the hippocampus in a rapid effort to match previously stored information with the new information to assess potential danger. The closeness of this memory match and the valence and intensity of the emotional tone attached to the memory prompts the amygdala to trigger the behavioral (via the basal ganglia and specific prefrontal cortex circuits), autonomic, and endocrine (via the hypothalamus and then the pituitary) responses to the stress.[123] The amygdala reciprocally innervates the dorsal raphe nucleus and the locus coeruleus. These serotonergic and noradrenergic sources, respectively, innervate CRH neurons in the hypothalamic paraventricular nucleus.[124] The CRH neurons also receive direct input from the amygdala.[125] In humans, the amygdala, hippocampus, and several prefrontal cortical circuits are dysfunctional in mood disorder (see below), and abnormalities in CRH receptors are reported in suicide victims.[126]

Prolonged exposure to high levels of glucocorticoids is associated with increased risk for hypertension, insulin-resistant diabetes mellitus, osteoporosis, and gastric ulcer.[127] Immunosuppression, impotency, and amenorrhea are associated signs. Learning and memory are disrupted and synaptic plasticity reduced. Impaired hippocampal neurogenesis with dendritic atrophy and volume reduction is reported. BDNF expression in the hippocampus is reduced. A neurotoxic effect occurs. The mesolimbic dopamine reward system is suppressed.[128]

Sympathetic arousal, a hallmark of an acute stress response, is also regulated by the hypothalamus. CRH neurons in the amygdala subserve classic fear conditioning. CRH receptors in many parts of the brain are involved in regulating flight/fight behaviors. [129] The locus coeruleus is activated during the early stages of the stress response. Through its widespread norepinephrine projections its action leads to decreased grooming, sleeping, and eating and increased sympathetic outflow.[130]

The stress response in melancholia

The behavioral and physiologic effects associated with a strong and sustained stress response are consistent with classic features of melancholia and offer face validity to the conclusion that an abnormal stress response is a core component of the syndrome.[131] The effects which are set in motion by HPA hyperactivity and the development of a hyperglucocorticoid state and its effects on noradrenergic and serotonergic systems are described in Table 14.1.

Excessive HPA activation is observed in over half of melancholic patients.[133] Persons who have experienced chronic stress in childhood are most likely to have abnormal cortisol functioning.[134] The abnormality is characterized by increased cortisol production with high serum levels (fourfold or more above norms) throughout the day rather than a morning peak followed by a decline in the afternoon. Despite this activation, serum ACTH levels remain normal. The high cortisol levels are not suppressed by exogenous steroids, with dexamethasone the conventionally administered steroid in test situations. ACTH responses are blunted to intravenous CRH, and the greater the hypercortisolemia, the more pronounced is this blunted response. Hypersecretion of CRH is also observed.[135] Depending on how subjects are selected, up to 90% will show HPA hyperactivity when the DST is combined with ACTH response to CRH.[136]

Table 14.1. Behavioral and physiologic effects of the stress response[132]

Acute stress	Chronic stress
Fearfulness	Fearfulness and irritability
Increased arousal and decreased sleep	Increased stereotyped fear-related and defensive behavior
Sympathetic arousal	Anhedonia from suppression of the mesolimbic dopamine reward system
Energy mobilization	Hypertension and tachycardia
Increased vascular tone	Decreased food intake and weight loss
Decreased food consumption	Decreased sleep
Suppression of sexual behavior	Decreased grooming
Suppression of tissue repair	Impotency
Immune suppression	Amenorrhea
Emotional memory for traumatic events emerges	
Working memory is less accessible	Immune suppression
Executive functioning is less involved than procedural memory	Acute learning and memory problems become entrenched
	Gastric ulcer
	Insulin resistance
	Osteoporosis
	Reduced synaptic plasticity
	Impaired hippocampal neurogenesis with dendritic atrophy and volume reduction

Other circadian processes are also disrupted in melancholia. Nighttime core body temperature[137] and heart rate[138] are elevated. Thyrotropin is decreased.[139] The abnormalities are corrected by electroconvulsive therapy (ECT)[140] and some antidepressant drugs.[141]

Postmortem data from persons who had depressive illness indicate increased CRH levels in the paraventricular nucleus of the hypothalamus with a corresponding reduction of CRH receptors.[142] These findings are also reported in rodents separated from their mothers early in life.[143] Centrally administered CRH induces an increase in arousal and vigilance, decreased appetite and sexual behavior, and increased heart rate and blood pressure.[144] Another postmortem study found decreased CRH receptors in the frontal cortex of persons who had depressive illness.[145] The reduction in CRH receptors may not be a receptor problem but dysfunction elsewhere in the feedback loop, perhaps in the pituitary or above.[146]

Melancholia is associated with increased glucocorticoid release and a decrease in $5HT_{1A}$ receptors in the hippocampus.[147] $5HT_{1A}$ receptor binding in the hippocampus is decreased in suicide victims.[148] Depressed patients who exhibit reduced glucocorticoid receptor binding also exhibit elevated serum cortisol levels and fail to respond to dexamethasone – findings that suggest that the $5HT_{1A}$ glucocorticoid receptor abnormality pertains to melancholia.[149] Cytosolic binding assays find reduced numbers of glucocorticoid receptors in cells of depressed patients.[150] Studies using whole-cell binding methods mostly find no differences between depressed and comparison subjects, suggesting nuclear compartmentalization or protein decoupling rather than changes in receptor affinity as an explanation for the reduced binding ability (or resistance to cortisol). Postmortem studies of suicide victims fail to show abnormalities in glucocorticoid messenger RNA.[151] Such findings reflect chronic exposure to cortisol, placing receptor resistance as a secondary phenomenon.[152] A more direct genetic predisposition for impaired glucocorticoid receptor function in depression has been suggested, but not established.[153]

A third possibility proposes that the glucocorticoid receptor resistance to cortisol is secondary to abnormalities in cyclic adenosine monophosphate (cAMP) and protein kinase cascades. Depressed patients have reduced G protein function[154] and reduced cAMP-dependent protein kinase activity in cultured cell lines.[155] Some antidepressant drugs affect this system.[156]

Further evidence for abnormal glucocorticoid receptor functioning in melancholia comes from observations that treatments for depression affect neurotransmitter systems modulating the stress response system. Norepinephrine alters the expression of genes involved in neural sprouting and differentiation. Increased norepinephrine activity alters neural placidity.[157] Pharmacodynamic broad-spectrum antidepressants, some selective serotonin reuptake inhibitors (SSRIs), and ECT increase norepinephrine transmission.[158] Norepinephrine and serotonin interact in the brain.[159] One site of action is the locus coeruleus where antidepressants inhibit CRH release.[160] Lithium decreases CRH mRNA expression in the amygdala and frontal cortex, while valproic acid increases CRH receptor expression in the cortex.[161] Chronic administration of antidepressants down-regulates CRH systems.[162]

Many antidepressants and ECT affect glucocorticoid receptor expression and feedback inhibition. The treatments up-regulate glucocorticoid protein and mRNA in the neural circuitry that mediates the stress response. This is true for tricyclic antidepressants (TCAs), lithium, $alpha_2$-adrenergic antagonists (idazoxan), norepinephrine reuptake inhibitors (reboxetine), mirtazepine (an $alpha_2$ and $5\text{-}HT_2$ antagonist), venlafaxine (a serotonin (5–HT) and norepinephrine reuptake inhibitor) and ECT. Monoamine oxidase inhibitors may not have a direct effect on this receptor system. SSRIs also do not directly affect glucocorticoid receptors.[163] Antidepressant drugs up-regulate glucocorticoid receptors via gene–protein changes, leading to enhancement of receptor negative feedback function and subsequent normalization of the HPA hyperactivity in melancholia.[164]

Abnormal neurochemical functioning

Neurochemical functions in depressive mood disorders have received intensive study. Changes in no single neurotransmitter system, however, explain the mechanism of disorders of mood, nor their relief. These systems are interactive. The neurotransmitter abnormalities that are widely reported contribute to the signs and symptoms of the illness, but are secondary to the abnormal stress response observed in patients with mood disorders. Antidepressant drugs are believed to work by increasing monoamine concentrations at the synapse that induce desensitization of pre- and postsynaptic receptors followed by a cascade of intraneuronal changes.[165]

Serotonin Dysfunction

For over 40 years the monoamine deficit theory has prevailed as the central mechanism underlying mood disorders, and it is standard practice to explain to patients that they are suffering from a "chemical imbalance" in their brain that can be corrected by medication. This understanding is based mainly on laboratory animal data, studies of depressed patients, and postmortem brain findings of suicide victims.

Abnormal 5-HT function is the most discussed neurotransmitter explanation for depressive illness. Extensive studies in laboratory animals find the primary brain source of 5-HT neurons is the midbrain raphe nuclei. Projections from the dorsal and medial raphe nuclei parallel and modulate dopaminergic and noradrenergic systems.[166] 5-HT plays a role in modulating sexual function, sleep, eating, and mood.[167] The prefrontal cortex (medial) projects fibers to the midbrain dorsal raphe nucleus. Stimulation of the medial prefrontal cortex has two effects on the dorsal raphe nucleus. Excitation is mediated by alpha-amino-3-hydroxy-5-methyl-4-isoxazolepropionic acid/kainate-mediated (AMPA/KA) and *N*-methyl-D-aspartate (NMDA) receptors, whereas inhibition is mediated by GABA-A and 5-HT (1A) receptors.[168]

The development of chemical agents that increase the availability of synaptic serotonin by inhibiting presynaptic serotonin reuptake (SSRIs) was encouraged by the explanation for depressed mood as a serotonin deficiency. Their efficacy in treating depressive mood disorders is offered as support for the concept. Additional support comes from reduced serotonin$_{1A}$ receptor binding in living and postmortem brain tissue of depressed persons, reduced serotonin binding in platelets, reduced cerebrospinal fluid serotonin metabolites (5-HIAA), and the induction of depressive symptoms following tryptophan depletion, the precursor necessary for serotonin production.[169] Table 14.2 summarizes these findings.[170]

The abnormalities in 5-HT metabolism in depressive illness, however, are inconsistent and initial claims are often based on small samples that are rarely expanded. For example, Drevets *et al.* (1999) state that 5-HT$_{1A}$ receptor-binding potential "is abnormally decreased in the depressed phase of familial mood disorders in multiple brain regions." This conclusion is based on the study of 4 bipolar and 4 unipolar depressed patients with bipolar relatives. Subtyping of depression is almost never done because of the small sample sizes. Thus, while neurochemical abnormality in melancholia is undoubtedly present, it is unclear exactly what abnormalities occur, and if any are specific to a type of depression.

It is also unlikely that a deficiency in one neurotransmitter system is the central problem in depressive illness. It is probable that the association between depressive

Table 14.2. Serotonin function in human depressive illness

Decreased 5-HIAA levels in the CSF
5-HT depletion induces depression
Inhibition of 5-HT presynaptic reuptake relieves some depressions
5-HT transporter sites are reduced in postmortem hippocampus
Functional brain imaging shows reduced 5-HT transporter sites in raphe nuclei
Reduced $5HT_{1a}$ receptor binding in hippocampus on PET in suicide victims
Platelet 5-HT-binding sites reduced
Increased frontal cortex and platelet postsynaptic 5-HT receptor-binding site density decreases with successful antidepressant treatment

mood disorders and abnormal serotonin function may not be causal. A reduction in monoamines does not invariably induce depression, nor does depletion exacerbate existing mood disorder.[171] Serotonin therapy resolves only about 30% of depressive illnesses.[172] Nortriptyline, for example, has minimal effects on serotonin receptors and yet is an excellent antidepressant. Serotonin abnormality is not a sufficient explanation for depressed mood, and may be a "downstream" effect of the process that leads to depressive illness rather than the initiating cause of the illness. As an example, glucocorticoids regulate serotonin activity from the raphe nuclei and serotonin is reduced in chronic states of elevated corticosteroids in laboratory animals and humans.[173] The abnormal stress response in depressive illness could account for the serotonin abnormalities observed in some depressed patients. Estrogen and progesterone modulate aspects of serotonin metabolism, and estrogen facilitates serotonergic transmission by enhancing synthesis and decreasing presynaptic reuptake.[174] Thus, serotonin abnormalities may be particularly pertinent in the pathophysiology of depressive illness in women. The effects of the menstrual cycle on serotonin in depressed women are not controlled in most studies and most samples are small.[175] The reduced serotonin function reported in depressed women could result from illness or from physiologically normal dips in estrogen levels.

Noradrenergic (norepinephrine) dysfunction

Norepinephrine projections primarily derive from the locus coeruleus. In laboratory animal studies, stimulation of the locus coeruleus inhibits neurovegetative functions, including sleep, feeding, and sexual behavior. The system mediates stress responses, and receives input from other neurotransmitter systems (5-HT, opioid, GABA, CRH, dopamine, and glutamate) in maintaining homeostasis.[176] Norepinephrine projections inhibit medial prefrontal cortex regions functioning in mood change in response to circumstances. Norepinephrine projections activate amygdala fear responses. Norepinephrine serves to establish vigilance, arousal, activation of the stress response, and modulation of memory systems that associate salient aversive stimuli.

The characteristics of norepinephrine dysfunction in depressive illness are uncertain. Increased cerebrospinal fluid norepinephrine levels are reported in melancholic patients, reflecting anxiety and hyperarousal.[177] Norepinephrine receptor sensitivity may occur in humans and in laboratory animals from increased norepinephrine turnover or depletion may occur.[178] Chronic antidepressant drug administration increases synaptic norepinephrine availability, which in turn leads to reduced neuronal firing in the locus coeruleus.[179] Table 14.3 summarizes these findings.[180]

Table 14.3. Norepinephrine (NE) function in human depressive illness

Increased CSF NE levels in depressed patients
Reserpine depletes NE in laboratory animals and is associated with depression in humans
3-methoxy-4-hydroxy-phenylglycol (MHPG) CSF and urinary levels, the major metabolite of NE, are reported to be abnormal in some depressed patients
Inhibiting NE synthesis may be associated with relapse
Increased tyrosine hydroxylase and alpha$_2$-adrenergic autoreceptor density in the locus coeruleus of suicide victims
Blunted growth hormone response to alpha$_2$-adrenergic agonist clonidine in depressed patients
Selective NE reuptake inhibitors are effective antidepressants

NE–5-HT interactions

Studies of individual neurotransmitters give the false impression that each functions independently. This is not the case and no one neurotransmitter system is likely to be the underlying neurochemical substrate of depressive disorders. Laboratory animal studies find that 5-HT projections from the raphe nuclei innervate the locus coeruleus, while norepinephrine fibers from the locus coeruleus project to the raphe nuclei. These interconnections are mutually inhibitory.[181] Alpha$_2$-adrenergic receptors on 5-HT nerve terminals modulate 5-HT release. Norepinephrine transmission is altered when specific SSRI drugs are administered and 5-HT transmission is altered following the administration of specific norepinephrine antidepressants.[182]

Mesolimbic and mesocortical dopamine pathways are also modulated by 5-HT projections from the raphe nuclei in laboratory animals. The likely involvement of multiple neurotransmitter systems in depressive illness is one explanation for the evidence that pharmacodynamically broad-spectrum antidepressants have a therapeutic advantage in the treatment of melancholia.

The concept that abnormal neuroplasticity occurs at some point in melancholia is based, in part, on laboratory animal studies demonstrating interactions between 5-HT and norepinephrine. Exposure to stress-related glucocorticoids, elevated in melancholia, is associated with loss of pyramidal neurons in the hippocampus, and prevents neurogenesis in laboratory animals.[183] Some antidepressant drugs and ECT inhibit this process by increasing the expression of BDNF. These salutary effects are likely mediated by 5-HT and beta-adrenergic receptors linked to AMP.[184] Norepinephrine and probably 5-HT alters gene expression involved in neuronal sprouting and differentiation.[185] These laboratory findings suggest that neural plasticity in melancholic patients may be affected at two levels. Gene transcription is altered because of aberrations in neurotransmission that lower the threshold for illness (probably by reducing the hippocampal ability to modulate stress responses). Once a depressive mood state ensues, further hippocampal damage occurs from persistently elevated levels of stress-related glucocorticoids.

Dopamine dysfunction

Dopamine systems function has also been studied for their role in depressive illness. The mesolimbic–mesocortical pathway links midbrain dopamine neurons with limbic and cortical regions. This system is implicated in several neuropsychiatric disorders. The nigrostriatal pathway has been studied for its role in Parkinson's disease and other basal ganglia disorders and the common co-occurring depression, and in depressions poststroke. The tuberoinfundibular pathway functions within the hypothalamus and its modulation of the pituitary. Studies generally find reduced levels of dopamine metabolites (homovanillic acid) in the CSF of depressed patients, and conclude that decreased dopamine turnover is the likely cause.[186] Dopamine reuptake is inhibited by some antidepressants (e.g., sertraline) and this is offered as indirect evidence for the depletion hypothesis.[187]

More recently, autopsy material from suicide victims who had been depressed at the time of their deaths showed a lower density of dopamine transporter binding and elevated D_2 and D_3 receptor binding, but not D_1 in basal and central nuclei of the amgydala. The authors interpreted these findings as consistent with the depletion theory.[188]

One brain system subserved by dopamine that has not been directly studied in depressive illness is the hedonistic reward system. Studies of laboratory animals show that this system arises in dopamine neurons in the ventral tegmental area of the midbrain.[189] These neurons innervate the amygdala and limbic regions of the neocortex and the nucleus accumbens in the forebrain. All physiologically addicting drugs increase dopamine transmission in the nucleus accumbens, which mediates the biochemical effects of these agents. Because response to reward is influenced by stress and depression is associated with anhedonia, the hedonistic reward system is a region of interest in the pathophysiology of melancholia.[190] BDNF potentiates drug reward mechanisms and is hypothesized to play a role in depressive illness.[191] Pregnant rats under stress have female offspring prone to abnormal adult behavior consistent with symptoms of depression. These offspring have permanent decreased dopamine function in the nucleus accumbens that correlates with the depressive-like behavior.[192]

Excitatory amino acids

The role of excitatory amino acids in the pathophysiology of depression is unknown. Results are often confounding. Increased *taurine* and decreased *glycine* and *glutamate* levels are reported in some depressed patients.[193] But surgical material from the frontal lobes of persons with a history of depressive illness does not show abnormalities in amino acid levels.[194] Some postmortem studies find reduced high-affinity binding to NMDA receptors in the frontal cortex of suicide victims[195], but others do not.[196] Glutamate transmission is reduced in the anterior cingulate region of depressed persons[197], but these measures could reflect effects of benzodiazepine and antidepressants.[198] Studies of *N*-acetyl-aspartate, myo-inositol, and choline have been conflicting, or consistently negative.[199]

Neurotrophic abnormalities

Neurotrophic factors influence neural growth and differentiation during development and regulate neural plasticity and neuronal and glial survival in the adult brain.[200] Based on laboratory animal studies, BDNF abnormalities are hypothesized in several neurologic diseases and in the pathophysiology of depressive illness.[201] Acute and chronic stress in rodents decreases BDNF expression in the dentate gyrus and pyramidal cell layer of the hippocampus. This reduction is partially mediated by glucocorticoids.[202] Genetically BDNF-deficient mice are aggressive, hyperphagic, and exhibit brain serotonergic abnormalities.[203] Chronic administration of antidepressant drugs in rodents and humans, and ECT increase BDNF in these regions.[204] These interventions prevent the stress-induced decreases and increases hippocampal neurogenesis.[205] Infusion of BDNF into laboratory animals produces behavioral responses similar to those seen from antidepressant drug administration.[206] BDNF is also said to be involved in the anxiolytic effect of SSRIs.[207] A proposed mechanism involves alterations in cAMP as a consequence of the abnormal stress response in depression. Antidepressant drugs up-regulate the cAMP signal transduction cascade, leading to increased expression of AMP response element-binding protein (CREB), which in turn increases the expression of BDNF. The expression of BDNF is reduced in depressed patients and increased by antidepressants. Electrical brain stimulation of rats to simulate ECT also increases BDNF in the hippocampus, and the entorhinal and frontal cortices.[208] A BDNF gene variant has been linked to personality traits that increase the risk for depression.[209]

Although the response of BDNF expression to stress and antidepressant drug administration is intriguing, there is little direct evidence that BDNF functioning is disturbed in depressive illness. One study of patients with major depression observed the most reduced BDNF serum levels in those who had the severest mood disorders.[210]

Neuropeptides

The role, if any, of neuropeptides in depressive illness is unknown. *Vasopressin* is a neuropeptide synthesized in the hypothalamus. Vasopressin release from the anterior pituitary potentiates the effect of corticotropin-releasing hormone (CRH) on ACTH release. In addition to its well-known antidiuretic effects, vasopressin also plays a role in emotional expression, learning, and memory.[211] Chronic stress increases vasopressin expression in the hypothalamus and its subsequent release. Although involved in the stress response, vasopressin has not been adequately studied in depressed patients.[212]

Substance P is an immunoreactive neuropeptide mediating pain and inflammatory responses. Substance P cells co-localize with 5-HT neurons.[213] Exposure to substance P elicits anxiety-like behavior in laboratory animals.[214] Antidepressant properties are reported for substance P antagonists.[215]

Vasoactive intestinal polypeptide (VIP) is widely distributed in hypothalamic, pituitary, and other limbic structures and co-localizes with CRH.[216] VIP is involved in the stress response. It potentiates CRH-induced release of ACTH[217], and acts synergistically with CRH to stimulate ACTH.[218]

Neuropeptide Y is synthesized in arcuate nucleus neurons projecting to paraventricular neurons of the hypothalamus.[219] Neuropeptide Y regulates feeding behavior, blood pressure, circadian rhythms, reproductive behavior, and the stress response.[220] It co-localizes with norepinephrine.[221]

Cholecystokinins (CCKs) are a group of neuropeptides that are involved in the stress response and anxiety-related behaviors.[222] The administration of one of its subtypes (CCK-4) precipitates panic attacks in normal persons and in patients with anxiety disorder.[223]

Abnormal brain structure

Clinicopathologic studies of stroke and brain-injury victims reveal depressive illness to be frequent when frontal structures are involved. Patients with degenerative disease of the basal ganglia are also prone to depressive moods that are not sadness responses to "bad news" but are episodes of illness. High rates of depressive illness are reported in patients with basal ganglia disease before motor symptoms are noted. The severity of mood disorder that follows the emergence of motor features is not correlated with the degree of motor impairment.[224] The relationship between mood disorder and frontal circuitry dysfunction has led to investigations of these brain systems in depressed patients that found an association with frontal circuitry and limbic system structures.

Left anterior cingulate cortex ventral to the genu of the corpus callosum is reduced in volume in magnetic resonance imaging and postmortem studies of depressed patients.[225] Hippocampal volume is also smaller.[226] A meta-analysis of 12 studies meeting criteria for suitability for analysis examined 351 patients with depressive illness and 279 controls, and found an average hippocampal volume loss in patients of 8% on the left and 10% on the right.[227] The hippocampus is the primary site for GR II glucocorticoid receptors and exhibits negative feedback following glucocorticoid release. Loss of hippocampal neurons and reduced hippocampal metabolic activity in melancholia is suggested as the explanation for the inability to inhibit the HPA axis and subsequent hypercortisolemia in these patients.[228] The left amygdala

Table 14.4. Structural brain abnormalities in depressed patients

Left anterior cingulate cortex volume loss ventral to the corpus callosum genu
Hippocampal volume loss
Amygdala volume loss
Gray-matter loss in orbital cortex
Gray-matter loss in posterior ventrolateral prefrontal cortex
Reduced density and size of neurons and glia in anterior dorsolateral prefrontal cortex

may also be smaller in persons with severe recurrent depression.[229] These findings correlate with the patients' cognitive problems.[230]

The amount of gray matter is reduced in the *orbital cortex* and *posterior ventrolateral prefrontal cortex* of depressed patients postmortem. The density and size of neurons and glia are reduced in the *anterior dorsolateral prefrontal cortex.*[231]

The structural changes reported in persons experiencing severe depressive illness (Table 14.4) are consistent with the brain metabolic abnormalities detailed below.

Abnormal brain metabolism

Functional neuroimaging studies in depressive illness, as with much technology-driven psychiatric research, are tempered by methodological limitations. Small sample size prevents most studies from comparing different forms of depressive illness, despite the recognition of within-sample heterogeneity in symptom pattern (e.g., anxious versus apathetic) and in other important ways (e.g., family illness pattern). Multivariate studies are rare. Methods vary in sensitivity. Controls are often lacking. Results are inconsistent.

Structural brain changes in patients with depressive illnesses modify functional images, making it unclear if what is observed represents a metabolic change or an abnormal structure. Medication effects are rarely accounted for and medication-free subjects are rarely assessed.[232] Studies in elderly patients are typically complicated by the high prevalence of vascular brain changes that may be unrelated to mood disorder, but which alter functional images. Early studies used technology with only modest resolution, preventing visualization of important, but small, brain structures, such as the amygdala.[233]

Despite these limitations, some interpretable findings have emerged. *Amygdala metabolism* is altered in unmedicated severely depressed patients. Resting blood flow and glucose metabolism increase with illness severity, with the left hemisphere showing greater elevations than the right.[234] Increased metabolic rate in the right amygdala is associated with negative mood in depressed patients.[235] The increase in amygdala metabolism is estimated to be 50–70% above that observed in controls.[236] This abnormality is not found in patients with anxiety disorder or schizophrenia, suggesting it may be specific to depressive illness.[237] Successful antidepressant drug treatment normalizes these elevations.[238]

The amygdala integrates aspects of emotional expression and the stress response. Deep brain electrical stimulation of the amygdala in humans induces anxiety and fear, and ruminations of past emotionally disturbing events in association with cortisol release, a pattern observed in melancholia.[239] In one study, glucose metabolism was elevated in the left amygdala of depressed patients, an increase that positively correlated with plasma cortisol levels.[240] These and other brain functional imaging studies have been interpreted to indicate that continuous amygdala overactivity accounts for the unremitting apprehension and ruminations of melancholia. Amygdala overflow to the periaqueductal gray area relates to social withdrawal, inactivity, and analgesia seen in severe melancholia, similar to behaviors observed in laboratory animals when this brain area is stimulated.[241] Amygdala overflow into the lateral hypothalamus and to the locus coeruleus accounts for the increased sympathetic tone observed in melancholia and the associated elevated resting heart rate, arousal, and insomnia.[242] Amygdala activity also elicits CRF hypersecretion, which suppresses appetite, interrupts sleep, and increases anxiety.[243]

Reduced metabolism in the *anterior cingulate cortex ventral to the genu of the corpus callosum* in mood disorder is accompanied by reduced volume. The metabolic measures accounting for volume reduction indicate increased metabolism. Thus, fewer glia cells are working harder.[244] Successful antidepressant treatment decreases the activity in these structures.[245] Anterior cingulate lesions in humans are associated with abnormal emotional responses to emotionally laden concepts, akinetic mutism, stupor, and catatonia. Severe melancholia is the second most common cause of catatonia.[246] Recently, decreased cerebral blood flow in the right anterior frontal cortex, temporal cortex, putamen, and thalamus of depressed patients was reported.[247]

Reduced *left hippocampal* metabolism is also observed in depressive illness, and is inversely related to severity. Reduced volume in this region only partially explains the decreased activity.[248] Hippocampal hypofunction is associated with hypercortisolemia[249] as it can no longer inhibit the hypothalamic–pituitary axis.[250] Its dysfunction also impairs new learning.[251]

Blood flow and glucose metabolism are decreased in the *dorsolateral prefrontal cortex anteriorly and medially* in depressed patients.[252] Dorsolateral prefrontal cortex abnormality has been reported in severely depressed preteens and young teens.[253] Lesions in these cortical regions and their corresponding subcortical circuitry produce avolitional and apathetic syndromes that mimic depression. Reduced metabolism in the dorsolateral prefrontal cortex in depression correlates with the degree of psychomotor retardation, anhedonia, and cognitive impairment.[254] Successful antidepressant drug therapy reverses the hypometabolism, although not all studies find this.[255]

In contrast, increased metabolism is reported in the *ventrolateral and posterior orbital cortex* and the *anterior insula* of some unmedicated depressed patients. The metabolic increase in ventrolateral prefrontal cortex appears greater on the left, while orbital metabolism is elevated bilaterally. The increases are normalized with successful antidepressant drug therapy[256] and ECT.[257] These increases, however, are also observed in patients with obsessive-compulsive and anxiety disorder, suggesting that the changes are not specific to depression but are an expression of anxiety. The increase in ventrolateral cortex metabolism is inversely related to depressive mood severity. The ventrolateral prefrontal, cortex posteriorly modulates behavioral, visceral, and cognitive responses in flight/fight situations and in reward responses. Lesions in this cortical area result in a disinhibited syndrome similar to mania.[258]

Overall, decreased dorsolateral, and increased anterior cingulate and ventrolateral frontal activity, and increased amygdala activity, are hallmarks of severe depressive illness. The greater the anxiety and severity of depression, the greater is the decrease in dorsolateral prefrontal cortex metabolism and the greater are the increases in ventrolateral and orbital prefrontal cortex metabolism. The greater the sadness, the greater is the decrease in the dorsolateral cortex and the greater the increase in the ventrolateral cortex. One hypothesis is that the ventrolateral and orbital cortices with their reduced gray matter have to work harder, but nevertheless unsuccessfully, to correct the behavioral effects that result from the reduced activity of the dorsolateral prefrontal cortex.[259] A prefrontal cortical pattern is triggered by limbic dysregulation, specifically in the amgydala (overactive) and the hippocampus (underactive). The downstream nature of the frontal pattern is consistent with findings that similar frontal metabolic changes occur in mania.[260] Table 14.5 summarizes the findings.

Table 14.5. Brain metabolic abnormalities in depressed patients

Amygdala resting blood flow and glucose metabolism increase, left > right
Anterior cingulate cortex increase ventral to the corpus callosum genu
Ventrolateral and orbital cortex increase, left > right
Anterior insular cortex increase
Left hippocampal decrease
Prefrontal cortex decrease anteriorly and medially

Electrophysiologic abnormalities

The discovery of the brain's electrical rhythms set off a spate of activity to find relations to psychiatric illness. The resting EEG and various methods to activate brain responses, including medication and sensory stimulation, were tested in populations of psychiatric patients and compared to normal subjects. After more than 75 years of effort, the principal contributions have been to identify seizure disorders.

Patients with melancholia, however, exhibit severe disturbances in sleep physiology and it is here that EEG measures have been fruitful in understanding depressive illness. The application of sleep EEG as a laboratory test of melancholia is discussed in Chapter 4. This chapter details the contributions of EEG studies to the understanding of the pathophysiology of melancholia.

EEG

EEG was described in 1929 by the psychiatrist Hans Berger, seeking an objective measure of psychiatric disorders.[261] He recorded oscillating electrical frequencies from 4 to 18 Hz from scalp electrodes in normal and psychiatric subjects. Brain waves varied with conscious cognitive processes (e.g., doing "mental arithmetic"), level of alertness (wakefulness through stages of sleep), and at rest with eyes opened or closed. The rhythms were not yet developed in the immature brain of the newborn infant and changed with age. The rhythms disappeared during chloroform anesthesia, were absent in postictal coma, and were slowed in patients with brain lesions.[262] Berger concluded that "in the alpha-waves we are dealing only with the concomitant phenomena of the material processes which are connected to the mental ones, but not with the processes themselves."

Although Berger failed to find unique brain wave patterns for patients with schizophrenia or manic-depressive illness, his technique is established as a distinct physiologic measure.[263]

Non-activated ("resting") EEG

The first successful clinical application of EEG was in the determination of dysrhythmias in patients with seizure disorders.[264] Epileptic patients exhibit bursts of higher-voltage slow waves mixed with spike activity.[265] The identification, classification, and monitoring of treatments of seizure disorders is the most successful application of EEG technology.[266]

EEG slowing and amplitude irregularities are also found during acute delirium, acute neurotoxic states, and dementia associated with degenerative brain disease. Berger's demonstration that the EEG was altered by pharmaceuticals led to studies of drug-enhanced EEG (pharmaco-EEG).[267]

In studies of depressed patients, some typical EEG characteristics have been identified. In one study, increased fast activity over the right and relative or absolute greater slow frequencies over the left frontal regions were observed.[268] Another report found more right hemisphere frontal fast activity (21.5–30.0 Hz) that was most pronounced in melancholic patients.[269] The more severe the mood disorder, the greater the right-hemisphere beta activity. High beta activity was correlated positively with anxiety.[270] Greater degrees of beta activity have been associated with higher amounts of cortisol secretion in normal subjects, interpreted as evidence of increased vigilance.[271] Other studies fail to find beta EEG asymmetry.[272]

Differences in frontal alpha (7.5–12.5 Hz) and right hemisphere slow frequencies (7 Hz and under) are reported in depressed patients compared to comparison groups but these reports are also inconsistent, with the former linked to measures of anxiety.[273] For example, in a study of 78 unmedicated right-handed male depressed outpatients compared to 23 control subjects, the patients showed increased beta power but no differences in alpha or slow frequencies.[274] Frequency coherence discriminated patients from controls with 91% correct classification. Beta power over the right hemisphere contributed to the discrimination. Increased beta power over the right frontal region was correlated with increased recurrence[275] and increased psychomotor disturbance.[276] Other studies fail to find beta EEG asymmetry.[277] Using three-dimensional electromagnetic tomography, investigators reported increased theta activity in the rostral anterior cingulate that seemed to correlate with the clinical response to nortriptyline.[278] These investigators also reported these EEG findings to be negatively correlated with prefrontal cortex gray-matter density (the greater the EEG slowing, the less the density), but only in melancholic patients.[279] Quantitative EEG studies in college students said to be "subclinically" depressed have been offered as indirect support for the EEG changes noted in patients, but these findings are inconsistent.[280]

Little use is made of scalp recorded EEG as a laboratory diagnostic aid in mood disorder, unless seizure disorder is suspected.[281] Psychomotor disturbance and response to TCAs are features of melancholia and the syndrome can be identified more simply by its clinical features and characteristic HPA abnormalities.

Approach–withdrawal theories of hemisphere specialization are offered as explanations for EEG asymmetries in depressive illness. The left hemisphere is identified as specialized in approach behavior and positive mood, and the right hemisphere as mediating withdrawal and negative mood.[282] When depressive mood is associated with behavioral withdrawal, the right hemisphere would be most engaged and more activated than the left, which would also be inhibited. This concept is supported by studies in normal subjects simulating various mood states, but this strategy is not applicable to patients with depressive illness.[283]

The failure to adequately control for medication effects is a common problem in studies of EEG in depressed patients.[284] Psychoactive drugs materially alter EEG rhythms in drug-specific and dose-related fashions.[285] For more than half a century, psychiatric patients come to clinical study with prescriptions of EEG-altering substances offered by general practitioners and family and friends. Few studies consider men and women separately, although EEG gender differences are defined in non-ill subjects.[286] As women often make up the majority of depressed subjects, gender and menstrual cycle phase confound findings. As an example, women with a history of childhood depression were reported to exhibit higher right mid-frontal EEG alpha suppression. The finding is interpreted as increased activation in that region. Men with a childhood history of depression had higher suppression on the left. These findings were most prominent for patients with a manic-depressive course.[287] Neither the point in menstrual cycle nor the degree of anxiety and agitation was considered.

Reference electrode placements are not consistent and affect symmetry analyses.[288] The focus on high-frequency EEG beta frequencies introduces the contamination from muscle potentials that are higher-voltage, faster frequencies at the upper range of recorded scalp EEG frequencies.[289] This interference is especially troublesome because facial muscle emotional expression is asymmetrical, with greater expression on the left than the right in right-handed individuals.[290] Depressed patients are in a state of intense emotional expression and would be expected to have asymmetrical electromyographic findings.

These concerns and the association of increased beta power with arousal and anxiety suggest that the reported patterns of scalp-recorded resting EEG differences in depressed subjects compared to comparison subjects may be an epiphenomenon representing severity of illness. Consistent with this view is the coupling of EEG in the higher frequencies with cortisol secretory pulses.[291] The implications of the EEG changes in depressed patients are further limited when attempting to correlate the EEG findings with positron emission tomography (PET) and SPECT results. Combining awake EEG and brain-imaging methods in the same patients is rarely reported. The studies generally show greater beta activity to be correlated with increased brain metabolism and increased cerebral blood flow.[292] Metabolic studies report abnormalities to be greater on the left than on the right (decreased dorsolateral and increased anterior cingulate loci) and to be associated with psychomotor disturbance. EEG beta power is reported to be greater on the right than on the left, indicating greater arousal on the right.[293] Greater absolute or relative EEG arousal over the right hemisphere is accompanied by increased, not decreased, metabolism on the right. Again, the most parsimonious explanation for such reports is that EEG frontal beta activity is muscle artifact and not a direct measure of the pathophysiologic process.

Activated EEG

Medication activation

Following Berger's report that the EEG was sensitive to medication effects, EEG changes during the course of insulin coma and ECT were examined. The interseizure EEG in ECT was related to treatment efficacy, with the early appearance of high-voltage slow-wave activity associated with better clinical outcomes.[294] Later, with the ability to record the seizure EEG, this measure became an index of treatment efficacy.[295]

The onset of EEG beta frequencies to a measured dose of intravenous amobarbital, labeled the "sedation threshold," was considered a diagnostic test to separate depressive and schizophrenic syndromes.[296] In depressed patients and in those with dementia the onset of beta activity occurred at lower doses of amobarbital. In patients with schizophrenia and anxiety syndromes, the onset required greater doses of amobarbital. A sleep threshold test was also developed.

The EEG changes with psychoactive drugs were found to be medication class-specific – that is, different EEG patterns were elicited with antidepressant, anxiolytic, and antipsychotic drugs. Attempts to separate patient samples by their quantitative EEG responses to antidepressant and anxiolytic medications were, however, unsuccessful.[297]

Sensory evoked potentials (SEP)

The ability to digitize electrophysiologic signals and to manipulate the data statistically with digital computer-based algorithms offered opportunities to examine the immediate responses of the brain to a sensory stimulus. In the somatosensory (SEP), auditory (AEP), and visual evoked potential response (VEP) tests, stimuli are applied as electrical stimulation of the median nerve, auditory clicks, or flashes of light. These are offered at frequent intervals and the succeeding EEG response to 50 or 200 stimuli is summed and a smooth curve of brain response is recorded. The peaks and troughs of the acquired averages are measured for height and location in milliseconds after the stimulus. The technology was developed to measure cortical excitability.

The reliability of each measure varies with the stimulus number and rate of presentation. As the responses are summed and presented as a single waveform, any waveform aberrations not from the brain will have little effect on the average. The anticipated benefit of AEP is that the artifacts are minimized. The limitation of AEP is that it reflects the brain's processing of repeated sensory stimulation and assumes a stable state over the minutes of stimulation.

Evoked potential studies were examined as measures of mood state.[298] When applied to patients with mood disorders, the SEP was reported to have smaller P_{300} wave amplitude or longer latency.[299] Longer P_{300} latency was related to a poorer response to antidepressant medication.[300] The P_{300} was assumed to be a cortically derived response that reflects the efficiency and speed of information processing. It is influenced by expectation.[301]

The evoked potential findings in mood disorders, however, are inconsistent and complicated by the inability to relate evoked potential measures to clinical signs and symptoms. For example, AEP P_{300} latencies are reported to correlate with psychomotor retardation.[302] Many observers, however, do not find this association.[303] P_{300} amplitudes have been related to suicide risk and hopelessness in some reports,[304] but not others.[305] A study of VEPs observed melancholic patients to have long N_{80} and P_{100} latencies while patients with atypical depression had shorter latencies. Melancholic patients were reported to have a positive correlation between latencies and age of first episode of mood disorder and a negative correlation with precipitating events.[306]

Several studies of psychotic melancholic patients found a negative correlation between psychotic features and P_{300} amplitude.[307] Delayed latencies in psychotic and non-psychotic patients were reported when compared to controls.[308] Successful treatment normalized these findings. The P_{300} response was reduced in amplitude and prolonged in latency, particularly over the left hemispheres, in psychotic patients; depressive symptoms were associated with amplitude reduction over the right temporal area.[309]

Overall, the tests do not demarcate depressed subjects and controls. The connections to mood and thought and motor functions, the principal interests in psychiatry, are unclear. It is best to consider evoked potential changes in mood disorders as epiphenomena reflecting severity, psychosis, or other clinical heterogeneity.[310] The effects of medication and of sleep on evoked responses do not offer better indices of diagnosis.

Sleep EEG

The EEG during sleep is a measurable reflection of brain physiology. As sleep is severely disturbed in patients with melancholia, the changes in sleep EEG have become a useful test of the presence and severity of melancholia. The relevant features are discussed in Chapter 4. The sleep EEG as a measure of pathophysiology of melancholia is discussed here.

Studies of EEG sleep parameters indicate increased arousal and less deep sleep.[311] Melatonin nighttime concentrations are higher, but do not correlate with sleep rhythms.[312] A meta-analysis of 115 sleep studies with over 3600 psychiatric patients concluded that patients with mood disorders differed most from normal subjects.[313] Rapid eye movement (REM) latency was the best sleep parameter to correlate with severity of depressive mood disorder. Patients who had an endogenous, melancholic, or psychotic depressive illness differed the most from controls. The findings in over 1400 depressed patients are summarized in Table 14.6. Also reported is the association of greater sleep disturbance with a greater likelihood of relapse.[314]

Table 14.6. Sleep disturbances in depressed patients

Total sleep time reduced
Sleep efficiency reduced
Sleep latency prolonged (time to fall asleep)
Slow wave sleep total and percentage time reduced
NREM total time reduced
REM latency shortened (time from sleep to first REM period)
All-night REM density increased
First REM period duration increased
REM as percentage of total sleep time increased

In both depressed and healthy subjects the degree of EEG arousal correlates positively with whole-brain glucose metabolism during non-REM (NREM) sleep.[315] Factors that affect sleep, such as age and overactivity of the hypothalamic–pituitary cortisol axis in depressive illness, play a role in this disturbance.[316] Adolescents who are deemed likely to make a suicide attempt exhibit elevated cortisol levels prior to the onset of sleep, a time when levels are typically at their lowest.[317] Melancholic patients have increased brain metabolism during NREM sleep, consistent with greater arousal, even during sleep.[318] However, unlike normal controls, there is less arousal during NREM sleep in the frontal regions of depressed patients, paralleling the metabolic studies in alert patients.[319]

Sleep EEG is influenced by gender-determined neuroendocrine findings, with low estrogen levels inversely related to sleep disturbance.[320] Depressed women have more marked disturbances than depressed men.[321] While depressed men (particularly those 20–40 years of age) have reduced NREM slow-wave sleep, there is no similar evidence in depressed women.[322] Thus, the studies show an interaction among age, gender, hormone levels, and cortisol activity and the sleep problems of depressed patients.[323]

Sleep difficulties are ubiquitous among psychiatric patients and most sleep EEG abnormalities observed in depressed patients reflect a severity or illness factor (anxiety and arousal) rather than a specific marker of depression. Some sleep abnormalities, however, may be biological markers for mood disorder.[324] Shortened REM latency is consistently observed in adult and adolescent depressed patients. It is an inconsistent finding in children. Such reports suggest a developmental process as a feature of the depressed illness state.[325]

Quantitative EEG studies reveal several mood-sensitive sleep variables that are gender-dependent. In adults, alpha and beta fast-frequency amplitudes and amounts are increased while delta slow-frequency amplitudes and amounts are decreased.[326] Synchronization in sleep EEG ultradian (90-min) rhythms is also disturbed with poor temporal coherence between hemispheres.[327] Low coherence is observed in depressed women, whereas depressed men have reduced slow-wave activity, particularly in the first NREM sleep period.[328] Low coherence is also observed in depressed adolescent girls, particularly after puberty.[329]

Low sleep phase coherence between hemispheres is considered a marker of the risk for depressive illness in girls. Among children with a family history of depressive illness who had never been depressed, 23% exhibited low coherence.[330] After comparing the sleep EEG rhythms in 41 adolescent girls with a maternal history of depressive illness to 40 healthy controls in a sample that was clinically assessed every six months for two years, the sleep phase coherence between hemispheres was lower in the high-risk girls and regression analysis correctly classified 70% of the high-risk group with a 5% false-positive rate among the controls.[331] Forty-one percent of the girls with the most abnormally low EEG sleep phase coherence developed depressive features during follow-up and six became depressed. Only one control participant became depressed. In a follow-up, 50% of the girls with low hemispheric EEG coherence had their first episode of depressive illness within 3–5 years from the study's onset.[332] Estrogen and progesterone effects on EEG and sleep have been proposed as an explanation for the gender difference in coherence.[333]

Sleep deprivation

Keeping a depressed patient awake for 24–36 h induces temporary modest relief from depressed mood in 40–60% of patients.[334] Permitting some sleep to occur or only awakening the patient when entering REM sleep (partial sleep deprivation) does not relieve depressive symptoms,[335] whereas advancing bedtimes after a night of sleep deprivation may have a modest effect at sustaining the antidepressant response.[336] Patients who respond to total sleep deprivation tend to be those with abnormal cortisol metabolism and abnormal brain glucose metabolism, suggesting the effect may be specific to melancholia.[337] Before sleep deprivation, responders have elevated metabolism compared with non-responders and normal controls on functional imaging in the orbital medial prefrontal cortex and the ventral portions of the anterior cingulated cortex. After sleep deprivation, these hyperactive areas normalize in the responders.[338] One study associates the presence of a stress response-related gene polymorphism (angiotensin-converting enzyme gene) with mood response to sleep deprivation.[339] Changes in serotonin function[340] and cholinergic activity[341] leading to a more normal ultradian rhythm are hypothesized, but unproven, explanations for the temporary antidepressant effect of sleep deprivation. Sleep deprivation also increases serum prolactin release to serotonin stimulation, and this is associated with the response to sleep deprivation.[342]

Cognitive deficits

Depressed patients commonly exhibit difficulties in memory, recall, and concentration. Their subjective self-assessment is typically worse than their performance, but deficits in cognitive functioning are measurable and substantial.[343] The difficulties vary with severity of illness and are state-dependent. Some cognitive difficulties, however, often persist even after remission, and are interpreted as evidence of the neurotoxic effects of depressive illness.

Among melancholic patients, explicit verbal and visual memory is impaired, while implicit memory appears to be spared.[344] Episodic memory (visual memory for events) is impaired.[345] Performance deficits are not due to poor effort but derive from intrinsic memory dysfunction. Equivalent deficits are found with tests requiring little effort (recognition rather than verbal recall). The impairments in memory of depressed patients have been directly linked to hippocampal volume loss on magnetic resonance imaging (MRI).[346]

Melancholic patients show deficits in executive and other frontal circuitry functions.[347] Both old,[348] and young[349] patients are affected. Melancholic patients also appear to have specific deficits not observed in other forms of depressive illness. These include poor working memory and focused attention, difficulty shifting from one set of problem-solving rules to another set, and increased perseverative responsiveness. Conceptual functions are spared. Severity of mood disorder partially explains the differences among depressed patients in frontal lobe-related tasks, with performance correlated with severity.[350] Melancholic patients, however, have a diurnal pattern in their performance, worse in the morning and better in the evening, opposite to the pattern seen in normal persons.[351]

Cognitive performance and the patient's subjective experience in concentration and memory typically improve after recovery with antidepressant therapy.[352] Concerns with cognition in some patients, however, persist after acute treatment, but these studies are confounded by methodologic shortcomings. Treatment response is defined as a 50% or greater drop in a severity rating-scale score rather than full remission. As a consequence, many patients are still symptomatic even with such a percentage decrease in symptoms. It is difficult to know if lower than expected performance is due to lingering depressed mood or the prolonged aftermath of a resolved depressive illness. Medication effects on cognition are not usually assessed and non-ill controls are rarely included for comparison. So, despite an improvement in performance from pretreatment levels, after treatment some depressed patients continue to perform below their age-expected range. About half of depressed patients continue to have cognitive deficits during the six months or so after they experience improvement in their disorder, and perhaps much longer.[353] These impairments are similar to those observed during the acute phase of the illness and are not treatment-related. Melancholic patients are particularly likely to have these problems.[354]

The study of cognitive function in depressed, and specifically melancholic, patients indicates two patterns of impairment. One pattern affects explicit memory and is related to hippocampal volume loss. This loss is associated with the hypercortisolemia of melancholia.[355] Exposure to exogenous glucocorticoids impairs memory in non-depressed persons.[356] Repeated and prolonged depressions increase the likelihood of hippocampal cell loss, and thus account for persistent cognitive deficits.[357] The second pattern of cognitive impairment is in frontal state-dependent functions related to frontal circuitry. Some dysfunction persists in older patients. Neither pattern of impairment is specific to melancholia, but both correlate with severity of the depressive mood disorder. Thus melancholic patients are more likely to exhibit measurable cognitive impairment.[358] Such impairment is a suicide risk factor.[359]

Why some melancholic patients have manic episodes

About 10% of patients with depressive mood disorders also have manic episodes. The association of these seemingly opposite disorders of mood and motor function is well documented. Are the pathophysiologies the same in melancholia accompanied by mania as those in which mania is not recorded? What are the processes that elicit depressed mood at one time and manic behavior at another, sometimes separated by years and sometimes by months, but also occurring within weeks, or days, or even within the same day or the same examination?[360]

The *sensitization model* of manic-depressive illness is the rationale for the use of anticonvulsants as mood stabilizers, but the model does not explain why patients with recurrent depressive mood disorders also have manic episodes.[361] The depressive moods associated with manic-depressive illness are melancholic, and these episodes cannot be clinically distinguished from melancholic episodes in patients who only have recurrent depressive mood disorders from studies in depressed patients.[362]

The *neurobiologic markers* of mania and depression are very much alike. For example, cortisol non-suppression to dexamethasone is observed with equivalent frequencies in manic-depressive and in recurrent depressive patients.[363] Both depressed and manic phases of manic-depressive illness are associated with increased cortisol levels.[364] Although less consistently observed, both forms have abnormal circadian phase shifts.[365] Abnormalities in HPT axis functioning occur in both forms of mood disorder, perhaps more so in manic-depressive patients than in patients experiencing only recurrent depression.[366] Neurochemically, serotonergic and dopaminergic responsiveness appear similar in both forms of illness.[367]

Brain structural and metabolic studies reveal substantial similarities between mania and depression. The literature in mania, however, is very limited. Structural studies report inconsistent findings difficult to reconcile, while metabolic studies are confounded by the inclusion of many medicated patients. Compared to studies of depressed patients, there are also relatively fewer investigations of manic-depressive patients, making reconciliation of differences in findings even more arduous.

Overall, the same brain structures are found to be abnormal in mania and depression.[368] The few differences reflect opposite regional activity. For example, in depressed phases of the illness increased ventral and decreased dorsal prefrontal cortex metabolism is reported in cerebral blood flow and PET investigations. In mania an opposite pattern is reported. In studies identifying asymmetrical abnormalities, depression is associated with increased metabolism on the left, while in mania homologous right-sided structures appear less active.[369] Hemispheric instability has been hypothesized to explain these differences and how a patient shifts from one form of mood disorder to another.

Cerebral hemispheric instability is an explanation offered for those melancholic patients who switch into mania. The explaining concept holds that the right and left cerebral hemispheres have different information-processing styles, responding differently to specific physical attributes of stimuli (e.g., the right hemisphere is better at processing low-frequency information, the left hemisphere better at processing high-frequency information), and different cognitive specialization (visual-spatial versus language, respectively). These hemisphere differences appear to be "hardwired" in adults.

Several researchers propose that the two hemispheres experience and express emotions differently. The left hemisphere mediates positive emotions (e.g., happiness) while the right hemisphere mediates negative emotions (e.g., sadness). Motor activation is also related to a propensity for signals of reward to reflect left hemisphere activity while the tendency to avoid signals of non-reward (e.g., pain) is mediated by right hemisphere activity. Mania is hypothesized to reflect overactivity in left hemisphere systems whereas depression reflects decreased left or increased right hemisphere activity, or both.[370]

When the left hemisphere is overactive, positive moods and approach behavior dominate. Stressful events may intensify the positive mood state, and mania occurs. When the right hemisphere is overactive negative emotions and avoidance behaviors predominate, and a depressive mood disorder results. The limbic generators of emotion and the abnormal stress-response mechanisms observed in mood disorder drive the illness, while the symmetry of hemisphere activation determines whether the patient will experience depression alone or experience depressive and manic episodes.[371] There is no evidence for these concepts from studies in depressed patients.

Which depressed patient will develop mania or hypomania cannot be predicted. One 11-year prospective study of over 500 patients, however, offers some clues.[372] Patients with recurrent depressive episodes who subsequently developed mania (so-called bipolar I) were not distinguished from those depressed patients who only experience depressive states. The depressed patients who subsequently experienced hypomania (so-called bipolar II) had early onsets of illness, mood-labile temperaments, high energy, excessive responsiveness, the propensity to daydream, high rates of illicit substance abuse and social and job disruptions, and were more likely to commit "minor" antisocial acts. Another study reported that depressed patients who switched into mania were more likely to have low levels of TSH than those who did not.[373]

Unstable temperament with mood lability leads to stormy life events and undue stress, pushing such a person over the illness threshold. A childhood or teen depressive illness develops. Thyroid instability increases such a risk. Early mood disorder episodes, chronic and severe stress, and the use of medications with seizure-inducing potential further influence this recurrent circle. An unstable mood system accentuates the interhemisphere imbalance proposed to explain shifts from one form of mood disorder to another.

A *genetic predisposition* is offered to explain unstable temperament, perhaps a reflection of the imbalance in interhemisphere function proposed in manic-depressive illness.[374] Severe depressive moods and psychomotor disturbances are most common in patients with manic-depressive illness.[375] Those with first episodes in their early 20s or even younger are likely to have the atypical forms of illness, but many others have classic recurrent melancholic episodes. The frequency of both manic-depressive and recurrent depressive illnesses in relatives of probands with manic-depressive illness is increased.[376] Twin studies show this overlap.[377] An analysis of 30 monozygotic and 37 dizygotic twin pairs is revealing.[378] Proband concordance was higher for the monozygotic than for the dizygotic twins, with heritability estimated at 89%. In almost 29% of the monozygotic pairs, one twin had both manic and depressive episodes while the other had recurrent depressive illnesses. Among the dizygotic pairs 13.5% exhibited mixed concordance. The investigators tested several liability models and concluded that manic-depressive illness was not simply a more severe form of recurrent depressive illness. The two forms exhibit a substantial genetic overlap (about 30%). That is, persons with mood disorder share a substantial genetic liability but those who experience mania or hypomania have an additional and distinct genetic predisposition. Thus, centuries of clinical experience and modern behavioral genetic strategies converge and lead to the conclusion that to understand fully the pathophysiology of recurrent melancholic illness the pathophysiology of mania must also be considered.

Conclusions

The etiology and pathophysiology of melancholia may be inferred from studies that carefully identify melancholic patients and from studies (the majority) that characterize their patients as "severely ill," "psychotic," or hospitalized with depressive illness. The more severely ill the depressed patients are, the more likely they will exhibit abnormalities on laboratory measures, have a family history of mood disorder, and meet criteria for melancholia. The findings in severely ill depressed patients are consistent with findings in melancholic patients. Viewed through this interpolation "lens," melancholia is a recurrent disorder with a substantial genetic vulnerability. Early, severe, and chronic stressful experiences increase the likelihood that a genetic vulnerability will be expressed as mood disorder. Acute stress precipitates episodes. Experiencing recurrent episodes lowers the threshold for future episodes. An episode of melancholia has characteristic behavioral and laboratory expressions and treatment-responsiveness.[379]

The literature, however, does not resolve the question whether melancholia is a stage of depressive illness or a distinct syndrome, although the evidence strongly favors a distinct syndrome. Multivariate studies following children at high risk for depressive illness and prospective studies of episodes as they unfold are needed to answer this question. While the following conclusions certainly apply to severe recurrent depressive illness and likely also to melancholia, further studies that focus on melancholia are needed.

Table 14.7. Genetic influences on the risk for depression

Suspected genetic predisposition	Association with depression
Specific genes for psychopathology	Weak for milder forms
	Moderate to substantial for severe melancholic forms
Temperament	Weak for milder forms
	No relationship to severe forms of recurrent depressive illness, but may reflect a manic-depressive course
Stress-responsiveness	Substantial in laboratory animals
	Unknown in humans

Genes and endophenotype

Genes play a definable role in the risk for developing melancholia (Table 14.7). The genes of vulnerability are of moderate strength (about 40–50% heritability) and are additive (multiple small genes of increasing "dose" rather than one or two genes with big effects). For most persons with the genotype, chronic severe stress, pregnancy, or aging are precipitants of the disease. Some persons with the genotype for melancholia do not become depressed because they do not experience sufficient precipitants. They may, however, transmit the genetic risk to their offspring.

Genes of vulnerability are expressed through a gene–environment interaction. Other than the chronic stress in childhood, factors that alter gene activity leading to clinical illness are unknown. Whatever the interaction, it results in an alteration in the sensitivity of the person to stress.[380] The genetic risk leads to an endophenotypic "prekindling" state. Repeated stress lowers the threshold for depressive illness, and at some point a clinical episode emerges. Repeated and prolonged episodes of depressed mood abnormally prolong stress responses. The episodes are themselves stressful experiences. Each episode sensitizes the limbic system and further lowers the threshold for depressive illness, leading to chronicity.

As an example, the association between stressful life events and the risk for depressive mood disorder decreases as the number of depressive episodes increases (i.e., the more episodes of depression, the less stress is needed to precipitate a disorder).[381]

Persons with high genetic risk begin with low thresholds for illness and become depressed with few or no stressors. Persons with lower genetic risk become depressed only under severe stress, but if depressive mood disorders recur, these persons subsequently become ill without a specific stressful precipitant. It is unclear whether these or other genes add risk for additional forms of psychopathology such as anxiety disorder and substance abuse. The overlap of recurrent depressive illness and manic-depressive illness has yet to be clarified.

Brain metabolic abnormalities that are observed in mood states reflect disrupted functions of the limbic system and frontal circuitry. A direct causal relationship, however, has not been established between abnormal mood and behavior and the structures that are metabolically abnormal. In part the failure is due to clinical heterogeneity, small samples, and technical differences across studies. EEG findings in severe depressive mood states are contaminated by anxiety, agitation, increased arousal, and the use of psychoactive agents. Neurotransmitter changes are considered to result from abnormal mood states as well as being contributory to them. Brain structural changes occur with chronic stress and with repeated, prolonged altered mood states; they are not the direct cause of those mood states. The cognitive problems seen in melancholia are the result of the illness, not its cause.

Temperament genes and genes affecting reactivity to stress play a modest role in altering an individual's liability for depression. When the genotypes are expressed in persons as high-risk temperaments and with excessive stress-responsiveness, they, along with the genes of illness vulnerability, are sufficient to overcome the illness threshold and depressive illnesses occur. Such persons are likely to have strong family histories of mood disorder, anxiety disorder, and anxious-fearful personality traits. Other genes that may affect temperament and mood lability add a risk factor for mania and hypomania. The social storminess experienced by persons with mood lability and maniform mood states are both stressors that adversely affect the limbic system and sensitizers to stress, increasing the risk for more episodes.

Women during the menstrual preluteal phase, immediately postpartum, and during the perimenopausal period experience substantial changes in estrogen levels. Such changes alter serotonergic activity and in a genetically vulnerable person initiate mood changes. A heightened stress response contributes to lowering the illness threshold and to the initiation of depressive illness. Age-related brain changes lower the illness threshold, resulting in late-life depression.

Cycle of stress

Environmental factors that increase the risk for depressive illness are elusive. Factors that are associated with increased risk have their greatest impact early in a person's life. Maternal mood disorders during pregnancy and in the postpartum period carry the biggest risks followed by maternal depressive and psychotic illness during childhood. The presence of a healthy father with good parenting skills modestly reduces these postpartum and childhood risks. Marital discord, child abuse, and other chronic stress increase risk and interact with maternal depression to increase risk substantially. Chronic stress in life increases risk for depression. These experiences lead to a state of chronic stress in the child with its associated brain changes and gene transcription effects.

Once begun, the pathophysiology of the depressive episode takes on a life of its own. Abnormal stress responses cascade without the feedback inhibition available to non-ill persons. Illness builds and fuels itself. A broad array of neurotransmitters and stress hormones interact synergistically, making focused pharmacologic interventions less effective. More symptoms emerge. The social, job, and health consequences of symptoms cause more stress, feeding the cycle. Starvation and weight loss, sleeplessness, stupor or fitful agitation, catatonia, psychosis, and self-injury are now more likely to occur. Heart rhythms are perturbed and immune system effectiveness is reduced. Morbidity and mortality increase. Melancholia is established.

NOTES

1 "Carrion comfort" in *Gerald Manley Hopkins, Poems and Prose*. London: Penguin Books, London (1985), p. 62.

2 In a Danish study of 352 inpatients and 581 outpatients assessed with the Hamilton Depression Rating Scale and the Newcastle Diagnostic Rating System, 76% of the inpatients and 40% of the outpatients met criteria for melancholia (Stage *et al.*, 1998).

3 A patient is identified as a proband when family members are studied. This identification is needed when considering ascertainment and other biases in the data. For example, beginning with ill probands insures that all families studied will have at least one ill member. Starting with ill parents yields different results than when starting with ill children, in assessing environmental and genetic variables.

4 Studies that include comparison groups typically examine children of parents with illness (high-risk children) versus children of well parents (low risk). See Puig-Antich *et al.* (1989); Kutcher and Marton (1991); Harrington *et al.* (1993, 1997); Todd *et al.* (1993, 1996); Weller *et al.* (1994); Williamson *et al.* (1995); Kovacs *et al.* (1997); Neuman *et al.* (1997); Klein *et al.* (2001).

For other family studies, see: Weissman *et al.* (1984b, 1987, 1988, 1992, 1997); Keller *et al.* (1986a, 1988); Klein *et al.* (1988); Merikangas *et al.* (1988a); Orvaschel *et al.* (1988); Mitchell *et al.* (1989); Downey and Coyne (1990); Fendrich *et al.* (1990); Hammen (1990); Hammen *et al.* (1990); Radke-Yarrow *et al.* (1992); Warner *et al.* (1995, 1999); Beardslee *et al.* (1996); Kendler *et al.* (1997); Wickramaratne and Weissman (1998); Dierker *et al.* (1999); Goodman and Gotlib (1999); Lieb *et al.* (2002).

Some studies, however, do not find an increased risk for depressive illness in the adult relatives of ill children (Livingston *et al.*, 1985; Mitchell *et al.*, 1989).

5 This figure represents an estimate of variance, i.e., how much of differences in the sample(s) is contributed by genes. Zero indicates no genetic influence while 1.00 indicates all the contribution is genetic.

6 Merikangas *et al.* (2002).
7 Ingraham and Wender (1992).
8 Huang *et al.* (2003) studied 394 depressed outpatients and 96 normal controls and report modest genetic linkage on a serotonin receptor gene (5-HT1B, G861C) for major depression and substance abuse. The odds, however, for a single polymorphism accounting for two complex and heterogeneous conditions is slim.

Lemonde *et al.* (2003) studied 129 persons with major depression and 102 suicide completers, each with a comparison group. They found the G(-1019) homozygous genotype to occur twice as often in depressed patients and four times as often in suicide victims than in controls. Frodl *et al.* (2004) examined 40 patients with depressive illness and report an association between the long variant of the serotonin transporter polymorphism and reduced hippocampal volumes. The former finding is consistent with resistance to antidepressant medication and the latter finding with the effects of prolonged depression. Many studies, however, fail to find linkage between depressive illness and specific polymorphisms (Koper *et al.*, 1997).
9 Community studies also underestimate the base rates for manic-depressive illness because many manic patients are in hospital or in other assisted living programs.
10 Moldin *et al.* (1991); Tsuang *et al.* (1994).
11 Tsuang and Faraone (1990).
12 Kendler *et al.* (1996); Klein *et al.* (2001).
13 Weissman *et al.* (1984a, 1988); Weissman (1988).
14 Modell *et al.* (1998).
15 Weissman *et al.* (1984a, b) report high rates of depression in the relatives of their most severely ill probands; severity was defined as "hospitalized," not by the patterns of psychopathology. Puig-Antich *et al.* (1989), examining the relatives of hospitalized depressed children, reported high rates of depression, particularly in the relatives of children with endogenous depression. There likely was a substantial proportion of persons with endogenous depression in Weissman *et al.*'s hospitalized adult patients (and similar studies).
16 Leckman *et al.* (1984).
17 Puig-Antich *et al.* (1989).
18 Price *et al.* (1984); Zimmerman *et al.* (1986a).
19 Sullivan *et al.* (2000).
20 Todd *et al.* (1993); Sanders *et al.* (1999).
21 Kovacs *et al.* (1997); Williamson *et al.* (2004).
22 Livingston *et al.* (1985); Kutcher and Marton (1991); Warner *et al.* (1995); Todd *et al.* (1996); Weissman *et al.* (1997); Klein *et al.* (2001); Preisig *et al.* (2001). Genetic linkage studies report inconsistent findings (Nurnberger *et al.*, 2001).
23 Prescott *et al.* (2000).
24 Brook *et al.* (2002); Chen *et al.* (2002); Patton *et al.* (2002).
25 Maher *et al.* (2002).
26 Fu *et al.* (2002b).
27 The depressed moods in recurrent depressive illness and manic-depressive illness are not distinguishable. There also appears to be some genetic overlap between what is presently defined as unipolar and bipolar mood disorders. Chapter 2.
28 Gershon *et al.* (1982); Coryell *et al.* (1984); Fieve *et al.* (1984); Tsuang *et al.* (1985); Andreasen *et al.* (1987).
29 Bertelsen *et al.* (1977); Torgersen (1986); McGuffin *et al.* (2003).

30 Taylor and Abrams (1980); Weissman *et al.* (1984c).
31 Rende *et al.* (1993); Harrington *et al.* (1996); McGuffin *et al.* (2003).
32 Murray and Sines (1996). Environmental influences on genetic predisposition that leads to individual differences can be shared (e.g., being raised in the same household, going to the same school) or non-shared (e.g., siblings going to different schools, one sibling suffering a head injury).
33 For a general discussion, see Taylor (1999) (Chapter 6). For more detailed supporting data, see Cloninger (1987); Costa and Widiger (1994); Livesley *et al.* (1993); Plomin *et al.* (1994).
34 Maier *et al.* (1992a, b); Ono *et al.* (2002).
35 Loehlin (1992); Goodman and Gotlib (1999).
36 Klein *et al.* (1995); Pepper *et al.* (1995).
37 Kendler *et al.* (1993b).
38 Sen *et al.* (2003).
39 van Eck *et al.* (1996).
40 Pruessner *et al.* (1997).
41 Adler *et al.* (1997).
42 Bossert *et al.* (1988).
43 Plomin *et al.* (1994); O'Connor *et al.* (1995).
44 Brown and Harris (1978); Kendler *et al.* (1991b); McGue and Lykken (1992).
45 Caspi *et al.* (2003).
46 Coste *et al.* (2000).
47 Veenema *et al.* (2003).
48 Bale *et al.* (2000).
49 Tannenbaum and Anisman (2003).
50 Ventura *et al.* (2002).
51 Pepin *et al.* (1992a, b); Stout *et al.* (2002).
52 Kalin *et al.* (2000).
53 Williamson *et al.* (2003).
54 Handley *et al.* (1980); Smith *et al.* (1990).
55 Field (1998).
56 Hammen (1990).
57 Glover *et al.* (1998).
58 Field *et al.* (2002a).
59 Hulshoff *et al.* (2000); Field *et al.* (2002a, b); O'Connor *et al.* (2002).
60 Glover (1997).
61 Field (1998).
62 Rahman *et al.* (2004).
63 Emory *et al.* (1983).
64 Milberger *et al.* (1996).
65 Watson *et al.* (1999).
66 Dunn *et al.* (1989).
67 Hedegaard *et al.* (1996).
68 Zuckerman *et al.* (1990).
69 Gotlib and Whiffen (1989).
70 Maternal–child interactions and their effect on child development have been extensively studied. Home observations and controlled studies in laboratory settings yield similar,

reproducible results. Among the many reviews, see Brockington and Kumar (1982); Keller *et al.* (1986a); Gotlib and Goodman (1999).

71 Dawson *et al.* (1994a).

72 Porges *et al.* (1994); Field *et al.* (1995).

73 Portales *et al.* (1992). These findings are supported by studies of laboratory primates undergoing early exposure to stress that is associated with persistent elevation of stress-related hormones (e.g., corticotropin-releasing factor) in cerebrospinal fluid, even after the stressors are removed (Coplan *et al.*, 1996; Ladd *et al.*, 1996).

74 Hay and Kumar (1995); Sharp *et al.* (1995).

75 Hay *et al.* (2001).

76 Goodman *et al.* (1993).

77 Sinclair and Murray (1998).

78 Field *et al.* (2001); Aalto-Setala *et al.* (2002).

79 Lyons *et al.* (1998).

80 Merikangas *et al.* (1988b); Mathews and Reus (2001).

81 Thomas and Forehand (1991); Goodman *et al.* (1993).

82 Carro *et al.* (1993).

83 Conrad and Hammen (1989).

84 Eiden and Leonard (1996).

85 Hossain *et al.* (1994).

86 Goodman and Gotlib (1999).

87 Brown and Moran (1994).

88 McCauley *et al.* (1997).

89 Parker *et al.* (1997, 1998b).

90 Canetti *et al.* (2000); Kendler *et al.* (2002); Gilman *et al.* (2003).

91 Harkness and Monroe (2002).

92 Harkness and Monroe (2002).

93 Holsinger *et al.* (2002).

94 Alonso *et al.* (1994); Bremner (2003).

95 McKittrick *et al.* (2000).

96 Sapolsky (2000).

97 Fahlke *et al.* (2000).

98 Sanchez *et al.* (1998).

99 De Bellis *et al.* (1999). Studies of chronic stress led to the concept of "learned helplessness" as a model for depressive illness. In this paradigm, a laboratory animal is exposed to inescapable stress and eventually stops trying to escape, even when escape is permitted. The animal becomes inactive. It may stop eating and drinking and these behaviors have been interpreted as depressive-like (Seligman, 1997).

100 Kendler *et al.* (1993a); Piccinelli and Wilkinson (2000); Bogner and Gallo (2004).

101 Kessler (2003).

102 Kendler *et al.* (2001b). Among women with depressive illnesses there is almost twice the risk of a suicide attempt during menses (Baca-Garcia *et al.*, 2003).

103 Fink G. *et al.* (1996); Seeman (1997).

104 Buckwalter *et al.* (2001).

105 Rubinow (1992).

106 Patchev and Almeida (1996).

107 Sheng *et al.* (2003).

108 Shors and Leuner (2003).
109 Altshuler *et al.* (2001a).
110 MacQueen and Joffe (2002).
111 Muller *et al.* (2001).
112 Holsboer *et al.* (1986).
113 Garbutt *et al.* (1994).
114 MacQueen and Joffe (2002).
115 Demonstrations of the HPA and HPT axis dysfunction in melancholia became the basis for the dexamethasane suppression test (DST), Dex/DST, TSH response to TRH, and similar tests that are useful indices of melancholia. These are discussed in Chapter 4.
116 Heim and Nemeroff (2001); Rothschild (2003b).
117 Young *et al.* (2000a); Chalmers *et al.* (1993); Heim and Nemeroff (2001).
118 Gold and Chrousos (1999).
119 Gold and Chrousos (1999).
120 Van de Kar and Blair (1999).
121 Meyer *et al.* (2001b).
122 Young *et al.* (2000a); Heim and Nemeroff (2001).
123 Van de Kar and Blair (1999).
124 Wallace *et al.* (1992); Petrov *et al.* (1993).
125 Gray (1993).
126 Hucks *et al.* (1997); Hiroi *et al.* (2001).
127 Sapolsky (1996, 2000); Sheline *et al.* (1996); Reagen and McEwen (1997); Bremner *et al.* (2000). Nestler *et al.* (2002); Carrasco and Van de Kar (2003).
128 Gold and Chrousos (1999).
129 Gold and Chrousos (1999).
130 Goldstein (1995).
131 Tests of neuroendocrine metabolism, including cortisol, are discussed in Chapter 4.
132 Hibberd *et al.* (2000); Keck and Holsboer (2001); Sheline *et al.* (2003).
133 Arborelius *et al.* (1999); Holsboer (2001).
134 Heim *et al.* (2000); Young *et al.* (2000a); Heim and Nemeroff (2001).
135 Meyer *et al.* (2001).
136 Souetre *et al.* (1985); Rybakowski and Twardowska (1999).
137 Daimon *et al.* (1992).
138 Stampfer (1998).
139 Peteranderl *et al.* (2002).
140 Szuba *et al.* (1997).
141 Beier *et al.* (2003).
142 Raadsheer *et al.* (1995).
143 Francis and Meaney (1999); Heim and Nemeroff (2001).
144 Arborelius *et al.* (1999); Holsboer (2001).
145 Nemeroff and Evans (1988).
146 Young *et al.* (1995).
147 Lopez *et al.* (1998); Sargent *et al.* (2000).
148 Cheetham *et al.* (1990); Gonzalez *et al.* (1994).
149 Gormley *et al.* (1985); Lowy *et al.* (1988).
150 Gormley *et al.* (1985); Yehuda *et al.* (1993).
151 Lopez *et al.* (1998).

152 Parianti and Miller (2001).
153 Koper *et al.* (1997); Modell *et al.* (1998).
154 Avissar *et al.* (1997).
155 Shelton *et al.* (1996).
156 Nibuya *et al.* (1996).
157 Laifenfeld *et al.* (2002).
158 Owens (1997).
159 Ben-Shacha *et al.* (1999).
160 Valentino *et al.* (1990); Curtis and Valentino (1994).
161 Gilmore *et al.* (2003).
162 Brady *et al.* (1991).
163 Lopez *et al.* (1998); Parianti and Miller (2001); Serra *et al.* (2002); Stout *et al.* (2002).
164 Pepin *et al.* (1992a, b); Parianti *et al.* (1997).
165 Elhwuegi (2004).
166 Azmitia and Segal (1978); Frazer and Hensler (1994).
167 Stahl (1998).
168 Stahl (1998); Celada *et al.* (2002).
169 Manji *et al.* (2001); Neumeister *et al.* (2004).
170 Ressler and Nemeroff (2000); Meyer *et al.* (2001); Nemeroff (2002b).
171 Delgado (2000b).
172 Nemeroff (2002a, b).
173 Meijer and de Kloet (1998); López-Ibor (1992).
174 Bethea *et al.* (1999).
175 Quantitative EEG studies of normal women find monthly variation in percentage time slow frequencies (theta/delta). Slowing precedes menses. For controlled pharmaco-EEG studies, women were excluded unless they were taking antiovulatory medication (Irwin and Fink, 1983; Corsi-Cabrera *et al.*, 1997a; Kaneda *et al.*, 1997).
176 Anand and Charney (2000).
177 Wong *et al.* (2000).
178 Anand and Charney (2000).
179 Le Doux (1992); Arnsten *et al.* (1999); Wong *et al.* (2000).
180 Freis (1954); Charney and Redmond (1983); Delgado *et al.* (1993); Ordway (1997); Ressler and Nemeroff (1999).
181 Ressler and Nemeroff (2000).
182 Cleare *et al.* (1997); Owens (1997).
183 Duman *et al.* (1999); Duman (2002).
184 Nibuya *et al.* (1996); Duman *et al.* (1999); Malberg *et al.* (2000); Hellsten *et al.* (2002).
185 Laifenfeld *et al.* (2002).
186 Delgado (2000b).
187 Corrigan *et al.* (2000).
188 Klimek *et al.* (2002). Supporting evidence comes from studies of laboratory animals that find an association between stress and abnormal dopamine metabolism in frontal lobe circuitry that is prevented by chronic administration of antidepressant agents (Dazzi *et al.*, 2001).
189 Naranjo *et al.* (2001).
190 Di Chiara *et al.* (1999).
191 Horger *et al.* (1999).

192 Alonso *et al.* (1994).
193 Altamura *et al.* (1995).
194 Francis *et al.* (1989).
195 Nowak *et al.* (1995).
196 Holemans *et al.* (1993).
197 Auer *et al.* (2000).
198 Cheetham *et al.* (1988).
199 Auer *et al.* (2000).
200 Thoenen (1995).
201 Duman *et al.* (1997); Karege *et al.* (2002).
202 Smith *et al.* (1995a).
203 Lyons *et al.* (1999).
204 Nibuya *et al.* (1995); Chen *et al.* (2001a, b).
205 Malberg *et al.* (2000).
206 Siuciak *et al.* (1997).
207 Pandey *et al.* (1999).
208 Altar *et al.* (2003). Russo-Neustadt *et al.* (1999).
209 Sen *et al.* (2003).
210 Karege *et al.* (2002).
211 Ebner *et al.* (2000).
212 Carrasco and Van de Kar (2003).
213 Hokfelt *et al.* (1980); Elliott (1988).
214 Carrasco and Van de Kar (2003).
215 Rupniak and Kramer (1999).
216 Ceccatelli *et al.* (1991).
217 Leonard *et al.* (1988).
218 Carrasco and Van de Kar (2003).
219 Baker and Herkenham (1995).
220 Rutkowski *et al.* (1999).
221 Lundberg *et al.* 1996.
222 Dauge and Lena (1998).
223 Bradwejn and Koszycki (1994, 2001).
224 Grafman *et al.* (1986); Starkstein *et al.* (1987, 1988); Mayberg (1994).
225 Drevets *et al.* (1997a); Ongur *et al.* (1998); Hirayasu *et al.* (1999).
226 Sheline *et al.* (1996); Shah *et al.* (1998); Bremner *et al.* (2000); Saxena *et al.* (2001).
227 Videbech and Ravnkilde (2004).
228 Young *et al.* (1991).
229 von Gunten *et al.* (2000).
230 Paradiso *et al.* (1997).
231 Rajkowska *et al.* (1999).
232 Maes *et al.* (1993a) assessed patients with various forms of recurrent depression and a comparison group using cerebral blood flow measured with single positron emission computed tomography (SPECT). They found no meaningful group differences for any brain region studied. They did find differences in frontal and parietal cortex in patients receiving benzodiazepines, suggesting that drug effects confounded earlier reports. Studies since then have focused on drug-free subjects.
233 Drevets (1998).

234 Drevets *et al.* (1992, 1995a, 1997b); Wu *et al.* (1992); Drevets (1999a).
235 Abercrombie *et al.* (1998).
236 Drevets *et al.* (1992). This is comparable to increases observed in laboratory animals during exposure to fear-conditioning stimuli (Le Doux *et al.*, 1983).
237 Drevets and Botteron (1997).
238 Ordway *et al.* (1991); Drevets (1999b); Brody *et al.* (2001b, c, 1999).
239 Gloor *et al.* (1982); Okun *et al.* (2003).
240 Drevets *et al.* (2002).
241 Price (1999).
242 Davis (1992); Veith *et al.* (1994).
243 Musselman and Nemeroff (1993).
244 Drevets (1999b). A recent study using magnetic resonance spectroscopy reports reduced glutamate in this region in children with depressive illness (Rosenberg *et al.* 2005).
245 Buchsbaum *et al.* (1997); Mayberg *et al.* (1999); Brody *et al.* (2001b, c).
246 Fink and Taylor (2003).
247 Murata *et al.* (2000).
248 Saxena *et al.* (2001).
249 Axelson *et al.* (1993).
250 Young *et al.* (1991).
251 Burt *et al.* (1995).
252 Cohen *et al.* (1992); Biver *et al.* (1994); Ring *et al.* (1994); Bremner *et al.* (1997); Brody *et al.* (2001a).
253 Farchione *et al.* (2002).
254 Dolan *et al.* (1992, 1993, 1994); Mayberg 1997; Galynker *et al.* (1998); See Brody *et al.* (2001b) for a detailed synthesis of this pattern.
255 Nobler *et al.* (1994); Bonne *et al.* (1996); Buchsbaum *et al.* (1997); Navarro *et al.* (2002, 2004).
256 Drevets *et al.* (1992, 1995a, 1999b); Biver *et al.* (1994); Rubin *et al.* (1994); Saxena *et al.* (2002).
257 Yathan *et al.* (2000); Nobler *et al.* (1994); Navarro *et al.* (2002, 2004); Michael *et al* (2003).
258 Rauch *et al.* (1994); Drevets *et al.* (1995b); Schneider *et al.* (1995).
259 Drevets (2000a, b).
260 Rubin *et al.* (1995).
261 Gloor (1969).
262 Gloor (1969). Hans Berger was born in 1873, and graduated in medicine from the University of Jena in 1893. After years on the faculty he was appointed chairman of the Department of Psychiatry, replacing Otto Binswanger in 1919, a position he retained until 1938. Berger undertook psychophysiologic studies in the psychiatrically ill, including patients with surgical skull defects. After finding electrical rhythms in these patients, he recorded brain waves through the intact skull. His first report in 1929 was followed by 12 successive reports that described the changes in brain waves with eye-opening, sleep, drugs (stimulants and depressants), age, epilepsy, and brain lesions. Berger's rhythms were widely acknowledged after Adrian and Matthews published a confirming report in 1934. During the Nazi era, Berger became melancholic and died by suicide at age 68 in 1941.
263 The EEG is a highly complex physiological signal that varies from moment to moment. It is sensitive to changes in vigilance (alertness), physiology (blood levels of glucose, oxygen, and carbon dioxide), and motor movement. Only the gross rhythms of seizures or

asymmetric differences between the hemispheres or localized lesions of the brain are identifiable by visual analysis. For quantitative analysis, the variations in electrical voltage are digitized, processed, and variations are calculated using complex mathematical algorithms. At one time the frequencies and amplitudes were measured by ruler. Then electronic frequency analyzers were introduced and these were useful during the Second World War in determining the severity of head injuries. The common analytic methods today are power spectral density analysis, period analysis, or amplitude analysis. Many programs for pattern analysis have been attempted but none is considered reliable. Sleep EEG records are usually recorded over 6–8 h of sleep. The records fluctuate with periods of REM, high-voltage slowing, and other patterns. Quantitative analysis has been attempted but the records must be hand-analyzed to remove artifact periods – those deemed by the observer to be secondary to motor movements. All in all, EEG analysis is highly complex and so sensitive to moment-to-moment changes in alertness, physiology, and motor movement that the data are of limited merit in clinical questions.

Technical modifications of the EEG, as in the averaged evoked potential, and more recently, magneto-EEG, suggest other opportunities for diagnostic studies. At present, none offers much optimism for an association with a psychiatric diagnosis and their characteristics have not been associated with depressive mood disorders.

264 Strauss *et al.* (1952); Hill and Parr (1963).

265 The same dysrhythmic patterns are recorded during an induced seizure, as in ECT or with chemicals, as pentylenetetrazol or flurothyl. In ECT the ictal EEG is now a measure of the efficacy of each seizure and remains integral to modern effective ECT. In a successful course of treatment, the EEG develops sustained measurable slowing of EEG frequencies, increased amplitudes, and the expression of seizure patterns. Failures to develop and sustain measurable EEG changes are signs of little physiologic effect of ECT and ineffective treatment trials. This interseizure EEG has limited clinical application (Fink, 1979).

266 In 56% of patients with well-defined epilepsy, single EEG recordings are abnormal. Repeated second and third samples increase the incidence of abnormal recordings by 26%, for an overall success rate of 82%. The yields vary with type of seizure disorder, age of the subject, time since a full seizure, medication, activation procedure (hyperventilation, photic stimulation, sleep), and with the use of 24-h video-EEG recording. Controlling for subjects with a history of head injury, medications, illicit substance abuse, and central nervous system infections, dysrhythmic EEG recordings are obtained in fewer than 2% of normal subjects (Kooi, 1971; Hill and Parr 1963; Scott, 1976).

267 For psychoactive medications the EEG offered a reliable and replicable classification of the clinical effects of the agents, predicted whether an agent would be clinically effective, suggested effective dosage ranges, and measured pharmacodynamic activity (Fink, 1969; Itil, 1974). When bolstered by digital computer methods to analyze EEG rhythms, quantitative pharmaco-EEG became highly successful in identifying and classifying putative central nervous system active agents. But the methods were never developed in relation to psychiatric diagnoses.

268 Davidson and Henriques (2000).

269 Pizzagalli *et al.* (2002).

270 Increased beta activity is interpreted as reflecting increased vigilance.

271 Chapotot *et al.* (1998).

272 Reid *et al.* (1998).

273 Knott and Lapierre (1987); Kwon *et al.* (1996); Bruder *et al.* (1997); Knott *et al.* (2001).

274 Knott *et al.* (2001).
275 Matousek (1991).
276 Nieber and Schlegel (1992).
277 Reid *et al.* (1998).
278 Pizzagalli *et al.* (2001).
279 Pizzagalli *et al.* (2002, 2004).
280 Henriques and Davidson (1991); Debener *et al.* (2000).
281 For a time in the 1980s, EEG frequency analyzer manufacturers offered programs for EEG diagnosis of psychiatric conditions. The analyses required age, gender, and duration of illness as part of the input data. The separation of psychotic and non-psychotic and mood disorder patients were based more on the age and duration of illness criteria than on EEG criteria. The programs are no longer offered.
282 Sackeim *et al.* (1982); Dawson (1994a); Davidson (1998).
283 Reid *et al.* (1998).
284 Knott *et al.* (2001).
285 Fink (1969).
286 Women have smaller overall absolute EEG power, but relatively higher-frequency alpha rhythms, larger absolute theta and relatively slower beta activity (Kaneda *et al.*, 1996; Martinovic *et al.*, 1998). Interhemispheric gender differences are reported (Corsi-Cabrera *et al.*, 1997b).
287 Miller *et al.* (2002a).
288 Reid *et al.* (1998).
289 Lieber and Newbury (1988).
290 Thompson (1985).
291 Chapotot *et al.* (1998).
292 Martinot *et al.* (1990); D'haenen *et al.* (1992); Bench *et al.* (1993); Drevets (2000b).
293 Martinot *et al.* (1990).
294 Fink and Kahn (1957).
295 Chapter 9.
296 Shagass (1954, 1957).
297 Itil (1974).
298 Shagass (1972, 1983).
299 Pfefferbaum *et al.* (1984); Gordon *et al.* (1986); Bruder *et al.* (1991); Schlegel *et al.* (1991); Vandoolaeghe *et al.* (1998); Imani *et al.* (1999).
300 Vandoolaeghe *et al.* (1998); Kalayam and Alexopoulos (1999).
301 The letters N and P before a number in evoked potential terminology indicate a negative and positive deflection, respectively, in the summed wave. The number that follows indicates the milliseconds from the stimulus. Thus, the P_{300} is the largest positive wave that occurs between 250 and 350 ms from the stimulus. Priming refers to the observation that the electrophysiologic response will be heightened if the subject is anticipating a stimulus to occur. Anticipation is elicited by presenting a stimulus that precedes the target stimulus or by "warming up" the system by engaging the subject in a task similar to the test task before the test task is presented.
302 Bruder *et al.* (1991); Schlegel *et al.* (1991).
303 Karaaslan *et al.* (2003).
304 Urcelay-Zaldua *et al.* (1995); Hansenne *et al.* (1996).
305 Karaaslan *et al.* (2003).

306 Fotiou *et al.* (2003).
307 Santosh *et al.* (1994); Karaaslan *et al.* (2003).
308 Karaaslan *et al.* (2003).
309 Kaustio *et al.* (2002).
310 Ford *et al.* (1994).
311 Jindal *et al.* (2002).
312 Szymanska *et al.* (2001).
313 Benca *et al.* (1992).
314 Benca *et al.* (1992); Nofzinger *et al.* (1999a).
315 Nofzinger *et al.* (1999b, 2000).
316 Antonijevic *et al.* (2003). Aging is not the only factor leading to sleep disturbances in depressed patients. Depressed adolescents with a unipolar course also have disturbed sleep with reduced REM latency, increased REM density, and more REM sleep time. Depressed adolescents who develop a manic-depressive course show more stage-1 sleep time and less deep sleep (Rao *et al.*, 2002).
317 Mathew *et al.* (2003).
318 Sleep analysis quantifies EEG rhythms and then identifies the principal frequencies during periods when REMs are recorded. Measures at other times are defined as NREM periods.
319 Nofzinger *et al.* (1999b).
320 Antonijevic *et al.* (2000a, b).
321 Liscombe *et al.* (2002).
322 Armitage *et al.* (2000b, c, d).
323 Antonijevic *et al.* (2000a, b, 2003).
324 Morehouse *et al.* (2002).
325 Birmaher *et al.* (1996a, b); Rao *et al.* (1996b).
326 The findings are interpreted as indicating increased "arousal" (Borbely *et al.*, 1984; Kupfer and Reynolds, 1992).
327 Coherence in quantitative EEG refers to the degree of correlation of EEG parameters within and among brain regions. In the sleep EEG literature assessing phases of sleep, the term is used to describe the degree of phase correlation between the left and right hemispheres.
328 Armitage *et al.* (1999).
329 Armitage *et al.* (2000c, d).
330 Fulton *et al.* (2000).
331 Morehouse *et al.* (2002).
332 Armitage *et al.* (2002).
333 Driver *et al.* (1996). Gender differences are also observed in evoked potentials, with women having shorter latencies and larger amplitudes than men (Kaneda *et al.*, 1996).
334 Giedke and Schwarzler (2002).
335 Giedke *et al.* (2003).
336 Voderholzer *et al.* (2003).
337 Clark *et al.* (2001).
338 Gillin *et al.* (2001); Smith *et al.* (2002b).
339 Baghai *et al.* (2003a, b).
340 Adrien (2002).
341 Berger *et al.* (2003).
342 Seifritz (2001).

343 Goodwin (1997).

344 Ilsley *et al.* (1995); Austin *et al.* (1999a, b). Other explanations have been offered to account for poor performance of depressed patients on cognitive tasks. One idea is that depression is a state of low hedonic capacity and that therefore depressed patients will not appropriately respond to reward. Doing well on one item does not motivate them to work harder on the next item, and performance declines. Another approach recognizes that depression is also a state of increased uncertainty and that depressed patients will therefore more likely hesitate to respond to a task, and performance on timed tests and multiple choice items will suffer (Henriques *et al.*, 1994). A third idea involves negative feedback. Here the depressed patient is hypothesized to be more likely to fail tasks that follow a failed task. The patient overresponds to negative feedback and failure escalates (Elliott *et al.*, 1997; Murphy *et al.*, 2003a). It is likely that all these state-dependent factors play some role in the cognitive performance of depressed patients.

345 Sheline *et al.* (1996).

346 Austin *et al.* (2001).

347 Beats *et al.* (1996); Austin *et al.* (1999a, b); Murphy *et al.* (1999).

348 Beats *et al.* (1996).

349 Channon (1996); Channon and Green (1999).

350 Austin *et al.* (1992, 1999a, b); Murphy *et al.* (1999, 2003a).

351 Moffoot *et al.* (1994).

352 Calev *et al.* (1986); Bazin *et al.* (1994).

353 Abas *et al.* (1990).

354 Abas *et al.* (1990); Beats *et al.* (1996); Paradiso *et al.* (1997).

355 Belanoff *et al.* (2001b).

356 Newcomer *et al.* (1994, 1999).

357 Sheline *et al.* (1999).

358 Kizilbash *et al.* (2002).

359 Chapter 7 on suicide.

360 Chapter 2.

361 Post and Weiss (1997); Ghaemi *et al.* (1999a).

362 Parker *et al.* (2000b); Chapter 5. Patients with recurrent melancholias are also more likely to respond to lithium enhancement and prophylaxis than are patients with other forms of depressive illness (Serretti *et al.*, 2000a).

363 Schmider *et al.* (1995); Rush *et al.* (1997); Rybakowski and Twardowska (1999); Matsunaga and Sarai (2000).

364 Linkowski *et al.* (1994); Cassidy *et al.* (1998); Cervantes *et al.* (2001).

365 Pepper and Krieger (1984); Halbreich *et al.* (1985); Cervantes *et al.* (2001).

366 Linkowski *et al.* (1981); Poirier *et al.* (1995); Rush *et al.* (1997); Matsunaga and Sarai (2000); Sassi *et al.* (2001).

367 Sobczak *et al.* (2002); McPherson *et al.* (2003); Sher *et al.* (2003).

368 The most consistent finding is mild lateral ventricular enlargement, particularly in older male patients. Less consistent abnormalities have been observed in the basal ganglia, thalamus, hippocampus, and amygdala. Functional MRI also suggests abnormality in the basal ganglia, and gray matter, and the hippocampus and anterior cingulate (Cecil *et al.*, 2002; Bertolino *et al.*, 2003). Studies of glucose metabolism indicate frontal cortex hypometabolism (Strakowski *et al.*, 2000a). Increased anterior cingulate and caudate cerebral blood flow are also reported (Blumberg *et al.*, 2000).

369 Blumberg *et al.* (2003a, b).
370 Heilman (1997); Pettigrew and Miller (1998); Taylor (1999); Harmon-Jones *et al.* (2002); Hirshfeld-Becker *et al.* (2003); The application of transcranial magnetic stimulation (TMS) to the left frontal regions of the head to treat depression is based in part on these formulations (Garcia-Toro *et al.*, 2001). Chapter 13 reviews the efficacy of TMS in psychiatric illness.
371 Pettigrew and Miller (1998).
372 Akiskal *et al.* (1995).
373 Bottlender *et al.* (2000).
374 McGuffin *et al.* (2003).
375 Mitchell and Malhi (2004).
376 Jones and Craddock (2001b); Jones *et al.* (2002a).
377 Bertelsen *et al.* (1977); McGuffin *et al.* (2003).
378 McGuffin *et al.* (2003).
379 Chapters 2, 4 and 8–11.
380 Kendler *et al.* (1995).
381 Kendler *et al.* (2001b).

15

Future directions

The madness of depression is . . . a storm of muck. Soon evident are the slowed-down responses, near paralysis, psychic energy throttled back close to zero. Ultimately, the body is affected and feels sapped, drained[1]

Melancholia, a severe disturbance of mood, movement, and thought, has been recognized for millennia. It is a brain disease with abnormalities in neurochemical, neurohormonal, metabolic, and electrophysiologic processes.

The syndrome is considered moderately heritable. Under circumstances of stress at critical phases of development, the genetic predisposition is expressed, and the mood disorder develops. A prominent feature of melancholia is an "abnormal stress response state." Recognizing melancholia is a clinical judgment that combines a signature psychopathology with identifiable hormonal and neurophysiologic perturbations.

Melancholia is well defined in the literature of medicine. Its characteristic psychopathology and laboratory testing are established in evidence, if not yet by consensus. Guidelines for the examination of melancholic patients and the differential diagnosis of depressive syndromes derive from the clinical experience and investigations of many authors. Suicide is a special risk for sufferers of melancholia, and prevention strategies are established.

Two effective treatment modalities for melancholic patients have been developed. Convulsive therapy is the oldest and the most effective intervention; guidelines for its effective application are well known. Medications are also delineated from the evidence, but the therapeutics has been distorted by the pharmaceutical industry. An objective consensus is needed. The efficacy of psychotherapies and other proposed treatment interventions has yet to be substantiated.

Modern neuroscience is heavily invested in the technologies of neurochemistry, neuroendocrinology, electrophysiology, brain imaging, and genetics. Much effort has been expended in studying the mood disorders and animal models of depression. These studies are exciting, but are limited by their adherence to the prevailing classifications of mood disorders and thus do not recognize sample heterogeneity. A synthesis of this literature provides some clarification, but much work remains.

Changing the DSM classification of depression

The present American Psychiatric Association classification of psychiatric disorders as codified in the *Diagnostic and Statistical Manual* (DSM) identifies many depressive mood disorders in several different sections of the taxonomy. The rationale is poor and this scattering is confusing. Melancholia warrants a separate category from other depressive syndromes – a home of its own. Uniting identifiable depressive mood disorders into the classification and into clinical practice will facilitate differential diagnosis.

The so-called "minor" depressive syndromes (e.g., adjustment disorder, brief depressive episode) are harbingers of future severe mood disorders. They are most probably early or mild phases of a recurrent depressive illness. These diagnoses carry increased suicide risks and require treatment. Rather than identifying them by an arbitrarily designated lesser number and severity of symptoms, they should be defined by the pattern of clinical features and classified as either "melancholic" or "non-melancholic."

The validity of a separate syndrome of dysthymia is in doubt. Patients with long-standing depressive mood disorders of moderate or mild severity do not qualify as having a distinct disease. Outcome is variable, as are treatment needs. The term should be eliminated or limited to a modifier of the course of illness.

Psychotic depression is best understood as a severe form of melancholia. It is a lethal disorder for which effective treatments have been discerned but poorly applied.

The separation of mood disorders by the expression of mania or hypomania is inconsistent with the experience of more than a century and a half of clinical psychopathology. Mania is recognized in 10% of severely depressed patients and hypomania and mania-like features are reported in over half of depressed patients. The bipolar–unipolar dichotomy is better eliminated. Organizing mood disorders by the presence or absence of melancholia fits the evidence and what has historically been recognized as manic-depressive illness is best included within melancholic illness.

Abnormal bereavement and puerperal depressions are melancholic depressions following specific events. The evidence for their distinction from melancholia is weak. To separate them from melancholia minimizes their lethality and encourages less effective treatments. Eliminating the categories of puerperal depression and abnormal bereavement would distinguish them from their non-illness counterparts of postpartum blues and grieving. Recognition that they are episodes of melancholia encourages effective treatment.

Several practical and heuristic reasons justify changing the classification of depressive syndromes.[2] The official recognition of "minor" depressive experiences as variants of depressive illness that can be melancholic will influence the choice of long-term treatments to prevent recurrence. Recognizing those minor depressions linked to melancholia would encourage more specific and effective treatment for these patients. Because prolonged episodes lead to more episodes, the early effective treatment of such depressions should reduce the number of episodes and their resistance to treatment. Suicide is the third leading cause of death among teenagers and "minor" depressions are particularly common in this age group. Recognizing that many minor depressions are early forms of melancholia would discourage the minimization of suicide risk in these episodes.

Genetic studies of clinical syndromes as complex as the mood disorders are challenged by the uncertainty in the recognition of the phenotype. What conditions should be counted as illness in pedigrees? Which mood disorders are likely to have a common genetic root? Recognizing melancholia as a single phenotypic syndrome increases the likelihood that a genotype will be identified.

The availability of effective treatments for melancholia – medications with a broad pharmacodynamic spectrum and electroconculsive therapy – encourages the recognition of the disorder and offers specific treatment algorithms, in the same manner as is now applied to manic-depressive illness. An analogy is the staging of cancers to choose the most effective treatments. Staging is critical in treatment choice, even though the different stages of the cancer still represent the same cell line. The responsiveness of melancholia to proper treatment and its lethality if less than optimal treatments are applied warrant similar consideration.

Changing the DSM diagnostic criteria for melancholia

The diagnostic criteria for mood disorders are cross-sectional and limited to a list of over-simplified features. There is no weighting of signs and symptoms. Persons who feel saddened by life events or who are disgruntled as an exaggeration of their personality traits meet the criteria for major depression if these moods are associated with decreased energy or interest. Their inclusion into a major depression category confounds the results of clinical treatment trials and laboratory searches for an understanding of mood disorders. The large numbers of placebo responders in treatment trials are testimony to the need for a higher threshold for identifying depressed persons that warrant somatic treatment. *Psychomotor disturbance* (agitation or bradykinesia), *vegetative signs* (two or more), *quality of mood* (unremitting apprehension and sadness), and *psychosis* best identify the single syndrome of melancholia. The present psychiatric classification does not require these features in the diagnosis of a depressive illness. All depressive mood disorders are viewed as expressions of the same pathophysiology. The present criteria permit the diagnosis in the absence of a depressed mood *if* anhedonia is present. Such poor criteria lead to false-positive diagnoses, confusing apathetic and other syndromes with depressive mood disorder.

Neuroendocrine tests and sleep electroencephatogram measures are indices of melancholia. Although developed heuristically and without a central theory, they are useful in assuring the melancholia diagnosis.

Regardless of the ultimate understanding of the independence of melancholia, giving it a separate category will increase its recognition and encourage the use of the most appropriate treatments. Table 15.1 offers a simplified classification.

The evidence for a single syndrome of melancholia and the conditions from which it needs to be differentiated are described in the earlier chapters. Table 15.2

Table 15.1. Proposed changes in the classification of mood disorder

Melancholia	Non-melancholic mood disorder
Psychotic depression	Characterological and other non-melancholic depressions
Manic-depression	
Puerperal depression	
Abnormal bereavement	

Table 15.2. Proposed diagnostic criteria for melancholia (all must be present)

1. An episode of illness with reduced functioning that compromises normal daily activities that persists for at least 2 weeks, and is characterized by an unremitting mood of apprehension and gloom
2. Psychomotor disturbance such as agitation, retardation, or both
3. Vegetative signs (at least 2)
4. At least one of the following:

(a) Abnormal DST and CRH tests* or high nighttime cortisol levels

(b) Decreased REM latency or other sleep abnormalities

*Chapter 4 offers the rationale for adding these laboratory tests as diagnostic criteria for melancholia.

offers proposed diagnostic criteria for melancholia. They have face validity for high specificity, making false-positive diagnoses unlikely.

Changing the standards of pharmacotherapy research

To improve remission rates with our available interventions and to encourage the development of better treatments, the standards in treatment research need to be changed.

Remission is the gold standard

The goal of the treatment of melancholia must be remission, not merely "better than placebo" or an arbitrary reduction in scores on depression-rating scales. Assessing an intervention as "effective" because it elicits a 50% reduction in a rating-scale score leaves many patients symptomatic. Such patients are likely to relapse, to make suicide attempts, and to develop a chronic course of illness. In a French survey of over 1700 depressed patients who received antidepressant drug treatment for 8–12 weeks, 20% achieved Hamilton Rating Scale scores of 18 or greater and 47% had scores between 8 and 18. Fully two-thirds of patients remained depressed, although only the 20% with scores above 18 were considered "non-responders" because they had experienced a drop in scores of 50% or more. Half or more of the patients remained substantially ill with depressed mood, psychic anxiety, loss of interest, and time away from work.[3] In a 2-year follow-up in a Spanish study, 15% of depressed patients who had achieved remission and 67% of those with a partial response to the index episode relapsed.[4]

When measured by the yardstick of remission, the common belief that all antidepressant treatments are of about equal efficacy is clearly untrue. For melancholia, ECT has the best efficacy. Tricyclic antidepressant drugs achieve better remission rates than do the selective serotonin reuptake inhibitors. Drugs with both serotonergic and noradrenergic-enhancing properties elicit better efficacy than do pure SSRIs. A recent analysis of depressive illness and its treatments in 14 world regions concluded that using the older agents was the most cost-effective strategy.[5]

Publication "noise" needs to be reduced

The publication of multiple small samples and open treatment trials is best discouraged. If two or more uncontrolled clinical treatment trials find a treatment to be safe and to benefit depressed patients, randomized, large-sample placebo-controlled studies are necessary as the standard for publication.

For example, a Medline search of citations to "bupropion" between 1977 and 2004 identifies 1320 citations. "Double-blind efficacy trials" yields 29 citations. Sixteen are review articles or concerned with smoking cessation. Thirteen studies, many with small samples, directly address the merits of bupropion in treating depressed patients. Other key word entries identify a handful of additional reports.[6] The few pertinent studies, however, are inconsistent in their report that bupropion is the least likely of antidepressant agents to induce mania, a feature that is the basis for the recommendation for its use. The reviews, small clinical trials, and anecdotal reports masked the weak evidence to assert that bupropion is an effective treatment for manic-depressive illness.[7]

Industry influence needs to be limited

Treatment trials sponsored and managed by the manufacturer and conducted under the imprimatur of academic faculty members receiving personal consultant fees are tainted. At best, the findings may be considered preliminary. They should not be considered definitive and not accepted in the rationale for a treatment's marketing or recommendation in algorithm guidelines. Journal editors and writers of review articles need to be particularly cautious in citing the data of such studies as evidentiary.

Sadly, the influence of industry goes beyond increased prescribing. US authorities favor SSRIs in treatment guidelines while European reviewers conclude that TCAs have advantages for the more severely affected. UK authorities view SSRIs as agents with increased suicide risk in children and adolescents and limit their use in those age groups, while US authorities offer warnings in package insert descriptions. Firewalls between industry and academia are needed. A pharmaceutical firm consultant helping to develop a new medication should not be the same person that reports its efficacy. The conflict of interest is patent.[8]

Changing treatment guidelines: endless drug trials elicit chronicity

The longer a depressive illness persists, the more likely the patient will have recurrences, respond poorly to treatments, and become chronically dysfunctional. Multiple drug treatment trials with multiple-medication combinations and augmentations are codified in expert treatment algorithms, but these recommendations are of questionable efficacy. Newer agents, often from the manufacturer sponsoring many of the panel members, are invariably recommended over older antidepressants. ECT is reserved as "the last resort" treatment, despite the evidence that for some situations it is the treatment of choice and the first-line treatment. The multiple-medication trial strategy, each of 4–6 weeks to ascertain efficacy or failure, requires months and sometimes years of inadequate treatments, leaving many patients with residual symptoms. Such patients are most likely to relapse. The practice that accepts *improvement* and not *remission* and tolerates multiple-medication trials increases chronicity of illness.[9]

Treatment guidelines need to reflect efficacy data. For melancholic patients who can be treated as outpatients, no more than two acute medication trials, at least the second with augmentation, is reasonable on medical, social, and economic grounds.[10] If remission is not achieved, ECT should be offered. For hospitalized melancholic patients, ECT is the treatment of choice. When antidepressant drugs are used, however, the choice should be for agents with the broadest pharmacodynamic spectrum, preferably TCAs.

Improving the education of medical practitioners in mood disorders

Medical student teaching of psychiatric illnesses fails to insure the early recognition and treatment of patients with mood disorders, and the adequate teaching of suicide prevention. A population analysis by the World Health Organization in 14 world regions concluded that better recognition and treatment could reduce the world's burden of depression by 10–30%.[11]

The accreditation requirements for residency training programs in primary care specialties and in internal medicine in the diagnosis and treatment of depressed patients or in suicide assessment are inadequate. As a consequence, competence in prescribing treatment and preventing suicide is widely recognized as inadequate.

Considering that ECT is the effective treatment for melancholia, the lack of training in ECT in psychiatry residency programs makes it likely that graduates are poorly able to identify patients for whom ECT is warranted. Only 10% of US psychiatrists referred patients for or administered ECT in 1988.[12] A survey of ECT practice in the metropolitan New York region found many psychiatric services to be without ECT, or to administer treatments that did not meet present standards of adequacy, or to adequately offer adequate continuation treatments.[13]

Inadequate training in ECT in psychiatric residency programs is ensured by the training guidelines offered by the Accreditation Council of Graduate Medical Education (ACGME) residency review committee. Programs are required to demonstrate that trainees are competent in specific diagnostic and treatment procedures. Each facility *must* provide experiences in various forms of psychotherapy, including long-term weekly psychodynamic supervision and specific training in cognitive and behavior therapy. Experience in psychological testing and interpretation *is required*. For ECT the standard reads: "Electroconvulsive therapy, a somatic therapy that is viewed as so important that its absence must be justified (examples of other somatic therapies include biofeedback and phototherapy)." The loophole of *justified absence*, not allowed in other aspects of psychiatric training, is commonly exercised; we know of no psychiatry residency program that has been criticized for not providing ECT training. Many do not. Lumping ECT with the marginal interventions of phototherapy and biofeedback further diminishes its perceived value.

Neither questions about ECT nor a record of experience in ECT is required for specialist certification in psychiatry, nor in the subspecialty of geriatric psychiatry.

To assure accreditation from the ACGME, training programs should be required to offer candidates hands-on experience with ECT, to demonstrate competency in evaluating patients for ECT, and competency in its administration. Tertiary care psychiatric facilities should require direct experience with ECT as part of their facility's accreditation requirements. Not to do so makes it unlikely that melancholic patients will have the maximum opportunity for effective and safe treatment.[14]

The failure to assure such competency forces physicians to obtain training electively in continuing medical education (CME) programs. Certification in attendance is offered for half-day and 1-day lecture courses and for a limited number of 5-day full-time fellowships. Only the latter offer hands-on experience that is essential for competency in this surgical-type intervention.[15]

Given the efficacy of ECT, its widespread unavailability is unacceptable.[16] In one survey of ECT practice covering over 300 US metropolitan regions, ECT was not available in 115 areas. In the remaining regions its variability of use was greater than that of most other medical procedures. In some regions its use was minimal.[17] Psychiatrists administering ECT in the USA are also more likely to be male, trained outside the USA, to be older, also to use pharmacotherapy, and to be in private practice near an academic center.[18] ECT practitioners are more likely to have been trained a decade or more ago, suggesting that ECT will likely be even less available than it is today. For most patients who receive ECT in the USA, the diagnoses and indications are within practice guidelines; where available, ECT, is not overused or misused.[19] The actual practice of ECT, however, is faulty, with many centers failing to meet minimal practice guidelines.[20] Because ECT practitioners also tend to be trained outside the USA it seems clear that US training programs are not meeting the need.

Studies of the mechanism of convulsive therapy

One of the most remarkable findings of twentieth-century medicine is that induced grand mal seizures have clinical merit. Equally remarkable is the safety of such inductions. In the 70 years since the introduction of ECT, its efficacy in reversing disorders of human mood, motor behavior, and thought has been well documented. ECT is an effective treatment for melancholia, catatonia, psychotic depression, and acute forms of schizophrenia.[21] Its superiority over medications in the treatment of patients with severe mood disorders has been repeatedly demonstrated.[22]

Its mechanism of action is well studied but no understanding is widely accepted. Psychological and memory-related theories that dominated thinking in the 1940s and 1950s are disproved. Neurophysiologic hypotheses formulated a relationship between EEG abnormalities and changes in seizure threshold. While highly correlated with outcome and useful as predictors of behavior change, the EEG changes induced with ECT are not explanatory because the intervening mechanisms between ECT-induced physiologic measures and clinical changes are obscure.

Changes in brain neurohumors, the chemical mediators of transmission, are the most common explanation offered for the action of psychoactive drugs. When these mechanisms are studied in ECT, no effective correlations or relationships can be discerned.[23]

A neuroendocrine hypothesis has been offered to explain the therapeutic effect of ECT. First enunciated in the 1940s with reports of the role of steroids in behavior, it received its principal impetus from descriptions of the neuroendocrine abnormalities in patients with severe mood disorders and observations that the seriously compromised cortisol physiology in such patients is rapidly and effectively relieved by ECT.[24]

Autonomic functions of feeding, sleep, vigilance, and sex are abnormal in melancholia. These functions are modulated by the endocrines produced by the hypothalamus and pituitary. Hormones are distributed to all body tissues (not limited to the interstitial spaces of brain cells) and their effects are measured in hours (not in milliseconds). The effects are systemic, not localized. During seizures the hypothalamus and pituitary release large boluses of their products. With repeated seizures, their functions are normalized. The return of neuroendocrine abnormality heralds a clinical relapse.

The neuroendocrine hypothesis is consistent with observations of the greater efficacy of bilateral over unilateral electrode placements and the need for "effective" seizures. It focuses our interest on the role of the brain's neuroendocrine products in psychiatric illnesses and their relief.

The neurohumoral theory dominated the development of psychoactive medications. As the endocrine and neuroendocrine mechanisms that control body physiology are elaborated, each compound is examined for its utility as an intervention for systemic relief of a disorder. Insulin, thyroid, cortisone, estrogens, androgens, progesterone, as well as their antagonists, have been tested.[25] But these studies have been hampered by the same problems that limit pharmacotherapy research (e.g., sample heterogeneity, small trials without adequate comparison groups). As an example, glucocorticoid receptor antagonists, in the form of mifepristone, are undergoing clinical trials in patients with psychotic depression.[26] Many motivations for this study have been suggested, including the neuroendocrine hypothesis of ECT, and the goal of these studies has been voiced as finding "ECT in a bottle" for patients with psychotic depression.[27] Reductions in psychosis (Brief Psychotic Rating Scale measures) and lesser reductions in mood disorder (HAMD measures) are reported with short-term treatment. Present data do not support their use as first-line monotherapy treatments.[28]

Assessing mood-disordered patients who meet criteria for melancholia will offer more homogeneous samples. Assessing the patients before and after a course of successful ECT will describe the processes that are altered by induced seizures and that change with recovery. Assessing hormone responses immediately after treatments offers information as to the direct effect of seizures. These studies have been done sporadically. Greater attention to the hormonal changes associated with ECT offers an opportunity for the development of new psychoactive treatments.

In patients who exhibit cortisol suppression before ECT, some exhibit cortisol nonsuppression at the end of a treatment course when the patients are assessed as improved. This finding and the changes in metabolism of dexamethasone are unexplained and warrant greater attention.

Optimal ECT efficacy is associated with a sustained seizure that ends in electrical silence. ECT has been likened to cardioversion, i.e., the shutting-down of an organ in a dysrhythmic state so that it can naturally "reboot."[29] For ECT, this process has been attributed in part to the treatment's antiseizure properties, and the electrical quiet after a treatment is thought to reflect the activation of the brain's antiseizure mechanisms. What ECT does to achieve this, and what this mechanism then does to relieve melancholia, have not been studied.

Preventive approaches to reduce the burden of melancholia

Early prevention

Prevention is much preferred to treating a developed syndrome. Factors that increase the risk for a first episode of melancholia are listed in Table 15.3.

Studying children at risk for depressive illness

The study of children at high risk for schizophrenia has increased our understanding of psychosis.[30] The examination of offspring of psychotic mothers from early childhood or from birth through young adult life is the focus of more than 40 studies. Differences in gestational and neonatal experience and in childhood neuromotor, emotional, and cognitive functioning are identified in children who subsequently develop psychoses. This strategy has recently been applied to the study of mood disorders. A retrospective study of over 700 persons found that childhood conduct problems were accompanied by depressive mood disorders.[31] The types of depressive illness were not identified. Another study of more than 3000 persons born in Finland between 1945 and 1965 who were separated at birth from mothers ill with

Table 15.3. Risk factors and predictors of the first depressive episode

Risk Factors
Family history of mood disorder[a]
Maternal depression during pregnancy and postpartum[b]
Severe and chronic stress in childhood and young adulthood[c]
Regular use of marijuana[d]
Predictors
Abnormal personality traits[e]
Anxiety attacks in childhood and adolescence[f]
Childhood and adolescent sleep EEG abnormalities[g]
Abnormal steroid levels[h]

[a] Kendler *et al.* (1997; 2001b).
[b] Parker *et al.* (1995c).
[c] Kendler *et al.* (1999, 2001a).
[d] Chen *et al.* (2002).
[e] Kendler *et al.* (1991a, 1993b). Childhood depressions adversely influence personality development, suggesting that aggressive treatment has preventive benefits (Ramklint and Ekselius, 2003).
[f] Tokuyama *et al.* (2003).
[g] Fulton *et al.* (2000); Goetz *et al.* (2001); Morehouse *et al.* (2002).
[h] Goodyer *et al.* (2000, 2003).

tuberculosis found no linkage between separation and the onset of a depressive illness.[32] A prospective 6-year follow-up of children divided into high familial and low familial risk based on the presence or absence of ill first-degree relatives found that the former was associated with childhood behavior problems and later depression.[33] A study of 13-year-old children who had been exposed to postnatal maternal depressive illness reported that the children had more variable morning serum cortisol levels than a comparison group.[34] Increased white-matter hyperintensities in children and adolescent inpatients with recurrent depressive illness and a history of a suicide attempt are also reported.[35] These findings suggest that children at high risk for mood disorder express their vulnerability early and may be more mutable to prevention strategies.[36]

Women in their child-bearing years who have recurrent depressive illness or a family history of mood disorder, along with their families, warrant investigation as they convey risk factors to their offspring. Preventing maternal illness and reducing exposure to severe stresses in childhood address the two identified principal risk factors for mood disorder in children. We lack effective prevention strategies. A study of pregnant women without a history of psychiatric illness who were thought to be at risk for postpartum depression reported some protection with counseling and cognitive-behavior therapy.[37] Bright-light therapy is said to achieve some benefit.[38]

Prophylactic medication treatment in women without a history of depressive illness, however, did not affect rates of depression during pregnancy or in the postpartum period.[39]

Sleep and prevention of depressive illness

Sleep is a novel area of interest in primary prevention of recurrent depressive illness. Sleep efficiency is compromised, rapid eye movement (REM) latency is shortened, and ultradian rhythms are perturbed in depressed persons, particularly melancholic patients.[40] Ultradian rhythm disturbances are observed during wakefulness as well as in sleep and contribute to more chronic behavioral and cognitive dysfunction for some patients even when no longer depressed.[41]

Although sleep disturbances in patients with mood disorders are state-related and resolve with clinical improvement, some aspects of ultradian and circadian rhythms may be biological markers for the illness.[42] In laboratory animals, neonatal suppression of REM sleep by pharmacologic agents (e.g., clomipramine)[43] or by being kept awake for prolonged periods is associated with adult "depressive-like" behavior, including reduced sexual activity, less motor activity, and increased aggression. Similar behaviors are reported in children and teens at high risk for depression.[44] The hypothesis from this work is that children with disturbed sleep architecture are at greater risk for mood disorders and that correcting or preventing sleep disturbances will reduce their risk for mood disturbances.

Several mutable environmental sources of sleep disturbances suggest prevention strategies. The first addresses the relationship between maternal depressive illness with abnormalities in infant arousal and sleep–wake cycles. The early identification of maternal illness and its immediate effective treatment to remission would minimize infant circadian and ultradian abnormalities.

A second strategy focuses on maximizing normal development of sleep–wake states. Studies in laboratory animals, including primates, identify the suprachiasmatic nucleus (SCN) in the anterior hypothalamus as the primary "biological clock" controlling periodic activity, cardiovascular functioning, glucose production, and cortisol release.[45] Through special cells in the retina and via the retinohypothalamic tract, light and darkness influence the modulation of melatonin release by the SCN.[46] Much of the neuroendocrine and autonomic nervous system effects of SCN activity are through its modulation of the paraventricular nucleus of the hypothalamus.[47] An involvement of the SCN in the pathophysiology of abnormal stress responses in depressive mood disorder has been proposed.[48]

During gestation, the developing fetus relies on maternal control of its circadian cycles.[49] At birth, humans do not exhibit circadian rhythms and the sleep–wake cycle and other circadian rhythms are shaped during the first 12 weeks after birth.[50] Depressed mood during pregnancy alters circadian rhythms and accounts for some of the adverse effects observed in the offspring of these women.

Normal sleep is essential for synaptic formation and remodeling in brain development.[51] An important influence in the development of normal sleep is infant self-soothing behavior – the ability to regulate the state of arousal – self-calming from crying to quiet wakefulness without parental assistance, settling to sleep at the beginning of the night, and going back to sleep upon awakening during the night.[52] Parental behavior affects infant self-soothing. Maternal psychiatric illness[53] and abnormal mother–infant attachment[54] disturb infant sleep and reduce the ability to self-soothe. Sleep deprivation has persistent behavioral effects.[55] Good neonatal sleep practice is a strategy to reduce risk for psychiatric illness.

Exposure to selective serotonin-enhancing drugs, but not drugs that primarily affect norepinephrine, adversely affects sleep architecture.[56] Because GABA mediates SCN function, GABAergic agents that improve mood are less disruptive to circadian systems.[57] Infants at greatest risk are the offspring of actively depressed women receiving SSRI antidepressants. Such families need to be educated in how to optimize the sleep environment of their infants. The practice of maintaining bright light in neonatal nurseries and intensive care units should be questioned, particularly in newborns with a family history of mood disorder.[58]

Chronic alcohol use adversely affects the functions of SCN and the paraventricular nucleus of the hypothalamus, interfering with circadian rhythms and the stress response.[59] Persons at risk for recurrent depressive illness and comorbidity for alcohol abuse will fare best by not using alcohol.

Early identification and aggressive treatment of puerperal mood disorder

Preventing maternal mood disorder and immediately and rapidly treating any emerging psychiatric symptoms during pregnancy and after delivery addresses the most obvious and the most critical non-genetic risk factors affecting the fetus and newborn. Rapidly and effectively treating parental symptoms reduces family turmoil and improves parenting skills.

Child abuse and neglect need to be identified early and stopped. Parental loss is not as great a risk factor for mood disorders in the child as is parental abuse. Removing the abusing parent or the victimized child from the home is less of a risk factor than permitting abuse to continue through omission or inadequate efforts.

Early recognition and aggressive treatment of first episode of mood disorder

Once an episode of depressive illness develops, early diagnosis and aggressive treatment are required. The earlier the age of onset of the first symptoms and the longer they linger, the more likely it is that the sufferer will have repeated episodes. From 4 to 5% of children under age 10 meet criteria for depressive illness.[60] One-third to one-half of such children experience recurrent mood disorders.[61] Anxiety disorder in a young child is associated with developing mood disorder and with both nicotine use and illicit substance abuse.[62] Half of young adolescents with depressive symptoms develop recurrent depressive illness.[63] Childhood and adolescent depressed moods occur frequently and predict future recurrent depressive illness.[64] Childhood depressive illness carries a substantial risk for suicide.[65] When properly treated, most young persons recover from their first episode of depressive illness.[66]

In present practice, even moderate to severe depressive mood disorders in adolescence are interpreted as psychosocial reactions, despite the evidence that more often the symptoms are early expressions of recurrent biological dysfunction. The first episodes are likely to be associated with a precipitating stress event.[67] Long-term or recent stressful life events are not associated with persistent depressive illness. Poor treatment, however, is associated with persistent illness.[68] Although women are at greater risk for a first episode of a depressed mood disorder, there are no gender differences in the treatment response or subsequent course when adequately treated.[69]

Depressive episodes are also often associated with anxiety which, with a predepression history of anxiety, engenders diagnostic ambiguity. A recent assessment study and treatment trial of anxious depressed patients reported that effective treatment for the depressed mood rather than the anxiety symptoms yielded the best opportunity for a good outcome. Patients had better outcomes with imipramine than with fluvoxamine prescription.[70]

Adult patients in a first episode of melancholia show brain dysfunction in amygdala bilaterally and in the left hippocampus on functional brain imaging.[71] An increased amygdala volume contrasts with the reduced volume seen in patients with recurrent episodes. Reduced hippocampal volume is a sign of a neurotoxic process with early onset in severe depressive illness. If these findings are confirmed, they support the need for early identification and vigorous treatment to remission of first depressive episodes. Depressed patients most likely to be diagnosed and treated tend to be older and married, more severely ill, and melancholic.[72]

Prevention of chronicity

Melancholic patients in remission have a high probability of relapse unless vigorous continuation management is applied. The structural and functional brain changes occur at increasingly shorter intervals during the few years after the first episode. Rapid remission and vigorous prevention of relapse after the first episode are key to tertiary prevention.[73]

Environmental factors influence risk of relapse. A home or treatment setting in which persons relate to the patient with high *expressed emotion* (interactions characterized by criticism, intrusion, and high verbal output) increases relapse rates. Efforts at understanding this process and correcting it have focused on schizophrenia, but the effects of expressed emotion apply equally to patients with mood disorders.[74] The expressed emotion triggers of abnormal stress in melancholia have not been studied. Nevertheless, interventions to reduce the expressed emotion in the environment of depressed patients need to be done following the same standards proposed for other treatments.

Compliance with medical prescription also affects relapse, yet systematic and demonstrably efficacious strategies to improve compliance are not routine components of treatment planning. Even a program of low-cost educational four telephone calls and five mailings to depressed patients during the continuation phase of treatment substantially increased compliance rates.[75] Table 15.4 summarizes prevention strategies.

Table 15.4. Prevention strategies

Early prevention
Rapid treatment of puerperal depressions
Good prenatal care and maternal nutrition
Good newborn sleep hygiene
Identifying and correcting abusive childhood households
Treating children with sleep disorders
Minimizing drug and alcohol use in children and adolescents at high risk for depression
Early identification and treatment to rapid remission of first depression
Prevention of chronicity
Continuation of medical management to prevent relapse
Maximizing compliance
Identifying and reducing major stressors
Identifying and reducing expressed emotion among families at risk
Early detection of relapse and vigorous treatment back to remission

Pharmacogenetics

This science seeks to identify gene variants that affect drug metabolism to minimize individual variability in response and side-effects. The goal is individualized treatment with improved outcome.[76] The method is to modify genes affecting the pharmacokinetics and dynamics of medications. The search is for multiple small genes with additive effects (polygenic) interacting at multiple sites (epistasis) that are modified by environmental influences.[77]

The metabolism of drugs by the liver is a topic of interest. A variation in the CYP2D6 gene alters antidepressant drug metabolism and is accompanied by higher plasma levels and more clinical effects.[78] Persons with two functional CYP2D6 alleles experience fewer pronounced TCA side-effects than those with only one.[79] Genes affecting the numbers and affinity of 5-HT2A receptors alter susceptibility to the physiological effects on sleep and circadian rhythm, and sexual and gastrointestinal functions of SSRI.[80] The goal of the studies is to match the patient's genetic susceptibilities (through gene identification or through its expression) to minimize the risk of side-effects.

Some genetic pedigree studies suggest a familial disposition to respond to a particular class of antidepressant agent.[81] Some investigations focus on transporter reuptake molecules and how they alter response to treatment.[82] One variant of the serotonin transporter molecule (SERT) is associated with a poor response to acute antidepressant medication treatment.[83] This SERT "short variant" is associated with an initial medication response that is not maintained despite continued treatment.[84]

Although the SERT variant and the 5-HT2A polymorphism influence treatment response, they are not considered influences on the expression of mood.[85] The

5-HT2A receptor gene, however, is associated with increased risk for suicide.[86] Of 12 published studies since 1998, the most consistent finding is an association between the serotonin transporter long genotype and better response to SSRI drugs.[87]

A gene for tryptophan hydroxylase, the rate-limiting enzyme of serotonin synthesis, is another candidate gene related to the response to SSRIs.[88] Polymorphisms of genes coding for MAO-A, G-protein, and serotonin receptors have also been identified.[89]

Transcription factors are also considered.[90] Cytoplasmic transcription factors link signals initiated at the cell surface with gene expression within the cell nucleus. This process permits the cell to change genetic coding in response to physiologic and environmental cues. Some abnormalities in this signal transduction pathway have been reported in melancholia. Fibroblasts from melancholic patients show a blunted protein kinase A (PKA) response to β-adrenoceptor agonists and to second messenger cyclic adenosine monophosphate cAMP.[91] PKA response is a critical step in the transduction pathway and its reduced response decreases the nuclear protein phosphorylated cAMP response element-binding (pCREB) protein essential in the energy functioning of the cell.[92] This finding is similar to that reported in postmortem brain tissues of persons with mood disorder and of suicide victims with a history of depression.[93] The glucocorticoid receptor (GR) transcription factor is also dysfunctional in depression.[94] Both CREB and GR abnormal functioning make cells less resistant to stress.[95]

All effective antidepressant treatments, including ECT, activate transcription cascades and this effect is offered as the final common pathway for their action.[96] CREB and GR are specifically targeted. The expression of genes for tyrosine hydroxylase, beta_1-adrenoreceptors, and corticotropin-releasing factor are down-regulated by long-term exposure to antidepressant drugs.[97] The effect counters the noradrenergic hyperactivity observed in melancholia.[98] The same observations have been offered as explanations for the therapeutic superiority of noradrenergic antidepressants like TCAs and venlafaxine over specific SSRIs.[99] Many other transcription factor cascades are affected by antidepressant drugs. How and to what degree these cascades affect treatment await study.[100]

The pathophysiology of melancholia

Depressive illness is lifelong. Vulnerabilities for mood disorder are present at birth and accrue over the first decades of life. Each episode increases the likelihood of future episodes. Investigators usually recruit patients during an episode of dysfunction and measure some putative biologic target of interest. Much has been learned by this approach, but it is artificial and limited. It does not adequately consider the multiple converging forces that lead to the illness. When a person is in an episode of behavioral dysfunction and has the biological derangements listed in Table 15.5, that person is likely to be actively depressed. What is unclear, however, is how the patient came to that state, why we can usually resolve it, and why it recurs.

Table 15.5. Laboratory indicators of melancholia

Abnormal HPA functioning (CRH/ACTH), elevated cortisol levels, loss of diurnal cortisol pattern
Shortened REM sleep latency

To answer questions about the pathophysiology of melancholia requires a change in focus from cross-sectional to longitudinal investigations and from univariate to multivariate analyses. This new focus requires a sea change in the attitudes of research-funding agencies because the challenges in obtaining grant support drive much research. Experts need to reach a consensus to shape the attitudes of government, industry, and private funding sources toward more synthesizing projects.[101] If the question, "What is the first step in the cascade that leads to an episode of depression?" can be answered, then direct preventive interventions can be devised.

Genetic predisposition – molecular *CLOCK* genes

Depressive disorders emerge in a roughly seasonal pattern with increased expression in the winter months. Circadian and ultradian rhythms are disturbed during these illnesses. Some patients experience a diurnal mood change with a worsening in the early morning and some relief in the late afternoon. Manic-depressive illness has been likened to a seasonal arousal and hibernation pattern.[102] Could the initiating trigger for an episode of depression be a genetically vulnerable biological clock that is aberrantly reset by stress?

Biological clock genes (*CLOCK*) that control circadian rhythms have been identified.[103] These are considered to be of ancient origin.[104] They are localized in the SCN of the hypothalamus, hippocampus, cerebellum, and piriform cortex.[105] Entrainment of the molecular clock to light/dark cycles is a critical early step in newborn development. Mutant *CLOCK* genes alter normal circadian rhythms.[106] Some *CLOCK* gene alleles are linked to sleep disturbances in humans.[107]

Circadian rhythm abnormalities in sleep, temperature, and cortisol secretion are hallmarks of melancholia.[108] Sudden shifts in circadian rhythms predispose to mood disorders in genetically vulnerable persons and may be considered the first step in an episode of depressive illness.[109] An examination of 143 persons with a history of major depression for two *CLOCK* gene alleles, however, found no difference from controls, although they observed differences between Euro-Americans and African-Americans.[110] A genetic predisposition for abnormal circadian rhythms is not well tested, and *CLOCK* and other genes regulating circadian rhythm need to be studied in pedigrees that include persons with mood disorder and circadian rhythm disturbances. Treatments are needed that are targeted to prevent the circadian clock's response to stress and to reset the abnormal clock once depression sets in. Bright-light therapy and manipulation of the sleep cycle are empirical efforts at this resetting, but their effects are weak and temporary.

Other genes of vulnerability

Although family and twin studies find recurrent depressive illness to have substantial heritability, the type of genetic transmission and the specific genes involved are unknown. The emerging picture of the human genome presents an opportunity to delineate a genetic contribution to depressive illness. In genome-wide linkage surveys for genetic loci connected to recurrent depressive illnesses, one study found chromosomal regions that met stringent linkage criteria.[111] Several loci related to the transcription factor CREB. Sex-specific effects were noted, with some loci more common in women, suggesting gender differences in the molecular pathophysiology of mood disorder and partially explaining the greater risk for mood disorder in women. Four of 19 susceptibility regions for depression overlapped with the risk for comorbid alcoholism. Only one region overlapped with a risk for manic-depressive illness, and there were no overlaps for schizophrenia.

Another study found a linkage for a region on chromosome 12, but this was stronger among men than women with a suggested relationship with manic-depressive illness.[112] Genome scans for manic-depressive illness, however, depend on how the phenotype is delineated.[113] The same is likely true for recurrent depressive illness.

Other susceptibility genes under consideration include the human opposite paired (HOPA) polymorphism, a thyroid receptor gene,[114] a nicotine-receptor variant,[115] and a tyrosine hydroxylase gene that affects serotonin metabolism.[116] No linkage is revealed for several other candidate genes, including G protein,[117] a number of serotonin-related genes,[118] and D_2 and D_3 receptor genes.[119] These studies reveal the complexity in the genetic contribution to depressive illness. Extensive work will be needed before any practical applications are likely.

Enhancing neuronal plasticity and reducing the neurotoxic effects of the prolonged stress response in depression

The brain characteristic that permits it to adapt and respond to stimuli throughout life is labeled *plasticity*. The processes of synaptic remodeling, axon sprouting, neurite extension, synaptogenesis, long-term potentiation, and neurogenesis, are the topics that are considered. The last, neurogenesis, is notable in the hippocampus. Without neuroplasticity, responses and problem-solving are limited and perseverative and new learning is compromised.[120]

Neuroplasticity is impaired in mood disorders. The brain regions that are structurally and functionally abnormal in depression subserve neuroplastic processes, and stress and glucocorticoids adversely affect neural plasticity.[121] The hippocampus is a particular focus of study.[122]

The hypothalamic–pituitary axis is activated in the stress response. High levels of glucocorticoids affect *N*-methyl-D-aspartate (NMDA) receptors, increasing glutaminergic transmission. A neurotoxic cascade with hippocampal pyramidal cell loss and morphologic change that is blocked by NMDA antagonists is postulated.[123] The findings mirror postmortem data from depressed and manic-depressive patients, and TCAs, ECT, and lithium ameliorate the proposed neurotoxic processes.[124] This salutary effect is linked to increased CREB expression and brain derived neurotrophic factor (BDNF) activity.[125]

Neurogenesis in the hippocampus is increased in laboratory animals by enriched environment, exercise, and by hippocampal-dependent learning.[126] Reducing glucocorticoid levels in older laboratory animals restores neurogenesis to levels observed in younger animals.[127]

The capacity for neurogenesis and its response to stress are heritable.[128] Acute and chronic stress decreases neurogenesis, as does aging. BDNF is a potent neuronal survival substance that modulates synaptic transmission.[129] Several classes of antidepressant drugs have neurotrophic-like effects[130] and increase neurogenesis.[131] Lithium administration increases neurogenesis.[132] Neurogenesis in laboratory animals is enhanced with induced seizures.[133]

Preventing the neurotoxic processes of depressive mood disorders may protect the neural plasticity of sufferers. Treating a depressed patient vigorously to a quick remission is essential, and the strategies detailed in Chapters 8–12 come closest to this ideal.[134] TCAs, lithium, and ECT provide the best treatment outcomes and they are the most potent antineurotoxic treatments available. Regular physical, verbal, and visual learning exercises should be part of continuation treatment.

Glutamate signaling modifiers are studied as potential treatments for the neurotoxic process in depressive disorders.[135] Investigations have focused on riluzole and memantine, presumptive neuroprotective agents with anticonvulsant properties, and felbamate, an anticonvulsant. The efficacy or safety of these agents in the treatment of depression is unknown.

Targeting the hypothalamic-pituitary–adrenal (HPA) axis is also under study with glucocorticoid antagonists as proposed treatments for depression.[136] Corticotropin-releasing factor-1 receptor antagonists are reported to reduce fear and anxiety responses in non-human primates and offered for development as an antidepressant.[137] The Corticotropin-releasing hormone antagonist R121919 was administered in low and high doses to 24 depressed patients and 8 of 10 patients in the high-dose group were reported to have responded. The agent, however, is hepatotoxic and no longer in development.[138]

Other strategies focus on the CREB/BDNF cascade. Inhibitors of cAMP breakdown enzymes are developed for this purpose.[139]

The inflammatory response[140]

The immune response system is activated in depressed patients. Melancholic and non-melancholic patients exhibit different immune responses. While non-melancholic patients exhibit increased leukocytes and lymphocytes,[141] melancholic patients have normal cell counts but a change in cytokine patterns that normalizes with successful treatment.[142] Cytokines are small-molecular-weight protein messengers (e.g., interferon) that mediate the immune response. Cytokine structures and receptors are highly heritable. Some are proinflammatory and others are anti-inflammatory. They serve as intermediates between immune and nerve cells. In this context, the immune system monitors the internal milieu and conveys information to the brain. Cytokines are produced in the glia, astrocytes, and neurons.[143] They interact with the hypothalamic–pituitary axis.[144] During injury and illness, increased cytokine levels affect sleep, eliciting increased fatigue, and also decrease appetite and libido.[145] Stress stimulates cytokine production, but this relationship is not understood.[146]

Plasma proinflammatory cytokines increase in depressed patients.[147] This increase occurs in other severe psychiatric conditions[148] and in general medical illnesses.[149] Chronicity of illness is a factor in the increase.[150] Reduced activity of cytokines accounts for the reported decrease in white blood cells in depressive disorders.[151]

While an increase in immune response is a consistent finding in depression, it may be a general response to illness and stress rather than a direct step in the development of depressive illness.[152] Nevertheless, proinflammatory cytokines adversely affect brain serotonin and norepinephrine metabolism.[153] The same changes are elicited by chronic HPA overactivity.[154] Treatments that prevent this response are likely to ameliorate the severity of a depressive illness, giving time for antidepressant therapies to work. For outpatients, such early easing of symptoms reduces suicide risk while increasing compliance. Considering the cytokine–HPA axis association and the salutary effects of antidepressant drugs on the immune system, the study of the immune system has particular relevance to melancholia.[155]

Regulation of emotion

Melancholia is an illness that is associated with prolonged and severe dysregulation of mood. Depressed patients have volume reductions in brain structures that subserve *emotional identification* and *appraisal* and the *generation of the emotional state* (the amygdala, ventral striatum, and subgenual cingulate gyrus). These, and related structures (the anterior insula and thalamus), are at the same time metabolically stimulated. Brain structures subserving *emotional regulation* also show reduced volume but also reduced activity (the dorsolateral and dorsomedial prefrontal cortex). After recovery, metabolic activity is re-established.[156] Exactly how these systems become perturbed and how our treatments normalize the dysfunction are unknown. Models of the generation and modulation of emotion have been proposed, but are untested.[157] Longitudinal studies using multiple assessments are needed to examine each step in the process of mood generation and modulation.[158]

Coda

Depressive mood disorders are recognized as many syndromes that are poorly separated from each other in present psychiatric classifications. Few markers assure homogeneity of patient samples for study and treatment. Many "treatments" are recommended but only a few are effective. Melancholia is a well-defined syndrome that allows the identification of more homogeneous patient groups for research and for applying effective treatment algorithms. A simplified treatment algorithm for melancholia that integrates ECT and pharmacotherapy with the broad pharmacodynamic spectrum antidepressants is defined by the evidence. Greater success in alleviating the more severely ill depressed patients is assured, including those now labeled as major depressed, bipolar disorder, and psychotic depressed, as well as the subgroups of delirious mania, rapid-cycling mania, and catatonic depression. Such an understanding and proper application offer the means to reduce suicide rates.

The limitations of the present classification of mood disorders are recognized by the American Psychiatric Association and the next iteration of the DSM is underway. Past efforts from DSM-II to DSM-IV, over 40 years, have resulted in increasing the number of identified syndromes without practical benefit to patients, researchers, or clinicians. In the history of psychiatric classifications, there has been a tension between "lumpers" and "splitters." The argument is reminiscent of the "nature–nurture" debate and is equally fruitless. A change in present thinking and a reorganization of the mood disorder category toward greater homogeneity within subgroups of patients is needed. We offer an image that favors redefining mood disorders by the presence or absence of melancholia. The syndrome is well delineated, is identified in 20–30% of clinical samples of depressed patients, is responsive to specific treatments, and incorporates some, but not all, of the present DSM-identified depressive syndromes. Until a better pathophysiology is discerned, our patients will be better served by separating melancholia from the large group of lifelong characterological dysfunctions that have a depressive component.

NOTES

1 Styron (1990).
2 Parker (2000).
3 Mouchabac *et al.* (2003).
4 Pintor *et al.* (2003).
5 Chisholm *et al.* (2004).
6 Goren and Levin (2000); Post *et al.* (2001); Erfurth *et al.* (2002); McIntyre *et al.* (2002); Ghaemi *et al.* (2004b).
7 Chapter 12 provides relevant citations. Detailed analyses of exaggerated claims and minimization of risks for the more recently introduced antidepressant and antipsychotic agents are to be found in Healy (1997, 2002) and in Medawar and Hardon (2004).
8 The connections between Food and Drug Administration (FDA) officers and industry led the US government to issue stringent guidelines on consulting appointments and income for federal appointees at the National Institute of Health and FDA. Calls for members of the Institute of Medicine to monitor FDA rulings meet the same conflicts of interest (Carroll, 2005). The close relationships of academia, industry, and government are discussed by Healy and Thase (2003) and Angell (2004), and further in Chapters 10 and 11.
9 The seemingly endless numbers of drug trials that have little benefit for patients with depressive illness is an international problem. An Israeli study of patients with psychotic

disorders found that women underwent fewer drug trials than did men, received ECT earlier in their illness course, and had a better long-term outcome (Bloch *et al.*, 2005).

10 Fink (1990, 1999a).

11 Chisholm *et al.* (2004).

12 The survey was of members of the American Psychiatric Association (Hermann *et al.* 1998). A recent survey of ECT practice in Belgium found ECT to be underused and, when used, treatment guidelines were often not followed (Sienaert *et al.*, 2005).

13 Prudic *et al.* (2001, 2004).

14 Ottosson and Fink (2004).

15 The check on licensed physicians administering ECT is the function of institutional medical boards to privilege physicians in the use of procedures at the institution. Physicians who administer ECT as outpatient procedures in non-institutional offices are under no community control. When institutional medical boards assess competency to administer ECT, they may ask for evidence of CME attendance. Such attendance in sessions that fail to offer hands-on experience is an inadequate standard for privileging. Minimal guidelines are provided by the American Psychiatric Association (1990, 2001). The guidelines are criticized by Ottosson and Fink (2004) and implicitly criticized by the findings of inadequate procedures in the surveys by Prudic *et al.* (2001, 2004). Also see Fink (1986b).

16 Ottosson and Fink (2004).

17 Hermann *et al.* (1995).

18 Hermann *et al.* (1998).

19 Hermann *et al.* (1999).

20 Prudic *et al.* (2001, 2004).

21 For melancholia and psychotic depression, see Chapters 8 and 9. For catatonia, see Fink and Taylor (2003). For schizophrenia, see Fink and Sackeim (1996).

22 A spate of assessments by independent commissions have been published in the past few years. These include the Agence d'Evaluation des Technologies et des modes d'Intervention en Santé (AETMIS) review in Quebec (2002), the UK ECT Review Group (National Institute for Clinical Excellence, 2003), the UK National Institute for Clinical Excellence review (2003), and the British HTA assessment (Greenhalgh *et al.*, 2005). Each review assesses the literature for the efficacy and safety of ECT. Each finds the use well documented in depression with greater benefits than medications. Each finds the evidence inadequate in schizophrenia, catatonia, and mania. The findings for technical factors in ECT, side-effects, and ethical considerations overlap. The major omission in each of these assessments is any mention of the benefits for individual patients.

23 Fochtmann (1994).

24 Fink (1979, 1999a, 2000a); Fink and Ottosson (1980); Ottosson and Fink (2004).

25 Insulin was introduced in 1922 and by 1928 its use in opiate withdrawal was described. A few years later, higher doses were used to induce periods of coma in patients with dementia praecox. Insulin coma therapy was widely used until it was replaced in the late 1950s by chlorpromazine. Reviews of the evidence of those experiences find the best results in patients with involutional depression and manic-depressive insanity, conditions that are subsumed in our concept of melancholia.

The efficacy of thyroid extract to relieve mental deficiency was demonstrated early. In the past few decades the neuroendocrine cycle of hypothalamic thyrotropin releasing hormone (TRH) influencing the release of pituitary thyrotropin-stimulating hormone (TSH) influencing the thyroid to release thyroxine, and thyroxine inhibiting the release of TRH has been well studied. Intravenous administration of TRH elicits an antidepressant response in normal volunteers and depressed patients. TRH levels in the cerebrospinal fluid increase with seizures. But the duration of clinical effect is short. Thyroid products triiodothyronine and thyroxine have been administered in antidepressant trials. Their efficacy is low but a role has been established as augmentations for antidepressant medications. The additional benefit of augmentation of ECT is small.

Administration of adrenocorticotropic hormone and steroids has wide systemic effects that limit their use in relieving psychiatric syndromes. Administration of sex hormones (testosterone, progesterone, estrogen) in severely depressed patients is reported to have transient benefits. The wider systemic effects limit their use.

Corticotropin-releasing hormone (CRH) and CRH antagonists are under study as antidepressants. The benefits have yet to be defined.

26 Parianti and Miller (2001); Belanoff *et al.* (2001a, b; 2002), Rothschild (2003b) Mifepristone is also known as RU-486, the abortifacient approved for use in some countries.

27 Belanoff *et al.* (2001a, b, 2002).

28 Chapter 13.

29 Chapter 9.

30 Erlenmeyer-Kimling and Cornblatt (1984); Fish *et al.* (1992); Olin *et al.* (1998).

31 Mason *et al.* (2004).

32 Veijola *et al.* (2004).

33 Williamson *et al.* (2004).

34 Halligan *et al.* (2004).

35 Ehrlich *et al.* (2004).

36 An additional indication of the early expression of the vulnerability for depression comes from an EEG study of newborns of apparently normal mothers. Relative right frontal activation in the newborn was associated with more disrupted sleep patterns and poorer performance on assessments of neonatal motor and behavioral responsiveness. These children had mothers with lower pre- and postnatal serotonin and higher postnatal cortisol levels, and more prepartum levels of moodiness, anxiety, and anger. These mothers also had greater right frontal EEG activation (Field *et al.*, 2002b). This EEG, cortisol, and behavioral pattern is exactly what is observed in newborns of women who were depressed during pregnancy.

37 Chabrol *et al.* (2002a, b).

38 Oren *et al.* (2002).

39 Wisner *et al.* (2001).

40 Benca *et al.* (1992); Armitage *et al.* (2000a, b, c, d). Low interhemispheric EEG coherence is reported.

41 Pollock and Schneider (1990); Teicher *et al.* (1993, 1997).

42 Birmaher *et al.* (1996a, b); Rao *et al.* (1996b); Morehouse *et al.* (2002).

43 Feng and Ma (2002).

44 Feng and Ma, (2003).

45 There are also peripheral clocks influenced by the SCN that have tissue-specific regulatory features (Shearman *et al.*, 1997; Zylka *et al.*, 1998).

46 Foster (1998); Lucas and Foster (1999).

47 Buijs *et al.* (2003).

48 Zhou *et al.* (2001).

49 In laboratory animals, maternal hormonal rhythms affect fetal growth rates and hormonal functions (Kennaway, 2002).

50 Menna-Barreto *et al.* (1996); Mirmiran *et al.* (2003).
51 Peirano *et al.* (2003).
52 Burnham *et al.* (2002).
53 Seifer *et al.* (1996).
54 Benoit *et al.* (1992).
55 Mirmiran and Van Someran (1993); Mirmiran (1995). Similar findings are reported in studies of laboratory animals. Prenatal stress in rats elicits enduring adverse effects on offspring behavior and sleep structure (Dugovic *et al.*, 1999), as does prenatal hypoxia (Joseph *et al.*, 2002) and protein restriction (Datta *et al.*, 2000). Repeated stress in rats also disrupts circadian rhythmicity and alters gene transcription (Amir and Stewart, 1998). Cocaine or D_1 receptor agonists also induce gene changes in the SCN (Weaver *et al.*, 1992).
56 Frank and Heller (1997); Feng and Ma (2002). SSRIs down-regulate 5-HT_7 receptors in the SCN that can lead to gene transcription changes in the SCN (Mullins *et al.*, 1999).
57 Wang *et al.* (2003).
58 Glotzbach *et al.* (1993); Kennaway *et al.* (1996).
59 Madeira *et al.* (1997); Shumake *et al.* (2001); Silva *et al.* (2002).
60 Kroes *et al.* (2001).
61 Geller *et al.* (2001).
62 Woodward and Fergusson (2001); Mathet *et al.* (2003).
63 Lewinsohn *et al.* (2000, 2001a).
64 Kovacs *et al.* (1994); Weissman *et al.* (1999).
65 Rao *et al.* (1993).
66 Birmaher *et al.* (2002).
67 Ezquiaga *et al.* (1987).
68 Goodyer *et al.* (1997).
69 Simpson *et al.* (1997).
70 de Kemp *et al.* (2002).
71 Frodl *et al.* (2002, 2003).
72 Coryell *et al.* (1995a).
73 MacQueen *et al.* (2003).
74 Bachmann *et al.* (2002).
75 Aubert *et al.* (2003).
76 Serretti *et al.* (2002).
77 Lerer and Macciardi (2002).
78 Murphy *et al.* (2003b).
79 Steimer *et al.* (2004).
80 Sindrup *et al.* (1992); Pullar *et al.* (2000).
81 O'Reilly *et al.* (1994); Serretti *et al.* (1998a).
82 Schafer (1999).
83 Lesch (2001); Serretti *et al.* (2002); Murphy *et al.* (2004).
84 Arias *et al.* (2001); Perlis *et al.* (2003).
85 Minov *et al.* (2001); Baghai *et al.* (2003b).
86 Du *et al.* (2001).
87 Lerer and Macciardi (2002).
88 Serretti *et al.* (2001a, b).
89 Serretti *et al.* (2002).

90 Sulser (2002).
91 Human fibroblasts exhibit receptor-mediated transduction cascades similar to those of brain cell, and so are used as models because any aberration in this process would extend to all cells dependent upon the specific transduction cascade.
92 Shelton *et al.* (1996, 1999).
93 Rahmann *et al.* (1997); Dwivedi *et al.* (2000).
94 Holsboer and Barden (1996).
95 Stone and Platt (1982).
96 Sulser (2002).
97 Nestler *et al.* (1990); Brady *et al.* (1991); Hosoda and Duman (1993).
98 Wong *et al.* (2000).
99 Sulser (2002).
100 Rossby *et al.* (2000).
101 The National Institutes of Mental Health have developed a strategic plan for research priorities (Charney and Babich, 2002). The plan is at website http://www.nimh.nih.hov/strategic/strategicplanningmenu.cfm. The American Psychiatric Association has offered a research agenda focused on formulations for the next iteration of the psychiatric disorders classification (Kupfer *et al.*, 2002). Another formulation has been proposed by the American Psychopathological Association (Helzer and Hudziak, 2002).
102 Avery *et al.* (1997).
103 Wehr (1996).
104 Bunney and Bunney (2000).
105 Abe *et al.* (1999).
106 Bunney and Bunney (2000).
107 Katzenberg *et al.* (1998); Jones *et al.* (1999a).
108 Benca *et al.* (1992); Duncan (1996).
109 Wirz-Justice (1998).
110 Desan *et al.* (2000).
111 Zubenko *et al.* (2003a).
112 Abkevich *et al.* (2003).
113 Rice *et al.* (1997); Segurado *et al.* (2003).
114 Philibert *et al.* (2002).
115 Lai *et al.* (2001).
116 Serretti *et al.* (2001b).
117 Zill *et al.* (2002).
118 Neiswanger *et al.* (1998).
119 Serretti *et al.* (2000b).
120 Mesulam (1999).
121 Watanabe *et al.* (1992); also see discussion in Chapter 14.
122 Manji *et al.* (2003).
123 Sapolsky (2000).
124 Holsboer (2001); Manji *et al.* (2003).
125 Duman *et al.* (1999).
126 Gould *et al.* (2000).
127 Cameron and McKay (1999).
128 Kempermann (2002).
129 Manji *et al.* (2003).

130 Czeh *et al.* (2001).
131 Jacobs *et al.* (2000).
132 Manji *et al.* (2003).
133 Madsen *et al.* (2000).
134 Kempermann (2002).
135 Zarate *et al.* (2003).
136 Chapter 13.
137 Habib *et al.* (2000). Antalarmin is one such agent under study.
138 Zobel *et al.* (2000).
139 Dyke and Montana (2002); Manji *et al.* (2003).
140 See references in end notes 156–160 for detailed discussion of the inflammatory response and how it relates to depressive illness.
141 This is a non-specific response seen in non-depressed persons with general medical illness.
142 Rothermundt *et al.* (2001a).
143 Kronfol and Remick (2000).
144 Rivier (1993); Rivest and Rivier (1993); Schuld *et al.* (2001).
145 Krueger and Majde (1994).
146 Maes *et al.* (1998).
147 Kronfol and House (1989); Maes *et al.* (1993b); (1995); Weizman *et al.* (1994); Kronfol *et al.* (1995); Maes and Smith (1998); Licinio and Wong (1999); van West and Maes (1999).
148 Maes *et al.* (1997).
149 Musselman *et al.* (2001b); Pasic *et al.* (2003).
150 Anisman *et al.* (1999).
151 Miller *et al.* (1999).
152 Kenis and Maes (2002).
153 Myint and Kim (2003).
154 Leonard (2001); Schuld *et al.* (2003).
155 Kubera *et al.* (2004).
156 Soares and Mann (1997); Davidson *et al.* (2000); Davidson and Slagter (2000); Mayberg (2003).
157 Phillips *et al.* (2003a, b).
158 A largely untested left–right cerebral hemisphere model with negative emotional stimuli activating the right hemisphere more than the left, and positive emotional stimuli activating the left hemisphere more than the right has been offered to explain shifts in mood states seen in manic-depressive illness (Borod, 1992; Heller, 1993; Lee *et al.*, 1993, 2004; Davidson, 1995; George *et al.*, 1995; Lane *et al.*, 1997).

References

Aalto-Setala, T., Marttunen, M., Ruulio-Henriksson, A., Poikolainen, K., and Lonnqvist, J. (2002). Depressive symptoms in adolescence as predictors of early adulthood depressive disorders and maladjustment. *Am. J. Psychiatry*, **159**, 1235–7.

Aarsland, D., Larsen, J. P., Waage, O., and Langeveld, J. H. (1997). Maintenance electroconvulsive therapy for Parkinson's disease. *Convuls. Ther.*, **13**, 274–7.

Abas, M. A., Sahakian, B. J., and Levy, R. (1990). Neuropsychological deficits and CT scan changes in elderly depressives. *Psychol. Med.*, **20**, 507–20.

Abe, H., Honma, S., Namithira, M., *et al.* (1999). Circadian rhythm and light responsiveness of *BMAL1* expression, a partner of mammalian clock gene, *Clock*, in the suprachiasmatic nucleus of rats. *Neurosci. Lett.*, **258**, 93–6.

Aben, I., Verhey, F., Lousberg, R., Lodder, J., and Honig, A. (2002). Validity of the Beck Depression Inventory, Hospital Anxiety and Depression Scale, SCL-90, and Hamilton Depression Rating Scale as screening instruments for depression in stroke patients. *Psychosom.*, **43**, 386–93.

Aben, I., Verhey, F., Strik, J., *et al.* (2003). A comparative study into the one year cumulative incidence of depression after stroke and myocardial infarction. *J. Neurol. Neurosurg. Psychiatry*, **74**, 581–5.

Abercrombie, H. C., Schaefer, S. M., Larson, C. L., *et al.* (1998). Metabolic rate in the right amygdala predicts negative affect in depressed patients. *Neuro. Report*, **9**, 3301–7.

Abkevich, V., Camp, N. J., Hensel, C. H., *et al.* (2003). Predisposition locus for major depression at chromosome 12q22–12q23. 2. *Am. J. Hum. Genet.*, **73**, 1271–81.

Ablon, J. S. and Jones, E. E. (2002). Validity of controlled clinical trials of psychotherapy: findings from the NIMH treatment of depression collaborative research program. *Am. J. Psychiatry*, **159**, 775–83.

Abraham, K. (1927). *Selected Papers of Karl Abraham*. Translated by Bryan D. and Strachey, A. London: Hogarth Press, pp. 503–10.

Abrams, R. (1982). ECT and tricyclic antidepressants in the treatment of endogenous depression. *Psychopharm. Bull.*, **18**, 73–5.

(ed.) (1989). ECT in the high-risk patient. *Convuls. Ther.*, **6**, 1–122.

(1997). The mortality rate with ECT. *Convuls. Ther.*, **3**, 125–7.

(2002a). *Electroconvulsive Therapy*, 4th edn. New York: Oxford University Press.

(2002b). Stimulus titration and ECT dosing. *J. ECT*, **18**, 3–9.

Abrams, R. and Swartz, C. M. (1985a). ECT and prolactin release: relation to treatment response in melancholia. *Convuls. Ther.*, **1**, 38–42.

(1985b). ECT and prolactin release: effect of stimulus parameters. *Convuls. Ther.*, **1**, 115–119.

Abrams, R. and Taylor, M. A. (1976). Catatonia: a prospective study. *Arch. Gen. Psychiatry*, **33**, 579–81.

(1980). A comparison of unipolar and bipolar depressive illness. *Am. J. Psychiatry*, **137**, 1084–7.

(1983). The importance of mood-incongruent psychotic symptoms in melancholia. *J. Affect. Disord.*, **5**, 179–81.

Abrams, R., Volavka, J., Roubicek, J., Dornbush, R., and Fink, M. (1970). Lateralized EEG changes after unilateral and bilateral electroconvulsive therapy. *Dis. Nerv. Syst.*, **31**, (suppl.) 28–33.

Abrams, R., Fink, M., Dornbush, R., *et al.* (1972). Unilateral and bilateral ECT: effects on depression, memory and the electroencephalogram. *Arch. Gen. Psychiatry*, **27**, 88–91.

Abrams, R., Volavka, J., and Fink, M. (1973). EEG seizure patterns during multiple unilateral and bilateral ECT. *Compr. Psychiatry*, **14**, 25–8.

Abrams, R., Taylor, M. A., Faber, R., *et al.* (1983). Bilateral versus unilateral ECT: efficacy in melancholia. *Am. J. Psychiatry*, **140**, 463–5.

Abrams, S. M., Field, T., Scafidi, F., and Prodromidis, M. (1995). Newborns of depressed mothers. *Infant Mental Health J.*, **16**, 233–9.

Abuzallouf, S., Dayes, I., and Lukka, H. (2004). Baseline staging of newly diagnosed prostate cancer: a summary of the literature. *J. Urol.*, **171**, 2122–7.

Accornero, F. (1988). An eyewitness account of the discovery of electroshock. *Convuls. Ther.*, **4**, 40–9.

Ackerman, D. L., Greenland, S., Bystritsky, A., and Small G. W. (1997). Characteristics of fluoxetine versus placebo responders in a randomized trial of geriatric depression. *Psychopharmacol. Bull.*, **33**, 707–14.

Adams, F. (ed.) (1939). *The Genuine Works of Hippocrates.* Baltimore: Williams & Wilkins.

Addington, D. and Addington, J. (1990). Depression, dexamethasone nonsuppression and negative symptoms in schizophrenia. *Can. J. Psychiatry*, **35**, 430–3.

Addington, D., Addington, J., Patten, S., *et al.* (2002). Double-blind, placebo-controlled comparison of the efficacy of sertraline as treatment for a major depressive episode in patients with remitted schizophrenia. *J. Clin. Psychopharmacol*, **22**, 20–5.

Adler, L., Wedekind, D., Pilz, J., Weniger, G., and Huether, G. (1997). Endocrine correlates of personality traits: a comparison between emotionally stable and emotionally labile healthy young men. *Neuropsychobiology*, **35**, 205–10.

Adrian, E. D. and Matthews, B. H. C. (1934). The Berger rhythm: potential changes from the occipital lobes in man. *Brain*, **57**, 355–85.

Adrien, J. (2002). Neurobiological bases for the relation between sleep and depression. *Sleep Med. Rev.*, **6**, 341–51.

Adson, D. E., Crow, S. J., Meller, W. H., and Magraw, R. M. (1998). Potential drug–drug interactions on a tertiary-care hospital consultation-liaison psychiatry service. *Psychosom.*, **39**, 360–5.

Affonso, D. D., Loven, S., Paul, S. M., and Sheptak, S. (1990). A standardized interview that differentiates pregnancy and postpartum symptoms from perinatal clinical depression. *Birth*, **17**, 121–30.

Agargun, M. Y., Kara, H., and Solmaz, M. (1997). Sleep disturbances and suicidal behavior inpatients with major depression. *J. Clin. Psychiatry*, **58**, 249–51.

Agence d'Évaluation des Technologies et des Modes d'Intervention en Santé (AETMIS) (2002). The use of electroconvulsive therapy in Quebec. AETMIS 02-05RE. Montreal: AETMIS.

Aharónovich, E., Liu, X., Nunes, E., and Hasin, D. S. (2002). Suicide attempts in substance abusers: effects of major depression in relation to substance use disorders. *Am. J. Psychiatry*, **159**, 1600–2.

Ahearn, E. P., Jamison, K. R., Steffens, D. C., *et al.* (2001). MRI correlates of suicide attempt history in unipolar depression. *Biol. Psychiatry*, **50**, 266–70.

Ahokas, A., Kaukoranta, J., and Aito, M. (1999). Effect of oestradiol on postpartum depression. *Psychopharmacology*, **146**, 108–10.

Ahokas, A., Aito, M., and Turiainen, S. (2000). Association between oestradiol and puerperal psychosis. *Acta Psychiatr. Scand.*, **101**, 167–9.

Ahokas, A., Kaukoranta, J., Wahlbeck, K., and Aito, M. (2001). Estrogen deficiency in severe postpartum depression: successful treatment with sublingual physiologic 17beta-estradiol: a preliminary study. *J. Clin. Psychiatry*, **62**, 332–6.

Ahrens, B., Grof, P., Möller, H. J., Muller-Oerlinghausen, B., and Wolf, T. (1995). Extended survival of patients on long-term lithium treatment. *Can. J. Psychiatry*, **40**, 241–6.

Akdemir, A., Turkvapar, M. H., Orsel, S. D., *et al.* (2001). Reliability and validity of the Turkish version of the Hamilton Depression Rating Scale. *Compr. Psychiatry*, **42**, 161–5.

Akechi, T., Nakano, T., Okamura, H., *et al.* (2001). Psychiatric disorders in cancer patients: descriptive analysis of 1721 psychiatric referrals at two Japanese cancer center hospitals. *Jpn J. Clin. Oncol.*, **31**, 188–94.

Akhondzadeh, S., Faraji, H., Sadeghi, M., *et al.* (2003). Double-blind comparison of fluoxetine and nortriptyline in the treatment of moderate to severe major depression. *J. Clin. Pharm. Ther.*, **28**, 379–84.

Akiskal, H. S. (1981) . Subaffective disorders: dysthymic, cyclothymic and bipolar II disorders in the "borderline" realm. *Psychiatr. Clin. North Am.*, **4**, 25–46.

(1983a). Dysthymic disorder: psychopathology of proposed chronic depressive subtypes. *Am. J. Psychiatry*, **140**, 11–20.

(1983b). Diagnosis and classification of affective disorders: new insights from clinical and laboratory approaches. *Psych Dev.*, **2**, 123–60.

(1990). Towards a definition of dysthymia: boundaries with personality and mood disorders. In Burton, S. W. and Akiskal, H. S. (eds) *Dysthymic Disorder.* London: Gaskell, pp. 1–12.

(ed.) (1999). Bipolarity: beyond classical mania. *Psychiatr. Clin. North Am.*, **22**, 517–703.

Akiskal, H. S. and Benazzi, F. (2003). Family history validation of the bipolar nature of depressive mixed states. *J. Affect. Disord.*, **73**, 113–22.

(2004). Validating Kraepelin's two types of depressive mixed states: "depression with flight of ideas" and "excited depression." *World J. Biol. Psychiatry*, **5**, 107–13.

Akiskal, H. S. and Katona, C. (eds) (2001). Millennial issue: the new bipolar era. *J. Affect. Disord.*, **67**, 1–292.

Akiskal, H. S. and Pinto, O. (1999). The evolving bipolar spectrum: prototypes I, II, III, and IV. *Psychiatr. Clin. North Am.*, **22**, 517–34.

Akiskal, H. S., Rosenthal, T. H., Haykal, R. F., Lemmi, H., and Scott-Strauss, A. (1980). Characterological depressions: clinical and sleep EEG findings separating 'subaffective dysthymias' from 'character spectrum' disorders. *Arch. Gen. Psychiatry*, **37**, 777–83.

Akiskal, H. S., Maser, J. D., Zeller, P. J., *et al.* (1995). Switching from 'unipolar' to bipolar II. An 11-year prospective study of clinical and temperamental predictors in 559 patients. *Arch. Gen. Psychiatry*, **52**, 114–23.

Akiskal, H. S., Benazzi, F., Perugi, G., and Rihmer, Z. (2005). Agitated "unipolar" depression reconceptualized as a depressive mixed state: implications for the antidepressant–suicide controversy. *J. Affect. Disord.*, **85**, 245–58.

Albala, A. A., Greden, J. F., Tarika, J., and Caroll, B. J. (1981). Changes in serial dexamethasone suppression tests among unipolar depressives receiving electroconvulsive treatment. *Biol. Psychiatry*, **16**, 551–60.

Alderton, H. R. (1995). Tricyclic medication in children and the QT interval: case report and discussion. *Can. J. Psychiatry*, **40**, 325–9.

Aldred, G. and Healy, D. (2004). Antidepressants and suicide. *Br. Med. J.*, **329**, (letter) 461.

Alexander, G. E. and Goldman, P. S. (1978). Functional development of the dorsolateral prefrontal cortex: an analysis utilizing reversible cryogenic depression. *Brain Res.*, **143**, 233–49.

Alexander, R. C., Salomon, M., Ionescu-Poggia, M., and Cole, J. (1988). Convulsive therapy in the treatment of mania: McLean Hospital 1973–1986. *Convuls. Ther.*, **4**, 1152–5.

Alexopoulos, G. S., Young, R. C., and Abrams, R. C. (1989). ECT in the high-risk geriatric patient. *Convuls. Ther.*, **5**, 75–87.

Alexopoulos, G. S., Meyers, B. S., Young, R. C., *et al.* (1997). 'Vascular depression' hypothesis. *Arch. Gen. Psychiatry*, **54**, 915–22.

Alexopoulos, G. S., Borson, S., Cuthbert, B. N., *et al.* (2002). Assessment of late life depression. *Biol. Psychiatry*, **52**, 164–74.

Allain, H., Lieury, A., Brunet-Bourgin, F., *et al.* (1992). Antidepressants and cognition: comparative effects of moclobemide, viloxazine and maprotiline. *Psychopharmacology*, **106**, S56–61.

Allain, H., Pollak, P., and Neukirch, H. C. (1993). Symptomatic effect of selegiline in de novo parkinsonian patients: the French Selegiline Multicenter Trial. *Move. Disord.*, **8** (suppl. 1), S36–40.

Allard, P. and Norlen, M. (2001). Caudate nucleus dopamine D (2) receptors in depressed suicide victims. *Neuropsychobiology*, **44**, 70–3.

Allen, J. M., Lam, R. W., Remick, R. A., and Sadovnick, A. D. (1993). Depressive symptoms and family history in seasonal and nonseasonal mood disorders. *Am. J. Psychiatry*, **130**, 443–8.

Almeida-Montes, L. G. Valles-Sanchez, V., Moreno-Aguilar, J., *et al.* (2000). Relation of serum cholesterol, lipid, serotonin and tryptophan levels to severity of depression and to suicide attempts. *J. Psychiatry Neurosci.*, **25**, 371–7.

Alonso, S. J., Navarro, E., and Rodriguez, M. (1994). Permanent dopaminergic alterations in the n. accumbens after prenatal stress. *Pharmacol. Biochem. Behav.*, **49**, 353–8.

Alpert, J. E., Übelacker, L. A., McLean, N. E., *et al.* (1997). Social phobia, avordant personality disorder and atypical depression: co-occurrence and clinical implications. *Psychol. Med.*, **27**, 627–33.

Altamura, C., Maes, M., Dai, J., and Meltzer, H. Y. (1995). Plasma concentrations of excitatory amino acids, serine, glycine, taurine and histidine in major depression. *Eur. Neuropsychopharmacol.*, **5** (suppl.), 71–5.

Altar, C. A., Whitehead, R. E., Chen, R., Wortwein, G., and Madsen, T. M. (2003). Effects of electroconvulsive seizures and antidepressant drugs on brain-derived neurotrophic factor protein in rat brain. *Biol. Psychiatry*, **54**, 703–9.

Altshuler, L., Post, R. M., Leverich, G. S., *et al.* (1995). Antidepressant-induced mania and cycle acceleration: a controversy revisited. *Am. J. Psychiatry*, **152**, 1130–8.

Altshuler, L., Kiriakos, L., Calcagno, J., *et al.* (2001c). The impact of antidepressant discontinuation versus antidepressant continuation on 1-year risk for relapse of bipolar depression: a retrospective chart review. *J. Clin. Psychiatry*, **62**, 612–16.

Altshuler, L. L., Devinsky, O., Post, R. M., and Theodore, W. (1990). Depression, anxiety, and temporal lobe epilepsy: laterality of focus and symptoms. *Arch. Neurol.*, **47**, 284–8.

Altshuler, L. L., Cohen, L., Szuba, M. P., *et al.* (1996). Pharmacologic management of psychiatric illness during pregnancy: dilemmas and guidelines. *Am. J. Psychiatry*, **153**, 592–606.

Altshuler, L. L., Bauer, M., Frye, M. A., *et al.* (2001a). Does thyroid supplementation accelerate tricyclic antidepressant response? A review and meta-analysis of the literature. *Am. J. Psychiatry*, **158**, 1617–22.

Altshuler, L. L., Cohen, L. S., Moline, M. L., *et al.* (2001b). Treatment of depression in women. *Postgrad. Med.*, (special no.), 1–107.

Altshuler, L. L., Frye, M. A., and Gitlin, M. J. (2003). Acceleration and augmentation strategies for treating bipolar depression. *Biol. Psychiatry*, **53**, 691–700.

Alvarez, E., Perez-Sola, V., Perez-Blanco, J., *et al.* (1997). Predicting outcome of lithium added to antidepressants in resistant depression. *J. Affect. Disord.*, **42**, 179–86.

Ambrosini, P. J., Bennett, D. S., Cleland, C. M., and Haslam, N. (2002). Taxonicity of adolescent melancholia: a categorical or dimensional construct? *J. Psychiatr. Res.*, **36**, 247–56.

American College of Obstetricians and Gynecologists (2004). Hormone therapy. *Obstet. Gynecol.*, **104**, S49–55.

American Psychiatric Association (1952). *Diagnostic and Statistical Manual of Mental Disorders.* Washington, DC: American Psychiatric Association Mental Health Service.

(1968). *DSM-II Diagnostic and Statistical Manual of Mental Disorders.* Washington, DC: American Psychiatric Association.

(1978). *Electroconvulsive Therapy.* Task force report 22. Washington, DC: American Psychiatric Association.

(1980). *DSM-III. Diagnostic and Statistical Manual of Mental Disorders.* Washington, DC: American Psychiatric Association.

(1990). *Electroconvulsive Therapy: Recommendations for Treatment, Training and Privileging.* Washington, DC: American Psychiatric Association.

(1994). *DSM-IV. Diagnostic and Statistical Manual of Mental Disorders.* Washington, DC: American Psychiatric Association.

(2001). *The Practice of Electroconvulsive Therapy. Recommendations for Treatment, Training, and Privileging.* 2nd edn. Washington, DC: American Psychiatric Association.

(2002). Practice guideline for the treatment of patients with bipolar disorder (revision). *Am. J. Psychiatry,* **159** (4 suppl.), 1–50.

Amir, S. and Stewart, J. (1998). Conditioned fear suppresses light-induced resetting of the circadian clock. *Neuroscience,* **86**, 345–51.

Amsterdam, J. D., Maislin, G., Winokur, A., *et al.* (1988). The DST/CRH stimulation test before and after clinical recovery from depression. *J. Affect. Disord.,* **14**, 213–22.

Anand, A. and Charney, D. S. (2000). Norepinephrine dysfunction in depression. *J. Clin. Psychiatry,* **61** (suppl. 1), 16–24.

Anderson, I. M. (2000). Selective serotonin reuptake inhibitors versus tricyclic antidepressants: a meta-analysis of efficacy and tolerability. *J. Affect. Disord.,* **58**, 19–36.

Andersen, G., Vestergaard, K., and Lauritzen, L. (1994). Effective treatment of poststroke depression with the selective serotonin reuptake inhibitor citalopram. *Stroke,* **25**, 1099–104.

Andersen, K., Balldin, J., Gottfries, C. G., *et al.* (1987). A double-blind evaluation of electroconvulsive therapy in Parkinson's disease with "on–off" phenomenon. *Acta. Neurol. Scand.,* **76**, 191–9.

(2001). Meta-analytical studies on new antidepressants. *Br. Med. Bull.,* **57**, 161–78.

Anderson, I. M. and Tomenson, B. M. (1994). The efficacy of selective serotonin re-uptake inhibitors in depression: a meta-analysis of studies against tricyclic antidepressants. *J. Psychopharmacol.,* **8**, 238–49.

Andreasen, N., Rice, J., Endicott, J., *et al.* (1987). Familial rates of affective disorder. *Arch. Gen. Psychiatry,* **44**, 461–9.

Andreasen, N. C. and Grove, W. M. (1982). The classification of depression: traditional versus mathematic approaches. *Am. J. Psychiatry,* **139**, 45–52.

Andreasen, N. C., Grove, W. M., and Maurer, R. (1980). Cluster analysis and the classification of depression. *Br. J. Psychiatry,* **137**, 256–65.

Andrew, B., Hawton, K., Fagg, J., and Westbrook, D. (1993). Do psychosocial factors influence outcome in severely depressed female psychiatric outpatients? *Br. J. Psychiatry,* **163**, 747–54.

Angell, M. (2004). *The Truth About the Drug Companies: How They Deceive Us and What to Do About It.* New York: Random House.

Angst, J. (1966). *Zur Atiologie and Nosologie endogener depressiver Psychosen.* Berlin: Springer.

(1978). The course of affective disorders: II: typology of bipolar manic-depressive illness. *Arch Psychiatr. Nevenkro,* **226**, 65–73.

(1985). Switch from depression to mania – a record study over decades between 1920 and 1982. *Psychopathology,* **18**, 140–54.

(1987). Switch from depression or mania, or from mania to depression: Role of psychotropic drugs. *Psychopharm. Bull.,* **23**, 66–7.

(1997). Minor and recurrent brief depression. In Akiskal, H. S., and Cassano, G. B. (eds) *Dysthymia and the Spectrum of Chronic Depressions.* New York: Guilford Press, pp. 183–90.

Angst, J. and Marneros, A. (2001). Bipolarity from ancient to modern times: conception, birth and rebirth. *J. Affect. Disord.,* **67**, 3–19.

Angst, J. and Perris, C. (1972). The nosology of endogenous depression: comparison of the results of two studies. *Int. J. Mental Health*, **1**, 145–58.

Angst, J. and Preisig, M. (1995). Outcome of a clinical cohort of unipolar, bipolar and schizoaffective patients. Results of a prospective study from 1959 to 1985. *Schweiz. Arch. Neurol. Psychiatr.*, **146**, 17–23.

Angst, J., Dittrich, A., and Grof, P. (1969). Course of endogenous affective psychoses and its modification by prophylactic administration of imipramine and lithium. *Int. Pharmacopsychiatry*, **2**, 1–11.

Angst, J., Angst, K., Baruffol, I., and Meinherz-Surbeck, R. (1992). ECT-induced and drug-induced hypomania. *Convuls. Ther.*, **8**, 179–85.

Angst, J., Gamma, A., Sellaro, R., Zhang, H., and Merikangas, K. (2002). Toward validation of atypical depression in the community: results of the Zurich cohort study. *J. Affect. Disord.*, **72**, 125–38.

Angst, J., Sellaro, R., Stassen, H. H., and Gamma, A. (2005). Diagnostic conversion from depression to bipolar disorders: results of a long-term prospective study of hospital admissions. *J. Affect. Disord.*, **84**, 149–57.

Anisman, H., Ravindran, A. V., Griffiths, J., and Merali, Z. (1999). Endocrine and cytokine correlates of major depression and dysthymia with typical or atypical features. *Mol. Psychiatry*, **4**, 182–8.

Anton, R. F., Moak, D. H., Waid, L. R., *et al.* (1999). Naltrexone and cognitive behavioral therapy for the treatment of outpatient alcoholics. *Am. J. Psychiatry*, **156**, 1758–64.

Anton, R. F., Moak, D. H., Latham, P. K., *et al.* (2001). Posttreatment results of combining naltrexone with cognitive-behavior therapy for the treatment of alcoholism. *J. Clin. Psychopharmacol.*, **21**, 72–7.

Antonijevic, I. A., Murck, H., Frieboes, R. M., and Steiger, A. (2000a). Sexually dimorphic effects of GHRH on sleep-endocrine activity inpatients with depression and normal controls – part II: hormone secretion. *Sleep Res. Online*, **3**, 15–21.

Antonijevic, I. A., Stalla, G. K., and Steiger, A. (2000b). Modulation of the sleep electroencephalogram by oestrogen replacement in postmenopausal women *Am. J. Obstet. Gynecol.*, **182**, 277–82.

Antonijevic, I. A., Murck, H., Frieboes, R.-M., Uhr, M., and Steiger, A. (2003). On the role of menopause for sleep-endocrine alterations associated with major depression. *Psychoneuroendocrinology*, **28**, 401–18.

APA Task Force on Laboratory Tests in Psychiatry (1987). The dexamethasone suppression test: an overview of its current status in psychiatry. *Am. J. Psychiatry*, **144**, 1253–62.

Apgar, V. (1953). A proposal for a new method of evaluation of the newborn infant. *Curr. Res. Anesth. Analg.*, **32**, 260–7.

(1962). Further observations on the newborn scoring system. *Am. J. Dis. Child.*, **104**, 419–28.

Appelhof, B. C., Brouwer, J. P., van Dyck, R., *et al.* (2004). Triiodothyronine addition to paroxetine in the treatment of major depressive disorder. *J. Clin. Endocrinol. Metab.*, **89**, 6271–6.

Arana, G. W., Baldessarini, R. J., and Ornsteen, M. (1985). The dexamethasone suppression test for diagnosis and prognosis in psychiatry. *Arch. Gen. Psychiatry*, **42**, 1193–204.

Arango, V., Underwood, M. D., and Mann, J. J. (2002). Serotonin brain circuits involved in major depression and suicide. *Prog. Brain Res.*, **136**, 443–53.

Arborelius, L., Owens, M. J., Plotsky, P. M., and Nemeroff, C. B. (1999). The role of corticotropin-releasing factor in depression and anxiety disorders. *J. Endocrinol*, **160**, 1–12.

Arciniegas, D. B. and Anderson, C. A. (2002). Suicide in neurologic illness. *Curr. Treat. Options Neurol.*, **4**, 457–68.

Arean, P. A. and Cook, B. L. (2002). Psychotherapy and combined psychotherapy/pharmacotherapy for late life depression. *Biol. Psychiatry*, **52**, 293–303.

Arias, B., Catalan, R., Gasto, C., *et al.* (2001). Genetic variability in the promoter region of the serotonin transporter gene is associated with clinical remission of major depression after long term treatment with citalopram. *World J. Biol. Psychiatry*, **2**, 9.

Armitage, R. (2000). The effects of antidepressants on sleep in patients with depression. *Can. J. Psychiatry*, **45**, 803–9.

Armitage, R., Emslie, G., and Rintelmann, J. (1997a). The effect of fluoxetine on sleep EEG in childhood depression: a preliminary report. *Neuropsychopharm.*, **17**, 241–5.

Armitage, R., Yonkers, K., Cole, D., and Rush, A. J. (1997b). A multicenter, double-blind comparison of the effects of nefazodone and fluoxetine on sleep architecture and quality of sleep in depressed outpatients. *J. Clin. Psychopharmacol.*, **17**, 161–8.

Armitage, R., Hoffmann, R. F., and Rush, A. J. (1999). Biological rhythm disturbance in depression: temporal coherence of ultradian sleep EEG rhythms. *Psychol. Med.*, **29**, 1435–48.

Armitage, R., Emslie, G. J., Hoffmann, R. F., *et al.* (2000a). Ultradian rhythms and temporal coherence in sleep EEG in depressed children and adolescents. *Biol. Psychiatry*, **47**, 338–50.

Armitage, R., Hoffmann, R. F., Fitch, T., Trivedi, M., and Rush, A. J. (2000b). Temporal characteristics of delta activity during NREM sleep in depressed outpatients and healthy adults: group and sex effects. *Sleep*, **23**, 607–17.

Armitage, R., Hoffmann, R., Trivedi, M., and Rush, A. J. (2000c). Slow-wave activity in NREM sleep: sex and age effects in depressed outpatients and healthy controls. *Psychiatry Res.*, **95**, 201–13.

Armitage, R., Hoffmann, R. F., Fitch, T., Trivedi, M., and Rush, A. J. (2000d). Temporal characteristics of delta activity during NREM sleep in depressed outpatients and healthy adults: group and sex effects. *Sleep*, **23**, 607–17.

Armitage, R., Emslie, G. J., Hoffmann, R. F., Rintelmann, J., and Rush, A. J. (2001). Delta sleep EEG in depressed adolescent females and healthy controls. *J. Affect. Disord.*, **63**, 139–48.

Armitage, R., Hoffmann, R. F., Emslie, G. J., *et al.* (2002). Sleep microarchitecture as a predictor of recurrence in children and adolescents with depression. *Int. J. Neuropsychopharmacol.*, **5**, 217–28.

Armitage, R., Husain, M., Hoffmann, R., and Rush, A. J. (2003). The effects of vagus nerve stimulation on sleep EEG in depression. *J. Psychosom. Res.*, **54**, 475–82.

Arnold, O. H. and Stepan, H. (1952). Untersuchungen zur Frage der akuten tödliche Katatonie. *Wr. Z. Nerven.*, **4**, 235–87.

Arnsten, A. F., Mathew, R., Ubriani, R., Taylor, J. R., and Li, B. M. (1999). Alpha-1 noradrenergic receptor stimulation impairs prefrontal cortical cognitive function. *Biol. Psychiatry*, **45**, 26–31.

Aronson, R., Offman, H. J., Joffe, R. T., and Naylor, C. D. (1996). Triiodothyronine augmentation in the treatment of refractory depression. *Arch. Gen. Psychiatry*, **53**, 842–8.

Aronson, T. (1987). Continuation therapy after ECT for delusional depression: a naturalistic study of prophylactic treatments and relapse. *Convuls. Ther.*, **3**, 251–9.

Ascher, E. (1951/52). A criticism of the concept of neurotic depression. *Am. J. Psychiatry*, **108**, 901–8.

Ashton, C. H., Marshall, E. F., Hassanyeh, F., Marsh, V. R., and Wright-Honari, S. (1994). Biological correlates of deliberate self-harm behaviour: a study of electroencephalographic, biochemical and psychological variables in parasuicide. *Acta Psychiatr. Scand.*, **90**, 316–23.

Attwood, A., Frith, U., and Hermelin, B. (1988). The understanding of interpersonal gestures by autistic and Down syndrome children. *J. Autism Dev. Disord.*, **18**, 241–57.

Aubert, R. E., Fulop, G., Xia, F., *et al.* (2003). Evaluation of a depression health management program to improve outcomes in first or recurrent episode depression. *Am. J. Manag. Care*, **9**, 374–80.

Auer, D. P., Putz, B., Kraft, E., *et al.* (2000). Reduced glutamate in the anterior cingulate cortex in depression: an in vivo proton magnetic resonance spectroscopy study. *Biol. Psychiatry*, **47**, 305–13.

Austin, M. C., Whitehead, R. E., Edgar, C. L., Janosky, J. E., and Lewis, D. A. (2002). Localized decrease in serotonin transporter-immunoreactive axons in the prefrontal cortex of depressed subjects committing suicide. *Neurosci.*, **114**, 807–15.

Austin, M. P., Ross, M., Murray, C., *et al.* (1992). Cognitive function in major depression. *J. Affect. Disord.*, **25**, 21–9.

Austin, M. P., Mitchell, P., Wilhelm, K., *et al.* (1999). Cognitive function in depression: a distinct pattern of frontal impairment in melancholia? *Psychol. Med.*, **29**, 73–85.

Austin, M. P., Mitchell, P., and Goodwin, G. M. (2001). Cognitive deficits in depression. *Br. J. Psychiatry*, **178**, 200–6.

Avery, D. and Lubrano, A. (1979). Depression treated with imipramine and ECT: the DeCarolis study reconsidered. *Am. J. Psychiatry*, **136**, 559–62.

Avery, D. and Winokur, G. (1977). The efficacy of electroconvulsive therapy and antidepressants in depression. *Biol. Psychiatry*, **12**, 507–23.

Avery, D. H., Dahl, K., Savage, M. V., *et al.* (1997). Circadian temperature and cortisol rhythms during a constant routine are phase-delayed in hypersomnic winter depression. *Biol. Psychiatry*, **41**, 1109–23.

Avery, D. H., Eder, D. N., Bolte, M. A., *et al.* (2001). Dawn simulation and bright light in the treatment of SAD: a controlled study. *Biol. Psychiatry*, **50**, 205–16.

Avissar, S., Nechamkin, Y., Roitman, G., and Schreiber, G., (1997). Reducecd. G protein functions and immunoreactive levels in mononuclear leukocytes of patients with depression. *Am. J. Psychiatry*, **154**, 211–17.

Axelson, D. A., Doraiswamy, P. M., McDonald, W. M., *et al.* (1993). Hypercortisolemia and hippocampal changes in depression. *Psychiatry Res.*, **47**, 163–73.

Ayuso-Gutierrez, J., Cabranes, J., Garcia-Camba, E., and Almoguera, I. (1987). Pituitary-adrenal disinhibition and suicide attempts in depressed patients. *Biol. Psychiatry*, **22**, 1409–12.

Ayuso-Mateos, J. L., Vazquez-Barquero, J. L., Dowrick, C., *et al.* (2001). Depressive disorders in Europe: prevalence figures from the ODIN study. *Br. J. Psychiatry,* **179**, 308–16.

Azmitia, E. C. and Segal, M. (1978). An autoradiographic analysis of the differential ascending projections of the dorsal and median raphe nuclei in the rat. *J. Comp. Neurol.,* **179**, 641–67.

Baca-Garcia, E., Blanco, C., Saiz-Ruiz, J., *et al.* (2001). Assessment of reliability in the clinical evaluation of depressive symptoms among multiple investigators in a multicenter clinical trial. *Psychiatry Res.,* **102**, 163–73.

Baca-Garcia, E., Diaz-Sastre, C., Ceverino, A., *et al.* (2003). Association between the menses and suicide attempts: a replication study. *Psychosom. Med.,* **65**, 237–44.

Bachmann, S., Bottmer, C., Jacob, S., *et al.* (2002). Expressed emotion in relatives of first-episode and chronic patients with schizophrenia and major depressive disorder – a comparison. *Psychiatry Res.,* **112**, 239–50.

Baethge, C., Salvatore, P., and Baldessarini, R. J. (2003a). "On cyclic insanity" by Karl Ludwig, Kahlbaum, MD: a translation and commentary. *Harv. Rev. Psychiatry,* **11**, 78–90.

(2003b). Cyclothymia, a circular mood disorder. *Hist. Psychiatry,* **14**, 377–99.

Baethge, C., Gruschka, P., Smolka, M. N., *et al.* (2003c). Effectiveness and outcome predictors of long-term lithium prophylaxis in unipolar major depressive disorder. *J. Psychiatry Neurosci.,* **28**, 355–61.

Bagby, R. M., Ryder, A. G., and Cristi, C. (2002). Psychosocial and clinical predictors of response to pharmacotherapy for depression. *J. Psychiatry Neurosci.,* **27**, 250–7.

Baghai, T. C., Schule, C., Zwanzger, P., *et al.* (2003a). Influence of a functional polymorphism within the angiotensin I-converting enzyme gene on partial sleep deprivation in patients with major depression. *Neurosci. Lett.,* **339**, 223–6.

(2003b). No influence of a functional polymorphism within the serotonin transporter gene on partial sleep deprivation in major depression. *World J. Biol. Psychiatry,* **4**, 111–4.

Bailine, S. H., Rifkin, A., Kayne, E., *et al.* (2000). Comparison of bifrontal and bitemporal ECT for major depression. *Am. J. Psychiatry,* **157**, 121–3.

Bailine, S. H., Petrides, G., Doft, M., and Lui, G. (2003). Indications for the use of propofol in electroconvulsive therapy. *J. ECT,* **19**, 129–32.

Baillerger, J. (1854). De la folie à double forme. *Ann. Med. Psychol.,* **6**, 367–91.

Baker, A. A., Morison, M., Game, J. A., and Thorpe, J. G. (1961). Admitting schizophrenic mothers with their babies. *Lancet,* **2**, 237–9.

Baker, C. B., Johnsrud, M. T., Crismon, M. L., Rosenheck, R. A., and Woods, S. W. (2003). Quantitative analysis of sponsorship bias in economic studies of antidepressants. *Br. J. Psychiatry,* **183**, 498–506.

Baker, R. A. and Herkenham, M. (1995). Arcuate nucleus neurons that project to the hypothalamic paraventricular nucleus: neuropeptidergic identity and consequences of adrenalectomy on mRNA levels in the rat. *J. Comp. Neurol.,* **358**, 518–30.

Bakish, D. (2001). New standard of depression treatment: remission and full recovery. *J. Clin. Psychiatry,* **62** (suppl. 26), 5–9.

Baldessano, C. F., Datto, S. M., Littman, L., and Lipari, M. A. (2003). What drugs are best for bipolar depression? *Ann. Clin. Psychiatry,* **15**, 225–32.

Baldessarini, R. J. (2001). Drugs and the treatment of psychiatric disorders: antidepressant and antianxiety agents. In Hardman, J. G., Limbird, L. E., and Gilman, A. G. (eds) *Goodman and Gilman's The Pharmacological Basis of Therapeutics*, 10th ed. New York: McGraw-Hill, pp. 447–83.

Baldessarini, R. J. and Tondo, L. (2003). Suicide risk and treatments for patients with bipolar disorder. *J.A.M.A.*, **290**, 1517–19.

Baldessarini, R. J., Tondo, L., Floris, G., and Hennen, J. (2000). Effects of rapid cycling on response to lithium maintenance treatment in 360 bipolar I and II disorder patients. *J. Affect. Disord.*, **61**, 13–22.

Baldessarini, R. J., Tondo, L., and Hennen, J. (2001). Treating the suicidal patient with bipolar disorder: reducing suicide risk with lithium. *Ann. N. Y. Acad. Sci.*, **932**, 24–38.

Baldwin, D. S., Hawley, C. J., Abed, R. T., *et al.* (1996). A multicenter double-blind comparison of nefazodone and paroxetine in the treatment of outpatients with moderate-to-severe depression. *J. Clin. Psychiatry*, **57** (suppl. 2), 46–52.

Baldwin, R. C. (2005). Is vascular depression a distinct sub-type of depressive disorder? A review of causal evidence. *Int. J. Geriatr. Psychiatry*, **20**, 1–11.

Baldwin, R. C. and O'Brien, J. (2002). Vascular basis of late-onset depressive disorder. *Br. J. Psychiatry*, **180**, 157–60.

Baldwin, R. C. and Tomenson, B. (1995). Depression in later life: a comparison of symptoms and risk factors in early- and late-onset cases. *Br. J. Psychiatry*, **167**, 649–52.

Bale, T. L., Contarino, A., Smith, G. W., *et al.* (2000). Mice deficient for corticotropin-releasing hormone receptor-2 display anxiety-like behaviour and are hypersensitive to stress. *Nat. Genet.*, **24**, 410–14.

Ballard, C., Banniester, C., Solis, M., Oyebode, F., and Wilcock, G. (1996). The prevalence, associations and symptoms of depression amongst dementia sufferers. *J. Affect. Disord.*, **36**, 135–44.

Ballon, N., Siobud-Dorocant, E., Even, C., Slama, F., and Dardennes, R. (2001) Tricyclic antidepressants dosage and depressed elderly inpatients: a retrospective pharmaco-epidemiologic study. *Encephale*, **27**, 373–6.

Ban, T. A., Healy, D., and Shorter, E. (1998). *The Triumph of Psychopharmacology and the Story of CINP.* Budapest: Animula.

(2000). *The Triumph of Psychopharmacology and the Story of CINP.* Budapest: Animula.

(2002). *The Rise of Psychopharmacology and the Story of CINP.* Budapest: Animula.

(2004).*Reflections on Twentieth-Century Psychopharmacology.* Budapest: Animula.

Banki, C., Arato, M., Papp, Z., and Kurcz, M. (1984). Biochemical markers in suicidal patients. *J. Affect. Disord.*, **6**, 341–50.

Baran, A. S. and Richert, A. C. (2003). Obstructive sleep apnea and depression. *CNS Spectr.*, **8**, 120–34.

Barbui, C. and Hotopf, M. (2001). Amitriptyline v. the rest: still the leading antidepressant after 40 years of randomised controlled trials. *Br. J. Psychiatry*, **178**, 129–44.

Barclay, M. L., Brownlie, B. E. W., Turner, J. G., and Wells, J. E. (1994). Lithium associated thyrotoxicosis: a report of 14 cases, with statistical analysis of incidence. *Clin. Endocrinol.*, **40**, 759–64.

Barden, N., Reul, J. M. H. M., and Holsboer, F. (1995). Do antidepressants stabilize mood through actions on the hypothalamic-pituitary-adrenocortical system? *Trends Neurosci.*, **18**, 6–11.

Bardwell, W. A., Moore, P., Ancoli-Israel, S., and Dimsdale, J. E. (2003). Fatigue in obstructive sleep apnea: driven by depressive symptoms instead of apnea severity? *Am. J. Psychiatry*, **160**, 350–5.

Barraclough, B., Bunch, J., Nelson, B., and Sainsbury, P. (1974). One hundred cases of suicide: clinical aspects. *Br. J. Psychiatry*, **125**, 355–73.

Bauer, M. and Dopfmer, S. (1999). Lithium augmentation in treatment-resistant depression: meta-analysis of placebo-controlled studies. *J. Clin. Psychopharmacol.*, **19**, 427–34.

Bauer, M., Bschor, T., Kunz, D., *et al.* (2000). Double-blind, placebo-controlled trial of the use of lithium to augment antidepressant medication in continuation treatment of unipolar major depression. *Am. J. Psychiatry*, **157**, 1429–35.

Baumhackl, U., Biziere, K., Fischbach, R., *et al.* (1989). Efficacy and tolerability of moclobemide compared with imipramine in depressive disorder (DSM-III): an Austrian double-blind, multicentre study. *Br. J. Psychiatry*, **155** (suppl.), 78–83.

Baxter, H., Singh, S. P., Standen, P., and Duggan, C. (2001). The attitudes of 'tomorrow's doctors' towards mental illness and psychiatry: changes during the final undergraduate year. *Med. Educ.*, **35**, 381–3.

Bazin, N., Perruchet, P., De Bonis, R., and Feline, A. (1994). The dissociation of explicit and implicit memory in depressed patients. *Psychol. Med.*, **24**, 239–45.

Beardslee, W. R., Keller, M. B., Seifer, R., *et al.* (1996). Prediction of adolescent affective disorder: effects of prior parental affective disorders and child psychopathology. *J. Am. Acad. Child Adolesc. Psychiatry*, **35**, 279–88.

Beats, B. C., Sahakian, B. J., and Levy, R. (1996). Cognitive performance in tests sensitive to frontal lobe dysfunction in the elderly depressed. *Psychol. Med.*, **26**, 591–603.

Beautrais, A. L. (2003). Suicide and serious suicide attempts in youth: a multiple-group comparison study. *Am. J. Psychiatry*, **160**, 1093–9.

Bech, P. and Rafaelsen, O. J. (1980). The use of rating scales exemplified by a comparison of the Hamilton and the Bech Rafaelsen Melancholia Scale. *Acta Psychiatr. Scand.*, **62** (suppl. 185), 128–32.

Bech, P., Cialdella, P., Haugh, M. C., *et al.* (2000). Meta-analysis of randomized controlled trial of fluoxetine v. placebo and tricyclic antidepressants in the short-term treatment of major depression. *Br. J. Psychiatry*, **176**, 421–8.

Beck, A. T., Ward, C. H., Mendelson, M., Mock, J., and Erbaugh, J. (1961). An inventory for measuring depression. *Arch. Gen. Psychiatry*, **4**, 53–63.

Beck, A. T., Brady, J. P., and Quen, J. M. (1977). The history of depression. *Psychiatr. Ann.*, **7**, 1–50.

Beck, C. T. (1996). A meta-analysis of predictors of postpartum depression. *Nurs. Res.*, **45**, 297–303.

Beekman, A. T. F., Copeland, J. R. M., and Prince, M. J. (1999). Review of community prevalence of depression in later life. *Br. J. Psychiatry*, **174**, 307–11.

Beer, A. M. and Ostermann, T. (2001). St. John's wort: interaction with cyclosporine increases risk of rejection for the kidney transplant and raises daily cost of medication. *Med. Klin.*, **96**, 480–3.

Beier, E. V., Arushanian, E. B., Titenok, A. L., and Alferor, V. V. (2003). The dorsal hippocampus injury influences chronobiological effects of depressants and antidepressants in rats. *Eksp. Klin. Farmakol.*, **66**, 9–12.

Belanoff, J., Flores, B., Kalezhan, M., Sund, B., and Schatzberg, A. (2001a). Rapid reversal of psychotic major depression using mifepristone. *J. Clin. Psychopharmacol.*, **21**, 516–54.

Belanoff, J. K., Kalehzan, M., Sund, B., Fleming Ficek, S. K., and Schatzberg, A. F. (2001b). Cortisol activity and cognitive changes in psychotic major depression. *Am. J. Psychiatry*, **158**, 1612–16.

Belanoff, J. K., Rothschild, A. J., Cassidy, F., *et al.* (2002). An open label trial of C-1073 (mifepristone) for psychotic major depression. *Biol. Psychiatry*, **52**, 386–92.

Bell, H., Tallaksen, C. M., Try, K., and Haug, E. (1994). Carbohydrate-deficient transferring and other markers of high alcohol consumption: a study of 502 patients admitted consecutively to a medical department. *Alcohol Clin. Exp. Res.*, **18**, 1103–8.

Bellini, L., Gatti, F., Gasperini, M., and Smeraldi, E. (1992). A comparison between delusional and nondelusional depressives. *J. Affect. Disord.*, **25**, 129–38.

Bellush, L. L. and Reid, S. G. (1994). Metabolic and neurochemical profiles in insulin-treated diabetic rats. *Am. J. Physiol.*, **266**, R87–94.

Benazzi, F. (1999). Atypical depression in private practice depressed outpatients: a 203-case study. *Compr. Psychiatry*, **40**, 80–3.

(1999c). Psychotic late-life depression: a 376-case study. *Int. Psychogeriatr.*, **11**, 325–32.

(2000). Late-life atypical major depressive episode. A 358-case study in outpatients. *Am. J. Geriatr. Psychiatry*, **8**, 117–22.

(2001). Prevalence and clinical correlates of residual depressive symptoms in bipolar II disorder. *Psychother. Psychosom.*, **70**, 232–8.

(2002). Psychomotor changes in melancholic and atypical depression: unipolar and bipolar-II subtypes. *Psychiatry Res.*, **112**, 211–20.

(2003a). Is there a link between atypical and early-onset "unipolar" depression and bipolar II disorder? *Compr. Psychiatry*, **44**, 102–9.

(2003b). Bipolar II disorder and major depressive disorder: continuity or discontinuity? *World J. Biol. Psychiatry*, **4**, 166–71.

(2004a). Melancholic outpatient depression in bipolar-II vs. unipolar. *Prog. Neuro-psychopharm. Biol. Psychiatry*, **28**, 481–5.

(2004b). Depressive mixed state: a feature of the natural course of bipolar II (and major depressive) disorder? *Psychopathology*, **7**, 207–12.

(2004c). Is depressive mixed state a transition between depression and hypomania? *Eur. Arch. Psychiatry Clin. Neurosci.*, **254**, 69–75.

(2004d). Agitated depression: a valid depression subtype? *Prog. Neuropsychopharmacol. Biol. Psychiatry*, **28**, 1279–85.

Benazzi, F. and Akiskal, H. S. (2001). Delineating bipolar II mixed states in the Ravenna-San Diego collaborative study: the relative prevalence and diagnostic significance of hypomanic features during major depressive episodes. *J. Affect. Disord.*, **67**, 115–22.

(2003). Refining the evaluation of bipolar II: beyond the strict SCID-CV guidelines for hypomania. *J. Affect. Disord.*, **73**, 33–8.

Benazzi, F., and Rihmer, Z. (2000). Sensitivity and specificity of DSM-IV atypical features for bipolar II disorder diagnosis. *Psychiatry Res.*, **93**, 257–62.

Benazzi, F., Koukopolous, A., and Akiskal, H. S. (2004). Toward a validation of a new definition of agitated depression as a bipolar mixed state (mixed depression). *Eur. Psychiatry*, **19**, 85–90.

Benbow, S. M., Benbow, J., and Tomenson, B. (2003). Electroconvulsive therapy clinics in the United Kingdom should routinely monitor electroencephalographic seizures. *J. ECT*, **19**, 217–20.

Benca, R. M., Obermeyer, W. H., Thisted, R. A., and Gillin, J. C. (1992). Sleep and psychiatric disorders: a meta-analysis. *Arch. Gen. Psychiatry*, **49**, 651–68.

Bench, C. J., Friston, K. J., Brown, R. G., *et al.* (1993). Regional cerebral blood flow in depression measured by positron emission tomography: the relationship with clinical dimensions. *Psychol. Med.*, **23**, 579–90.

Benedetti, F., Colombo, C., Pontiggia, A., *et al.* (2003a). Morning light treatment hastens the antidepressant effect of citalopram: a placebo-controlled trial. *J. Clin. Psychiatry*, **64**, 648–53.

Benedetti, F., Colombo, C., Serretti, A., *et al.* (2003b). Antidepressant effects of light therapy combined with sleep deprivation are influenced by a functional polymorphism within the promoter of the serotonin transporter gene. *Biol. Psychiatry*, **54**, 687–92.

Bennett, A. E. (1938). Convulsive (pentamethyline-tetrazol) shock therapy in depressive psychosis: preliminary report of results obtained in ten cases. *Am. J. Med. Sci.*, **196**, 420–8.

(1939). Metrazol convulsive shock therapy in affective psychoses; follow-up report of results in 61 depressive and 9 manic cases. *Am. J. Med. Sci.*, **198**, 695–701.

(1972). *Fifty Years in Neurology and Psychiatry.* New York: Intercontinental Medical Book.

Benoit, D., Zeanah, C. H., Boucher, C., and Minde, K. (1992). Sleep disorders in early childhood: association with insecure maternal attachment. *J. Am. Acad. Child Adolesc. Psychiatry*, **31**, 86–93.

Ben-Shachar, D., Gawawi, H., Riboyad-Levin, J., and Klein, E. (1999). Chronic repetitive transcranial magnetic stimulation alters β-adrenergic and 5-HT_2 receptor characteristics in rat brain. *Brain Res.*, **81**, 678–83.

Bent-Hansen, J., Lauritzen, L., Clemmesen, L., Lunde, M., and Korner, A. (1995). A definite and a semidefinite questionnaire version of the Hamilton/melancholia (HDS/MES) scale. *J. Affect. Disord.*, **33**, 143–50.

Bent-Hansen, J., Lunde, M., Klysner, R., *et al.* (2003). The validity of the depression rating scales in discriminating between citalopram and placebo in depression recurrence in the maintenance therapy of elderly unipolar patients with major depression. *Pharmacopsychiatry*, **36**, 313–16.

Berenbaum, S. A., Abrams, R., Rosenberg, S., and Taylor, M. A. (1987). The nature of emotional blunting: a factor-analytic study. *Psychiatry Res.*, **20**, 57–67.

Berger, M., Pirke, K.-M., Doerr, P., Krieg, J.-C., and von Zerssen, D. (1984). The limited utility of the dexamethasone suppression test for the diagnostic process in psychiatry. *Br. J. Psychiatry*, **145**, 372–82.

Berger, M., Van Calker, D., and Riemann, D. (2003). Sleep and manipulations of the sleep-wake rhythm in depression. *Acta Psychiatr. Scand. Suppl.*, **418**, 83–91.

Berman, R. L., Darnell, A. M., Miller, H. L., Anand, A., and Charney, D. S. (1997). Effect of pindolol in hastening response to fluoxetine in the treatment of major depression: a double-blind, placebo-controlled trial. *Am. J. Psychiatry*, **154**, 37–43.

Berns, G. S., Martin, M., and Proper, S. M. (2002). Limbic hyperreactivity in bipolar II disorder. *Am. J. Psychiatry*, **159**, 304–6.

Berrios, G. and Porter, R. (1995). *A History of Clinical Psychiatry.* London: Athlone Press.

(1995b). Cotard's syndrome: analysis of 100 cases. *Acta Psychiatr Scand.*, **91**, 185–8.

Berrios, G. E. and Luque, R. (1995a). Cotard's delusion or syndrome? A conceptual history. *Compr. Psychiatry*, **36**, 218–23.

Bertelsen, A., Harvald, B., and Hauge, M. (1977). A Danish twin study of manic-depressive disorders. *Br. J. Psychiatry*, **130**, 330–51.

Bertolino, A., Frye, M., Callicott, J. H., *et al.* (2003). Neuronal pathology in the hippocampal area of patients with bipolar disorder: a study with proton magnetic resonance spectroscopic imaging. *Biol. Psychiatry*, **53**, 906–13.

Bethea, C. L., Pecins-Thompson, M., Schutzer, W. E., Gundlah, C., and Lu, Z. N. (1999). Ovarian steroids and serotonin neural function. *Mol. Neurobiol.*, **18**, 87–123.

Beyer, J. L., Weiner, R. D., and Glenn, M. D. (1998). *Electroconvulsive Therapy. A Programmed Text.* Washington, DC: American Psychiatric Press.

Bhandari, M., Busse, J. W., Jackowski, D., *et al.* (2004). Association between industry funding and statistically significant pro-industry findings in medical and surgical randomized trials. *C.M.A.J.*, **170**, 477–80.

Bianchi, J. A. and Chiarello, C. J. (1944). Shock therapy in the involutional and manic-depressive psychoses. *Psych. Q.*, **18**, 118–26.

Bielski, R. J., Mayor, J., and Rice, J. (1992). Phototherapy with broad spectrum white fluorescent light: A comparative study. *Psychiatry Res.*, **43**, 167–75.

Bilikiewicz, A. (1999). Medical student curriculum in psychiatry in Poland. *Psychiatr. Pol.*, **33**, 169–77.

Birchwood, M., Iqbal, Z., Chadwick, P., and Trower, P. (2000). Cognitive approach to depression and suicidal thinking in psychosis. I. Ontogeny of post-psychotic depression. *Br. J. Psychiatry*, **117**, 516–21.

Birkenhäger, T. K., Pluijms, E. M., and Lucius, S. A. P. (2003). ECT response in delusional versus non-delusional depressed inpatients. *J. Affect. Disord.*, **74**, 191–5.

Birmaher, B., Arbelaez, C., and Brent, D. (2002). Course and outcome of child and adolescent major depressive disorder. *Child Adolesc. Psychiatr. Clin. North Am.*, **11**, 619–37.

Birmaher, B., Ryan, N. D., Williamson, D. E., *et al.* (1996a). Childhood and adolescent depression: a review of the past 10 years. Part I. *J. Am. Acad. Child Adolesc. Psychiatry*, **35**, 1427–39.

Birmaher, B., Williamson, D. E., Dahl, R. E., *et al.* (2004). Clinical presentation and course of depression in youth: does onset in childhood differ from onset in adolescence? *J. Am. Acad. Child Adolesc. Psychiatry*, **43**, 63–70.

Birmaher, B., Ryan, N. D., Williamson, D. E., Brent, D. A., and Kaufman, J. (1996b). Childhood and adolescent depression. A review of the past 10 years. Part II. *J. Am. Acad. Child Adolesc. Psychiatry*, **35**, 1575–83.

Biro, M., and Till, E. (1989). Factor analytic study of depressive disorders. *J. Clin. Psychol.*, **45**, 369–73.

Bissessur, S., Tissingh, G., Wolters, E. C., and Scheltens, P. (1997). rCBF SPECT in Parkinson's disease with mental dysfunction. *J. Neural Transm.*, **50** (suppl.), 25–30.

Biver, F., Goldman, S., Delvenne, V., *et al.* (1994). Frontal and parietal metabolic disturbances in unipolar depression. *Biol. Psychiatry*, **36**, 381–8.

Black, D. W., Winokur, G., and Nasrallah, A. (1987a). The treatment of depression: electroconvulsive therapy vs antidepressants: a naturalistic evaluation of 1495 patients. *Compr. Psychiatry*, **26**, 169–82.

(1987b). Suicide on subtypes of major affective disorder. A comparison with general population suicide mortality. *Arch. Gen. Psychiatry*, **44**, 878–80.

(1988). Effect of psychosis on suicide risk in 1593 patients with unipolar and bipolar affective disorders. *Am. J. Psychiatry*, **145**, 849–52.

Black, D. W., Monohan, P. O., and Winokur, G. (2002). The relationship between DST results and suicidal behavior. *Ann. Clin. Psychiatry*, **14**, 83–8.

Black, D. W. G., Wilcox, J. A., and Stewart, M. (1985). The use of ECT in children: case report. *J. Clin. Psychiatry*, **46**, 98–9.

Blair-West, G. W., Cantor, C. H., Mellsop, G. W., and Eyeson-Annan, M. L. (1999). Lifetime suicide risk in major depression: sex and age determinants. *J. Affect. Disord.*, **55**, 171–8.

Blanco, C., Laje, G., Olfson, M., Marcus, S. C., and Pincus, H. A. (2002). Trends in the treatment of bipolar disorder by outpatient psychiatrists. *Am. J. Psychiatry*, **15a**, 1005–10.

Blashfield, R. K. and Morey, L. C. (1979). The classification of depression through cluster analysis. *Compr. Psychiatry*, **20**, 516–27.

Blazer, D., Swartz, M., Woodbury, M., *et al.* (1988). Depressive symptoms and depressive diagnoses in a community population. Use of a new procedure for analysis of psychiatric classification. *Arch. Gen. Psychiatry*, **45**, 1078–84.

Blazer, D. G., Kessler, R. L., McGonagle, K. A., and Swartz, M. S. (1994). The prevalence and distribution of major depression in a national community sample: the National Comorbidity Survey. *Am. J. Psychiatry*, **151**, 979–86.

Blier, P. and Ward, N. M. (2003). Is there a role for 5-HT1A agonists in the treatment of depression? *Biol. Psychiatry*, **53**, 193–203.

Bligh-Glover, W., Kolli, T. N., Shapiro-Kulnane, L., *et al.* (2000). The serotonin transporter in the midbrain of suicide victims with major depression. *Biol. Psychiatry*, **47**, 1015–24.

Blinder, M. G. (1969). Classification and treatment of depression. *Int. Psychiatry Clin.*, **6**, 3–26.

Bloch, M., Schmidt, P. J., Danaceau, M., *et al.* (2000). Effects of gonadal steroids in women with a history of postpartum depression. *Am. J. Psychiatry*, **157**, 924–30.

Bloch, M., Daly, R. C., and Rubinow, D. R. (2003). Endocrine factors in the etiology of postpartum depression. *Compr. Psychiatry*, **44**, 234–46.

Bloch, Y., Ratzoni, G., Sobol, D., *et al.* (2005). Gender differences in electroconvulsive therapy: a retrospective chart review. *J. Affect. Disord.*, **84**, 99–102.

Block, M., Schwartzman, Y., Bonne, O., and Lerer, B. (1977). Concurrent treatment of nonresistant major depression with desipramine and lithium: a double-blind, placebo-controlled study. *J. Clin. Psychopharmacol.*, **17**, 44–8.

Block, S. D. (1994). The primary care imperative: challenges and opportunities for medical student education in psychiatry. *Harv. Rev. Psychiatry*, **2**, 52–4.

Blumberg, A. G., Cohen, L., and Miller, J. S. A. (1956). The relation of mecholyl induced hypotension to the classification of psychiatric patients and its prognostic significance with electroshock therapy. *J. Hillside Hosp.*, **5**, 216–31.

Blumberg, H. P., Stern, E., Martinez, D., *et al.* (2000). Increased anterior cingulate and caudate activity in bipolar mania. *Biol. Psychiatry*, **48**, 1045–52.

Blumberg, H. P., Leung, H.-C., Skudlarski, P., *et al.* (2003a). A functional magnetic resonance imaging study of bipolar disorder. *Arch. Gen. Psychiatry*, **60**, 601–9.

Blumberg, H. P., Martin, A., Kaufman, J., *et al.* (2003b). Frontostriatal abnormalities in adolescents with bipolar disorder: preliminary observations from functional MRI. *Am. J. Psychiatry*, **160**, 1345–7.

Blumer, D. and Zielinski, J. (1988). Pharmacologic treatment of psychiatric disorders associated with epilepsy. *J. Epilepsy*, **1**, 135–50.

Bocchetta, A. Ardau, R., Burrai, C., *et al.* (1998). Suicidal behavior on and off lithium prophylaxis in a group of patients with prior suicide attempts. *J. Clin. Psychopharmacol.*, **18**, 384–9.

Bodkin, J. A. and Amsterdam, J. D. (2002). Transdermal selegiline in major depression: a double-blind, placebo-controlled, parallel-group study in outpatients. *Am. J. Psychiatry*, **159**, 1869–75.

Bodkin, J. A., Zornberg, G. L., Lukas, S. E., and Cole, J. C. (1995). Buprenorphine treatment of refractory depression. *J. Clin. Psychopharm.*, **15**, 49–57.

Boerlin, H. L., Gitlin, M. J., Zoellner, L. A., and Hammen, C. L. (1998). Bipolar depression and antidepressant-induced mania: a naturalistic study. *J. Clin. Psychiatry*, **59**, 374–9.

Bogner, H. R. and Gallo, J. J. (2004). Are higher rates of depression in women accounted for by differential symptom reporting? *Soc. Psychiatry Psychiatr. Epidemiol.*, **39**, 126–32.

Bolwig, T. G. and Rafaelson, O. J. (1972). Salivation in affective disorders. *Psychol. Med.*, **2**, 232–8.

Bonanno, G. A. and Kaltman, S. (2001). The varieties of grief experience. *Clin. Psychol. Rev.*, **21**, 705–34.

Bondy, B., Kuznik, J., Baghai, T., *et al.* (2000). Lack of association of serotonin-2A receptor gene polymorphism (T102C) with suicidal ideation and suicide. *Am. J. Med. Genet.*, **96**, 831–5.

Bonne, O., Krausz, Y., Shapira, B., *et al.* (1996). Increased cerebral blood flow in depressed patients responding to electroconvulsive therapy. *J. Nucl. Med.*, **37**, 1075–80.

Bonnet, U. (2003). Moclobemide: therapeutic use and clinical studies. *CNS Drug Rev.*, **9**, 97–140.

Booker, J. M. and Hellekson, C. J. (1992). Prevalence of seasonal affective disorder in Alaska. *Am. J. Psychiatry*, **149**, 1176–82.

Borbely, A. A., Tobler, I., Loepfe, M., *et al.* (1984). All-night spectral analysis of the sleep EEG in untreated depressives and normal controls. *Psychiatry Res.*, **12**, 27–33.

Borod, J. (1992). Interhemispheric and intrahemispheric control of emotion: a focus on unilateral brain damage. *J. Consult. Clin. Psychol.*, **60**, 339–48.

Bossert, S., Berger, M., Krieg, J. C., *et al.* (1988). Cortisol response to various stressful situations: relationship to personality variables and coping styles. *Neuropsychobiology*, **20**, 36–42.

Bostwick, J. M. and Chozinski, J. P. (2002). Temporal competency in catatonia. *J. Am. Acad. Psychiatry Law*, **30**, 371–6.

Bostwick, J. M. and Pankratz, V. S. (2000). Affective disorders and suicide risk: a reexamination. *Am. J. Psychiatry*, **157**, 1925–32.

Bottlender, R., Rudolf, D., Strauss, A., and Moller, H. J. (2000). Are low basal serum levels of the thyroid stimulating hormone (TSH) a risk factor for switches into states of expansive syndrome known in Germany as "maniform syndromes" in bipolar I depression? *Pharmacopsychiatry*, **33**, 75–7.

Bourgon, L. N. and Kellner, C. H. (2000). Relapse of depression after ECT: a review. *J. ECT*, **16**, 19–34.

Bowden, C. (2004). The effectiveness of divalproate in all forms of mania and the broader bipolar spectrum: many questions, few answers. *J. Affect. Disord.*, **79** (suppl. 1), S9–S14.

Bowden, C. L., Mitchell, P., and Suppes, T. (1999). Lamotrigine in the treatment of bipolar depression. *Eur. Neuropsychopharm*, **9** (suppl. 4), S113–S117.

Bowden, C. L., Calabrese, J. R., Sachs, G., *et al.* (2003). A placebo-controlled 18-month trial of lamotrigine and lithium maintenance treatment in recently manic or hypomanic patients with bipolar I disorder. *Arch. Gen. Psychiatry*, **60**, 392–400; erratum in *Arch. Gen. Psychiatry*, **61**, 680.

Bowden, C. L., Asnis, G. M., Ginsberg, L. D., *et al.* (2004). Safety and tolerability of lamotrigine for bipolar disorder. *Drug Safety*, **27**, 173–84.

Bowen, A., Neumann, V., Conner, M., Tennant, A., and Chamberlain, M. A. (1998). Mood disorders following traumatic brain injury: identifying the extent of the problem and the people at risk. *Brain Inj.*, **12**, 177–90.

Bower, W. H. and Altschule, D. (1956). Use of progesterone in the treatment of postpartum psychosis. *N. Engl. J. Med.*, **254**, 157–60.

Boyer, W. F. and Feighner, J. P. (1994). Clinical significance of early non-response in depressed patients. *Depression*, **2**, 32–5.

Bozikas, V., Petrikis, P., and Karavatos, A. (2001). Urinary retention caused after fluoxetine-risperidone combination. *J. Psychopharmacol.*, **15**, 142–3.

Braconnier, A., Le Coent, R., and Cohen, D. (2003). Paroxetine versus clomipramine in adolescents with severe major depression: a double-blind, randomized, multicenter trial. *Child Adolesc. Psychiatry*, **42**, 22–9.

Bradvik, L. (2002). The occurrence of suicide in severe depression related to the months of the year and the days of the week. *Eur. Arch. Psychiatry Clin. Neurosci.*, **252**, 28–32.

(2003). Suicide after suicide attempt in severe depression: a long-tem follow-up. *Suicide Life-Threat. Behav.*, **33**, 381–8.

Bradwejn, J. and Koszycki, D. (1994). The cholecystokinin hypothesis of anxiety and panic disorder. *Ann. N. Y. Acad. Sci.*, **713**, 273–82.

(2001). Cholecystokinin and panic disorder: past and future clinical research strategies. *Scand. J. Clin. Lab. Invest.*, **234** (suppl.), 19–27.

Brady, L. S., Whitfield, H. J., Fox, R. J., Gold, P. W., and Herkenham, M. (1991). Long-term antidepressant administration alters corticotropin-releasing hormone, tyrosine hydroxylase, and mineralocorticoid receptor gene expression in rat brain. *J. Clin. Invest.*, **87**, 831–7.

Braga, R. J. and Petrides, G. (2005). The combined use of electroconvulsive therapy and antipsychotics in patients with schizophrenia. *J. ECT*, **21**, 75–83.

Braslow, J. (1997). *Mental Ills and Bodily Cures.* Berkeley, CA: University of California Press.

Bräunig, P., Krüger, S., and Shugar, G. (1998). Prevalence and clinical significance of catatonic symptoms in mania. *Compr. Psychiatry*, **39**, 35–46.

(1999). Prävalenz und klinische Bedeutung katatoner Symptome bei Manien. [Prevalence and clinical significance of catatonic symptoms in mania.] *Fortschr. Neurol. Psychiatr.*, **67**, 306–17.

Breier, A., Charney, D. S., and Heninger, G. R. (1985). The diagnostic validity of anxiety disorders and their relationship to depressive illness. *Am. J. Psychiatry*, **142**, 787–97.

Bremner, J. D. (2003). Long-term effects of childhood abuse on brain and neurobiology. *Child Adolesc. Psychiatr. Clin. North Am.*, **12**, 271–92.

Bremner, J. D., Innis, R. B., Salomon, R. M., *et al.* (1997). Positron emission tomography measurement of cerebral metabolic correlates of tryptophan depletion-induced depressive relapse. *Arch. Gen. Psychiatry*, **54**, 364–74.

Bremner, J. D., Naraya, M., Anderson, E. R., *et al.* (2000). Hippocampal volume reduction in major depression. *Am. J. Psychiatry*, **157**, 115–18.

Brenner, I. (1978). Apathetic hyperthyroidism. *J. Clin. Psychiatry*, **39**, 479–80.

Brent, D. A. (2004). Paroxetine and the FDA. *Child Adolesc. Psychiatry*, **43**, 127–8.

Brent, D. A., Perper, J. A., Moritz, G., *et al.* (1993). The validity of diagnoses obtained through the psychological autopsy procedure in adolescent suicide victims: use of family history. *Acta Psychiatr. Scand.*, **87**, 118–22.

(1994). Major depression or uncomplicated bereavement? A follow-up of youth exposed to suicide. *J. Am. Acad. Child Adolesc. Psychiatry*, **33**, 231–9.

Brent, D. A., Bridge, J., Johnson, B. A., and Connolly, J. (1996). Suicidal behavior runs in families. *Arch. Gen. Psychiatry* **53**, 1145–52.

Brent, D. A., Baugher, M., Birmaher, B., Kolko, D. J., and Bridge, J. (2000). Compliance with recommendations to remove firearms in families participating in a clinical trial for adolescent depression. *J. Am. Acad. Child Adolesc. Psychiatry*, **39**, 1220–26.

Brent, D. A., Oquendo, M., Birmaher, B., *et al.* (2002). Familial pathways to early-onset suicide attempts: a high-risk study. *Arch. Gen. Psychiatry*, **59**, 801–7.

Brent, D. A., Oquendo, M., Birmaher, B., *et al.* (2003). Peripubertal suicide attempts in offspring of suicide attempters with siblings concordant for suicidal behavior. *Am. J. Psychiatry*, **160**, 1486–93.

Bressan, R. A., Chaves, A. C., Pilowsky, L. S., Shirakawa, I., and Mari, J. J. (2003). Depressive episodes in stable schizophrenia: critical evaluation of the DSM-IV and ICD-10 diagnostic criteria. *Psychiatry Res.*, **117**, 47–56.

Bright, T. (1586). *A Treatise of Melancholie.* London: T. Vautrollier.

Bright-Long, L. and Fink, M. (1993). Reversible dementia and affective disorder: The Rip van Winkle Syndrome. *Convuls. Ther.*, **9**, 209–16.

Broadley, A. J., Korszun, A., Jones, C. J., and Frenneaux, M. P. (2002). Arterial endothelial function is impaired in treated depression. *Heart*, **88**, 521–3.

Brockington, I. F. and Kumar, R. (1982). *Motherhood and Mental Illness.* London: Academic Press.

Brockington, I. F., Winokur, G., and Dean, C. (1982). Puerperal psychosis. In Brockington, I. F. and Kumar, R. (eds) *Motherhood and Mental Illness*, vol. 3. London: Academic Press. pp. 37–69.

Brodaty, H., Luscombe, G., Parker, G. *et al.* (1997). Increased rate of psychosis and psychomotor change in depression with age. *Psychol. Med.*, **27**, 1205–13.

Brodersen, A., Licht, R. W., Vestergaard, P., Olesen, A. V., and Mortensen, P. B. (2000). Sixteen-year mortality in patients with affective disorder commenced on lithium. *Br. J. Psychiatry*, **176**, 429–33.

Brodsky, B. S., Oquendo, M., Ellis, S. P., *et al.* (2001). The relationship of childhood abuse to impulsivity and suicidal behavior in adults with major depression. *Am. J. Psychiatry*, **158**, 1871–77.

Brody, A. L., Saxena, S., Silverman, D. H. S., *et al.* (1999). Brain metabolic changes in major depressive disorder from pre- to post-treatment with paroxetine. *Psychiatry Res.*, **91**, 127–39.

Brody, A. L., Barsom, M. W., Bota, R. G., and Saxena, S. (2001a). Prefrontal-subcortical and limbic circuit mediation of major depressive disorder. *Semin. Clin. Neuropsychiatry*, **6**, 102–12.

Brody, A. L., Saxena, S., Mandelkern, M. A., *et al.* (2001b). Brain metabolic changes associated with symptom factor improvement in major depressive disorder. *Biol. Psychiatry*, **50**, 171–8.

Brody, A. L., Saxena, S., Stoessel, P., *et al.* (2001c). Regional brain metabolic changes in patients with major depression treated with either paroxetine or interpersonal therapy. *Arch. Gen. Psychiatry*, **58**, 631–40.

Bromet, E. J., Dunn, L. O., Connell, M. M., Dew, M. A., and Schulberg, H. C. (1986). Long-term reliability of diagnosing lifetime major depression in a community sample. *Arch. Gen. Psychiatry*, **43**, 435–40.

Brook, D. W., Brook, J. S., Zhang, C., Cohen, P., and Whiteman, M. (2002). Drug use and the risk of major depressive disorder, alcohol dependence, and substance use disorders. *Arch. Gen. Psychiatry*, **59**, 1039–44.

Brown, G. W. and Harris, T. (1978). *Social Origins of Depression.* New York: Free Press.

Brown, W. A. (1990). What happened to the DST? *Curr. Contents S&BS*, **22**, 12–13.

Brown, W. A., and Shuey, I. (1980). Response to dexamethasone and subtype of depression. *Arch. Gen. Psychiatry*, **37**, 747–51.

Brown, W. A., Johnston, R., and Mayfield, D. (1979). The 24-hour dexamethasone suppression test in a clinical setting: relationship to diagnosis, symptoms, and response to treatment. *Am. J. Psychiatry*, **136**, 543–7.

Brown, R. P., Mason, B., Stoll, P., *et al.* (1986). Adrenocortical function and suicidal behavior in depressive disorders. *Psychiatry Res.*, **17**, 317–23.

Brown, G. K., Beck, A. T., Steer, R. A., and Grisham, J. R. (2000). Risk factors for suicide in psychiatric outpatients: a 20-year prospective study. *J. Consult. Clin. Psychol.*, **68**, 371–7.

Brown, G. W. and Moran, P. (1994). Clinical and psychosocial origins of chronic depressive episodes I: a community survey. *Br. J. Psychiatry*, **165**, 447–56.

Brown, R. P., Stoll, P. M., Stokes, P. E., *et al.* (1988). Adrenocortical hyperactivity in depression: effects of agitation, delusions, melancholia, and other illness variables. *Psychiatry Res.*, **23**, 167–78.

Brown, S. J., Fann, J. R., and Grant, I. (1994). Post-concussion disorder: time to acknowledge a common source of neurobehavioral morbidity. *J. Neuropsychiatry Clin. Neurosci.*, **6**, 15–22.

Brown, T. A., Chorpita, B. F., and Barlow, D. H. (1998). Structural relationships among dimensions of the DSM-IV anxiety and mood disorders and dimensions of negative affect, positive affect, and autonomic arousal. *J. Abnorm. Psychol.*, **107**, 179–92.

Bruce, M. L. (2002). Psychosocial risk factors for depressive disorders in late life. *Biol. Psychiatry*, **52**, 175–84.

Bruder, G., Fong, R., Tenke, C., *et al.* (1997). Regional brain asymmetries in major depression with or without an anxiety disorder: a quantitative electroencephalographic study. *Biol. Psychiatry*, **41**, 939–48.

Bruder, G. E., Towey, J. P., Stewart, J. W., *et al.* (1991). Event-related potentials in depression: influence of task, stimulus hemifield and clinical features on P3 latency. *Biol. Psychiatry*, **30**, 233–46.

Bruijn, J. A., Moleman, P., Mulder, P. G., and van den Broek, W. W. (2001). Treatment of mood-congruent psychotic depression with imipramine. *J. Affect. Disord.*, **66**, 165–74.

Brunello, N., Armitage, R., Feinberg, I., *et al.* (2000). Depression and sleep disorders: clinical relevance, economic burden and pharmacological treatment. *Neuropsychobiology* **42**, 107–19.

Brymer, C. and Winograd, C. H. (1992). Fluoxetine in elderly patients: is there cause for concern? *J. Am. Geriatr. Soc.*, **40**, 902–5.

Bschor, T., Berghofer, A., Strohle, A., *et al.* (2002). How long should the lithium augmentation strategy be maintained? A 1-year follow-up of a placebo controlled study in unipolar refractory depression. *J. Clin. Psychopharmacol.*, **22**, 427–30.

Bschor, T., Baethge, C., Adli, M., *et al.* (2003). Association between response to lithium augmentation and the combined DEX/CRH test in major depressive disorder. *J. Psychiatr. Res.*, **37**, 135–43.

Buchan, H., Johnstone, E., McPherson, K., *et al.* (1992). Who benefits from electroconvulsive therapy? Combined results of the Leicester and Northwick Park trials. *Br. J. Psychiatry*, **160**, 355–9.

Buchholtz-Hansen, P. E., Wang, A. G., and Kragh-Sorensen, P. (1993). Mortality in major affective disorder: relationship to subtype of depression. The Danish University Antidepressant Group. *Acta Psychiatr. Scand.*, **87**, 329–35.

Buchkowsky, S. S. and Jewesson, P. J. (2004). Industry sponsorship and authorship of clinical trials over 20 years. *Ann. Pharmacother.*, **38**, 579–85.

Buchsbaum, M. S., Wu, J., Siegel, B. V., *et al.* (1997). Effect of sertraline on regional metabolic rate in patients with affective disorder. *Biol. Psychiatry*, **41**, 15–22.

Buckwalter, J. G., Buckwalter, D. K., Bluestein, B. W., and Stanczyk, F. Z. (2001). Pregnancy and postpartum: changes in cognition and mood. *Prog. Brain Res.*, **133**, 303–19.

Buerger, K., Zinkowski, R., Teipel, S. J., *et al.* (2003). Differentiation of geriatric major depression from Alzheimer's disease with CSF tau protein phosphorylated at threonine 231. *Am. J. Psychiatry*, **160**, 376–93.

Buijs, R. M., van Eden, C. G., Goncharuk, V. D., and Kalsbeek, A. (2003). Circadian and seasonal rhythms. The biological clock tunes the organs of the body: timing by hormones and the autonomic nervous system. *J. Endocrinol.*, **177**, 17–26.

Bukstein, O. G., Brent, D. A., Perper, J. A., *et al.* (1993). Risk factors for completed suicide among adolescents with a lifetime history of substance abuse: a case-control study. *Acta Psychiatr. Scand.*, **88**, 403–8.

Bull, S. A., Hu, X. H., Hunkeler, E. M., *et al.* (2002). Discontinuation of use and switching of antidepressants: influence of patient–physician communication. *J.A.M.A.*, **288**, 1403–9.

Bunney, W. E. and Bunney, B. G. (2000). Molecular clock genes in man and lower animals: possible implications for circadian abnormalities in depression. *Neuropsychopharmacol.*, **22**, 335–45.

Burg, M. M. and Abrams, D. (2001). Depression in chronic medical illness: the case of coronary heart disease. *J. Clin. Psychol.*, **57**, 1323–37.

Burke, W. J. (2004). Selective versus multi-transmitter antidepressants: are two mechanisms better than one? *J. Clin. Psychiatry*, **65** (suppl. 4), 37–45.

Burnham, M. M., Goodlin-Jones, B. L., Gaylor, E. E., and Anders, T. F. (2002). Nighttime sleep-wake patterns and self-soothing from birth to one year of age: a longitudinal intervention study. *J. Child Psychol. Psychiatry*, **43**, 713–25.

Burt, D. B., Zembar, M. J., and Niederehe, G. (1995). Depression and memory impairment: a meta-analysis of the association, its pattern, and specificity. *Psychol. Bull.*, **117**, 285–305.

Burt, T., Lisanby, S. H., and Sackeim, H. A. (2002). Neuropsychiatric applications of transcranial magnetic stimulation: a meta analysis. *Int. J. Neuropsychopharmacol.*, **5**, 73–103.

Burt, V. K., Suri, R., Altshuler, L., *et al.* (2001). The use of psychotropic medications during breast-feeding. *Am. J. Psychiatry*, **158**, 1001–9.

Burton, R. (1904). *The Anatomy of Melancholy.* London: George Bell.

Busch, K. A., Fawcett, J., and Jacobs, D. G. (2003). Clinical correlates of inpatient suicide. *J. Clin. Psychiatry*, **64**, 14–19.

Buysse, D. J., Reynolds, C. F. 3rd, Hoch, C. C., *et al.* (1996). Longitudinal effects of nortriptyline on EEG sleep and the likelihood of recurrence in elderly depressed patients. *Neuropsychopharmacology*, **14**, 243–52.

Byrne, S. E., and Rothschild, A. J. (1998). Loss of antidepressant efficacy during maintenance therapy: possible mechanisms and treatments. *J. Clin. Psychiatry*, **59**, 279–88.

Byron (1970). *The Lament of Tasso, The Complete Poetical Works.* Oxford: Oxford University Press.

Calabrese, J. R. (2004). Depression mood stabilisation: novel concepts of clinical management. *Eur. Neuropsychopharmacol.*, **14**, (suppl. 2), S100–S107.

Calabrese, J. R., Bowden, C. L., McElroy, S. L., *et al.* (1999a). Spectrum of activity of lamotrigine in treatment-refractory bipolar disorder. *Am. J. Psychiatry*, **156**, 1019–23.

Calabrese, J. R., Bowden, C. L., Sachs, G. S., *et al.* (1999b). A double-blind placebo-controlled study of lamotrigine monotherapy in outpatients with bipolar I depression. Lamictal 602 Study Group. *J. Clin. Psychiatry*, **60**, 79–88.

Calabrese, J. R., Elhaj, O., Gajwani, P., and Gao, K. (2005). Clinical highlights in bipolar depression: focus on atypical antipsychotics. *J. Clin. Psychiatry*, **66** Suppl 5, 26–33.

Calev, A., Korin, Y., Shapira, B., Kugelmass, S., and Lerer, B. (1986). Verbal and nonverbal recall by depressed and euthymic affective patients. *Psychol. Med.*, **16**, 789–94.

Caley, C. F. and Friedman, J. H. (1992). Does fluoxetine exacerbate Parkinson's disease? *J. Clin. Psychiatry*, **53**, 278–82.

Cameron, H. A. and McKay, R. D. (1999). Restoring production of hippocampal neurons in old age. *Nat. Neurosci.*, **2**, 894–7.

Cameron, O. G., Kerber, K., and Curtis, G. C. (1986). Obsessive-compulsive disorder and the DST (letter). *Psychiatry Res.*, **19**, 329–30.

Campbell, J., Nickel, E. J., Penick, E. C., *et al.* (2003a). Comparison of desipramine or carbamazepine to placebo for crack cocaine-dependent patients. *Am. J. Addict.*, **12**, 122–36.

Campbell, L. C., Clauw, D. J., and Keefe, F. J. (2003b). Persistent pain and depression: a biopsychosocial perspective. *Biol. Psychiatry*, **54**, 399–409.

Campbell, S. and Whitehead, M. (1977). Oestrogen therapy and the menopause syndrome. *Clin. Obstet. Gynecol.*, **4**, 31–47.

Candido, C. L. and Romney, D. M. (2002). Depression in paranoid and nonparanoid schizophrenic patients compared with major depressive disorder. *J. Affect. Disord.*, **70**, 261–71.

Canetti, L., Bachar, E., Bonne, O., *et al.* (2000). The impact of parental death versus separation from parents on the mental health of Israeli adolescents. *Compr. Psychiatry*, **41**, 360–8.

Cannon, W. B. (1929). *Bodily Changes in Pain, Hunger, Fear, and Rage*, 2nd edn. New York: D. Appleton.

(1939). *The Wisdom of the Body.* New York: WW Norton.

Cantor, C. H., Neulinger, K., and De Leo, D. (1999). Australian suicide trends 1964–1997: youth and beyond? *Med. J. Aust.*, **171**, 137–41.

Capps, L., Kasari, C., Yirmiya, N., and Sigman, M. (1993). Parental perception of emotional expressiveness in children with autism. *J. Consult. Clin. Psychol.*, **61**, 475–84.

Cardenas, L., Tremblay, L. K., Naranjo, C. A., *et al.* (2002). Brain reward system activity in major depression and comorbid nicotine dependence. *J. Pharmacol. Exp. Ther.*, **302**, 1265–71.

Carlson, G. A. (1998). Mania and ADHD: comorbidity or confusion. *J. Affect. Disord.*, **51**, 177–87.

Carlson, G. A. and Cantwell, D. P. (1980a). A survey of depressive symptoms syndrome and disorder in a child psychiatry population. *J. Child Psychol. Psychiatry*, **21**, 19–25.

(1980b). Unmasking masked depression in children and adolescents. *Am. J. Psychiatry*, **137**, 445–9.

Carmanico, S. J., Erickson, M. T., Singh, N. N., *et al.* (1998). Diagnostic subgroups of depression in adolescents with emotional and behavioral disorders. *J. Emotion Behav. Disord.*, **6**, 222–32.

Carney, R. M. and Jaffe, A. S. (2002). Treatment of depression following acute myocardial infarction. *J.A.M.A.*, **288**, 750–1.

Carney, M. W. P., Roth, M., and Garside, R. F. (1965). The diagnosis of depressive syndromes and the prediction of ECT response. *Br. J. Psychiatry*, **111**, 659–74.

Carney, R. M., Freedland, K. E., Veith, R. C., and Jaffe, A. S. (1999). Can treating depression reduce mortality after an acute myocardial infarction? *Psychosom. Med.*, **61**, 666–75.

Carpenter, L. L., Yasmin, S., and Price, L. H. (2002). A double-blind, placebo-controlled study of antidepressant augmentation with mirtazapine. *Biol. Psychiatry*, **51**, 183–8.

Carr, V., Dorrington, C., Schrader, G., and Wale, J. (1983). The use of ECT for mania in childhood bipolar disorder. *Br. J. Psychiatry*, **143**, 411–15.

Carrasco, G. A. and Van de Kar, L. D. (2003). Neuroendocrine pharmacology of stress. *Eur. J. Pharmacol.*, **463**, 235–72.

Carro, M. G., Grant, K. E., Gotlib, I. H., and Compas, B. E. (1993). Postpartum depression and child development: an investigation of mothers and fathers as sources of risk and resilience. Milestones in the development of resilience. *Dev. Psychopathol.*, **5**, 567–79.

Carroll, B. (1972a). The hypothalamic–pituitary–adrenal axis: functions, control mechanisms and methods of study. In Davies, B., Carroll, B. J., and Mowbray, R. M. (eds) *Depressive Illness: Some Research Studies*, vol. 3. Springfield, IL: C. C. Thomas, pp. 23–68.

(1972b). Plasma cortisol levels in depression. In: Davies, B., Carroll, B. J., and Mowbray, R. M. (eds) *Depressive Illness: Some Research Studies*, vol. 4. Springfield, IL: C. C. Thomas, pp. 69–86.

(1972c). Control of plasma cortisol levels in depression: studies with the dexamethasone suppression test. In Davies, B., Carroll, B. J., and Mowbray, R. M. (eds) *Depressive Illness: Some Research Studies*, vol. 5. Springfield, IL: C. C. Thomas, pp. 87–149.

(1972d). Studies with hypothalamic–pituitary–adrenal stimulation tests in depression. In Davies, B., Carroll, B. J., and Mowbray, R. M.. (eds) *Depressive Illness: Some Research Studies*, vol. 6. Springfield, IL: C. C. Thomas, pp. 149–201.

(1977). The hypothalamus–pituitary–adrenal axis in depression. In Burrows, G. D. (ed.) *Handbook of Studies on Depression*, vol. 18. Amsterdam: Excerpta Medica, pp. 325–42.

(1982a). The dexamethasone suppression test for melancholia. *Br. J. Psychiatry*, **140**, 292–304.

(1982b). Clinical applications of the dexamethasone suppression test for endogenous depression. *Pharmacopsychiatry*, **15**, 19–25.

(1989a). Diagnostic validity and laboratory studies: rules of the game. In Robins, L. N. and Barrett, J. E. (eds) *The Validity of Psychiatric Diagnosis.* New York: Raven Press, pp. 229–45.

(1989b). Combining laboratory and clinical criteria for depression. *Curr. Contents*, **41**, 14.

(2005). Can the Institute of Medicine review the FDA? *Nature Med.*, **11**, 369.

Carroll, B. J. and Mendels, J. (1978). Neuroendocrine regulation in affective disorders. In Sachar, E. J. (ed.) *Hormones, Behavior and Psychopathology.* New York: Raven Press, pp. 193–224.

Carroll, B. J., Martin, F. I. R., and Davies, B. (1968). Resistance to suppression by dexamethasone of plasma 11-OHCS levels in severe depressive illness. *Br. Med. J.*, 285–7.

Carroll, B. J., Curtis, G. C., and Mendels, J. (1976a). Neuroendocrine regulation in depression. I. Limbic system–adrenocortical dysfunction. *Arch. Gen. Psychiatry*, **33**, 1039–44.

(1976b). Neuroendocrine regulation in depression. II. Discrimination of depressed from nondepressed patients. *Arch. Gen. Psychiatry*, **33**, 1051–58.

Carroll, B. J., Feinberg, M., Greden, J. F., *et al.* (1980a). Diagnosis of endogenous depression. Comparison of clinical, research and neuroendocrine criteria. *J. Affect. Disord.*, 177–94.

Carroll, B. J., Greden, J. F., and Feinberg, M. (1980b). Suicide, neuroendocrine dysfunction and CSF 5-HIAA concentrations in depression. In Angrist, B. (ed.) *Recent Advances in Neuropsychopharmacology: Proceedings of the 12th CINP Congress.* Oxford, UK: Pergamon Press, pp. 307–13.

Carroll, B. J., Feinberg, M., Greden, J. F., *et al.* (1981a). A specific laboratory test for the diagnosis of melancholia. *Arch. Gen. Psychiatry*, **38**, 15–22.

Carroll, B. J., Feinberg, M., Smouse, P. E., Rawson, S. G., and Greden, J. F. (1981b). The Carroll rating scale for depression. I. Development, reliability and validation. *Br. J. Psychiatry*, **138**, 194–200.

Carroll, L. (2002). *Alice's Adventures in Wonderland and Through the Looking Glass.* New York: Modern Library, p. 186.

Carson, A. J., MacHale, S., Allen, K., *et al.* (2000). Depression after stoke and lesion location: a systematic review. *Lancet*, **356**, 122–6.

Casacalenda, N., Perry, J. C., and Looper, K. (2002). Remission in major depressive disorder: a comparison of pharmacotherapy, psychotherapy, and control conditions. *Am. J. Psychiatry*, **159**, 1354–60.

Casey, B. J., Giedd, J. N., and Thomas, K. M. (2000). Structural and functional brain development and its relation to cognitive development. *Biol. Psychol.*, **54**, 241–57.

Casey, P., Dowrick, C., and Wilkinson, G. (2001). Adjustment disorders. Fault line in the psychiatric glossary. *Br. J. Psychiatry*, **179**, 479–81.

Caspi, A., Sugden, K., Moffitt, T. E., *et al.* (2003). Influence of life stress on depression: moderation by a polymorphism in the 5-HTT gene. *Science*, **301**, 386–9.

Cassano, G. B., Rucci, P., Frank, E., *et al.* (2004). The mood spectrum in unipolar and bipolar disorder: arguments for a unitary approach. *Am. J. Psychiatry*, **161**, 1264–9.

Cassidy, F., Ritchie, J. C., and Carroll, B. J. (1998). Plasma dexamethasone concentration and cortisol response during manic episodes. *Biol. Psychiatry*, **43**, 747–54.

Catalano, G., Catalano, M. C., Epstein, M. A., and Tsambiras, P. E. (2001). QTc interval prolongation associated with citalopram overdose: a case report and literature review. *Clin. Neuropharmacol.*, **24**, 158–62.

Catapano, F., Monteleone, P., Maj, M., and Kemali, D. (1990). Dexamethasone suppression test in patients with primary obsessive-compulsive disorder and in healthy controls. *Neuropsychobiology*, **23**, 53–6.

Cavanagh, J. T. O., Carson, A. J., Sharpe, M., and Lawrie, S. M. (2003). Psychological autopsy studies of suicide: a systematic review. *Psychol. Med.*, **33**, 395–405.

Ceccatelli, S., Fahrenkrug, J., Villar, M. J., and Hokfelt, T. (1991). Vasoactive intestinal polypeptide/peptide histidine isoleucine immunoreactive neuron systems in the basal hypothalamus of the rat with special reference to the portal vasculature: an immunohistochemical and in situ hybridization study. *Neuroscience*, **43**, 483–502.

Cecil, D. (1988). *The Stricken Deer: The Life of Cowper* (1929 reprint). London: Constable.

Cecil, K. M., DelBello, M. P., Morey, R., and Strakowski, S. M. (2002). Frontal lobe differences in bipolar disorder as determined by proton MR spectroscopy. *Bipolar Disord.*, **4**, 357–65.

Celada, P., Puig, M. V., Martin-Ruiz, R., Casanovas, J. M., and Artigas, F. (2002). Control of the serotonergic system by the medial prefrontal cortex: potential role in the etiology of PTSD and depressive disorders. *Neurotox. Res.*, **4**, 409–19.

Cervantes, P., Gelber, S., Kin, F., Nair, V. N. P., and Schwartz, G. (2001). Circadian secretion of cortisol in bipolar disorder. *J. Psychiatry Neurosci.*, **26**, 411–16.

Chabrol, H., Teissedre, F., Saint-Jean, M., *et al.* (2002a). Prevention and treatment of postpartum depression: a controlled randomized study on women at risk. *Psychol. Med.*, **32**, 1039–47.

(2002b). Detection, prevention and treatment of postpartum depression: controlled study of 859 patients. *Encephale*, **28**, 65–70.

Chae, J. H., Nahas, Z., Lomarev, M., *et al.* (2003). A review of functional neuroimaging studies of vagus nerve stimulation (VNS). *J. Psychiatr. Res.*, **37**, 443–55.

Chalmers, D. T., Kwak, S. P., Mansow, A., Akil, H., and Watson, S. J. (1993). Corticosteroids regulate brain hippocampal 5-HTIA receptor mRNA expression. *J. Neurosci.*, **13**, 914–23.

Chamberlain, S., Hahn, P. M., Casson, P., and Reid, R. L. (1990). Effect of menstrual cycle phase and oral contraceptive use on serum lithium levels after a loading dose of lithium in normal women. *Am. J. Psychiatry*, **147**, 907–9.

Chambers, C. D., Johnson, K. A., Dick, L. M., Felix, R. J., and Jones, K. L. (1996). Birth outcomes in pregnant women taking fluoxetine. *N. Engl. J. Med.*, **335**, 1010–15.

Chan, C. H., Janicak, P. G., Davis, J. M., *et al.* (1987). Response of psychotic and nonpsychotic depressed patients to tricyclic antidepressants. *J. Clin. Psychiatry*, **48**, 197–200.

Channon, S. (1996). Executive dysfunction in depression: the Wisconsin Card Sorting Test. *J. Affect. Disord.*, **39**, 107–14.

Channon, S. and Green, P. S. (1999). Executive function in depression: the role of performance strategies in aiding depressed and nondepressed participants. *J. Neurol. Neurosurg. Psychiatry*, **66**, 162–71.

Chapotot, F., Gronfier, C., Jouny, C., Muzet, A., and Bradenberger, G. (1998). Cortisol secretion is related to electroencephalographic alertness in human subjects during daytime wakefulness. *J. Clin. Endocrinol. Metab.*, **83**, 4263–8.

Charlson, M. and Peterson, J. C. (2002). Medical comorbidity and late life depression: what is known and what are the unmet needs? *Biol. Psychiatry*, **52**, 226–35.

Charney, D. (1996). Double-blind study on the effects of pindolol addition to accelerate the antidepressant response (abstract). *Eur. Neuropsychopharmcol.*, **6**, 17.

Charney, D. S. and Babich, K. S. (2002). Foundation for the NIMH strategic plan for mood disorders research. *Biol. Psychiatry*, **52**, 455–6.

Charney, D. and Nelson, J. C. (1981). Delusional and nondelusional unipolar depression: further evidence for distinct subtypes. *Am. J. Psychiatry*, **138**, 328–33.

Charney, D. S. and Redmond, D. E. (1983). Neurobiological mechanisms in human anxiety. Evidence supporting central noradrenergic hyperactivity. *Neuropharmacology*, **22**, 1531–6.

Chaudron, L. H., Klein, M. H., Remington, P., *et al.* (2001). Predictors, prodromes and incidence of postpartum depression. *J. Psychosom. Obstet. Gynaecol.*, **22**, 103–12.

Cheetham, S. C., Crompton, M. R., Katona, C. L., Parker, S. J., and Horton, R. W. (1988). Brain GABA A/benzodiazepine binding sites and glutamic acid decarboxylase activity in depressed suicide victims. *Brain Res.*, **460**, 114–23.

Cheetham, S. C., Crompton, M. R., Katone, C. L., and Horton, R. W. (1990). Brain 5-HT 1 binding sites in depressed suicides. *Psychopharmacol.* **102**, 544–8.

Chen, A. C., Shin, K. H., Duman, R. S., and Sanacora, G. (2001a). ECS-induced mossy fiber sprouting and BDNF expression are attenuated by ketamine pretreatment. *J. ECT.*, **17**, 27–32.

Chen, B., Dowlatshahi, D., MacQueen, G. M., Wang, J. F., and Young, L. T. (2001b). Increased hippocampal BDNF immunoreactivity in subjects treated with antidepressant medication. *Biol. Psychiatry*, **50**, 260–5.

Chen, C. Y., Wagner, F. A., and Anthony, J. C. (2002). Marijuana use and the risk of major depressive episode. Epidemiological evidence from the United States National Comorbidity Survey. *Soc. Psychiatry Psychiatr. Epidemiol.*, **37**, 199–206.

Chen, L., Eaton, W. W., Gallo, J. J., and Nestadt, G. (2000). Understanding the heterogeneity of depression through the triad of symptoms, course, and risk factors; a longitudinal population-based study. *j. Affect. Disord.*, **59**, 1–11.

Chen, Y. W. and Dilsaver, S. C. (1996). Lifetime rates of suicide attempts among subjects with bipolar and unipolar disorders relative to subjects with other axis I disorders. *Biol. Psychiatry*, **39**, 896–9.

Cheng, A. T., Chen, T. H. H., Chen, C. C., and Jenkins, R. (2000). Psychosocial and psychiatric risk factors for suicide: case-control psychological autopsy study. *Br. J. Psychiatry*, **177**, 360–5.

Chisholm, D., Sanderson, K., Ayuso-Mateos, J. L., and Saxena, S. (2004). Reducing the global burden of depression. Population-level analysis of intervention cost-effectiveness in 14 world regions. *Br. J. Psychiatry*, **184**, 393–403.

Choudhry, N. K., Stelfox, H. T., and Detsky, A. S. (2002). Relationships between authors of clinical practice guidelines and the pharmaceutical industry. *J.A.M.A.*, **287**, 612–17.

Chu, J. W., Matthias, D. F., Belanoff, J., *et al.* (2001). Successful long-term treatment of refractory Cushing's disease with high-dose mifepristone (RU 486). *J. Clin. Endocrinol. Metab.*, **86**, 3568–73.

Chung, T. K., Lau, T. K., Yip, A. S., Chiu, H. F., and Lee, D. T. (2001). Antepartum depressive symptomatology is associated with adverse obstetric and neonatal outcomes. *Psychosom. Med.*, **63**, 830–4.

Cipriani, A., Barbui, C., and Geddes, J. R. (2005). Suicide, depression, and antidepressants (editorial). *Br. Med. J.*, **330**, 373–4.

Cizadlo, B. C. and Wheaton, A. (1995). ECT treatment of a young girl with catatonia: a case study. *J. Am. Acad. Child Adolesc. Psychiatry*, **34**, 332–5.

Clark, C. P., Frank, L. R., and Brown, G. G. (2001). Sleep deprivation, EEG, and functional MRI in depression: preliminary results. *Neuropsychopharm.*, 25 (suppl. 5), S79–S84.

Clark, L. A. and Watson, D. (1991). Tripartite model of anxiety and depression: psychometric evidence and taxonomic implications. *J. Abnorm. Psychol.*, **100**, 316–36.

Clark, N. A. and Alexander, B. (2000). Increased rate of trazodone prescribing with bupropion and selective serotonin-reuptake inhibitors versus tricyclic antidepressants. *Ann. Pharmacother.*, **34**, 1007–12.

Claxton, A. J., Li, Z., and McKendrick, J. (2000). Selective serotonin reuptake inhibitor treatment in the UK: risk of relapse or recurrence of depression. *Br. J. Psychiatry*, **177**, 163–8.

Clayton, P. (1982). Bereavement. In Paykel, E. S. (ed.) *Handbook of Affective Disorders*. New York: Guilford Press, pp. 403–15.

Cleare, A. J., Murray, R. M., and O'Keane, V. (1997). Do noradrenergic reuptake inhibitors affect serotonergic function in depression? *Psychopharmacology*, **134**, 406–10.

Clerc, G. E., Ruimy, P., and Verdeau-Palles, J. (1994). A double-blind comparison of venlafaxine and fluoxetine in patients hospitalized for major depression and melancholia. The Venlafaxine French Inpatient Study Group. *Int. Clin. Psychopharmacol.*, **9**, 139–43.

Cloninger, C. R. (1987). A systematic method for clinical description and classification of personality variants: a proposal. *Arch. Gen. Psychiatry*, **44**, 573–88.

Cohen, D., Paillère-Martinot, M. L., and Basquin, M. (1997). Use of electroconvulsive therapy in adolescents. *Convuls. Ther.*, **13**, 25–31.

Cohen, D., Taieb, O., Flament, M., *et al.* (2000a). Absence of cognitive impairment at long term follow-up in adolescents treated with ECT for severe mood disorders. *Am. J. Psychiatry*, **157**, 460–2.

Cohen, L. S., Friedman, J. M., Jefferson, J. W., Johnson, M., and Weiner, M. L. (1994). A reevaluation of risk of in utero exposure to lithium. *J.A.M.A.*, **271**, 146–50.

Cohen, L. S., Heller, V. L., Bailey, J. W., *et al.* (2000b). Birth outcomes following prenatal exposure to fluoxetine. *Biol. Psychiatry*, **48**, 996–1000.

Cohen, L. S., Soares, C. N., Poitras, J. R., *et al.* (2003). Short-term use of estradiol for depression in perimenopausal and postmenopausal women: a preliminary report. *Am. J. Psychiatry*, **160**, 1519–22.

Cohen, O., Rais, T., Lepkifker, E., and Vered, I. (1998). Lithium carbonate therapy is not a risk factor for osteoporosis. *Horm. Metab. Res.*, **30**, 594–7.

Cohen, R. M., Gross, M., Nordahl, T. E., *et al.* (1992). Preliminary data on the metabolic brain pattern of patients with winter seasonal affective disorder. *Arch. Gen. Psychiatry*, **49**, 545–52.

Cohn, J. B., Collins, G., Ashbrook, E., and Wernicke, J. F. (1989). A comparison of fluoxetine, imipramine and placebo in patients with bipolar depressive disorder. *Int. Clin. Psychopharmacol.*, **4**, 313–22.

Cole, J. O., Branconnier, R., Solomon, M., and Dessain, E. (1983). Tricyclic use in the cognitively impaired elderly. *J. Clin. Psychiatry*, **44**, 14–19.

Cole, M. G., Elie, L. M., McCusker, J., Bellavance, F., and Mansour, A. (2001). Feasibility and effectiveness of treatments for post-stroke depression in elderly inpatients: systematic review. *J. Geriatr. Psychiatry Neurol.*, **14**, 37–41.

Cole, M. G. and Dendukuri, N. (2003). Risk factors for depression among elderly community subjects: a systematic review and meta-analysis. *Am. J. Psychiatry*, **160**, 1147–56.

Combes, A., Peytavin, G., and Theron, D. (2001). Conduction disturbances associated with venlafaxine. *Ann. Intern. Med.*, **134**, 166–7.

Conca, A., Hrubos, W., Di Pauli, J., König, P., and Hausmann, A. (2004). ECT response after relapse during continuation repetitive transcranial magnetic stimulation. A case report. *Eur. Psychiatry*, **19**, 118–19.

Condon, J. T. (1993). The premenstrual syndrome: a twin study. *Br. J. Psychiatry*, **162**, 481–6.

Conner, K. R., Duberstein, P. R., Conwell, Y., *et al.* (2000). After the drinking stops: completed suicide in individuals with remitted alcohol use disorders. *J. Psychoact. Drugs*, **32**, 333–7.

Conrad, M. and Hammen, C. (1989). Role of maternal depression in perceptions of child maladjustment. *J. Consult. Clin. Psychol.*, **57**, 663–7.

Consensus Conference (1985). Electroconvulsive therapy. *J.A.M.A.*, **254**, 103–8.

Conwell, Y., Olsen, K., Caine, E. D., and Flannery, C. (1991). Suicide in later life: psychological autopsy findings. *Int. Psychogeriatr.*, **3**, 59–66.

Conwell, Y., Duberstein, P. R., Cox, and C., *et al.* (1996). Relationships of age and axis I diagnoses in victims of completed suicide: a psychological autopsy study. *Am. J. Psychiatry*, **153**, 1001–8.

Conwell, Y., Lyness, J. M., Duberstein, P., *et al.* (2000). Completed suicide among older patients in primary care practices: a controlled study. *J. Am. Geriatr. Soc.*, **48**, 23–9.

Conwell, Y., Duberstein, P. R., and Caine, E. D. (2002). Risk factors for suicide in later life. *Biol. Psychiatry*, **52**, 193–204.

Cook, L. C. (1938). The range of mental reaction states influenced by cardiozol convulsions. *J. Ment. Sci.*, **84**, 664–7.

Cooper, J. (1981). Is oestrogen therapy effective in the treatment of menopausal depression? *J. R. Coll. Gen. Pract.*, **31**, 134–40.

Cooper, J. E., Kendell, R. E., Gurland, B. J., *et al.* (1972). *Psychiatric Diagnosis in New York and London: A Comparative Study of Mental Hospital Admissions.* Maudsley monograph 20. London: Oxford University Press.

Cooper, P. J., Murray, L., Wilson, A., and Romaniuk, H. (2003). Controlled trial of the short- and long-term effect of psychological treatment of post-partum depression. I. Impact on maternal mood. *Br. J. Psychiatry*, **182**, 412–19.

Cooper-Patrick, L., Crum, R. M., and Ford, D. E. (1994). Identifying suicidal ideation in general medical patients. *J.A.M.A.*, **272**, 1757–62.

Copeland, J. R. (1985). Depressive illness and morbid distress. Onset and development data examined against five-year outcome, *Br. J. Psychiatry*, **146**, 297–307.

Coplan, J., Andrews, M., Rosenbaum, L., *et al.* (1996). Persistent elevations of CSF concentrations of CRF in adult non-human primates exposed to early life stressors: implications for the pathophysiology of mood and anxiety disorders. *Proc. Natl Acad. Sci. USA*, **93**, 1619–23.

Copper, R. L., Goldenberg, R. L., Das, A., *et al.* (1996). The preterm prediction study: maternal stress is associated with spontaneous preterm birth at less than thirty-five weeks gestation. *Am. J. Obstet. Gynecol.*, **175**, 1286–92.

Corey-Lisle, P. K., Nash, R., Stang, P., and Swindle, R. (2004). Response, partial reresponse, and nonresponse in primary care treatment of depression. *Arch. Intern. Med.*, **164**, 1197–204.

Cornelius, J. R., Salloum, I. M., Mezzich, J., *et al.* (1995). Disproportionate suicidality in patients with comorbid major depression and alcoholism. *Am. J. Psychiatry*, **152**, 358–64.

Cornelius, J. R., Salloum, I. M., Ehler, J. G., *et al.* (1997a). Double-blind fluoxetine in depressed alcoholic smokers. *Psychopharmacol. Bull.*, **33**, 165–70.

(1997b). Fluoxetine treatment in depressed alcoholics: a double-blind, placebo-controlled study. *Arch. Gen. Psychiatry*, **54**, 700–5.

Cornelius, J. R., Salloum, I. M., Lynch, K., Clark, D. B., and Mann, J. J. (2001). Treating the substance-abusing suicidal patient. *Ann. NY Acad. Sci.*, **932**, 78–90.

Corral, M., Kuan, A., and Kostaras, D. (2000). Bright light therapy's effect on postpartum depression. *Am. J. Psychiatry*, **157**, 303–4.

Correa, H., Campi-Azevedo, A. C., De Marco, L., *et al.* (2004). Familial suicide behaviour: association with probands suicide attempt characteristics and 5-HTTLPR polymorphism. *Acta Psychiatr. Scand.*, **110**, 459–64.

Corrigan, M. H., Denahan, A. Q., Wright, C. E., Ragual, R. J., and Evans, D. L. (2000). Comparison of pramipexole, fluoxetine, and placebo in patients with major depression. *Depress. Anxiety*, **11**, 58–65.

Corruble, E., Berlin, I., Lemoine, A., and Hardy, P. (2004). Should major depression with 'high normal' thyroid-stimulating hormone be treated preferentially with tricyclics? *Neuropsychobiology*, **50**, 144–6.

Corsi-Cabrera, M., Arce, C., Ramos, J., and Guevera, M. (1997a). Effects of spatial ability and sex on inter- and intrahemispheric correlation of EEG activity. *Electroencephalogr. Clin. Neurophysiol.*, **102**, 5–11.

Corsi-Cabrera, M., Solis-Ortiz, S., and Guevara, M. A. (1997b). Stability of EEG inter- and intrahemispheric correlation in women. *Electroencephalogr. Clin. Neurophysiol.*, **102**, 248–55.

Corya, S. A., Andersen, S. W., Detke, H. C., *et al.* (2003). Long-term antidepressant efficacy and safety of olanzapine/fluoxetine combination: a 76-week open-label study. *J. Clin. Psychiatry*, **64**, 1349–56.

Coryell, W. (1982). Hypothalamic–pituitary–adrenal axis abnormality and ECT response. *Psychiatry Res.*, **6**, 283–91.

(1986). Are serial dexamethasone suppression tests useful in electroconvulsive therapy? *J. Affect. Disord.*, **10**, 59–66.

(1990). DST abnormality as a predictor of course in major depression. *J. Affect. Disord.*, **19**, 163–9.

Coryell, W. and Schlesser, M. A. (1981). Suicide and the dexamethasone suppression test in unipolar depression. *Am. J. Psychiatry*, **138**, 1120–11.

(2001). The dexamethasone suppression test and suicide prediction. *Am. J. Psychiatry*, **158**, 748–53.

Coryell, W. and Winokur, G. (1992). Course and outcome. In Paykel, E. S. (ed.) *Handbook of Affective Disorders, 2nd ed.* Edinburgh: Churchill Livingstone, pp. 89–108.

Coryell, W. and Young, W. A. (2005). Clinical predictors of suicide in primary major depressive disorder. *J. Clin. Psychiatry*, **66**, 412–17.

Coryell, W. and Zimmerman, M. (1983). The dexamethasone suppression test and ECT outcome: a six-month follow-up. *Biol. Psychiatry*, **18**, 21–7.

(1984). Outcome following ECT for primary unipolar depression: a test of newly proposed response predictors. *Am. J. Psychiatry*, **141**, 862–7.

Coryell, W., Endicott, J., Reich, T., Andreasen, N., and Keller, M. (1984). A family study of bipolar II disorder. *Br. J. Psychiatry*, **145**, 49.

Coryell, W., Endicott, J., Andreasen, N., and Keller, M. (1985a). Bipolar I, bipolar II, and nonpolar major depression among the relatives of affectively ill probands. *Am. J. Psychiatry*, **142**, 817–21.

Coryell, W., Noyes, R. Jr., Clancy, J., Crowe, R., and Chaudhry, D. (1985b). Abnormal escape from dexamethasone suppression in agoraphobia with panic attacks. *Psychiatry Res.*, **15**, 301–11.

Coryell, W., Noyes, R. J. R.., and Schlechte, J. (1989b). The significance of HPA axis disturbance in panic disorder. *Biol. Psychiatry*, 1989b; **25**, 989–1002.

Coryell, W., Endicott, J., and Winokur, G. (1992). Anxiety syndromes as epiphenomena of primary major depression. Outcome and familial psychopathology. *Am. J. Psychiatry*, **149**, 100–7.

(1995a). Characteristics and significance of untreated major depressive disorder. *Am. J. Psychiatry*, **152**, 1124–9.

Coryell, W., Endicott, J., Maser, J. D., *et al.* (1995b). Long-term stability of polarity distinctions in the affective disorders. *Am. J. Psychiatry*, **152**, 385–90.

Coryell, W. H., Black, D. W., Kelly, M. W., and Noyes, R. Jr. (1989a). HPA axis disturbance in obsessive-compulsive disorder. *Psychiatry Res.*, **30**, 243–51.

Costa, P. T. and Widiger, T. A. (eds) (1994). *Personality Disorders and the Five-Factor Model of Personality.* Washington, DC: American Psychological Association.

Costa e Silva, J. (1998). Randomized, double-blind comparison of venlafaxine and fluoxetine in outpatients with major depression. *J. Clin. Psychiatry*, **59**, 352–7.

Coste, S. C., Kesterson, R. A., Heldwein, K. A., *et al.* (2000). Abnormal adaptations to stress and impaired cardiovascular function in mice lacking corticotropin-releasing hormone receptor-2. *Nat. Genet.*, **24**, 403–9.

Costei, A. M., Kozer, E., Ho, T., Ito, S., and Koren, G. (2002). Perinatal outcome following third trimester exposure to paroxetine. *Arch. Pediatr. Adolesc. Med.*, **156**, 1129–32.

Costello, E. J., Angold, A., and Sweeney, M. E. (1998). Comorbidity with depression in children and adolescents. In Tohen, M. (ed.) *Comorbidity in Affective Disorders.* New York: Marcel Dekker, pp. 179–96.

Courtney, D. B. (2004). Selective serotonin reuptake inhibitor and venlafaxine use in children and adolescents with major depressive disorder: a systematic review of published randomized controlled trials. *Can. J. Psychiatry*, **49**, 557–63.

Couturier, J. L. (2005). Efficacy of rapid-rate repetitive transcranial magnetic stimulation in the treatment of depression: a systematic review and meta-analysis. *J. Psychiatry Neurosci.*, **30**, 83–90.

Covey, L., Glassman, A. H., and Stetner, F. (1998). Cigarette smoking and major depression. *J. Addict. Disord.*, **17**, 35–46.

Covey, L. S., Glassman, A. H., Stetner, F., Rivelli, S., and Stage, K. (2002). A randomized trial of sertraline as a cessation aid for smokers with a history of major depression. *Am. J. Psychiatry*, **159**, 1731–7.

Cox, B. J., Enns, M. W., and Larsen, D. K. (2001). The continuity of depression symptoms: use of cluster analysis for profile identification in patient and student samples. *J. Affect. Disord.*, **65**, 67–73.

Craufurd, D., Thompson, J. C., and Snowden, J. S. (2001). Behavioral changes in Huntington disease. *Neuropsychiatry Neuropsychol. Behav. Neurol.*, **14**, 219–26.

Critchley, M. (1953). *The Parietal Lobes.* New York: Hafner.

Critchlow, D. G., Bond, A. J., and Wingrove, J. (2001). Mood disorder history and personality assessment in premenstrual dysphoric disorder. *J. Clin. Psychiatry*, **62**, 688–93.

Croop, R. S., Faulkner, E. B., Labriola, D. F., for The Naltrexone Usage Study Group (1997). The safety profile of naltrexone in the treatment of alcoholism. Results from a multicenter usage study. *Arch. Gen. Psychiatry*, **54**, 1130–5.

Cross-National Collaborative group (1992). The changing rate of depression: Cross-national comparisons. *J.A.M.A.*, **268**, 3098–105.

Crow, S., Meller, W., Christenson, G., and Mackenzie, T. (1996). Use of ECT after brain injury. *Convuls. Ther.*, **12**, 113–16.

Curtis, A. L. and Valentino, R. J. (1994). Corticotropin-releasing factor neurotransmission in locus ceruleus: a possible site of antidepressant action. *Brain Res. Bull.*, **35**, 581–7.

Cushing, H. (1932). The basophil adenomas of the pituitary body and their clinical manifestations (pituitary basophiliom). *Johns Hopkins Bull.*, **50**, 177.

Cuthill, F. M., Espie, C. A., and Cooper, S. A. (2003). Development and psychometric properties of the Glasgow Depression Scale for people with a learning disability. *Br. J. Psychiatry*, **182**, 347–53.

Czeh, B., Michaelis, T., Watanabe, T., *et al.* (2001). Stress-induced changes in cerebral metabolites, hippocampal volume, and cell proliferation are prevented by antidepressant treatment with tianeptine. *Proc. Natl Acad. Sci.*, **98**, 12796–801.

Daimon, K., Yamada, N., Tsujimoto, T., and Takahashi, S. (1992). Circadian rhythm abnormalities of deep body temperature in depressive disorders. *J. Affect. Disord.*, **26**, 191–8.

Dalton, K. (1989). Successful prophylactic progesterone for idiopathic postnatal depression. *Int. J. Prenat. Perinat. Stud.*, **1**, 323–7.

Dalton, S. O., Johansen, C., Mellemkjaer, L., *et al.* (2003). Use of selective serotonin reuptake inhibitors and risk of upper gastrointestinal tract bleeding: a population-based cohort study. *Arch. Intern. Med.*, **163**, 59–64.

Daly, J. M. and Wilens, T. (1998). The use of tricyclic antidepressants in children and adolescents. *Pediatr. Clin. Am.*, **45**, 1123–35.

Dam, H. (2001). Depression in stroke patients 7 years following stroke. *Acta Psychiatr. Scand.*, **103**, 287–93.

Danish University Antidepressant Group (1986). Citalopram: clinical effect profile in comparison with clomipramine: a controlled multicenter study. *Psychopharmacology (Berl).*, **90**, 131–8.

(1990). Paroxetine: a selective serotonin reuptake inhibitor showing better tolerance, but weaker antidepressant effect than clomipramine in a controlled multicenter study. *J. Affect. Disord.*, **18**, 289–99.

(1993). Moclobemide: a reversible MAO-A-inhibitor showing weaker antidepressant effect than clomipramine in a controlled multicenter study. *J. Affect. Disord.*, **28**, 105–16.

(1999). Clomipramine dose–effect study in patients with depression: clinical end points and pharmacokinetics. *Clin. Pharmacol. Ther.*, **66**, 152–65.

Dannon, P. N., Dolberg, O. T., Schreiber, S., and Grunhaus, L. (2002). Three and six-month outcome following courses of either ECT or rTMS in a population of severely depressed individuals – preliminary report. *Biol. Psychiatry*, **51**, 687–90.

Das, A. K., Olfson, M., Gameroff, M. J., *et al.* (2005). Screening for bipolar disorder in a primary care practice. *J.A.M.A.*, **293**, 956–63.

Datta, S., Patterson, E. H., Vincitore, M., *et al.* (2000). Prenatal protein malnourished rats show changes in sleep/wake behavior as adults. *J. Sleep Res.*, **9**, 71–9.

Dauge, V. and Lena, I. (1998). CCK in anxiety and cogniture processes. *Neurosci. Behav. Res.*, **2**, 815–25.

Davidson, J., Lipper, S., Zung, W. W., *et al.* (1984a). Validation of four definitions of melancholia by the dexamethasone suppression test. *Am. J. Psychiatry*, **141**, 1220–3.

Davidson, J., Strickland, R., Turnbull, C., Belyea, M., and Miller, R. D. (1984b). The Newcastle Endogenous Depression Diagnostic Index: validity and reliability. *Acta Psychiatr. Scand.*, **69**, 220–30.

Davidson, J., Turnbull, C. D., Strickland, R., Miller, R., and Graves, K. (1986). The Montgomery-Asberg Depression Scale: reliability and validity. *Acta Psychiatr. Scand.*, **73**, 544–8.

Davidson, J., Zisook, S., Giller, E., and Helms, M. (1989). Symptoms of interpersonal sensitivity in depression. *Compr. Psychiatry*, **30**, 357–68.

Davidson, J. R., Meoni, P., Haudiquet, V., Cantillon, M., and Hackett, D. (2002). Achieving remission with venlafaxine and fluoxetine in major depression: its relationship to anxiety symptoms. *Depress. Anxiety*, **16**, 4–13.

Davidson, K. M. and Blackburn, I. M. (1998). Co-morbid depression and drinking outcome in those with alcohol dependence. *Alcohol Alcohol.*, **33**, 482–7.

Davidson, R. (1998). Affective style and affective disorders: perspectives from affective neuroscience. *Cognition Emotion*, **12**, 307–30.

Davidson, R. J. (1995). Cerebral asymmetry, emotion, and affective style. In Davidson, R. J., and Hugdahl, K. (eds) *Brain Asymmetry*. Cambridge, MA: MIT Press, pp. 361–87.

Davidson, R. J. and Henriques, J. B. (2000). Regional brain function in sadness and depression. In Borod, J. (ed.) *The Neuropsychology of Emotion*. New York: Oxford University Press, pp. 269–97.

Davidson, R. J. and Slagter, H. A. (2000). Probing emotion in the developing brain: functional neuroimaging in the assessment of the neural substrates of emotion in normal and disordered children and adolescents. *Ment. Retard. Dev. Disabil. Res. Rev.*, **6**, 166–70.

Davidson, R. J., Putnam, K. M., and Larson, C. L. (2000). Dysfunction in the neural circuitry of emotion regulation – a possible prelude to violence. *Science*, **289**, 591–4.

Davies, B. J., Carroll, B. J., and Mowbray, R. M. (1972). *Depressive Illness: Some Research Studies*. Springfield, IL: C. C. Thomas.

Davis, M. (1992). The role of the amygdala in conditioned fear. In Aggleton, J. P. (ed.) *The Amygdala: Neurobiological Aspects of Emotion*. New York: Wiley-Liss, pp. 255–305.

Davis, L. L., Kabel, D., Patel, D., *et al.* (1996). Valproate as an antidepressant in major depressive disorder. *Psychopharmacol. Bull.*, **32**, 647–52.

Dawson, G. (1994). Frontal electroencephalographic correlates of individual differences in emotion expression in infants: a brain systems perspective on emotion. *Monogr. Soc. Res. Child Dev.*, **59**, 135–51.

Dawson, G., Klinger, L. G., Panagiotides, H., Hill, D., and Spieker, S. (1992). Frontal lobe activity and affective behavior of infants of mothers with depressive symptoms. *Child Dev.*, **63**, 725–37.

Dawson, G., Hessl, D., and Frey, K. (1994). Social influences on early developing biological and behavioral systems related to risk for affective disorder. *Dev. Psychopathology*, **6**, 759–79.

Dazzi, L., Serra, M., Spiga, F., *et al.* (2001). Prevention of the stress-induced increase in frontal cortical dopamine efflux of freely moving rats by long-term treatment with antidepressant drugs. *Eur. Neuropsychopharmacol.*, **11**, 343–9.

Deas, D., Randall, C. L., Roberts, J. S., and Anton, R. F. (2000). A double-blind, placebo-controlled trial of sertraline in depressed adolescent alcoholics: a pilot study. *Hum. Psychopharmacol.*, **15**, 461–9.

DeBattista, C. and Mueller, K. (2001). Is electroconvulsive therapy effective for the depressed patient comorbid with borderline personality disorder? *J. ECT*, **17**, 91–8.

DeBattista, C., Solvason, H. B., and Spiegel, D. (1998). ECT in dissociative disorder and comorbid depression. *J. ECT*, **14**, 275–9.

DeBellis, M. D., Dahl, R. E., Perel, J. M., *et al.* (1996). Nocturnal ACTH, cortisol, growth hormone, and prolactin secretion in prepubertal depression. *J. Am. Acad. Child Adolesc. Psychiatry*, **35**, 1130–8.

DeBellis, M. D., Keshavan, M. S., Clark, D. B., *et al.* (1999). Developmental traumatology: part II. Brain development. *Biol. Psychiatry*, **45**, 1271–84.

Debener, S., Beauducel, A., Nessler, D., *et al.* (2000). Is resting anterior EEG alpha asymmetry a trait marker for depression? *Neuropsychobiology*, **41**, 31–7.

De Carolis, V., Gubert, F., Roccataguata, G., *et al.* (1964). Imipramina ed electroshock nella terapia delle depression: analysi clinico-statistica dei resultati in 437 casi. *Sistema Nervosó*, **1**, 29–42.

DeGiorgio, C. M., Schachter, S. C., Handforth, A., *et al.* (2000). Projective long-term study of vagus nerve stimulation for the treatment of refractory seizures. *Epilepsia*, **41**, 1195–200.

de Jonghe, F., Hendriksen, M., van Aalst, G., *et al.* (2004). Psychotherapy alone and combined with pharmacotherapy in the treatment of depression. *Br. J. Psychiatry*, **185**, 37–45.

de Kemp, E. C. M., Moleman, P., Hoogduin, C. A. L., *et al.* (2002). Diagnosis at the first episode to differentiate antidepressant treatment responses in patients with mood and anxiety disorders. *Psychopharmacology*, **160**, 67–73.

de la Fuente-Fernandez, R. and Stoessl, A. J. (2002). The placebo effect in Parkinson's disease. *Trends Neurosci.*, **25**, 302–6.

Delay, J. (1946). *L'Electro-Choc et la Psycho-Physiologie.* Paris: Masson.

DelBello, M. P., Carlson, G. A., Tohen, M., *et al.* (2003). Rates and predictors of developing a manic or hypomanic episode 1 to 2 years following a first hospitalization for major depression with psychotic features. *J. Child Adolesc. Psychopharmacol.*, **13**, 173–85.

Delgado, P. L. (2000a). Approaches to the enhancement of patient adherence to antidepressant medication treatment. *J. Clin. Psychiatry*, **61** (suppl. 2), 6–9.

(2000b). Depression: the case for a monoamine deficiency. *J. Clin. Psychiatry*, **61**, 7–11.

Delgado, P. L., Miller, H. L., Salomon, R. M., *et al.* (1993). Monoamines and the mechanism of antidepressant action: effects of catecholamine depletion on mood of patients treated with antidepressants. *Psychopharmacol. Bull.*, **29**, 389–96.

D'Elia, G. and Raotma, H. (1975). Is unilateral ECT less effective than bilateral ECT? *Br. J. Psychiatry*, **126**, 83–9.

Delmas-Marsalet, P. (1943). *L'Electro-Choc Therapeutique et la Dissolution-Reconstruction.* Paris: J-B Bailliere.

Delva, N. J., Brunet, D., Hawken, E., *et al.* (2000). Electrical dose and seizure threshold: relations to clinical outcome and cognitive effects of bifrontal, bitemporal, and right unilateral ECT. *J. ECT*, **16**, 361–9.

Demitrack, M. A. (1997). Neuroendocrine correlates of chronic fatigue syndrome: a brief review. *J. Psychiatr. Res.*, **31**, 69–82.

de Montigny, C., Silverstone, P. H., Debonnel, G., Blier, P., and Bakish, D. (1995). Venlafaxine in treatment-resistant major depression: a Canadian multicenter, open-label study. *J. Clin. Psychopharmitacol.*, **19**, 401–6.

Demyttenaere, K. and De Fruyt, J. (2003). Getting what you ask for: on the selectivity of depression rating scales. *Psychother. Psychosom.*, **72**, 61–70.

Denihan, A., Kirby, M., Bruce, I., *et al.* (2000). Three-year prognosis of depression in the community-dwelling elderly. *Br. J. Psychiatry*, **176**, 453–7.

Depression Guideline Panel (1993). *Depression in Primary Care*, vol. 2. Treatment of Major Depression. Clinical practice guideline number 5: AHCPR publication 93–0551. Rockville, MD: US Department of Health and Human Services. Public Health Service, Agency for Health Care Policy and Research.

DeRubeis, R., Gelfand, L., Tang, T., and Simons, A. (1999). Medications versus cognitive behavioral therapy for severely depressed outpatients: mega-analysis of four randomized comparisons. *Am. J. Psychiatry*, **156**, 1007–13.

Desan, P. H., Oren, D. A., Malison, R., *et al.* (2000). Genetic polymorphism at the *CLOCK* gene locus and major depression. *Am. J. Med. Genet.*, **96**, 418–21.

Devanand, D. P. (2002). Comorbid psychiatric disorders in late life depression. *Biol. Psychiatry*, **52**, 236–42.

Devanand, D. P., Decina, P., Sackeim, H. A., *et al.* (1987). Serial dexamethasone suppression tests in initial suppressors and nonsuppressors treated with electroconvulsive therapy. *Biol. Psychiatry*, **22**, 463–72.

Devanand, D. P., Sackeim, H. A., Lo, E. S., *et al.* (1991). Serial dexamethasone suppression tests and plasma dexamethasone levels. Effects of clinical response to electroconvulsive therapy in major depression. *Arch. Gen. Psychiatry*, **48**, 525–33.

Devanand, D. P., Nobler, M. S., Singer, T., *et al.* (1994). Is dysthymia a different disorder in the elderly? *Am. J. Psychiatry*, **151**, 1592–9.

Dew, M. A., Reynolds, C. F. 3rd, Buysse, D. J., *et al.* (1996). Electroencephalographic sleep profiles during depression. Effects of episode duration and other clinical and psychosocial factors in older adults. *Arch. Gen. Psychiatry*, **53**, 148–56.

De Wied, D. and Weijnen, J. A. W. M. (eds) (1970). *Pituitary, Adrenal and the Brain.* Amsterdam: Elsevier.

D'haenen, H., Bossuyt, A., Mertens, J., *et al.* (1992). SPECT imaging of serotonin2 receptors in depression. *Psychiatry Res.*, **45**, 227–37.

Dhossche, D. M., Ulusarac, A., and Syed, W. (2001). A retrospective study of general hospital patients who commit suicide shortly after being discharged from the hospital. *Arch. Intern. Med.*, **161**, 991–4.

Di Chiara, G., Loddo, P., and Tanda, G. (1999). Reciprocal changes in prefrontal and limbic dopamine responsiveness to adverse and rewarding stimuli after chronic mild stress: implications for the psychobiology of depression. *Biol. Psychiatry*, **46**, 1624–33.

Dickens, C., McGowan, L., Clark-Carter, D., and Creed, F. (2002). Depression in rheumatoid arthritis: a systematic review of the literature with meta-analysis. *Psychosom. Med.*, **64**, 52–60.

Diego, M. A., Field, T., Hernandez-Reif, M., *et al.* (2004). Prepartum, postpartum, and chronic depression effects on newborns. *Psychiatry*, **67**, 63–80.

Dierick, M., Ravizza, L., Realini, R., and Martin, A. (1996). A double-blind comparison of venlafaxine and fluoxetine for treatment of major depression in outpatients. *Prog. Neuropsychopharmacol. Biol. Psychiatry*, **20**, 57–71.

Dierker, L. C., Merikangas, K. R., and Szatmari, P. (1999). Influence of parental concordance for psychiatric disorders on psychopathológy in offspring. *J. Am. Acad. Child Adolesc. Psychiatry*, **38**, 280–8.

Dierker, L. C., Avenevoli, S., Stolar, M., and Merikangas, K. R. (2002). Smoking and depression: an examination of mechanisms of comorbidity. *Am. J. Psychiatry*, **159**, 947–53.

Dietrich, D. E. and Emrich, H. M. (1998). The use of anticonvulsants to augment antidepressant medication. *J. Clin. Psychiatry*, **59** (suppl. 5), 51–8.

Ding, Z. and White, P. F. (2002). Anesthesia for electroconvulsive therapy. *Anesth. Analg.*, **94**, 1351–64.

Dixit, A. R. and Crum, R. M. (2000). Prospective study of depression and the risk of heavy alcohol use in women. *Am. J. Psychiatry*, **157**, 751–8.

Dolan, R. J., Bench, C. J., Brown, R. G., *et al.* (1992). Regional cerebral blood flow abnormalities in depressed patients with cognitive impairment. *J. Neurol. Neurosurg. Psychiatry*, **55**, 678–773.

Dolan, R. J., Bench, C. J., Liddle, P. F., *et al.* (1993). Dorsolateral prefrontal cortex dysfunction in the major psychoses: symptom or disease specificity? *J. Neurol. Neurosurg. Psychiatry*, **56**, 1290–4.

Dolan, R. J., Bench, C. J., Brown, R. G., Scott, L. C., and Frackowiak, R. S. (1994). Neuropsychological dysfunction in depression: the relationship to regional cerebral blood flow. *Psychol. Med.*, **24**, 849–57.

Donovan, S., Clayton, A., Beeharry, M., *et al.* (2000). Deliberate self-harm and antidepressant drugs. Investigation of a possible link. *Br. J. Psychiatry*, **177**, 551–6.

Dorpat, T. L., Anderson, W. F., and Ripley, H. S. (1968). The relationship of physical illness to suicide. In Resnik, H. P. L. (ed.) *Suicidal Behaviors: Diagnosis and Management.* Boston: Little, Brown, pp. 209–19.

Dorz, S., Borgherini, G., Conforti, D., Scarso, C., and Magni, G. (2003). Depression in inpatients: bipolar vs unipolar. *Psychol. Rep.*, **92**, 1031–9.

Doucet, J., Chassagne, P., Trivalle, C., *et al.* (1996). Drug–drug interactions related to hospital admissions in older adults: a prospective study of 1000 patients. *J. Am. Geriatr. Soc.*, **44**, 944–8.

Downey, G. and Coyne, J. C. (1990). Children of depressed parents: an integrative review. *Psychol. Bull.*, **108**, 50–76.

Downing, R. W. and Rickels, K. (1974). Mixed anxiety–depression. Fact or myth? *Arch. Gen. Psychiatry*, **30**, 312–17.

Dowrick, C., Lehtinen, V., Dalgard, O. S., *et al.* (2001). Depressive disorders in Europe: prevalence figures from the ODIN study. *Br. J. Psychiatry*, **179**, 308–16.

Drevets, W. C. (1998). Functional neuroimaging studies of depression: the anatomy of melancholia. *Annu. Rev. Med.*, **49**, 341–61.

(1999a). Prefrontal cortical-amygdalar metabolism in major depression. *In Advancing from the Ventral Striatum to the Extended Amygdala: Implications for Neuropsychiatry and Drug Abuse.* New York: New York Academy of Science, pp. 614–37.

(1999b). Integration of structural and functional neuroimaging in depression research. In Dougherty, D., and (ed.) *Psychiatric Neuroimaging Strategies: Research and Clinical Applications.* Washington, DC: American Psychiatric Press.

(2000a). Neuroimaging studies of mood disorders. *Biol. Psychiatry*, **48**, 813–29.

(2000b). Functional anatomical abnormalities in limbic and prefrontal cortical structures in major depression. *Prog. Brain Res.*, **126**, 413–31.

Drevets, W. C. and Botteron, K (1997). Neuroimaging in psychiatry. In Guze, S. B. (ed.) *Adult Psychiatry.* St. Louis, MO: Mosby, pp. 53–81.

Drevets, W. C., Videen, T. O., Price, J. L., *et al.* (1992). A functional anatomical study of unipolar depression. *J. Neurosci.*, **12**, 3628–41.

Drevets, W. C., Simpson, J. R. Jr, and Raichle, M. E. (1995). Regional blood flow changes in response to phobic anxiety and habituation (abstract). *J. Cerebral Blood Flow Metab.*, **15** (suppl. 1), S856.

Drevets, W. C., Sptiznagel, E., and Raichle, M. E. (1995b). Functional anatomical differences between major depressive subtypes. *J. Cerebral Blood Flow Metab.*, **15**, S93.

Drevets, W. C., Price, J. L., Simpson, J. R., *et al.* (1997a). Subgenual prefrontal cortex abnormalities in mood disorders. *Nature*, **386**, 824–7.

Drevets, W. C., Price, J. L., Todd, R. D., *et al.* (1997b). PET measures of amygdala metabolism in bipolar and unipolar depression: correlation with plasma cortisol. *Soc. Neurosci. Abstr.*, **23**, 1407.

Drevets, W. C., Frank, E., Price, J. C., *et al.* (1999). PET imaging of serotonin 1A receptor binding in depression. *Biol. Psychiatry*, **46**, 1375–87.

Drevets, W. C., Price, J. L., Bardgett, M. E., *et al.* (2002). Glucose metabolism in the amygdala in depression: relationship to diagnostic subtype and plasma cortisol levels. *Pharmacol. Biochem. Behav.*, **71**, 431–47.

Driver, H. S., Dijk, D.-J., Werth, E., Biedermann, K., and Borbely, A. A. (1996). Sleep and the sleep electroencephalogram across the menstrual cycle in young healthy women. *J. Clin. Endocrinol. Metab.*, **81**, 728–35.

Du, L., Faludi, G., Palkovits, M., Bakish, D., and Hrdina, P. D. (2001). Serotonergic genes and suicidality. *Crisis*, **22**, 54–60.

Duberstein, P. R. (2001). Are closed-minded people more open to the idea of killing themselves? *Suicide Life Threat Behav.*, **31**, 9–14.

Duffy, A., Grof, P., Robertson, C., and Alda, M. (2000). The implications of genetic studies of major mood disorders in clinical practice. *J. Clin. Psychiatry*, **61**, 630–7.

Duffy, J. D. (1995). General paralysis of the insane: neuropsychiatry's first challenge. *J. Neuropsychiatry Clin. Neurosci.*, **7**, 243–9.

Dugovic, C., Maccari, S., Weibel, L., Turek, F. W., and Van Reeth, O. (1999). High corticosterone levels in prenatally stressed rats predict persistent paradoxical sleep alterations. *J. Neurosci.*, **19**, 8656–64.

Duman, R. S. (2002). Synaptic plasticity and mood disorders. *Mol. Psychiatry*, **7**, S29–S34.

Duman, R. S., Heninger, G. R., and Nestler, E. J. (1997). A molecular and cellular hypothesis of depression. *Arch. Gen. Psychiatry*, **54**, 597–606.

Duman, R. S., Malberg, J., and Thome, J. (1999). Neural plasticity to stress and antidepressant treatment. *Biol. Psychiatry*, **46**, 1181–91.

Duncan, W. C. Jr. (1996). Circadian rhythms and the pharmacology of affective illness. *Pharmacol Ther.*, **71**, 253–312.

Dunn, A. J., Powell, M. L., Meitin, C., and Small, P. A. Jr. (1989). Virus infection as a stressor: influenza virus elevates plasma concentrations of corticosterone, and brain concentrations of MHPG and tryptophan. *Physiol. Behav.*, **45**, 591–4.

Dunn, C. G. and Quinlan, D. (1978). Indicators of ECT response and non-response in the treatment of depression. *J. Clin. Psychiatry*, **39**, 620–2.

Dunner, D. L. and Dunbar, G. C. (1992). Optimal dose regimen for paroxetine. *J. Clin. Psychiatry*, **53** (suppl.), 21–6.

Dunner, D. L., Gershon, E. S., and Goodwin, G. K. (1976). Heritable factors in the severity of affective illness. *Biol. Psychiatry*, **11**, 31–42.

Dwivedi, Y., Roberts, R., Conley, R. C., Tamminga, C., and Pandey, G. N. (2000). Protein kinase A in the postmortem brain of suicide victims. *Biol. Psychiatry*, **47**, 248.

Dyke, H. J. and Montana, J. G. (2002). Update on the therapeutic potential of PDE4 inhibitors. *Expert Opin. Inves. Drugs*, **11**, 1–13.

Eastman, C. I., Lahmeyer, H. W., Watell, L. G., Good, G. D., and Young, M. A. (1992). A placebo-controlled trial of light treatment for winter depression. *J. Affect. Disord.*, **26**, 211–21.

Eastman, C. I., Young, M. A., Fogg, L. F., Liu, L., and Meaden, P. M. (1998). Bright light treatment of winter depression: a placebo-controlled trial. *Arch. Gen. Psychiatry*, **55**, 883–9.

Eaton, W. W. and Kessler, L. G. (eds) (1985). *Epidemiologic Field Methods in Psychiatry: The NIMH Epidemiologic Catchment Area Program*. New York: Academic Press.

Eaton, W. W., Dryman, A., Sorenson, A., and McCutcheon, A. (1989). DSM-III major depressive disorder in the community. A latent class analysis of data from the NIMH epidemiologic catchment area program. *Br. J. Psychiatry*, **155**, 48–54.

Eberhard-Gran, M., Eskild, A., Tambs, K., Schei, B., and Opjordsmoen, S. (2001). The Edinburgh Postnatal Depression Scale: validation in a Norwegian community sample. *Nord. J. Psychiatry*, **55**, 113–17.

Eberhard-Gran, M., Eskild, A., Tambs, K., Samuelsen, S. O., and Opjordsmoen, S. (2002). Depression in postpartum and non-postpartum women: prevalence and risk factors. *Acta Psychiatr. Scand.*, **106**, 426–33.

Ebner, K., Wotjak, C. T., Landgraf, R., and Engelmann, M. (2000). A single social defeat experience selectively stimulates the release of oxytocin, but not vasopressin, within the septal brain area of male rats. *Brain Res.*, **872**, 87–92.

Echevarria, M. M., Martin, M. J., Sanchez, V. J., and Vazquez, G. T. (1998). Electroconvulsive therapy in the first trimester of pregnancy. *J. ECT*, **14**, 251–4.

Egeland, J. and Sussex, J. (1985). Suicide and family loading for affective disorders. *J.A.M.A.*, **254**, 915–18.

Ehrlich, S., Noam, G. G., Lyoo, I. K., *et al.* (2004). White matter hyperintensities and their associations with suicidality in psychiatrically hospitalized children and adolescents. *J. Am. Acad. Child Adolesc. Psychiatry*, **43**, 770–6.

Eiden, R. D. and Leonard, K. E. (1996). Paternal alcohol use and the mother–infant relationship. *Dev. Psychopathol.*, **8**, 307–23.

Eiler, K., Schaefer, M. R., Salstrom, D., and Lowery, R. (1995). Double-blind comparison of bromocriptine and placebo in cocaine withdrawal. *Am. J. Drug Alcohol Abuse*, **21**, 65–79.

Einarson, A., Fatoye, B., Sarkar, M., *et al.* (2001). Pregnancy outcome following gestational exposure to venlafaxine: a multicenter prospective controlled study. *Am. J. Psychiatry*, **158**, 1728–30.

Elger, G., Hoppe, C., Falkai, P., Rush, A. J., and Elger, C. E. (2000). Vagus nerve stimulation is associated with mood improvements in epilepsy patients. *Epilepsy Res.*, **42**, 203–10.

Elhwuegi, A. S. (2004). Central monoamines and their role in major depression. *Prog. Neuropsychopharm. Biol. Psychiatry*, **28**, 435–51.

Elkin, I. R., Shea, M. T., Watkins, J. T., *et al.* (1989). National Institute of Mental Health Treatment of Depression Collaborative Research Program. General effectiveness of treatments. *Arch. Gen. Psychiatry*, **46**, 971–82; discussion 983.

Elliott, H. (2002). Premenstrual dysphoric disorder. A guide for the treating clinician. *N. C. Med. J.*, **63**, 72–5.

Elliott, P. J. (1988). Place aversion induced by the substance P analogue, dimethyl-C7, is not state dependent: implication of substance P in aversion. *Exp. Brain Res.*, **73**, 354–6.

Elliott, R., Sahakian, B. J., Herrod, J. J., Robbins, T. W., and Paykel, E. S. (1997). Abnormal response to negative feedback in unipolar depression: evidence for a diagnostic specific impairment. *J. Neurol. Neurosurg. Psychiatry*, **63**, 74–82.

Elsehety, A. and Bertorini, T. E. (1997). Neurologic and neuropsychiatric complications of Crohn's disease. *South Med. J.*, **90**, 606–10.

Emilien, G., Maloteaux, J. M., Seghers, A., and Charles, G. (1995). Lithium therapy in the treatment of manic-depressive illness. Present status and future perspectives: a critical review. *Arch. Int. Pharmacodyn.*, **330**, 251–78.

Emory, E., Walker, E., and Cruz, A. (1983). Fetal heart rate: II. Behavioral correlates *Psychophysiology*, **19**, 680–6.

Emslie, G. J., Rush, A. J., Weinberg, W. A., *et al.* (1997). A double-blind, randomized, placebo-controlled trial of fluoxetine in children and adolescents with depression. *Arch. Gen. Psychiatry*, **54**, 1031–7.

Endicott, J., Nee, J., Andreasen, N., *et al.* (1985). Bipolar, II. Combine or keep separate? *J. Affect. Disord.*, **8**, 17–28.

Endler, N. S. (1982). *Holiday of Darkness. A Psychologist's Personal Journey Out of His Depression.* New York: John Wiley.

Engstrom, E. L. (2003). *Clinical Psychiatry in Imperial Germany.* Ithaca, NY: Cornell University Press.

Enns, M. W., Larsen, D. K., and Cox, B. J. (2000). Discrepancies between self and observer ratings of depression. The relationship to demographic, clinical and personality variables. *J. Affect. Disord.*, **60**, 33–41.

Enoch, M. D., Trethowan, W. H., and Barker, J. C. (1967). *Some Uncommon Psychiatric Syndromes.* Bristol: John Wright.

ENRICHD Investigators (2000). Enhancing recovery in coronary heart disease patients (ENRICHD): study design and methods. *Am. Heart J.*, **139**, 1–9.

(2001). Enhancing Recovery in Coronary Heart Disease (ENRICHD) study intervention: rationale and design. *Psychosom. Med.*, **63**, 747–55.

Entsuah, A. R., Rudolph, R. L., Hackett, D., and Miska, S. (1996). Efficacy of venlafaxine and placebo during long-term treatment of depression: a pooled analysis of relapse rates. *Int. Clin. Psychopharm.*, **11**, 137–45.

Entsuah, A. R., Huang, H., and Thase, M. E. (2001). Response and remission rates in different subpopulations with major depressive disorder administered venlafaxine, selective serotonin reuptake inhibitors, or placebo. *J. Clin. Psychiatry*, **62**, 869–77.

Epperson, C. N., Terman, M., Terman, J. S., *et al.* (2004). Randomized clinical trial of bright light therapy for antepartum depression: preliminary findings. *J. Clin. Psychiatry*, **65**, 421–5.

Epperson, N., Czarkowski, K. A., Ward-O'Brien, D., *et al.* (2001). Maternal sertraline treatment and serotonin transport in breast-feeding mother–infant pairs. *Am. J. Psychiatry*, **158**, 1631–7.

Erfurth, A., Michael, N., Stadtland, C., and Arolt, V. (2002). Bupropion as add-on strategy in difficult-to-treat bipolar depressive patients. *Neuropsychobiology*, **45**, 33–6.

Ericson, A., Kullen, B., and Wilholm, B. E. (1999). Delivery outcome after the use of antidepressants in early pregnancy. *Eur. J. Clin. Pharmacol.*, **55**, 503–8.

Erlenmeyer-Kimling, L. and Cornblatt, B. (1984). Biobehavioral risk factors in children of schizophrenic parents. *J. Autism Dev. Disord.*, **14**, 357–74.

Evans, C. L., Ha, Y., Saisch, S., Ellison, Z., and Fombonne, E. (1998). Tricyclic antidepressants in adolescent depression. A case report. *Eur. Child Adolesc. Psychiatry*, **7**, 166–71.

Evans, D. L. and Nemeroff, C. B. (1983). The dexamethasone suppression test in mixed bipolar disorder. *Am. J. Psychiatry*, **140**, 615–17.

(1987). The clinical use of the dexamethasone suppression test in DSM-III affective disorders: correlation with the severe depressive subtypes of melancholia and psychosis. *J. Psychiatr. Res.*, **21**, 185–94.

Evans, D. L., Pedersen, C. A., and Tancer, M. E. (1987). ECT in the treatment of organic psychosis in Huntington's disease. *Convuls. Ther.*, **3**, 145–50.

Everitt, B. S. (1981). Biomodality and the nature of depression. *Br. J. Psychiatry*, **138**, 336–9.

Evins, A. E. (2003). Efficacy of newer anticonvulsant medications in bipolar spectrum mood disorders. *J. Clin. Psychiatry*, **64** (suppl. 8), 9–14.

Eysenck, H. J., Wakefield, J. A., and Friedman, A. F. (1983). Diagnosis and clinical assessment: the DSM-III. *Annu. Rev. Psychol.*, **34**, 167–93.

Ezquiaga, E., Ayuso Gutierrez, J. L., and Garcia Lopez, A. (1987). Psychosocial factors and episode number in depression. *J. Affect. Disord.*, **12**, 135–8.

Faber, R. and Trimble, M. R. (1991). Electroconvulsive therapy in Parkinson's disease and other movement disorders. *Move. Disord.*, **6**, 293–303.

Faber, R. A. (2003). Suicide in neurological disorders. *Neuroepidemiology*, **222**, 103–5.

Faedda, G. L., Tondo, L., Teicher, M. H., *et al.* (1993). Seasonal mood disorders. Patterns of seasonal recurrence in mania and depression. *Arch. Gen. Psychiatry*, **50**, 17–23.

Fagiolini, A. and Kupfer, D. J. (2003). Is treatment-resistant depression a unique subtype of depression? *Biol. Psychiatry*, **53**, 640–8.

Fahlke, C., Lorenz, J. G., Long, J., *et al.* (2000). Rearing experiences and stress-induced plasma cortisol as early risk factors for excessive alcohol consumption in nonhuman primates. *Alcohol Clin. Exp. Res.*, **24**, 644–50.

Fahy, S. and Lawlor, B. A. (2001). Lithium use in octogenarians. *Int. J. Geriatr. Psychiatry*, **16**, 1000–3.

Fallon, B. A. and Nields, J. A. (1994). Lyme disease: a neuropsychiatric illness. *Am. J. Psychiatry*, **151**, 1571–83.

Falret, J. P. (1854). Mémoire sur la folie circulaire. *Bull. Acad. Méd.*, **19**, 382–415.

Faltermaier-Temizel, M., Laakmann, G., Baghai, T., and Kuhn, K. (1997). Predictive factors for therapeutic success in depressive syndrome. *Nervenarzt*, **68**, 62–6.

Fann, J. R., Uomoto, J. M., and Katon, W. J. (2000). Sertraline in the treatment of major depression following mild traumatic brain injury. *J. Neuropsychiatry Clin. Neurosci.*, **12**, 226–32.

Farchione, T. R., Moore, G. J., and Rosenberg, D. R. (2002). Proton magnetic resonance spectroscopic imaging in pediatric major depression. *Biol. Psychiatry*, **52**, 86–92.

Farvolden, P., Kennedy, S. H., and Lam, R. W. (2003). Recent developments in the psychobiology and pharmacotherapy of depression: optimizing existing treatments and novel approaches for the future. *Exp. Opin. Invest. Drugs*, **12**, 65–86

Fava, G., Grandi, S., Zielezny, M., Rafanelli, C., and Canestrari, R. (1996). Four year outcome of cognitive behavioral treatment of residual symptoms in major depression. *Am. J. Psychiatry*, **153**, 945–7.

Fava, M. (2001). Augmentation and combination strategies in treatment-resistant depression. *J. Clin. Psychiatry*, **62** (suppl. 18), 4–11.

(2003). Diagnosis and definition of treatment-resistant depression. *Biol. Psychiatry*, **53**, 649–59.

Fava, M., Labbate, L. A., Abraham, M. E., and Rosenbaum, J. F. (1995). Hypothyroidism and hyperthyroidism in major depression revisited. *J. Clin. Psychiatry*, **56**, 186–92.

Fava, M., Alpert, J., Nierenberg, A., *et al.* (2002a). Double-blind study of high-dose fluoxetine versus lithium or desipramine augmentation of fluoxetine in partial responders and nonresponders to fluoxetine. *J. Clin. Psychopharmacol.*, **22**, 379–87.

Fava, M., Farabaugh, A. H., Sickinger, A. H., *et al.* (2002b). Personality disorders and depression. *Psychol. Med.*, **32**, 1049–57.

Fawcett, J., Scheftner, W. A., Fogg, L., *et al.* (1987). Time-related predictors of suicide in patient with major affective disorders: a controlled prospective study. *Am. J. Psychiatry*, **144**, 35–40.

Feifel, D., Moutier, C. Y., and Swerdlow, N. R. (1999). Attitudes toward psychiatry as a prospective career among students entering medical school. *Am. J. Psychiatry*, **156**, 1397–402.

Feighner, J. P., Robins, E., Guze, S. B., *et al.* (1972). Diagnostic criteria for use in psychiatric research. *Arch. Gen. Psychiatry*, **26**, 47–63.

Feighner, J. P., Ehrensing, R. H., Kastin, A. J., *et al.* (2000). A double-blind, placebo-controlled, efficacy, safety, and pharmacokinetic study of INN 00835, a novel antidepressant peptide, in the treatment of major depression. *J. Affect. Disord.*, **61**, 119–26.

Feinberg, M. and Carroll, B. J. (1982). Separation of subtypes of depression using discriminant analysis. I. Separation of unipolar endogenous depression from nonendogenous depression. *Br. J. Psychiatry*, **140**, 384–91.

(1984). Biological markers for endogenous depression in series and parallel. *Biol. Psychiatry*, **19**, 3–11.

Feinberg, M., Carroll, B. J., Smouse, P. E., and Rawson, S. G. (1981a). The Carroll rating scale for depression. I. Development, reliability and validation. *Br. J. Psychiatry*, **138**, 194–200.

Feinberg, M., Carroll, B. J., Smouse, P. E., and Rawson, S. G. (1981b). The Carroll rating scale for depression. III. Comparison with other rating instruments. *Br. J. Psychiatry*, **138**, 205–9.

Feinstein, A. and Feinstein, K. (2001). Depression associated with multiple sclerosis. Looking beyond diagnosis to symptom expression. *J. Affect. Disord.*, **66**, 193–8.

Fendrich, M., Warner, V., and Weissman, M. M. (1990). Family risk factors, parental depression, and psychopathology in offspring. *Dev. Psychol.*, **26**, 40–50.

Feng, P. and Ma, Y. (2002). Clomipramine suppresses postnatal REM sleep without increasing wakefulness: implications for the production of depressive behaviors. *Sleep*, **25**, 177–84.

(2003). Instrumental REM sleep deprivation in neonates leads to adult depression-like behaviors in rats. *Sleep*, **26**, 990–6.

Ferrell, M. J., Kehoe, W. A., and Jacisin, J. J. (1992). ECT during pregnancy; physiologic and pharmacologic considerations. *Convul. Ther.*, **8**, 186–200.

Feske, U., Mulsant, B. H., Pilkonis, P. A., *et al.* (2004). Clinical outcome of ECT in patients with major depression and comorbid borderline personality disorder. *Am. J. Psychiatry*, **161**, 2073–80.

Field, T., Diego, M., and Sanders, C. (2001). Adolescent depression and risk factors. *Adolescence*, **36**, 491–8.

Field, T., Fox, N., Pickens, J., Nawrocki, T., and Soutullo, D. (1995). Right frontal EEG activation in 30 to 6-month-old infants of "depressed" mothers. *Dev. Psychol.*, **31**, 358–63.

Field, T., Diego, M., Hernandez-Reif, M., *et al.* (2002a). Prenatal anger effects on the fetus and neonate. *J. Obstet. Gynaecol.*, **22**, 260–6.

Field, T., Diego, M., Hernandez-Reif, M., Schanberg, S., and Kuhn, C. (2002b). Relative right versus left frontal EEG in neonates. *Dev. Psychobiol.*, **41**, 147–55.

Field, T. M. (1998). Early interventions for infants of depressed mothers. *Pediatrics*, **102**, 1305–10.

Fieve, R. R., Platman, S. R., and Plutchik, R. R. (1968). The use of lithium in affective disorders. I. Acute endogenous depression. *Am. J. Psychiatry*, **125**, 487–91.

Fieve, R. R., Go, R., Dunner, D. L., and Elston, R. (1984). Search for biological/genetic markers in a long-term epidemiological and morbid risk study of affective disorders. *J. Psychiatr. Res.*, **18**, 425.

Figiel, G. S., Epstein, C., McDonald, W. M., *et al.* (1998). The use of rapid-rate transcranial magnetic stimulation (rTMS) in refractory depressed patients. *J. Neuropsychiatry Clin. Neurosci.*, **10**, 20–5.

Findling, R. L., Reed, M. D., and Blumer, J. L. (1999). Pharmacological treatment of depression in children and adolescents. *Paediatr. Drugs*, **1**, 161–82.

Fink, G., Sumner, B. E. H., Rosie, R., Grace, O., and Quinn, J. P. (1996). Estrogen control of central neurotransmission: effect on mood, mental state and memory. *Cell Mol. Neurobiol.*, **16**, 325–44.

Fink, M. (1969). EEG and human psychopharmacology. *Annu. Rev. Pharmacol.*, **9**, 241–58.

(1978). EEG response strategies in psychiatric diagnosis. In Spitzer, R. L. and Klein, D. F. (eds) *Critical Issues in Diagnosis*. New York: Raven Press, pp. 253–64.

(1979). *Convulsive Therapy: Theory and Practice*. New York: Raven Press.

(1986a). Neuroendocrine predictors of ECT outcome: DST and prolactin. *Ann. NY Acad. Sci.*, **462**, 30–6.

(1986b). Training in ECT. *Convuls. Ther.*, **2**, 227–30.

(1987a). ECT: as last resort treatment for resistant depression? In Zohar, J. and Belmaker, R. (eds) *Treating Resistant Depression*. New York: PMA, pp. 163–73.

(1987b). Neuroendocrine aspects of convulsive therapy. In Nemeroff C. B. and P. T. Loosen, (eds) *Handbook of Clinical Psychoneuroendocrinology*, vol. 11. New York: Guilford Press, pp. 255–65.

(1989). Electroconvulsive therapy: the forgotten option in the treatment of therapy-resistant depression. In Extein, I. (ed.) *Treatment of Tricyclic Resistant Depression*. Washington, DC: APA Press, pp. 135–50.

(1990). A trial of ECT is essential before a diagnosis of refractory depression is made. In Amsterdam, J. D. (ed.) *Refractory Depression*, vol. 2. New York: Raven Press, pp. 87–92.

(1991). Impact of the anti-psychiatry movement on the revival of ECT in the US. *Psychiatric Clin. North Am.*, **14**, 793–801.

(1993). Who should get ECT? In Coffey, C. E. (ed.) *The Clinical Science of Electroconvulsive Therapy*, vol. 1. Washington, DC: APA, pp. 3–16.

(1997). The decision to use ECT: for whom? When? In Rush, A. J. (ed.) *Mood Disorders Systematic Medication Management. Modern Problems in Pharmacopsychiatry*, vol. 25. Basel, Switzerland: Karger, pp. 203–14.

(1999a). *Electroshock: Restoring the Mind*. New York: Oxford University Press; reissued 2002 (paperback) as *Electroshock: Healing Mental Illness*.

(1999b). Delirious mania. *Bipolar Disord.*, **1**, 54–60.

(2000a). Electroshock revisited. *Am. Scientist*, **88**, 162–7.

(2000b). The interaction of delirium and seizures. *Semin. Clin. Neuropsychiatry*, **5**, 31–5.

(2000c). A clinician-researcher and ECDEU: 1959–1980. In Ban, T., Healy, D., and Shorter, E., (eds) *The Triumph of Psychopharmacology and the Story of the CINP.* Budapest: Animula, pp. 82–96.

(2001). Electroconvulsive therapy in medication-resistant depression. In Amsterdam, J., Hornig-Rohan, M., and Nierenberg, A. (eds) *Treatment-resistant Mood Disorders.*, vol. 11. Cambridge, UK: Cambridge University Press, pp. 223–38.

(2002a). The 21st century clinical evaluation of psychoactive drugs. In Ban, T., Healy, D., and Shorter, E. (eds) *From Psychopharmacology to Neuropsychopharmacology in the 1980s and the Story of CINP as Told in Autobiography.* Budapest: Animula, pp. 21–6.

(2002b). Move on! Commentary on R. Abrams: stimulus titration and ECT dosing. *J. ECT*, **18**, 11–12.

(2003a). *A Beautiful Mind* and insulin coma: social constraints on psychiatric diagnosis and treatment. *Harv. Rev. Psychiatry*, **11**, 284–90.

(2003b). ECT update: recognizing and treating psychotic depression. *J. Clin. Psychiatry*, **64**, 232–4.

(2003c). Therapy-resistant depression: when to consider ECT. Algorithm seeks respect for neglected therapy. *Curr. Psychiatry*, **2**, 49–54.

(2004). Induced seizures as psychiatric therapy: Ladislas Meduna's contributions in modern neuroscience. *J. ECT*, **20**, 133–6.

Fink, M. (2005). Should the dexamethasone suppression test be resurrected? *Acta Psychiatr. Scand.*, **112**, 245–9.

Fink, M. and Johnson, L. (1982). Monitoring the duration of electroconvulsive therapy seizures: 'cuff' and EEG methods compared. *Arch. Gen. Psychiatry*, **39**, 1189–91.

Fink, M. and Kahn, R. L. (1957). Relation of EEG delta activity to behavioral response in electroshock: quantitative serial studies. *Arch. Neurol. Psychiatry*, **78**, 516–25.

(1961). Behavioral patterns in convulsive therapy. *Arch. Neurol. Psychiatry*, **5**, 30–6.

Fink, M. and Ottosson, J. O. (1980). A theory of convulsive therapy in endogenous depression: significance of hypothalamic functions. *Psychiatry Res.*, 49–61.

Fink, M. and Sackeim, H. A. (1996). Convulsive therapy in schizophrenia. *Schizophr. Bull.*, **22**, 27–39.

Fink, M. and Taylor, M. A. (2001). The many varieties of catatonia. *Eur. Arch. Psychiatry Clin. Neurosci.*, **251**, (suppl. 1), 8–13.

(2003). *Catatonia: A Clinician's Guide to Diagnosis and Treatment.* Cambridge, UK: Cambridge University Press.

Fink, M., Klein, D. F., and Kramer, J. (1965). Clinical efficacy of chlorpromazine–procyclidine combination, imipramine and placebo in depressive disorders. *Psychopharmacologia*, **7**, 27–36.

Fink, M., Abrams, R., Bailine, S., and Jaffe, R. (1996). Ambulatory electroconvulsive therapy: report of a task force of the Association of Convulsive Therapy. *Convuls. Ther.*, **12**, 41–55.

Finkel, S. I., Richter, E. M., Clary, C. M. (1999). Comparative efficacy and safety of sertraline versus nortriptyline in major depression in patients 70 and older. *Int. Psychogeriatr.*, **11**, 85–99.

Fish, B., Marcus, J., Hans, S. L., Auerbach, J. G., and Perdue, S. (1992). Infants at risk for schizophrenia: sequelae of a genetic neurointegrative defect: a review and replication analysis of pandysmaturation in the Jerusalem infant development study. *Arch. Gen. Psychiatry*, **409**, 221–35.

Fishbain, D. A. (1999). The association of chronic pain and suicide. *Semin. Clin. Neuropsychiatry*, **4**, 221–7.

Fishbain, D. A. (2000). Evidence-based data on pain relief with antidepressants. *Ann. Med.*, **325**, 305–16.

Fitzgerald, P. B., Brown, T. L., Marston, N. A. U., *et al.* (2003). Transcranial magnetic stimulation in the treatment of depression. *Arch. Gen. Psychiatry*, **60**, 1002–8.

Flament, M. F., Lane, R. M., Zhu, R., and Ying, Z. (1999). Predictors of an acute antidepressant response to fluoxetine and sertraline. *Int. Clin. Psychopharmacol.*, **14**, 259–75.

Fleck, M. P., Poirier-Littre, M. F., Guelfi, J. D., Bourdel, M. C., and Loo, H. (1995). Factorial structure of the 17-item Hamilton Depression Rating Scale. *Acta Psychiatr. Scand.*, **92**, 168–72.

Fleiss, J. L. (1972). Classification of the depressive disorders by numerical typology. *J. Psychiatr. Res.*, **9**, 141–53.

Flint, A. J. (1998). Choosing appropriate antidepressant therapy in the elderly. A risk–benefit assessment of available agents. *Drugs Aging*, **4**, 269–80.

Flint, A. J. and Rifat, S. L. (1998a). The treatment of psychotic depression in later life: a comparison of pharmacotherapy and ECT. *Int. J. Geriatr. Psychiatry*, **13**, 23–8.

(1998b). Two-year outcome of psychotic depression in late life. *Am. J. Psychiatry*, **155**, 178–83.

(2001). Nonresponse to first-line pharmacotherapy may predict relapse and recurrence of remitted geriatric depression. *Depress. Anxiety*, **13**, 125–31.

Fochtmann, L. J. (1994). Animal studies of electroconvulsive therapy: foundation for future research. *Psychopharmacol. Bull.*, **30**, 321–444.

Folk, J. W., Kellner, C. H., Beale, M. D., Conroy, J. M., and Duc, T. A. (2000). Anesthesia for electroconvulsive therapy: a review. *J. ECT*, **16**, 157–70.

Folkerts, H. W., Michael, N., Tolle, R., *et al.* (1997). Electroconvulsive therapy vs. paroxetine in treatment-resistant depression: a randomized study. *Acta Psychiatr. Scand.*, **96**, 334–42.

Fonagy, P., Moran, G. S. and Higgitt, A. C. (1989). Insulin-dependent diabetes in children and adolescents. In Pearce, S. and Wardle, J. (eds) *The Practice of Behavioral Medicine*. Oxford, UK British Psychological Society, 1989.

Forbes, E. E., Williamson., D. E., Ryan, N. D., *et al.* (2005). Peri-sleep-onset cortisol levels in children and adolescents with affective disorders. *Biol. Psychiatry*, (in press).

Ford, M. F. (1986). Treatment of depression in Huntington's disease with monoamine oxidase inhibitors. *Br. J. Psychiatry*, **149**, 654–66.

Ford, J. M., White, P. M., Csernansky, J. G., *et al.* (1994). ERPs in schizophrenia: effects of antipsychotic medication. *Biol. Psychiatry*, **36**, 153–70.

Forsell, Y., Jorm, A. F., and Winblad, B. (1994). Association of age, sex, cognitive dysfunction, and disability with major depressive symptoms in an elderly sample. *Am. J. Psychiatry*, **151**, 1600–4.

Fossey, L., Papiernik, E., and Bydlowski, M. (1997). Postpartum blues: a clinical syndrome and predictor of postnatal depression? *J. Psychosom. Obstet. Gynaecol.*, **18**, 17–21.

Fossion, P., Staner, L., Dramaix, M., *et al.* (1998). Does sleep EEG data distinguish between UP, BPI or BPII major depressions? An age and gender controlled study. *J. Affect. Disord.*, **49**, 181–7.

Foster, R. G. (1998). Shedding light on the biological clock. *Neuron*, **20**, 829–32.

Fotiou, F., Fountoulakis, K. N., Iacovides, A., and Kaprinis, G. (2003). Pattern-reversed visual evoked potentials in subtypes of major depression. *Psychiatry Res.*, **118**, 259–71.

Fountoulakis, K. N., Iacovides, A., Nimatoudis, I., Kaprinis, G., and Lerodiakonou, C. (1999). Comparison of the diagnosis of melancholic and atypical features according to DSM-IV and somatic syndrome according to ICD-10 in patients suffering from major depression. *Eur. Psychiatry*, **14**, 426–33.

Fountoulakis, K. N., Iacovides, A., Fotiou, F., *et al.* (2004). Neurobiological and psychological correlates of suicidal attempt and thoughts of death in patients with major depression. *Neuropsychobiology*, **49**, 42–52.

Fox, H. (2001). Extended continuation and maintenance ECT for long-lasting episodes of major depression. *J. ECT*, **17**, 60–4.

Francis, D. D. and Meaney, M. J. (1999). Maternal care and the development of stress responses. *Curr. Opin. Neurobiol.*, **9**, 128–34.

Francis, P. T., Poynton, A., Lowe, S. L., *et al.* (1989). Brain amino acid concentrations and Ca^{2+}-dependent release in intractable depression assessed antemortem. *Brain Res.*, **494**, 315–44.

Frank, E., Kupfer, D. J., and Perel, J. M. (1989). Early recurrence in unipolar depression. *Arch. Gen. Psychiatry*, **46**, 397–400.

Frank, E., Kupfer, D. J., Perel, J. M., *et al.* (1990). Three-year outcomes for maintenance therapies in recurrent depression. *Arch. Gen. Psychiatry*, **47**, 1093–9.

Frank, E., Swartz, H., and Kupfer, D. (2000). Interpersonal and social rhythm therapy: managing the chaos of bipolar disorder. *Biol. Psychiatry*, **48**, 593–604.

Frank, M. G. and Heller, H. C. (1997). Neonatal treatments with the serotonin uptake inhibitors clomipramine and zimelidine, but not the noradrenaline uptake inhibitor desipramine, disrupt sleep patterns in adult rats. *Brain Res.*, **678**, 287–93.

Frankle, W. G., Perlis, R. H., Deckersbach, T., *et al.* (2002). Bipolar depression: relationship between episode length and antidepressant treatment. *Psychol. Med.*, **32**, 1417–23.

Fras, I., Litin, E. M., and Bartholomew, L. G. (1968). Mental symptoms as an aid in the early diagnosis of carcinoma of the pancreas. *Gastroenterology*, **55**, 191–8.

Frazer, A. and Hensler J. (1994). Serotonin. In Siegel, G., Agranoff, B., Albers, R., and Molinoff, P. (eds) *Basic Neurochemistry*, 5th ed. New York: Raven Press, pp. 283–308.

Freedland, K. E., Skala, J. A., Carney, R. M., *et al.* (2002). The Depression Interview and Structured Hamilton (DISH): rationale, development, characteristics, and clinical validity. *Psychosom. Med.*, **64**, 897–905.

Freedland, K. E., Rich, M. W., Skala, J. A., *et al.* (2003). Prevalence of depression in hospitalized patients with congestive heart failure. *Psychosom. Med.*, **65**, 119–28.

Freeman, C. P. (1995). *The ECT Handbook*. London: Royal College of Psychiatrists.

Freeman, E. W. (2004). Luteal phase administration of agents for the treatment of premenstrual dysphoric disorder. *CNS Drugs*, **18**, 453–68.

Freeman, L. N., Poznanski, E. O., Grossman, J. A., Buchsbaum, Y. Y., and Banegas, M. E. (1985). Psychotic and depressed children: a new entity. *J. Am. Acad. Child Psychiatry*, **24**, 95–102.

Freeman, M. P., and Stoll, A. L. (1998). Mood stabilizer combinations: a review of safety and efficacy. *Am. J. Psychiatry*, **155**, 12–21.

Freeman, M. P., Smith, K. W., Freeman, S. A., *et al.* (2002). The impact of reproductive events on the course of bipolar disorder in women. *J. Clin. Psychiatry*, **63**, 284–7.

Freemantle, N., Anderson, I. M., and Young, P. (2000). Predictive value of pharmacological activity for the relative efficacy of antidepressant drugs. Meta-regression analysis. *Br. J. Psychiatry*, **177**, 292–302.

Freis, E. (1954). Mental depression in hypertensives treated for long periods with large doses of reserpine. *N. Engl. J. Med.*, **251**, 1006–8.

Freud, S. (1984). Mourning and melancholia. In Richards, A. (ed.) *The Pelican Freud Library, 11; On Metapsychology: The Theory of Psychoanalysis*. London: Penguin, pp. 245–68.

Friedman, L. S. and Richter, E. D. (2004). Relationship between conflicts of interest and research results. *J. Gen. Intern. Med.*, **19**, 51–6.

Frodl, T., Meisenzahl, E. M., Zetzsche, T., *et al.* (2002). Hippocampal changes in patients with a first episode of major depression. *Am. J. Psychiatry*, **159**, 1112–18.

(2003). Larger amygdala volumes in first depressive episode as compared to recurrent major depression and healthy control subjects. *Biol. Psychiatry*, **53**, 338–44.

Frodl, T., Meisenzahl, E. M., Zill, P., *et al.* (2004). Reduced hippocampal volumes associated with the long variant of the serotonin transporter polymorphism in major depression. *Arch. Gen. Psychiatry*, **61**, 177–83.

Fromm, G., Amores, C., and Thies, W. (1972). Imipramine in epilepsy. *Arch. Neurol.*, **27**, 198–204.

Frommer, E. A. (1967). Treatment of childhood depression with antidepressant drugs. *Br. Med. J.*, **1**, 729–32.

Fu, Q., Heath, A. C., Bucholz, K. K., *et al.* (2002a). A twin study of genetic and environmental influences on suicidality in men. *Psychol. Med.*, **32**, 11–24.

(2002b). Shared genetic risk of major depression, alcohol dependence, and marijuana dependence: contribution of antisocial personality disorder in men. *Arch. Gen. Psychiatry*, **59**, 1125–32.

Fulton, M. K., Armitage, R., and Rush, A. J. (2000). Sleep electroencephalographic coherence abnormalities in individuals at high risk for depression: a pilot study. *Biol. Psychiatry*, **47**, 618–25.

Funkenstein, D. H., Greenblatt, M., and Solomon, H. C. (1952). An autonomic nervous system test of prognostic significance in relation to electroshock treatment. *Psychosom. Med.*, **4**, 347–62.

Furukawa, T. and Sumita, Y. (1992). A cluster-analytically derived subtyping of chronic affective disorders. *Acta Psychiatr. Scand.*, **85**, 177–82.

Furukawa, T., McGuire, H., and Barbui, C. (2002). Meta-analysis of effects and side effects of low dosage tricyclic antidepressants in depression: systematic review. *Br. Med. J.*, **325**, 991–5.

Gaab, J., Huster, D., Peisen, R., *et al.* (2002). Low-dose dexamethasone suppression test in chronic fatigue syndrome and health. *Psychosom. Med.*, **64**, 311–18.

Galynker, I. I., Cai, J., Ongseng, F., *et al.* (1998). Hypofrontality and negative symptoms in major depressive disorder. *J. Nucl. Med.*, **39**, 608–12.

Gangadhar, B. N., Kapur, R. L., and Kalyanasundram, S. (1982). Comparison of electroconvulsive therapy with imipramine in endogenous depression: a double blind study. *Br. J. Psychiatry*, **141**, 367–71.

Garbutt, J. C., Mayo, J. P., Little, K. Y., *et al.* (1994). Dose–response studies with protirelin. *Arch. Gen. Psychiatry*, **51**, 875–83.

Garcia-Toro, M., Montes, J. M., and Talavera, J. A. (2001). Functional cerebral asymmetry in affective disorders: new facts contributed by transcranial magnetic stimulation. *J. Affect. Disord.*, **66**, 103–9.

Gardner, D. M., Shulman, K. I., Walker, S. E., and Tailor, S. A. (1996). The making of a user friendly MAOI diet. *J. Clin. Psychiatry*, **57**, 99–104.

Gareri, P., Stilo, G., Bevacqua, I., *et al.* (1998). Antidepressant drugs in the elderly. *Gen. Pharmacol.*, **30**, 465–75.

Garland, A. and Scott, J. (2002). Cognitive therapy for depression in women. *Psychiatr. Ann.*, **32**, 465–76.

Gastpar, M., Singer, A., and Zeller, K. (2005). Efficacy and tolerability of hypericum extract STW3 in long-term treatment with a once-daily dosage in comparison with sertraline. *Pharmacopsychiatry*, **38**, 78–86.

Gatti, F., Bellini, L., Gasperini, M., *et al.* (1996). Fluvoxamine alone in the treatment of delusional depression. *Am. J. Psychiatry*, **153**, 414–16.

Geddes, J., Freemantle, N., Mason, J., Eccles, M. P., and Boynton, J. (2000). SSRIs versus other antidepressants for depressive disorder. *Cochrane Database Syst. Rev.* CD001851.

Gelenberg, A. J., Shelton, R. C., Crits-Christoph, P., *et al.* (2004). The effectiveness of St. John's wort in major depressive disorder in naturalistic phase 2 follow-up in which nonresponders were provided alternate medication. *J. Clin. Psychiatry*, **65**, 1114–19.

Geller, B., Farooki, Z. Q., Cooper, T. B., Chestnut, E. C., and Abel, A. S. (1985). Serial ECG measurements at controlled plasma levels of nortriptyline in depressed children. *Am. J. Psychiatry*, **142**, 1095–7.

Geller, B., Cooper, T. B., McCombs, H. G., Graham, D., and Wells, J. (1989). Double-blind, placebo-controlled study of nortriptyline in depressed children using a "fixed plasma level" design. *Psychopharm. Bull.*, **25**, 101–8.

Geller, B., Cooper, T. B., Graham, D. L., Marsteller, F. A., and Bryant, D. M. (1990). Double-blind placebo-controlled study of nortriptyline in depressed adolescents using a "fixed plasma level" design. *Psychopharm. Bull.*, **26**, 85–90.

Geller, B., Zimerman, B., Williams, M., Bolhofner, K., and Craney, J. L. (2001). Bipolar disorder at prospective follow-up of adults who had prepubertal major depressive disorder. *Am. J. Psychiatry*, **158**, 125–7.

Gelman, S. (1999). *Medicating Schizophrenia: A History.* New Brunswick, NJ: Rutgers University Press.

George, M. S. and Belmaker, R. H. (2000). *Transcranial Magnetic Stimulation in Neuropsychiatry.* Washington, DC: American Psychiatric Press.

George, M. S., Ketter, T. A., Parekh, P. I., *et al.* (1995). Brain activity during transient sadness and happiness in healthy women. *Am. J. Psychiatry*, **152**, 341–51.

George, M. S., Nahas, Z., Bohning, D. E., *et al.* (2002). Vagus nerve stimulation therapy. A research update. *Neurology*, **59**, S56–61.

Gershon, A. A., Dannon, P. N., and Grunhaus, L. (2003). Transcranial magnetic stimulation in the treatment of depression. *Am. J. Psychiatry*, **160**, 835–45.

Gershon, E. S., Hamovit, J., Guroff, J. J., *et al.* (1982). A family study of schizoaffective, bipolar I, bipolar II, unipolar and normal control probands. *Arch. Gen. Psychiatry*, **39**, 1157.

(1999a). Kindling and second messengers: an approach to the neurobiology of recurrence in bipolar disorder. *Biol. Psychiatry*, **45**, 137–44.

Ghaemi, S. N., Sachs, G. S., Chiou, A. M., Pandurangi, A. K., and Goodwin, K. (1999b). Is bipolar disorder still underdiagnosed? Are antidepressants overutilized? *J. Affect. Disord.*, **52**, 135–44.

Ghaemi, S. N., Boiman, E. E., and Goodwin, F. K. (2000). Diagnosing bipolar disorder and the effect of antidepressants: a naturalistic study. *J. Clin. Psychiatry*, **61**, 804–8.

Ghaemi, S. N., Lenox, M. S., and Baldessarini, R. J. (2001). Effectiveness and safety of long-term antidepressant treatment in bipolar disorder. *J. Clin. Psychiatry*, **62**, 565–9.

Ghaemi, S. N., Hsu, D. J., Soldani, F., and Goodwin, F. K. (2003). Antidepressants in bipolar disorder: the case for caution. *Bipolar Disord.*, **5**, 421–33.

Ghaemi, S. N., Hsu, D. J., Ko, J. Y., *et al.* (2004a). Bipolar spectrum disorder: a pilot study. *Psychopathology*, **37**, 222–6.

Ghaemi, S. N., Rosenquist, K. J., Ko, J. Y., *et al.* (2004b). Antidepressant treatment in bipolar versus unipolar depression. *Am. J. Psychiatry*, **161**, 163–5.

Ghaziuddin, M., Wiedmer-Mikhail, E., and Ghaziuddin, N. (1998). Comorbidity of Asperger syndrome: a preliminary report. *J. Intellect. Disabil. Res.*, **4**, 279–83.

Ghaziuddin, M., Ghaziuddin, N., and Greden, J. (2002a). Depression in persons with autism: implications for research and clinical care. *J. Autism Dev. Disord.*, **32**, 299–306.

Ghaziuddin, N. (1998). Use of electroconvulsive therapy in childhood psychiatric disorders. *Child Adolesc. Psychopharm. News*, **3**, 1–8.

Ghaziuddin, N., Alkhouri, I., Champine, D., *et al.* (2002b). ECT treatment of malignant catatonia/NMS in an adolescent: a useful lesson in delayed diagnosis and treatment. *J. ECT*, **18**, 95–8.

Gibbons, R. D., Clark, D. C., and Kupfer, D. J. (1993). Exactly what does the Hamilton Depression Rating Scale measure? *J. Psychiatr. Res.*, **27**, 259–73.

Giedke, H. and Schwarzler, F. (2002). Therapeutic use of sleep deprivation in depression. *Sleep Med. Rev.*, **6**, 361–77.

Giedke, H., Klingberg, S., Schwarzler, F., and Schweinsberg, M. (2003). Direct comparison of total sleep deprivation and late partial sleep deprivation in the treatment of major depression. *J. Affect. Disord.*, **76**, 85–93.

Gilbody, S., Whitty, P., Grimshaw, J., and Thomas, R. (2003). Educational and organizational interventions to improve the management of depression in primary care. A systematic review. *J.A.M.A.*, **289**, 3145–51.

Gill, D. and Hatcher, S. (2000). Antidepressants for depression in people with physical illness. *Cochrane Database Syst. Rev.*, CD001312.

Gillespie, R. D. (1926). Discussion on manic-depressive psychosis. *Br. Med. J.*, **2**, 878–9.

(1929). The clinical differentiation of types of depression. *Guy's Hosp. Rep.*, **2**, 306–44.

Gillin, J. C., Buchsbaum, M., Wu, J., Clark, C., and Bunney, W. Jr. (2001). Sleep deprivation as a model experimental antidepressant treatment: findings from functional brain imaging. *Depress. Anxiety*, **14**, 37–49.

Gillis, M. C. (ed.) (1998). *Compendium of Pharmaceuticals and Specialties, 31st Edn. Ottawa, Ontario: Canadian Pharmaceutical Association.*

Gilman, S. E., Kawachi, I., Fitzmaurice, G. M., and Buka, S. L. (2003). Family disruption in childhood and risk of adult depression. *Am. J. Psychiatry*, **160**, 939–46.

Gilmore, M. L., Skelton, K. H., Nemeroff, C. B., and Owens, M. J. (2003). The effects of chronic treatment with mood stabilizers valproic acid and lithium on corticotropin-releasing factor neuronal systems. *J. Pharmacol. Exp. Ther.*, **305**, 434–9.

Gilmore, W. S. (2001). Anticonvulsants in the treatment of mood disorders: assessing current and future roles. *Exp. Opin. Pharmacother.*, **2**, 1597–608.

Gitlin, M. J. and Pasnau, R. O. (1989). Psychiatric syndromes linked to reproductive function in women: a review of current knowledge. *Am. J. Psychiatry*, **146**, 1413–22.

Gladstone, G. L., Mitchell, P. B., Parker, G., *et al.* (2001). Indicators of suicide over 10 years in a specialist mood disorders unit sample. *J. Clin. Psychiatry*, **62**, 945–51.

Glassman, A., Kantor, S. J., and Shostak, M. (1975). Depression, delusions and drug response. *Am. J. Psychiatry*, **132**, 716–19.

Glassman, A. H. (2005). Does treating post-myocardial infarction depression reduce medical mortality? *Arch. Gen. Psychiatry*, **62**, 711–12.

Glassman, A. H. and Roose, S. P. (1981). Delusional depression: a distinct clinical entity? *Arch. Gen. Psychiatry*, **38**, 424–7.

Glassman, A. H., Covey, L. S., Dalack, G. W., *et al.* (1993). Smoking cessation, clonidine, and vulnerability to nicotine among dependent smokers. *Clin. Pharmacol. Ther.*, **54**, 670–9.

Glassman, A. H., O'Connor, C. M., Califf, R. M., *et al.* (2002). Sertraline treatment of major depression in patients with acute MI or unstable angina. *J.A.M.A.*, **288**, 701–9.

Glaxo-SmithKline (1997). *Data on file.* Study 603, file RM1997/00712/00. Durham, NC: Glaxo-Smithkline.

Glazener, C. M., Evans, J. H., and Peto, R. E. (2003). Tricyclic and related drugs for nocturnal enuresis in children. *Cochrane Database Syst. Rev.* CD002117.

Gloor, P. (1969). Hans Berger and the electroencephalogram of man. *Electroencephalogr. Clin. Neurophysiol.*, (suppl. 28): 1–350.

Gloor, P., Olivier, A., Quesney, L. F., Andermann, F., and Horowitz, S. (1982). The role of the limbic system in experiential phenomena of temporal lobe epilepsy. *Ann. Neurol.*, **12**, 129–44.

Glotzbach, S. F., Rowlett, E. A., Edgar, D. M., Moffat, R. J., and Ariagno, R. L. (1993). Light variability in the modern neonatal nursery: chronobiologic issues. *Med. Hypotheses*, **41**, 217–24.

Glover, V. (1997). Maternal stress or anxiety in pregnancy and emotional development of the child. *Br. J. Psychiatry*, **171**, 105–6.

Glover, V., Teixeira, J., Gitau, R., and Fisk, N. (1998). Links between antenatal maternal anxiety and the fetus. Paper presented at the 11th Biennial Conference on Infant Studies, Atlanta, GA.

Godwin, C. D. (1984). The dexamethasone suppression test in acute mania. *J. Affect. Disord.*, **7**, 281–7.

Goel, N., Terman, M., Terman, J. S., Macchi, M. M., and Stewart, J. W. (2005). Controlled trial of bright light and negative air ions for chronic depression. *Psychol. Med.*, **35**, 945–55.

Goetz, R. R., Puig-Antich, J., Dahl, R. E., *et al.* (1991). EEG sleep of young adults with major depression: a controlled study. *J. Affect. Disord.*, **22**, 91–100.

Goetz, R. R., Wolk, S. I., Coplan, J. D., Ryan, N. D., and Weissman, M. M. (2001). Premorbid polysomnographic signs in depressed adolescents: a reanalysis of EEG sleep after longitudinal follow-up in adulthood. *Biol. Psychiatry*, **49**, 930–42.

Goh, S. E., Salmons, P. H., and Whittington, R. M. (1989). Hospital suicides: are there preventable factors? Profile of the psychiatric hospital suicide. *Br. J. Psychiatry*, **154**, 247–9.

Gold, M. S. and Pottash, A. L. C. (eds) (1986). *Diagnostic and Laboratory Testing in Psychiatry.* New York: Plenum Medical Book Publishing.

Gold, M. S., Pottash, A. L. C., and Extein, I. (1981). Hypothyroidism and depression: evidence from complete thyroid function evaluation. *J.A.M.A.*, **242**, 1919–22.

Gold, P. W. and Chrousos, G. P. (1999). The endocrinology of melancholic and atypical depression: relation of neurocircuitry and somatic consequences. *Prod. Assoc. Am. Phys.*, **111**, 22–34.

Gold, P. W., Gabry, K. E., Yasuda, M. R., and Chrousos, G. P. (2002). Divergent endocrine abnormalities in melancholic and atypical depression: clinical and pathophysiologic implications. *Endocrinol. Metab. Clin. North Am.*, **31**, 37–62.

Goldberg, J. F., Wankmuller, M. M., and Sutherland, K. H. (2004). Depression with versus without manic features in rapid-cycling bipolar disorder. *J. Nerv. Ment. Dis.*, **192**, 602–6.

Golden, R. N., McCartney, C. F., Haggerty, J. J. Jr, *et al.* (1991). The detection of depression by patient self-report in women with gynecologic cancer. *Int. J. Psychiatry Med.*, **21**, 17–27.

Golden, R. N., Gaynes, B. N., Ekstrom, R. D., *et al.* (2005). The efficacy of light therapy in the treatment of mood disorders: a review and meta-analysis of the evidence. *Am. J. Psychiatry*, **162**, 656–62.

Goldman-Rakic, P. S. and Brown, R. M. (1982). Postnatal development of monoamine content and synthesis in the cerebral cortex of rhesus monkeys. *Brain Res.*, **256**, 339–49.

Goldney, R. D. and Fisher, L. J. (2004). Double depression in an Australian population. *Soc. Psychiatry Psychiatr. Epidemiol.*, **39**, 921–6.

Goldstein, D. S. (1995). *Stress, Catecholamines, and Cardiovascular Disease.* New York: Oxford University Press.

Goldstein, D. S., Holmes, C. S., Dendi, R., Bruce, S. R., and Li, S. T. (2002). Orthostatic hypotension from sympathetic denervation in Parkinson's disease. *Neurology*, **58**, 1247–55.

Golomb, B. A., Tenkanen, L., Alikoski, T., *et al.* (2002). Insulin sensitivity markers: predictors of accidents and suicides in Helsinki Heart Study screenees. *J. Clin. Epidemiol.*, **55**, 767–73.

Gonzalez, A. M., Pascual, J., Meana, J. J., *et al.* (1994). Autoradiographic demonstration of increased alpha 2-adrenoceptor binding sites in the hippocampus and frontal cortex of depressed suicide victims. *J. Neurochem.*, **63**, 256–65.

Goodman, S. H. and Gotlib, I. H. (1999). Risk for psychopathology in children of depressed mothers: a developmental model of understanding mechanisms of transmission. *Psychol. Rev.*, **106**, 458–90.

Goodman, S. H., Brogan, D., Lynch, M. E., and Fielding, B. (1993). Social and emotional competence in children of depressed mothers. *Child Dev.*, **64**, 516–31.

Goodnick, P. J. (2001). Use of antidepressants in treatment of comorbid diabetes mellitus and depression as well as in diabetic neuropathy. *Ann. Clin. Psychiatry*, **13**, 31–41.

Goodnick, P. J., Jerry, J., and Parra, F. (2002). Psychotropic drugs and the ECG: focus on the QTc interval. *Exp. Opin. Pharmacother.*, **3**, 479–98.

Goodwin, F. K. (2002). Rationale for long-term treatment of bipolar disorder and evidence for long-term lithium treatment. *J. Clin. Psychiatry*, **63** (suppl. 10), 5–12.

Goodwin, F. K., Murphy, D. L., Dunner, D. L., and Bunney, W. E. Jr. (1972). Lithium response in unipolar versus bipolar depression. *Am. J. Psychiatry*, **129**, 44–7.

Goodwin, F. K. and Jamison, K. R. (1990). Suicide. In Goodwin, F. K., and Jamison, R. (eds) *Manic-Depressive Illness*. New York, NY: Oxford University Press, pp. 227–44.

Goodwin, F. K., Fireman, B., Simon, G. E., *et al.* (2003). Suicide risk in bipolar disorder during treatment with lithium and divalproex. *J.A.M.A.*, **290**, 1467–73.

Goodwin, G. M. (1997). Neuropsychological and neuroimaging evidence for the involvement of the frontal lobes in depression. *J. Psychopharm.*, **11**, 115–22.

Goodyer, I. M., Herbert, J., Altham, P. M., *et al.* (1996). Adrenal secretion during major depression in 8- to 16-year-olds, I. Altered diurnal rhythms in salivary cortisol and dehydroepiandrosterone (DHEA) at presentation. *Psychol. Med.*, **26**, 245–56.

Goodyer, I. M., Herbert, J., Tamplin, A., Secher, S. M., and Pearson, J. (1997). Short-term outcome of major depression: II. Life events, family dysfunction, and friendship difficulties as predictors of persistent psychiatric disorder. *J. Am. Acad. Child Adolesc. Psychiatry*, **36**, 474–80.

Goodyer, I. M., Herbert, J., Tamplin, A., and Altham, P. M. E. (2000). First-episode major depression in adolescents. *Br. J. Psychiatry*, **176**, 142–9.

Goodyer, I. M., Park, R. J., and Herbert, J. (2001). Psychosocial and endocrine features of chronic first-episode major depression in 8–16 year olds. *Biol. Psychiatry*, **50**, 351–7.

Goodyer, I. M., Herbert, J., and Tamplin, A. (2003). Psychoendocrine antecedents of persistent first-episode major depression in adolescents: a community-based longitudinal enquiry. *Psychol. Med.*, **33**, 601–10.

Gordon, E., Kraiuhin, C., Harris, A., Meares, R., and Howson, A. (1986). The differential diagnosis of dementia using P300 latency. *Biol. Psychiatry*, **21**, 1123–32.

Gorelick, D. A. and Paredes, A. (1992). Effect of fluoxetine on alcohol consumption in male alcoholics. *Alcoholism Clin. Exp. Res.*, **16**, 261–5.

Goren, J. L. and Levin, G. M. (2000). Mania with bupropion: a dose-related phenomenon? *Ann. Pharmacother*, **34**, 619–21.

Gorman, M. (1992). *Simulating Science*. Bloomington, IN: Indiana University Press.

Gormley, G. J., Loury, M. T., Reider, A. T., Hospethorn, V. D., and Antel, J. P. (1985). Glucocorticoid receptors in depression: Relationship to the dexamethasone suppression test. *Am. J. Psychiatry*, **142**, 1278–84.

Gotlib, I. H. and Goodman, S. H. (1999). Children of parents with depression. In Silverman, W. K. and Ollendick, T. H. (eds) *Developmental Issues in the Clinical Treatment of Children and Adolescents*. New York: Allyn & Bacon, pp. 415–32.

Gotlib, I. H. and Whiffen, V. E. (1989). Depression and marital functioning: an examination of specificity and gender differences. *J. Abnorm. Psychol.*, **98**, 23–30.

Gould, E., Tanapat, P., Rydel, T., and Hastings, N. (2000). Regulation of hippocampal neurogenesis in adulthood. *Biol. Psychiatry*, **48**, 715–20.

Graae, F., Tenke, C., Bruder, G., *et al.* (1996). Abnormality of EEG alpha asymmetry in female adolescent suicide attempters. *Biol. Psychiatry*, **40**, 706–13.

Graff, L. A., Dyck, D. G., and Schallow, J. R. (1991). Predicting postpartum depressive symptoms: a structural modeling analysis. *Percept. Motor Skills*, **73**, 1137–8.

Grafman, J., Vance, S. C., Weingartner, H., Salazar, A. M., and Amin, D. (1986). The effects of lateralized frontal lesions on mood regulation. *Brain*, **109**, 1127–48.

Granger, A. C. P. and Underwood, M. R. (2001). Review of the role of progesterone in the management of postnatal mood disorders. *J. Psychosom. Obstet. Gynecol.*, **22**, 49–55.

Grant, B. F. (1997). The influence of comorbid major depression and substance use disorders on alcohol and drug treatment: results of a national survey. *NIDA Res. Monogr.*, **172**, 4–15.

Grant, B. F. and Harford, T. C. (1995). Comorbidity between DSM-IV alcohol use disorders and major depression: results of a national survey. *Drug Alcohol Depend.*, **39**, 197–206.

Gray, T. S. (1993). Amygdaloid CRF pathways. Role in autonomic, neuroendocrine, and behavioral responses to stress. *Ann. NY Acad. Sci.*, **697**, 53–60.

Greenberg, D. B. (1997). Beyond neurasthenia and chronic fatigue. In Akiskal, H. S. and Cassano, G. B. (eds) *Dysthymia and the Spectrum of Chronic Depressions*. New York: Guilford Press, pp. 148–64.

Greenberg, L. B. (1985). Detection of prolonged seizures during electroconvulsive therapy: a comparison of electroencephalogram and cuff monitoring. *Convuls. Ther.*, **1**, 32–7.

Greenberg, L. B. and Gujavarty, K. (1985). The neuroleptic malignant syndrome: Review and report of three cases. *Compr. Psychiatry*, **26**, 63–70.

Greenblatt, M., Grosser, G. H., and Wechsler, H. (1964). Differential response of hospitalized depressed patients to somatic therapy. *Am. J. Psychiatry*, **120**, 935–43.

Greenfield, T. K., Rehm, J., and Rogers, J. D. (2002). Effects of depression and social integration on the relationship between alcohol consumption and all-cause mortality. *Addiction*, **97**, 29–38.

Greenhalgh, J., Knight, C., Hind, D., Beverley, C., and Walters, S. (2005). Clinical annual cost-effectiveness of electroconvulsive therapy for depressive illness, schizophrenia, catatonia and mania: systematic reviews and economic modeling studies. *Health Technol. Assess.*, **9**, 1–170.

Gregoire, A. J., Kumar, R., Everitt, B., Henderson, A. F., and Studd, J. W. (1996). Transdermal oestrogen for treatment of severe postnatal depression. *Lancet*, **347**, 930–3.

Grigoriadis, S. and Kennedy, S. H. (2002). Role of estrogen in the treatment of depression. *Am. J. Ther*, **9**, 503–9.

Gross, C. P., Gupta, A. R., and Krumholz, H. M. (2003). Disclosure of financial competing interests in randomized controlled trials: cross sectional review. *Br. Med. J.*, **326**, 526–7.

Gross-Isseroff, R., Biegon, A., Voet, H., and Weizman, A. (1998). The suicide brain: a review of postmortem receptor/transporter binding studies. *Neurosci. Biobehav. Rev.*, **22**, 653–61.

Grote, N. K. and Frank, E. (2003). Difficult-to-treat depression: the role of contexts and comorbidities. *Biol. Psychiatry*, **53**, 660–70.

Grove, W. M., Andreasen, N. C., Young, M., *et al.* (1987). Isolation and characterization of a nuclear depressive syndrome. *Psychol. Med.*, **17**, 471–84.

Grunebaum, M. F., Oquendo, M. A., Harkavy-Friedman, J. M., *et al.* (2001). Delusions and suicidality. *Am. J. Psychiatry*, **158**, 742–7.

Grunebaum, M. F., Ellis, S. P., Li, S., Oquendo, M. A., and Mann, J. J. (2004a). Antidepressants and suicide risk in the United States, 1985–1999. *J. Clin. Psychiatry*, **65**, 1456–62.

Grunebaum, M. F., Galfalvy, H. C., Oquendo, M. A., Burke, A. K., and Mann, J. J. (2004b). Melancholia and the probability and lethality of suicide attempts. *Br. J. Psychiatry*, **184**, 534–5.

Grunhaus, L., Zelnik, T., Albala, A. A., *et al.* (1987). Serial dexamethasone suppression tests in depressed patients treated only with electroconvulsive therapy. *J. Affect. Disord.*, **13**, 233–40.

Grunhaus, L., Schreiber, S., Dolbert, O. T., Polak, D., and Dannon, P. N. (2003). A randomized controlled comparison of electroconvulsive therapy and repetitive transcranial magnetic stimulation in severe and resistant nonpsychotic major depression. *Biol. Psychiatry*, **53**, 324–31.

Grunze, H. (2003). Lithium in the acute treatment of bipolar disorders: a stocktaking. *Eur. Arch. Psychiatry Clin. Neurosci.*, **253**, 115–19.

Grunze, H., Kasper, S., Goodwin, G., *et al.* (2002). WFSBP Task Force on Treatment Guidelines for Bipolar Disorders: World Federation of Societies of Biological Psychiatry (WFSBP) guidelines for biological treatment of bipolar disorders, part I: treatment of bipolar depression. *World J. Biol. Psychiatry*, **3**, 115–24.

Grunze, H., Marcuse, A., Scharer, L. O., Born, C., and Walden, J. (2004). Nefazodone in psychotic unipolar and bipolar depression: a retrospective chart analysis and open prospective study on its efficacy and safety versus combined treatment with amitriptyline and haloperidol. *Neuropsychobiology*, **46** (suppl. 1), 31–5.

Guberman, A. H., Besag, F. M. C., Brodie, M. J., *et al.* (1999). Lamotrigine-associated rash: risk/benefit considerations in adults and children. *Epilepsia*, **40**, 985–91.

Guelfi, J. D., White, C., Hackett, D., Guichoux, J. Y., and Magni, G. (1995). Effectiveness of venlafaxine in patients hospitalized for major depression and melancholia. *J. Clin. Psychiatry*, **56**, 450–8.

Guillemin, R. (2005). Hypothalamic hormones a.k.a. hypothalamic releasing factors. *J. Endocrinol.*, **184**, 11–28.

Gulley, L. R. and Nemeroff, C. B. (1993). The neurobiological basis of mixed depression–anxiety states. *J. Clin. Psychiatry*, **54** (suppl. 1), 16–19.

Gunderson, J. G. and Ridolfi, M. E. (2001). Borderline personality disorder. Suicidality and self-mutilation. *Ann. NY Acad. Sci.*, **932**, 61–77.

Gunnell, D. and Ashby, D. (2004). Antidepressants and suicide: what is the balance of benefit and harm? *Br. Med. J.*, **329**, 34–8.

Gurevitz, S. and Helme, W. H. (1954). Effects of electroconvulsive therapy on personality and intellectual functioning of the schizophrenic child. *J. Nerv. Ment. Dis.*, **120**, 213–26.

Guscott, R. and Grof, P. (1991). The clinical meaning of refractory depression: a review for the clinician. *Am. J. Psychiatry*, **148**, 695–704.

Gutgesell, H., Atkins, D., Barst, R., *et al.* (1999). AHA scientific statement: cardiovascular monitoring of children and adolescents receiving psychotropic drugs. *J. Am. Acad. Child Adolesc. Psychiatry*, **38**, 1047–50.

Guttmacher, L. B. and Cretella, H. (1988). Electroconvulsive therapy in one child and three adolescents. *J. Clin. Psychiatry*, **49**, 20–3.

Guze, S. B. (1967). The occurrence of psychiatric illness in systemic lupus erythematosus. *Am. J. Psychiatry*, **123**, 1562–70.

(1988). Psychotherapy and the etiology of psychiatric disorders. *Psychiatr. Dev.*, **3**, 183–93.

Guze, S. B. and Murphy, G. E. (1963). An empirical approach to psychotherapy: the agnostic position. *Am. J. Psychiatry*, **120**, 53–7.

Guze, S. B. and Robins, E. (1970). Suicide and primary affective disorders. *Br. J. Psychiatry*, **117**, 437–8.

Habib, K. E., Weld, K. P., Rice, K. C., *et al.* (2000). Oral administration of a corticotropin-releasing hormone receptor antagonist significantly attenuates behavioral, neuroendocrine, and autonomic responses to stress in primates. *Proc. Natl. Acad. Sci.*, **97**, 6079–84.

Habib, K. E., Gold, P. W., and Chrousos, G. P. (2001). Neuroendocrinology of stress. *Endocrinol. Metab. Clin. North Am.*, **30**, 695–728.

Hackett, M., Anderson, C., and House, A. (2004). Interventions for treating depression after stroke. *Cochrane Database Syst. Rev.*, **3**, CD003437.

Hagebeuk, E. E., Tans, J. T., and de Regt, E. W. (2002). A stroke patient with a non-convulsive status epilepticus during citalopram therapy. *Eur. J. Neurol.*, **9**, 319–20.

Haggerty, J. J. Jr., and Prange, A. J. Jr (1995). Borderline hypothyroidism and depression. *Annu. Rev. Med.*, **46**, 37–46.

Halbreich, U., Asnis, G. M., Shindledecker, R., Zumoff, B., and Nathan, R. S. (1985). Cortisol secretion in endogenous depression. II. Time-related functions. *Arch. Gen. Psychiatry*, **42**, 909–14.

Hall, S. D., Wang, Z., Huang, S. M., *et al.* (2003a). The interaction between St. John's wort and an oral contraceptive. *Clin. Pharmacol. Ther.*, **74**, 525–35.

Hall, W. and Solowij, N. (1998). Adverse effects of cannabis. *Lancet*, **352**, 1611–16.

Hall, W. D., Mant, A., Mitchell, P. B., *et al.* (2003b). Association between antidepressant prescribing and suicide in Australia, 1991–2000: trend analysis. *Br. Med. J.*, **326**, 1008–11.

Halligan, S. L., Herbert, J., Goodyer, I. M., and Murray, L. (2004). Exposure to postnatal depression predicts elevated cortisol in adolescent offspring. *Biol. Psychiatry*, **55**, 376–81.

Hamalainen, J., Kaprio, J., Isometsa, E., *et al.* (2001). Cigarette smoking, alcohol intoxication and major depressive episode in a representative population sample. *J. Epidemiol. Commun. Health*, **55**, 573–6.

Hameed, U., Schwartz, T. L., Malhotra, K., West, R. L., and Bertone, F. (2005). Antidepressant treatment in the primary care office: outcomes for adjustment disorder versus major depression. *Ann. Clin. Psychiatry*, **17**, 77–81.

Hamilton, J. A. (1982). The identity of postpartum psychosis. In Brockington, I. F. and Kumar, R. (eds) *Motherhood and Mental Illness*. London: Academic Press, pp. 1–20.

(1989). Psychiatric illness after childbearing. In Howels, J. G. (ed.) *Modern Perspectives in the Psychiatry of the Affective Disorders*, vol. 15. New York: Brunner/Mazel, pp. 275–91.

Hamilton, M. (1960). A rating scale for depression. *J. Neurol. Neurosurg. Psychiatry*, **23**, 56–62.

(1967). Development of a rating scale for primary depressive illness. *Br. J. Soc. Clin. Psychol*, **6**, 278–96.

(1982). Prediction of the response of depressions to ECT. In Abrams, R., and Essman, W. B. (eds) *Electroconvulsive Therapy: Biological Foundations and Clinical Applications.* New York: Spectrum, pp. 113–28.

Hammen, C. (1990). Vulnerability to depression: personal, situational, and family aspects. In Ingram, R. (ed), *Contemporary Approaches to Depression: Treatment, Research, and Theory.* New York, Plenum, pp. 59–69.

(1991). Generation of stress in the course of unipolar depression. *J. Abnorm. Psychol.* **100**, 555–61.

Hammen, C., Burge, D., Burney, E., and Cheri, A. (1990). Longitudinal study of diagnoses in children of women with unipolar and bipolar affective disorder. *Arch. Gen. Psychiatry,* **47**, 1112–17.

Handforth, A., DeGiorgius, C. M., Schacater, S. C., *et al.* (1998). Vagus nerve stimulastion therapy for partial-onset seizures: a randomized active-control trial. *Neurology,* **51**, 48–55.

Handley, S. L., Dunn, T. L., Waldron, G., and Baker, J. M. (1980). Tryptophan, cortisol and puerperal mood. *Br. J. Psychiatry,* **136**, 498–508.

Hansen, E. S. and Bolwig, T. G. (1998). Cotard syndrome: an important manifestation of melancholia. *Nord. J. Psychiatry,* **52**, 459–64.

Hansenne, M., Pitchot, W., Gonzalez Moreno, A., Zaldua, I. U., and Ansseau, M. (1996). Suicidal behavior in depressive disorder: an event-related potential study. *Biol. Psychiatry,* **40**, 116–22.

Hansten, P. D. and Horn, J. R. (2002). *The Top 100 Drug Interactions: A Guide to Patient Management.* Seattle, WA: University of Washington, H&H Publications.

Hapgood, C. C., Elkind, G. S., and Wright, J. J. (1988). Maternity blues: phenomena and relationship to later post-depression. *Aust. NZ J. Psychiatry,* **22**, 299–306.

Harden, C. L. (2002). The co-morbidity of depression and epilepsy. Epidemiology, etiology, and treatment. *Neurology,* **59**, S48–S55.

Harden, C. L. and Goldstein, M. A. (2001). Mood disorders in patients with epilepsy: epidemiology and management. *CNS Drugs,* **16**, 291–302.

Harden, C. L., Pulver, M. C., Ravdin, L. D., *et al.* (2000). A pilot study of mood and epilepsy patients treated with vagus nerve stimulation. *Epilepsy Behav.,* **1**, 93–9.

Harkness, K. L. and Monroe, S. M. (2002). Childhood adversity and the endogenous versus non-endogenous distinction in women with major depression. *Am. J. Psychiatry,* **159**, 387–93.

Harkness, K. L., Frank, E., Anderson, B., *et al.* (2002). Does interpersonal psychotherapy protect women from depression in the fact of stressful life events? *J. Consult. Clin. Psychol.,* **70**, 908–15.

Harmon-Jones, E., Abramson, L. Y., Sigelman, J., *et al.* (2002). Proneness to hypomania/mania symptoms or depression symptoms and asymmetrical frontal cortical responses to an anger-evoking event. *J. Pers. Soc. Psychol.,* **82**, 610–18.

Harney, J. H., Fulton, C., Ross, E. D., and Rush, A. J. (1993). Dexamethasone suppression test and onset of poststroke depression in patients with ischemic infarction. *J. Clin. Psychiatry,* **54**, 343–8.

Harrington, R. C., Fudge, H., Rutter, M. L., *et al.* (1993). Child and adult depression: a test of continuities with data from a family study. *Br. J. Psychiatry,* **162**, 627–33.

Harrington, R., Rutter, M., and Fombonne, E. (1996). Developmental pathways in depression: multiple meanings, antecedents, and endpoints. *Dev. Psychopathol.*, **8**, 601–16.

Harris, E. C. and Barraclough, B. M. (1994). Suicide as an outcome for medical disorders. *Medicine*, **73**, 281–96.

Hartling, O. J., Marving, J., Knudsen, P., *et al.* (1987). The effect of the tricyclic antidepressant drug, nortriptyline on left ventricular ejection fraction and left ventricular volumes. *Psychopharmacology (Berl.)*, **91**, 381–3.

Harvey, S. A. and Black, K. J. (1996). The dexamethasone suppression test for diagnosing depression in stroke patients. *Ann. Clin. Psychiatry*, **8**, 35–9.

Harwood, D. G., Barker, W. W., Ownby, R. L., and Duara, R. (1999). Association between premorbid history of depression and current depression in Alzheimer's disease. *J. Geriatr. Psychiatry. Neurol.*, **12**, 72–5.

Hashioka, S., Monji, A., Sasaki, M., *et al.* (2002). A patient with Cotard syndrome who showed an improvement in single photon emission computed tomography findings after successful treatment with antidepressants. *Clin. Neuropharmacol.*, **25**, 276–9.

Hasin, D., Liu, X., Nunes, E., *et al.* (2002). Effects of major depression on remission and relapse of substance dependence. *Arch. Gen. Psychiatry*, **59**, 375–80.

Hasin, D. S., Tsai, W. Y., Endicott, J., *et al.* (1996). Five-year course of major depression: effects of comorbid alcoholism. *J. Affect. Disord.*, **41**, 63–70.

Haslam, N. and Beck, A. T. (1993). Categorization of major depression in an outpatient sample. *J. Nerv. Ment. Dis.*, **181**, 725–31.

Hatotani, N., Nishikuba, M., and Kitayama, I. (1979). Periodic psychoses in the female and the reproductive process. In Zichella, L. and Panchevi, P. (eds) *Psychoneuroendocrinology in Reproduction*. Amsterdam: Elsevier, pp. 55–68.

Hatzinger, M., Hemmeter, U. M., Baumann, K., Brand, S., and Holsboer-Trachsler, E. (2002). The combined DEX-CRH test in treatment course and long-term outcome of major depression. *J. Psychiatr. Res.*, **36**, 287–97.

Hatzinger, M., Hemmeter, U. M., Brand, S., Ising, M., and Holsboer-Trachsler, E. (2004). Electroencephalographic sleep profiles in treatment course and long-term outcome of major depression: association with DEX/CRH-test response. *J. Psychiatry. Res.*, **38**, 453–65.

Hauser, R. A. and Zesiewicz, T. A. (1997). Sertraline for the treatment of depression in Parkinson's disease. *Move. Disord.*, **12**, 756–99.

Hausmann, A., Kemmler, G., Walpoth, M., *et al.* (2004a). No benefit derived from repetitive transcranial magnetic stimulation in depression: a prospective, single centre, randomized, double blind, sham controlled "add on" trial. *J. Neurol. Neurosurg. Psychiatry*, **75**, 320–2.

Hausmann, A., Pascual-Leone, A., Kemmler, G., *et al.* (2004b). No deterioration of cognitive performance in an aggressive unilateral and bilateral antidepressant rTMS add-on trial. *J. Clin. Psychiatry*, **65**, 772–82.

Hawley, C. J., Gale, T. M., Sivakumaran, T., and Hertfordshire Neuroscience Research Group. (2002). Defining remission by cut off score on the MADRS: selecting the optimal value. *J. Affect. Disord.*, **72**, 177–84.

Hay, D. F. and Kumar, R. (1995). Interpreting the effects of mothers' postnatal depression on children's intelligence: a critique and reanalysis. *Child Psychiatry Hum. Dev.*, **25**, 165–81.

Hay, D. F., Pawlby, S., Sharp, D., *et al.* (2001). Intellectual problems shown by 11-year-old children whose mothers had postnatal depression. *J. Child Psychol. Psychiatry*, **42**, 871–89.

Hay, D. P. (1989). Electroconvulsive therapy for the medically ill elderly. *Convuls. Ther.*, **5**, 8–16.

Hayden, M. R. (1981). *Huntington's Chorea.* New York, NY: Springer-Verlag.

Hayhurst, H., Cooper, Z., Paykel, E. S., Vearnals, S., and Ramana, R. (1997). Expressed emotion and depression: a longitudinal study. *Br. J. Psychiatry*, **171**, 439–43.

Healy, D. (1996). *The Psychopharmacologists.* London: Altman.

(1997). *The Anti-Depressant Era.* Cambridge, MA: Harvard University Press.

(1988). *The Psychopharamcologists II.* London: Altman.

(2000). *The Psychopharmacologists III.* London: Altman.

(2002). *The Creation of Psychopharmacology.* Cambridge, MA: Harvard University Press.

(2004). *Let Them Eat Prozac: The Unhealthy Relationship Between the Pharmaceutical Industry and Depression.* New York: New York University Press.

Healy, D. and Sheehan, D. V. (2001). Have drug companies hyped social anxiety disorder to increase sales? *West. J. Med.*, **175**, 364–5.

Healy, D. and Thase, M. E. (2003). Is academic psychiatry for sale? *Br. J. Psychiatry*, **182**, 388–90.

Hedegaard, M., Henriksen, T. B., Secher, N. J., Hatch, M. C., and Sabroe, S. (1996). Do stressful life events affect duration of gestation and risk of preterm delivery? *Epidemiology*, **7**, 339–45.

Hefferman, C. F. (1995). *The Melancholy Muse.* Pittsburgh, PA: Duquesne University Press.

Heikkinen, T., Ekblad, U., Kero, P., Ekblad, S., and Laine, K. (2003). Citalopram in pregnancy and lactation. *Clin. Pharmacol. Ther.*, **72**, 184–91.

Heikkinen, T., Ekblad, U., Palo, P., and Laine, K. (2003). Pharmacokinetics of fluoxetine and norfluoxetine in pregnancy and lactation. *Clin. Pharmacol. Ther.*, **73**, 330–7.

Heilman, K. M. (1997). The neurobiology of emotional experience. *J. Neuropsychiatry Clin. Neurosci.*, **9**, 439–48.

Heim, C. and Nemeroff, C. B. (2001). The role of childhood trauma in the neurobiology of mood and anxiety disorders: preclinical and clinical studies. *Biol. Psychiatry*, **49**, 1023–39.

Heim, C., Newport, D. J., Heit, S., *et al.* (2000). Pituitary–adrenal and autonomic responses to stress in women after sexual and physical abuse in childhood. *J.A.M.A*, **284**, 592–7.

Heinonen, O. P., Slone, D., and Shapiro, S. (1977). *Birth Defects and Drugs in Pregnancy.* Littleton, MA, Publishing Science Group.

Heiser, P. and Remschmidt, H. (2002). Selective serotonin reuptake inhibitors and newer antidepressive substances in child and adolescent psychiatry. *Z. Kinder Jugendpsychiatr. Psychother.*, **30**, 173–83.

Heller, W. (1993). Neuropsychological mechanisms of individual differences in emotion, personality, and arousal. *Neuropsychology*, **7**, 476–89.

Hellsten, J., Wennstrom, M., Mohapel, P., *et al.* (2002). Electroconvulsive seizures increase hippocampal neurogenesis after chronic corticosterone treatment. *Eur. J. Neurosci.*, **16**, 283–90.

Helmus, T. C., Downey, K. K., Wang, L. M., Rhodes, G. L., and Schuster, C. R. (2001). The relationship between self-reported cocaine withdrawal symptoms and history of depression. *Addict. Behav.*, **26**, 461–7.

Helzer, J. E. and Hudziak, J. J. (eds) (2002). *Defining Psychopathology in the 21st Century: DSM-V and Beyond.* Washington, DC: American Psychiatric Press.

Hemels, M. E., Vicente, C., Sadri, H., Masson, M. J., and Einarson, T. R. (2004). Quality assessment of meta-analysis of RCTs of pharmacotherapy in major depressive disorder. *Curr. Med. Res. Opin.*, **20**, 477–84.

Hemenway, D. and Miller, M. (2000). Firearm availability and homicide rates across 26 high-income countries. *J. Trauma*, **49**, 985–8.

(2002). Association of rates of household handgun ownership, lifetime major depression, and serious suicidal thoughts with rates of suicide across US census regions. *Inj. Prev.*, **8**, 313–16.

Hendrick, V. and Altshuler, L. L. (1998). Recurrent mood shifts of premenstrual dysphoric disorder can be mistaken for rapid-cycling bipolar II disorder. *J. Clin. Psychiatry*, **59**, 479–80.

(2002). Management of major depression during pregnancy. *Am. J. Psychiatry*, **159**, 1667–73.

Hendrick, V., Altshuler, L., Strouse, T., and Grosser, S. (2000). Postpartum and nonpostpartum depression: differences in presentation and response to pharmacologic treatment. *Depress. Anxiety*, **11**, 66–72.

Hendrick, V., Fukuchi, A., Altshuler, L., *et al.* (2001). Use of sertraline, paroxetine and fluvoxamine by nursing women. *Br. J. Psychiatry*, **179**, 163–6.

Hendrick, V., Stowe, Z. N., Altshuler, L. L., *et al.* (2003). Placental passage of antidepressant medications. *Am. J. Psychiatry*, **160**, 993–6.

Henriques, J. and Davidson, R. (1991). Left frontal hypoactivation in depression. *J. Abnorm. Psychol.*, **100**, 535–45.

Henriques, J. B., Glowacki, J. M., and Davidson, R. J. (1994). Reward fails to alter response bias in depression. *J. Abnorm. Psychol.*, **103**, 460–6.

Henry, J. A. (1997). Epidemiology and relative toxicity of antidepressant drugs in overdose. *Drug Safety*, **16**, 374–90.

Hermann, R. C., Dorwart, R. A., Hoover, C. W., and Brody, J. (1995). Variation in ECT use in the United States. *Am. J. Psychiatry*, **152**, 869–75.

Hermann, R. C., Ettner, S. L., Dorwart, R. A., Hoover, C. W., and Yeung, E. (1998). Characteristics of psychiatrists who perform ECT. *Am. J. Psychiatry*, **155**, 889–94.

Hermann, R. C., Ettner, S. L., Dorwart, R. A., Langman-Dorwart, N., and Kleinman, S. (1999). Diagnoses of patients treated with ECT: a comparison of evidence-based standards with reported use. *Psychiatr. Serv.*, **50**, 1059–65.

Herzog, A. G., Seibel, M. M., Schomer, D. L., Vaitukaitis, J. L., and Geschwind, N. (1986). Reproductive endocrine disorders in men with partial seizures of temporal lobe origin. *Arch. Neurol.*, **43**, 347–50.

Heuser, I., Yassouridis, A., and Holsboer, F. (1994). The combined dexamethasone/CRH test: a refined laboratory test for psychiatric disorders. *J. Psychiatry Res.*, **28**, 341–56.

Hibberd, C., Yau, J. L., and Seckl, J. R. (2000). Glucocorticoids and the ageing hippocampus. *J. Anat.*, **197**, 553–62.

Hickie, I. and Scott, E. (1998). Late-onset depressive disorders: a preventable variant of cerebrovascular disease? *Psychol. Med.*, **28**, 1007–13.

Hickie, I., Mason, C., Parker, G., and Brodaty, H. (1986). Prediction of ECT response: validation of a refined sign-based (CORE) system for defining melancholia. *Br. J. Psychiatry*, **169**, 68–74.

Hickie, I., Bennett, B., Mitchell, P., Wilhelm, K., and Orlay, W. (1996). Clinical and subclinical hypothyroidism in patients with chronic and treatment-resistant depression. *Aust. NZ J. Psychiatry*, **30**, 246–52.

Hickie, I., Scott, E., Naismith, S., *et al.* (2001). Late-onset depression: genetic, vascular and clinical contributions. *Psychol. Med.*, **31**, 1403–12.

Hickie, I. B. (2004). Commentary on 'evaluating treatments for the mood disorders: time for the evidence to get real.' *Aust. NZ J. Psychiatry*, **38**, 415–18.

Hickie, I. B., Scott, E. M., and Davenport, T. A. (1999). Are antidepressants all the same? Surveying the opinions of Australian psychiatrists. *Aust. NZ J. Psychiatry*, **33**, 642–9.

Hildebrandt, M. G., Steyerberg, E. W., Stage, K. B., Passchier, J., Kragh-Soerensen, P., The Danish University Antidepressant Group (2003). Are gender differences important for the clinical effects of antidepressants? *Am. J. Psychiatry*, **160**, 1643–50.

Hill, D. (1968). Depression: disease, reaction, or posture? *Am. J. Psychiatry*, **125**, 445–57.

Hill, D. and Parr, G. (eds) (1963). *Electroencephalography*. New York: Macmillan.

Hindmarch, I. and Kerr, J. S. (1994). Effects of paroxetine on cognitive function in depressed patients, volunteers and elderly volunteers. *Med. Sci. Res.*, **22**, 669–70.

Hindmarch, I., Shillingford, J., and Shillingford, C. (1990). The effects of sertraline on psychomotor performance in elderly volunteers. *J. Clin. Psychiatry*, **51** (suppl. B), 34–6.

Hippisley-Cox, J., Pringle, M., Hammersley, V., *et al.* (2001). Antidepressants as risk factor for ischaemic heart disease: case-control study in primary care. *Br. Med. J.*, **323**, 666–9.

Hirayasu, Y., Shenton, M. E., Salisbury, D. F., *et al.* (1999). Subgenual cingulate cortex volume in first-episode psychosis. *Am. J. Psychiatry*, **156**, 1091–3.

Hiroi, N., Wong, M. L., Licinio, J., *et al.* (2001). Expression of corticotropin releasing hormone receptors type I and type II mRNA in suicide victims and controls. *Mol. Psychiatry*, **6**, 540–6.

Hirose, S. and Ashby, C. R. (2002). An open pilot study combining risperidone and a selective serotonin reuptake inhibitor as initial antidepressant therapy. *J. Clin. Psychiatry*, **63**, 733–6.

Hirschfeld, R. M. (1999). Efficacy of SSRIs and newer antidepressants in severe depression: comparison with TCAs. *J. Clin. Psychiatry*, **60**, 326–35.

Hirschfeld, R. M. (2001). Clinical importance of long-term antidepressant treatment. *Br. J. Psychiatry*, **42** (suppl.), S4–8.

Hirschfeld, R. M. and Vornik, L. A. (2004). Newer antidepressants: review of efficacy and safety of escitalopram and duloxetine. *J. Clin. Psychiatry*, **65** (suppl.), 46–52.

Hirschfeld, R. M., Koslow, S. H., and Kupfer, D. J. (1983) The clinical utility of the dexamethasone suppression test in psychiatry. Summary of a National Institute of Mental Health Workshop. *J.A.M.A.*, **250**, 1983.

Hirschfeld, R. M., Montgomery, S. A., Aguglia, E., *et al.* (2002b). Partial response and nonresponse to antidepressant therapy: current approaches and treatment options. *J. Clin. Psychiatry*, **63**, 826–37.

Hirschfeld, R. M. A., Koslow, S. H., and Kupfer, D. J. (1985). *Clinical Utility of the Dexamethasone Suppression Test*. Rockville, MD: US DHHS.

Hirschfeld, R. M. A., Bowden, C. L., Gitlin, M. J., *et al.* (2002a). Practice guideline for the treatment of patients with bipolar disorder (revision). *Am. J. Psychiatry*, **159** (suppl. 4), 1–50.

Hirshfeld-Becker, D. R., Biederman, J., Calltharp, S., *et al.* (2003). Behavioral inhibition and disinhibition as hypothesized precursors to psychopathology: implications for pediatric bipolar disorder. *Biol. Psychiatry*, **53**, 985–99.

Hlatky, M. A., Boothroyd, D., Vittinghoff, E., *et al.* (2002). Quality-of-life and depressive symptoms in postmenopausal women after receiving hormone therapy: results from the Heart and Estrogen/Progestin Replacement Study (HERS) trial. *J.A.M.A.*, **287**, 191–7.

Hobson, R. F. (1953). Prognostic factors in electric convulsive therapy. *J. Neurol. Neurosurg. Psychiatry*, **16**, 275–81.

Hoch, A. (1921). *Benign Stupors: A Study of a New Manic-Depressive Reaction Type*. New York: Macmillan.

Hoffbrand, S., Howard, L., and Crawley, H. (2001). Antidepressant drug treatment for post-natal depression. *Cochrane Database Syst. Rev.*, **2**, CD002018.

Hoffman, R. E. and Cavus, I. (2002). Slow transcranial magnetic stimulation, long-term depotentiation, and brain hyperexcitability disorders. *Am. J. Psychiatry*, **159**, 1093–102.

Hokfelt, T., Lundberg, J. M., Schultzberg, M., *et al.* (1980). Cellular localization of peptides in neural structures. *Proc. R. Soc. Lond. B. Biol. Sci.*, **210**, 63–77.

Holemans, S., De Paermentier, F., Horton, R. W., *et al.* (1993). NMDA glutamatergic receptors, labeled with [^{3}H]MK-801, in brain samples from drug-free depressed suicides. *Brain Res.*, **616**, 138–43.

Holliday, S. M. and Plosker, G. L. (1993). Paroxetine. A review of its pharmacology, therapeutic use in depression and therapeutic potential in diabetic neuropathy. *Drugs Aging*, **3**, 278–99.

Hollon, S. D., DeRubeis, R. J., Evans, M. D., *et al.* (1992). Cognitive therapy and pharmacotherapy for depression. Singly and in combination. *Arch. Gen. Psychiatry*, **49**, 774–81.

Holmberg, G. (1953a). The influence of oxygen administration on electrically induced convulsions in man. *Acta Psychiatr. Neurol.*, **28**, 365–86.

(1953b). The factor of hypoxemia in electroshock therapy. *Am. J. Psychiatry*, **110**, 115–18.

Holmberg, G. and Thesleff, S. (1952). Succinylcholine-iodide as a muscular relaxant in electroshock therapy. *Am. J. Psychiatry*, **108**, 842–6.

Holsboer, F. (2001). Stress, hypercortisolism and corticosteroid receptors in depression: implications for therapy. *J. Affect. Disord.*, **62**, 77–91.

Holsboer, F. and Barden, N. (1996). Antidepressants and hypothalamic–pituitary–adrenocortical regulation. *Endocrinol. Rev.*, **17**, 187–203.

Holsboer, F., Gerken, A., von Bardeleben, U., *et al.* (1986). Human corticotropin-releasing hormone in depression-correlation with thyrotropin secretion following thyrotropin-releasing hormone. *Biol. Psychiatry*, **21**, 601–11.

Holsboer, F., von Bardeleben, U., Wiedemann, K., Müller, O. A., and Stalla, G. K. (1987). Serial assessment of corticotropin-releasing hormone response after dexamethasone in depression: implications for pathophysiology of DST nonsuppression. *Biol. Psychiatry*, **22**, 228–34.

Holsinger, T., Steffens, D. C., Phillips, C., *et al.* (2002). Head injury in early adulthood and the lifetime risk of depression. *Arch. Gen. Psychiatry*, **59**, 17–22.

Homan, S., Lachenbruch, P. A., Winokur, G., and Clayton, P. (1982). An efficacy study of electroconvulsive therapy and antidepressants in the treatment of primary depression. *Psychol. Med.*, **12**, 615–24.

Hopewell-Ash, E. L. (1934). *Melancholia in Everyday Practice.* London: John Bale.

Hordern, A., Holt, N. F., Burt, C. G., and Gordon, W. F. (1963). Amitriptyline in depressive states: Phenomenology and prognostic considerations. *Br. J. Psychiatry*, **109**, 815–25.

Horger, B. A., Iyasere, C. A., Berhow, M. T., *et al.* (1999). Enhancement of locomotor activity and conditioned reward to cocaine by brain-derived neurotrophic factor. *J. Neurosci.*, **19**, 4110–22.

Hori, M., Shiraishi, H., and Koizumi, J. (1993). Delusional depression and suicide. *Jpn J. Psychiatry Neurol.*, **47**, 811–17.

Horwath, E., Johnson, J. K., Weissman, M. M., and Hornig, C. D. (1992). The validity of major depression with atypical features based on a community sample. *J. Affect. Disord.*, **26**, 117–26.

Hosoda, K. and Duman, R. S. (1993). Regulation of $ß_1$-adrenergic receptor mRNA and ligand binding by antidepressant treatments and norepinephrine depletion in rat frontal cortex. *J. Neurochem.*, **69**, 1335–43.

Hossain, Z., Field, T., Gonzalez, J., *et al.* (1994). Infants of depressed mothers interact better with their nondepressed fathers. *Infant Men. Health J.*, **15**, 348–57.

Houlihan, D. J. (2004). Serotonin syndrome resulting from coadministration of tramadol, venlafaxine, and mirtazapine. *Ann. Pharmacother.*, **38**, 411–13.

Howland, R. H. (1993). Thyroid dysfunction in refractory depression: implications for pathophysiology and treatment. *J. Clin. Psychiatry*, **54**, 47–54.

(1996). Induction of mania with serotonin reuptake inhibitors. *J. Clin. Psychopharmacol.*, **16**, 425–7.

Hrdlicka, M. (2002). Combination of clozapine and maprotiline in refractory psychotic depression. *Euro. Psychiatry*, **17**, 484.

Huang, Y. Y., Oquendo, M. A., Friedman, J. M., *et al.* (2003). Substance abuse disorder and major depression are associated with the human 5-HT1B receptor gene (HTR1B) G861C polymorphism. *Neuropsychopharm.*, **28**, 163–9.

Hubain, P. P., Staner, L., Dramaix, M., *et al.* (1994). TSH response to TRH and EEG sleep in non-bipolar major depression: a multivariate approach. *Eur. Neuropsychopharmacol.*, **4**, 517–25.

Hubain, P. P., Staner, L., Dramaix, M., *et al.* (1998). The dexamethasone suppression test and sleep electroencephalogram in nonbipolar major depressed inpatients: a multivariate analysis. *Biol. Psychiatry*, **43**, 220–9.

Hucks, D., Lowther, S., Crompton, M. R., Katona, C. L., and Horton, R. W. (1997). Corticotropin-releasing factor binding sites in cortex of depressed suicides. *Psychopharmacology (Berl.)*, **134**, 174–8.

Hughes, C. W., Preskorn, S. H., Weller, E., Weller, R., and Hassanein, R. (1988). Imipramine vs. placebo studies of childhood depression: baseline predictors of response to treatment and factor analysis of presenting symptoms. *Psychopharm. Bull.*, **24**, 275–9.

Hughes, C. W., Preskorn, S. H., Weller, E., *et al.* (1990). The effect of concomitant disorders in childhood depression on predicting treatment response. *Psychopharm. Bull.*, **26**, 235–8.

Hughes, C. W., Emslie, G., Crismon, M. L., *et al.* (1999). Report of the Texas consensus conference panel on medication treatment of childhood major depressive disorder. *Child Adolesc. Psychiatry*, **38**, 1442–54.

Hulshoff, P. H. E., Hoek, H. W., Susser, E., *et al.* (2000). Prenatal exposure to famine and brain morphology in schizophrenia. *Am. J. Psychiatry*, **157**, 1170–2.

Hunter, R. and Macalpine, I. (1982). *Three Hundred Years of Psychiatry 1535–1860.* Hartsdale, NY: Carlisle.

Hurley, S. C. (2002). Lamotrigine update and its use in mood disorders. *Ann. Pharmacother.*, **36**, 860–73.

Husain, S. S., Kevan, I. M., Linnell, R., and Scott, A. I. F. (2004). Electroconvulsive therapy in depressive illness that has not responded to drug treatment. *J. Affect. Disord.*, **83**, 121–6.

Huston, P. E. and Locher, L. M. (1948). Involutional psychosis. Course when untreated and when treated with electric shock. *Arch. Neurol. Psychiatry*, **59**, 385–94.

Hypericum Depression Trial Study Group (2002). Effect of *Hypericum perforatum* (St. John's wort) in major depressive disorder: a randomized controlled trial. *J.A.M.A.*, **287**, 1807–14.

Ilsley, J. E., Moffoot, A. P. R., and O'Carroll, R. E. (1995). An analysis of memory dysfunction in major depression. *J. Affect. Disord.*, **35**, 1–9.

Imani, A., Tandon, O. P., and Bhatia, M. S. (1999). A study of P300-event related evoked potential in the patients of major depression. *Ind. J. Physiol. Pharmacol.*, **43**, 367–72.

Ingraham, L. J. and Wender, P. H. (1992). Risk for affective disorder and alcohol and other drug abuse in the relatives of affectively ill adoptees. *J. Affect. Disord.*, **26**, 45–52.

Inman, W. H. W. (1988). Blood disorders and suicide in patients taking minanserin or amitriptyline. *Lancet*, **2**, 90–2.

Inoue, T., Tsuchiya, K., Miura, J., *et al.* (1996). Bromocriptine treatment of tricyclic and heterocyclic antidepressant-resistant depression. *Biol. Psychiatry*, **40**, 151–3.

Insel, T. R., Kalin, N. H., Guttmacher, L. B., Cohen, R. M., and Murphy, D. L. (1982). The dexamethasone suppression test in patients with primary obsessive-compulsive disorder. *Psychiatry Res.*, **6**, 153–60.

Inskip, H. M., Harris, E. C., and Barraclough, B. (1998). Lifetime risk of suicide for affective disorder, alcoholism and schizophrenia. *Br. J. Psychiatry*, **172**, 35–7.

Irwin, P. and Fink, M. (1983). Familiarization session and placebo control in EEG studies of drug effects. *Neuropsychobiol.*, **10**, 173–7.

Isacsson, G., Bergman, U., and Rich, C. L. (1994). Antidepressants, depression and suicide: an analysis of the San Diego study. *J. Affect. Disord.*, **32**, 277–86.

Isacsson, G., Bergman, U., and Rich, C. L. (1996). Epidemiological data suggest antidepressants reduce suicide risk among depressives. *J. Affect. Disord.*, **41**, 1–8.

Isacsson, G., Holmgren, P., Druid, H., and Bergman, U. (1999). Psychotropics and suicide prevention: implications from toxicological screening of 5281 suicides in Sweden 1992–1994. *Br. J. Psychiatry*, **174**, 259–65.

Isacsson, G., Holmgrem, P., and Ahlner, J. (2005). Selective serotonin reuptake inhibitor antidepressants and the risk of suicide: a controlled forensic database study of 14 857 suicides. *Acta Psychiat. Scand.*, **111**, 286.

Isbister, G. K., Prior, F. H., and Foy, A. (2001). Citalopram-induced bradycardia and presyncope. *Ann. Pharmacother.*, **35**, 1552–5.

Ismail, K., Murray, R. M., Wheeler, M. J., and O'Keane, V. (1998). The dexamethasone suppression test in schizophrenia. *Psychol. Med.*, **28**, 311–17.

Isometsa, E., Henriksson, M., Aro, H., *et al.* (1994b). Suicide in psychotic major depression. *J. Affect. Disord.*, **31**, 187–91.

Isometsa, E. T., Henriksson, M. M., Aro, H. M., *et al.* (1994a). Suicide in major depression. *Am. J. Psychiatry*, **151**, 530–6.

Isometsa, E. T., Aro, H. M., Henriksson, M. M., Heikkinen, M. E., and Lonnqvist, J. K. (1994c). Suicide in major depression in different treatment settings. *J. Clin. Psychiatry*, **55**, 523–7.

Isometsa, E. T., Henriksson, M. M., Aro, H. M., and Lonnqvist, J. K. (1994d). Suicide in bipolar disorder in Finland. *Am. J. Psychiatry*, **151**, 1020–4.

Isometsa, E. T., Henriksson, M. M., Heikkinen, M. E., and Lonnqvist, J. K. (1996). Completed suicide and recent electroconvulsive therapy in Finland. *Convuls. Ther.*, **12**, 152–5.

Itil, T. M. (ed.) (1974). *Psychotropic Drugs and the Human EEG. Modern Problems in Pharmacopsychiatry*, vol. 8. Basel: S. Karger.

Iverson, G. L. (2002). Screening for depression in systemic lupus erythematosus with British Columbia Major Depression Inventory. *Psychol. Rep.*, **90**, 1091–6.

Jackson, J. L., O'Malley, P. G., Tomkins, G., Sanoro, J., and Kroenke, K. (2002). Treatment of functional gastrointestinal disorders with antidepressant medications: a meta-analysis. *Am. J. Med.*, **108**, 65–72.

Jackson, S. W. (1986). *Melancholia and Depression. From Hippocrates to Modern Times.* New Haven: Yale University Press.

Jacobs, B. L., Praag, H., and Gage, F. H. (2000). Adult brain neurogenesis and psychiatry: a novel theory of depression. *Mol. Psychiatry*, **5**, 262–9.

Jainer, A. K. and Chawala, M. (2003). Randomized controlled trials (letter). *Am. J. Psychiatry*, **160**, 1188–9.

Jainer, A. K. Singh, A. N., and Soni, N. (2001). Light therapy for seasonal affective disorder: a type II error. *Br. J. Psychiatry*, **179**, 270.

Jamison, K. R. (2000). Suicide and bipolar disorder. *J. Clin. Psychiatry*, **61** (suppl. 9), 47–51.

Janicak, P. G., Davis, J. M., Gibbons, R. D., *et al.* (1985). Efficacy of ECT: a meta-analysis. *Am. J. Psychiatry*, **142**, 297–302.

Janicak, P. G., Dowd, S. M., Martis, B., *et al.* (2002). Repetitive transcranial magnetic stimulation versus electroconvulsive therapy for major depression: preliminary results of a randomized trial. *Biol. Psychiatry*, **51**, 659–67.

Jansen Steur, E. N. H. and Ballering, L. A. P. (1999). Combined and selective monoamine oxidase inhibition in the treatment of depression in Parkinson's disease. In Stern, G. M. (ed.) *Parkinson's Disease: Advances in Neurology*, vol. 80. Philadelphia: Lippincott, Williams & Wilkins, pp. 505–8.

Janssen, H. J. E. M., Cuisinier, M. C. J., Hoogduin, K. A. L., and deGraaw, K. P. (1996). Controlled prospective study on the mental health of women following pregnancy loss. *Am. J. Psychiatry*, **153**, 226–30.

Januel, D., Benadhira, R., Saba, G., *et al.* (2004). Recurrent episode in three older patients suffering from chronic depression: positive response to TMS treatment. *Int. J. Geriatr. Psychiatry*, **19**, 493–4.

Jenike, M. A., Baer, L., Brotman, A. W., *et al.* (1987). Obsessive-compulsive disorder, depression, and the dexamethasone suppression test. *J. Clin. Psychopharmacol.*, **7**, 182–4.

Jennings, K. D., Ross, S., Popper, S., and Elmore, M. (1999). Thoughts of harming infants in depressed and nondepressed mothers. *J. Affect. Disord.*, **54**, 21–8.

Jessner, L. and Ryan, V. G. (1941). *Shock Treatment in Psychiatry: A Manual.* New York: Grune & Stratton.

Jick, H., Kaye, J. A., and Jick, S. S. (2004). Antidepressants and the risk of suicidal behaviors. *J.A.M.A.*, **292**, 379–81.

Jindal, R. D., Thase, M. E., Fasiczka, A. L., *et al.* (2002). Electroencephalographic sleep profiles in single-episode and recurrent unipolar forms of major depression: II. Comparison during remission. *Biol. Psychiatry*, **51**, 230–6.

Joffe, R. and Levitt, A. (1992). Major depression and subclinical (grade 2) hypothyroidism. *Psychoneuroendocrinology*, **17**, 215–21.

(1993). *The Thyroid Axis and Psychiatric Illness.* Washington, DC: American Psychiatric Press.

Joffe, R. T. and Marriott, M. (2000). Thyroid hormone levels and recurrence of major depression. *Am. J. Psychiatry*, **157**, 1689–91.

Joffe, R. T., Roy-Byrne, P. P., Uhde, T. W., and Post, R. M. (1984). Thyroid function and affective illness: a reappraisal. *Biol. Psychiatry*, **19**, 1685–91.

Joffe, R. T., Lippert, G. P., Gray, T. A., Sawa, G., and Horvath, Z. (1987). Mood disorder and multiple sclerosis. *Arch. Neurol.*, **44**, 376–8.

Joffe, R. T., Singer, W., Levitt, A. J., and MacDonald, C. (1993). A placebo-controlled comparison of lithium and triiodothyronine augmentation of tricyclic antidepressants in unipolar refractory depression. *Arch. Gen. Psychiatry*, **50**, 387–93.

Joffe, R. T., Levitt, A. J., Sokolov, S. T., and Young, L. T. (1996). Response to an open trial of a second SSRI in major depression. *J. Clin. Psychiatry*, **57**, 114–15.

Joffe, R. T., MacQueen, G. M., Marriott, M., *et al.* (2002). Induction of mania and cycle acceleration in bipolar disorder. *Acta Psychiatr. Scand.*, **105**, 427–30.

Johnson, B. A., Brent, D. A., Bridge, J., *et al.* (1998). The familial aggregation of adolescent suicide attempt. *Acta Psychiatr. Scand.*, **97**, 18–24.

Johnson, B. A., Roache, J. D., Javors, M. A., *et al.* (2000). Ondansetron for reduction of drinking among biologically predisposed alcoholic patients. A randomized controlled trial. *J.A.M.A.*, **284**, 963–71.

Johnson, F. N. (1987). *Depression and Mania, Modern Lithium Therapy.* Oxford, UK: IRL Press.

Johnson, J., Horwath, E., and Weissman, M. M. (1991). The validity of major depression with psychotic features based on a community study. *Arch. Gen. Psychiatry*, **48**, 1075–81.

Johnstone, S. J., Boyce, P. M., Hickey, A. R., Morris-Yates, A. D., and Harris, M. G. (2001). Obstetric risk factors for postnatal depression in urban and rural community samples. *Aust. NZ J. Psychiatry*, **35**, 69–74.

Jolliffe, T., Lansdown, R., and Robinson, T. (1992). *Autism: A Personal Account.* London: National Autistic Society.

Jones, C. R., Campbell, S. S., Zone, S. E., *et al.* (1999a). Familial advanced sleep-phase syndrome: a short period circadian rhythm variant in humans. *Nat. Med.*, **5**, 1062–5.

Jones, I. and Craddock, N. (2001a). Familiality of the puerperal trigger in bipolar disorder: results of a family study. *Am. J. Psychiatry*, **158**, 913–17.

(2001b). Candidate gene studies of bipolar disorder. *Ann. Med.*, **33**, 248–56.

Jones, I., Kent, L., and Craddock, N. (2002a). The genetics of affective disorders. In McGuffin, P., Owen, M. J., and Gottesman, I. I. (eds) *Psychiatric Genetics and Genomics*. Oxford, UK: Oxford University Press.

Jones, R., Yates, W. R., Williams, S., Zhou, M., and Hardman, L. (1999b). Outcome for adjustment disorder with depressed mood: comparison with other mood disorders. *J. Affect. Disord.*, **55**, 55–61.

Jones, R., Yates, W. R., and Zhou, M. H. (2002b). Readmission rates for adjustment disorders: comparison with other mood disorders. *J. Affect. Disord.*, **71**, 199–203.

Jorge, R. E., Robinson, R. G., Arndt, S. V., Starkstein, S. E., Forrester, A. W., and Geisler, F. (1993). Depression following traumatic brain injury: a 1 year longitudinal study. *J. Affect. Disord.*, **27**, 233–43.

Jorge, R. E., Robinson, R. G., Arndt, S., and Starkstein, S. (2003). Mortality and post-stroke depression: a placebo-controlled trial of antidepressants. *Am. J. Psychiatry*, **160**, 1823–9.

Jorge, R. E., Robinson, R. G., Moser, D., *et al.* (2004). Major depression following traumatic brain injury. *Arch. Gen. Psychiatry*, **61**, 42–50.

Josefsson, A., Berg, G., Nordin, C., and Sydsjo, G. (2001). Prevalence of depressive symptoms in late pregnancy and postpartum. *Acta Obstet. Gynecol. Scand.*, **80**, 251–5.

Joseph, V., Mamet, J., Lee, F., Dalmaz, Y., and Van Reeth, O. (2002). Prenatal hypoxia impaired circadian synchronization and response of the biological clock to light in adult rats. *J. Physiol.*, **543**, 387–95.

Jouvent, R., Abensour, P., Bonnet, A. M., *et al.* (1983). Antiparkinsonian and antidepressant effects of high doses of bromocriptine. *J. Affect. Disord.*, **5**, 141–5.

Joyce, P. R., Mulder, R. T., Luty, S. E., *et al.* (2002). Melancholia: definitions, risk factors, personality, neuroendocrine markers and differential antidepressant response. *Aust. NZ J. Psychiatry*, **36**, 376–83.

Judd, L. L., Akiskal, H. S., Schettler, P. J., *et al.* (2003). A prospective investigation of the natural history of the long-term weekly symptomatic status of bipolar II disorder. *Arch. Gen. Psychiatry*, **60**, 261–9.

Kahlbaum, K. L. (1882). Über cyclischen Irresein. *Irrenfreund*, **10**, 145–57.

(1874). *Die Katatonie oder das Spannungsirresein*. Berlin: Verlag August Hirshwald. Translated by Mora, G. (1973). *Catatonia*. Baltimore, MD: Johns Hopkins University Press.

Kahn, R. L. and Fink, M. (1960). Prognostic value of Rorschach criteria in clinical response to convulsive therapy. *J. Neuropsychiatry*, **1**, 242–5.

Kahn, R. L., Pollack, M., and Fink, M. (1960a). Figure-ground discrimination after induced altered brain function. *Arch. Neurol.*, **2**, 547–51.

(1960b). Social attitude (California F scale) and convulsive therapy. *J. Nerv. Ment. Dis.*, **130**, 187–92.

Kalayam, B. and Alexopoulos, G. S. (1989). Nifedipine in the treatment of blood pressure rise after ECT. *Convuls. Ther.*, **5**, 110–13.

(1999). Prefrontal dysfunction and treatment response in geriatric depression. *Arch. Gen. Psychiatry*, **56**, 713–18.

Kalin, N. H., Shelton, S. E., and Davidson, R. J. (2000). Cerebrospinal fluid corticotrophin-releasing hormone levels are elevated in monkeys with patterns of brain activity associated with fearful temperament. *Biol. Psychiatry*, **47**, 579–85.

Kalinowsky, L. B. (1943). Electric convulsive therapy, with emphasis on importance of adequate treatment. *Arch. Neurol. Psychiatry*, **50**, 652–60.

Kalinowsky, L. B. and Hoch, P. H. (1946). *Shock Treatments and Other Somatic Treatments in Psychiatry.* New York: Grune & Stratton.

Kallen, B. (2004). Neonate characteristics after maternal use of antidepressants in late pregnancy. *Arch. Pediatr. Adolesc. Med.*, **158**, 312–16.

Kallner, G., Lindelius, R., Petterson, U., Stockman, O., and Tham, A. (2000). Mortality in 4987 patients with affective disorders attending a lithium clinic or after having left it. *Pharmacopsychiatry*, **33**, 8–13.

Kamali, M., Oquendo, M. A., and Mann, J. J. (2001). Understanding the neurobiology of suicidal behavior. *Depress. Anxiety*, **14**, 164–76.

Kaneda, Y., Nakayama, H., Kagawa, K., Furuta, M., and Ikuta, T. (1996). Sex differences in visual evoked potential and electroencephalograms of healthy adults. *Tokushima J. Exp. Med.*, **43**, 143–52.

Kaneda, Y., Ikuta, T., Nakayama, H., Kagawa, K., and Furuta, N. (1997). Visual evoked potential and electroencephalogram of healthy females during the menstrual cycle. *J. Med. Invest.*, **44**, 41–6.

Kanetani, K., Kimura, M., and Endo, S. (2003). Therapeutic effects of milnacipran (serotonin noradrenalin reuptake inhibitor) on depression following mild and moderate traumatic brain injury. *J. Nippon Med. Sch.*, **70**, 313–20.

Kanner, A. M. and Nieto, J. C. (1999). Depressive disorders in epilepsy. *Neurology*, **53** (suppl. 2), S26–32.

Kanner, A. M., Kozak, A. M., and Frey, M. (2000). The use of sertraline in patients with epilepsy: is it safe? *Epilepsy Behav.*, **1**, 100–5.

Kantor, S. J. and Glassman, A. H. (1977). Delusional depressions: natural history and response to treatment. *Br. J. Psychiatry*, **131**, 351–60.

Kaplan, E. M. (2002). Efficacy of venlafaxine in patients with major depressive disorder who have unsustained or no response to selective serotonin reuptake inhibitors: an open-label, uncontrolled study. *Clin. Ther.*, **24**, 1194–200.

Kapur, S., Mieczkowski, T., and Mann, J. J. (1992). Antidepressant medications and the relative risk of suicide attempt and suicide. *J. A. M. A.*, **268**, 3441–5.

Karaaslan, F., Gonul, A. S., Oguz, A., Erdinc, E., and Esel, E. (2003). P300 changes in major depressive disorders with and without psychotic features. *J. Affect. Disord.*, **73**, 283–7.

Karam, E. G., Howard, D. B., Karam, A. N., *et al.* (1998). Major depression and external stressors: the Lebanon wars. *Eur. Arch. Psychiatry Clin. Neurosci.*, **248**, 225–30.

Karege, F., Perret, G., Bondolfi, G., *et al.* (2002). Decreased serum-derived neurotrophic factor levels in major depressed patients. *Psychiatry Res.*, **109**, 143–8.

Karliner, W. and Wehrheim, H. K. (1965). Maintenance convulsive treatments. *Am. J. Psychiatry*, **121**, 113–15.

Karpyak, V. M., Rasmussen, K. G., Hammill, S. C., and Mrazek, D. A. (2004). Changes in heart rate variability in response to treatment with electroconvulsive therapy. *J. ECT*, **20**, 81–8.

Kashani, J. H., Shekim, W. O., and Reid, J. C. (1984). Amitriptyline in children with major depressive disorder: a double-blind crossover pilot study. *J. Am. Acad. Child Psychiatry*, **23**, 348–51.

Kasper, S. (1995). Clinical efficacy of mirtazapine: a review of meta-analyses of pooled data. *Int. Clin. Psychopharmacol.*, **10** (suppl. 4), 25–35.

Katon, W. (1998). The effect of major depression on chronic medical illness. *Semin. Clin. Neuropsychiatry*, **3**, 82–6.

Katon, W., Rutter, C., Ludman, E. J., *et al.* (2001). A randomized trial of relapse prevention of depression in primary care. *Arch. Gen. Psychiatry*, **58**, 241–7.

Katzenberg, D., Young, T., Finn, L., *et al.* (1998). A *CLOCK* polymorphism associated with human diurnal preference. *Sleep*, **21**, 569–76.

Kaufman, J. and Charney D. (2003). The neurobiology of child and adolescent depression. In Cicchetti, D. and Walker, E. F. (eds) *Neurodevelopmental Mechanisms in Psychopathology.* Cambridge: Cambridge University Press, pp. 461–90.

Kaufman, J. and Ryan, N. (1999). The neurobiology of child and adolescent depression. In Charney, D., Nestler, E., and Bunny, B. (eds) *The Neurobiological Foundation of Mental Illness.* New York: Oxford University Press, pp. 810–22.

Kaustio, O., Partanen, J., Valkonen-Korhonen, M., Viinamaki, H., and Lehtonen, J. (2002). Affective and psychotic symptoms relate to different types of P300 alteration in depressive disorder. *J. Affect. Disord.*, **71**, 43–50.

Keck, M. E. and Holsboer, F. (2001). Hyperactivity of CRH neuronal circuits as a target for therapeutic interventions in affective disorders. *Peptides*, **22**, 835–44.

Keck, P. E. Jr. (2004). Evaluation and management of breakthrough depressive episodes. *J. Clin. Psychiatry*, **65** (suppl. 10), 11–15.

Keck, P. E. Jr., Hudson, J. I., Dorsey, C. M., and Campbell, P. I. (1991). Effect of fluoxetine on sleep. *Biol. Psychiatry*, **29**, 618–19.

Keck, P. E., McElroy, S. L., Havens, J. R., *et al.* (2003a). Psychosis in bipolar disorder: phenomenology and impact on morbidity and course of illness. *Compr. Psychiatry*, **44**, 263–9.

Keck, P. E. Jr., Nelson, E. B., and McElroy, S. L. (2003b). Advances in the pharmacologic treatment of bipolar depression. *Biol. Psychiatry*, **53**, 671–9.

Keilp, J. G., Sackeim, H. A., Brodsky, B. S., *et al.* (2001). Neuropsychological dysfunction in depressed suicide attempters. *Am. J. Psychiatry*, **158**, 735–41.

Keitner, G. I., Ryan, C. E., Miller, I. W., Kohn, R., and Epstein, N. B. (1991). 12-month outcome of patients with major depression and comorbid psychiatric or medical illness (compound depression). *Am. J. Psychiatry*, **148**, 345–50.

Keller, M. B. (1999). The long-term treatment of depression. *J. Clin. Psychiatry*, **60** (suppl. 17), 41–5.

(2004). Remission versus response: the new gold standard of antidepressant care. *J. Clin. Psychiatry*, **65** (suppl. 4), 53–9.

Keller, M. B., Klerman, G. L., Lavori, P. W., *et al.* (1982). Treatment received by depressed patients. *J. A. M. A*, **248**, 1848–55.

Keller, M. B., Beardslee, W. R., Dorer, D. J., *et al.* (1986a). Impact of severity and chronicity of parental affective illness on adaptive functioning and psychopathology in children. *Arch. Gen. Psychiatry*, **43**, 930–7.

Keller, M. B., Lavori, P. W., Klerman, G. L., *et al.* (1986b). Low levels and lack of predictors of somatotherapy and psychotherapy received by depressed patients. *Arch. Gen. Psychiatry*, **43**, 458–66.

Keller, M. B., Beardslee, W., Lavori, P. W., Wunder, J., and Samuelson, H. (1988). Course of major depression in non-referred adolescents: a retrospective study. *J. Affect. Disord.*, **15**, 235–43.

Keller, M. B., Harrison, W., Fawcett, J. A., *et al.* (1995). Mood disorders: treatment of chronic depression with sertraline or imipramine: preliminary blinded response rates and high rates of undertreatment in the community. *Psychopharmacol. Bull.*, **31**, 205–12.

Keller, M. B., Gelenberg, A. J., Hirschfeld, R. M., *et al.* (1998). The treatment of chronic depression, part 2: a double-blind, randomized trial of sertraline and imipramine. *J. Clin. Psychiatry*, **59**, 598–607.

Keller, M. B., Ryan, N., Strober, M., *et al.* (2001). Efficacy of paroxetine in the treatment of adolescent major depression: a randomized, controlled study. *J. Am. Acad. Child Adolesc. Psychiatry*, **40**, 762–72.

Kellner, C. H. (ed.) (1991). Electroconvulsive therapy. *Psychiatr. Clin. North Am.*, **14**, 793–1035.

Kellner, C. H. and Bernstein, H. J. (1993). ECT as a treatment for neurologic illness. In Coffey, C. E. (ed.) (1993). *The Clinical Science of Electroconvulsive Therapy.* Washington, DC: American Psychiatric Press, pp. 183–210.

Kellner, C. H. and Fink, M. (1996). Seizure adequacy: does EEG hold the key? *Convuls. Ther.*, **12**, 203–6.

Kellner, C. H., Pritchett, J. T., Beale, M. D., and Coffey, C. E. (1997). *Handbook of ECT.* Washington, DC: American Psychiatric Press.

Kellner, C. H., Husain, M., Petrides, G., Rummans, T., and Fink, M. (2002). Equivalency of rTMS and ECT unproven. *Biol. Psychiatry*, **52**, 1032–3.

Kellner, C. H., Fink, M., Knapp, R., *et al.* (2005). Relief of expressed suicidal intent by ECT. A consortium for research in ECT study. *Am. J. Psychiatry*, **162**, 977–82.

Kellner, C. H., Knapp, R. G., Petrides, G., *et al.* (2005). Continuation ECT versus pharmacotherapy for relapse prevention in major depression: a multi-site study from CORE. *Arch. Gen. Psychiatry* (submitted).

Kelly, T. M., Cornelius, J. R., and Lynch, K. G. (2002). Psychiatric and substance use disorders as risk factors for attempted suicide among adolescents: a case control study. *Suicide Life Threat Behav.*, **32**, 301–12.

Kempermann, G. (2002). Regulation of adult hippocampal neurogenesis – implications for novel theories of major depression. *Bipolar Disord.*, **4**, 17–33.

Kendell, R. E. (1968). *The Classification of Depressive Illness.* London: Oxford University Press.

(1976). The classification of depressions: a review of contemporary confusion. *Br. J. Psychiatry*, **129**, 15–28.

(1990). Clinical validity. In Robins, L. N. and Barrett, J. E. (eds) *The Validity of Psychiatric Diagnosis.* New York: Raven Press, pp. 305–23.

Kendler, K. S. (1991). Mood-incongruent psychotic affective illness. *Arch. Gen. Psychiatry*, **48**, 362–9.

(1998). Anna-Monika-Prize paper: major depression and the environment: a psychiatric genetic perspective. *Pharmacopsychiatry*, **31**, 5–9.

Kendler, K. S. and Gardner, C. O. (1998). Boundaries of major depression: an evaluation of DSM-IV criteria. *Am. J. Psychiatry*, **155**, 172–7.

Kendler, K. S., Kessler, R. C., Heath, A. C., Neale, M. C., and Eaves, L. J. (1991a). Coping: a genetic epidemiological investigation. *Psychol. Med.*, **21**, 337–46.

Kendler, K. S., Neale, M. C., Heath, A. C., Kessler, R. C., and Eaves, L. J. (1991b). Life events and depressive symptoms: a twin study perspective. In McGuffin, P. and Murray, R. M. (eds) *The New Genetics of Mental Illness*. Stoneham, MA: Butterworth-Heinemann, pp. 146–64.

Kendler, K. S., Silberg, J. L., Neale, M. C., *et al.* (1992). Genetic and environmental factors in the aetiology of menstrual, premenstrual and neurotic symptoms: a population-based twin study. *Psychol. Med*, **22**, 85–100.

Kendler, K. S., Kessler, R. C., Neale, M. C., Heath, A. C., and Eaves, L. J. (1993a). The prediction of major depression in women: toward an integrated etiologic model. *Am. J. Psychiatry*, **150**, 1139–48.

Kendler, K. S., Neale, M., Kessler, R. C., Heath, A. C., and Eaves, L. I. (1993b). A longitudinal twin study of personality and major depression in women. *Arch. Gen. Psychiatry*, **50**, 853–62.

Kendler, K. S., Kessler, R. C., Walters, E. E., *et al.* (1995). Stressful life events, genetic liability, and onset of an episode of major depression in women. *Am. J. Psychiatry*, **152**, 833–42.

Kendler, K. S., Eaves, L. J., Walters, E. E., *et al.* (1996). The identification and validation of distinct depressive syndromes in a population-based sample of female twins. *Arch. Gen. Psychiatry*, **53**, 391–9.

Kendler, K. S., Davis, C. G., and Kessler, R. C. (1997). The familial aggregation of common psychiatric and substance use disorders in the National Comorbidity Survey: a family history study. *Br. J. Psychiatry*, **170**, 541–8.

Kendler, K. S., Karkowski, L. M., and Prescott, C. A. (1999). Causal relationship between stressful life events and the onset of major depression. *Am. J. Psychiatry*, **156**, 837–41.

Kendler, K. S., Gardner, C. O., Neale, M. C., and Prescott, C. A. (2001a). Genetic risk factors for major depression in men and women: similar or different heritabilities and same or partly distinct genes? *Psychol. Med.*, **31**, 605–16.

Kendler, K. S., Thornton, L. M., and Gardner, C. O. (2001b). Genetic risk, number of previous depressive episodes, and stressful life events in predicting onset of major depression. *Am. J. Psychiatry*, **158**, 582–6.

Kendler, K. S., Sheth, K., Gardner, C. O., and Prescott, C. A. (2002). Childhood parental loss and risk for first-onset of major depression and alcohol dependence: the time-decay of risk and sex differences. *Psychol. Med.*, **32**, 1187–94.

Kenis, G. and Maes, M. (2002). Effects of antidepressants on the production of cytokines. *Int. J. Neuropsychopharmacol*, **5**, 401–12.

Kennaway, D. J. (2002). Programming of the fetal suprachiasmatic nucleus and subsequent adult rhythmicity. *Trends Endocrinol. Metab.*, **13**, 398–402.

Kennaway, D. J., Goble, F. C., and Stamp, G. E. (1996). Factors influencing the development of melatonin rhythmicity in humans. *J. Clin. Endocrinol. Metab.*, **81**, 1525–32.

Kennedy, N. and Paykel, E. S. (2004). Treatment and response in refractory depression: results from a specialist affective disorders service. *J. Affect. Disord.*, **81**, 49–53.

Kessing, L. V. (2003). Subtypes of depressive episodes according to ICD-10: prediction of risk and relapse and suicide. *Psychopathology*, **36**, 285–91.

(2004a). Severity of depressive episodes according to ICD-10: prediction of risk of relapse and suicide. *Br. J. Psychiatry*, **184**, 153–6.

(2004b). Endogenous, reactive and neurotic depression – diagnostic stability and long-term outcome. *Psychopathology*, **37**, 124–30.

Kessler R. (1998). Comorbidity of unipolar and bipolar depression with other psychiatric disorders in a general population survey. In Tohen, M. (ed). *Comorbidity in Affective Disorders*. New York: Marcel Dekker, pp. 1–25.

Kessler, R. C. (1997). The effects of stressful life events on depression. *Annu. Rev. Psychol.*, **48**, 191–214.

Epidemiology of women and depression. *J. Affect. Disord.*, **74**, 5–13.

Kessler, R. C., Berglund, P., Borges, G., Nock, M., and Wang, P. S. (2003). Epidemiology of women and depression. *J. Affect. Disord.*, **74**, 5–13.

Kessler, R. C. and Magee, W. J. (1993). Childhood adversities and adult depression: basic patterns of association in a US national survey. *Psychol. Med.*, **23**, 679–90.

Kessler, R. C., Nelson, C. B., McGonagle, K. A., *et al.* (1996). The epidemiology of co-occurring addictive and mental disorders: implications for prevention and service utilization. *Am. J. Orthopsychiatry*, **66**, 17–31.

Kessler, R. C., Crum, R. M., Warner, L. A., *et al.* (1997). Lifetime co-occurrence of DSM-III-R alcohol abuse and dependence with other psychiatric disorders in the National Comorbidity Survey. *Arch. Gen. Psychiatry*, **54**, 313–21.

Kessler, R. C. and Walters, E. E. (1998). Epidemiology of DSM-III-R major depression and minor depression among adolescents and young adults in the National Comorbidity Survey. *Depress. Anxiety*, **7**, 3–14.

Kessler, R. C., Berglund, P., Demler, O., *et al.* (2003a). The epidemiology of major depressive disorder: results from the National Comorbidity Survey Replication (NCS-R). *J. A. M. A.*, **289**, 3095–105.

Kessler, R. C., Merikangas, K. R., Berglund, P., *et al.* (2003b). Mild disorders should not be eliminated from the DSM-V. *Arch. Gen. Psychiatry*, **60**, 1117–22.

Kessler, R. C., Berglund, P., Borges, G., Nock, M., and Wang, P. S. (2005). Trends in suicide ideation, plans, gestures, and attempts in the United States, 1990–1992 to 2001–2003. *J. A. M. A.*, **293**, 2487–95.

Kety, S. S., Evarts, E. V., and Williams, H. L. (eds) (1967). *Sleep and Altered States of Consciousness*. Baltimore, MD: Williams & Wilkins.

Khan, A., Noonan, C., and Healey, W. (1991). Is a single tricyclic antidepressant trial an active treatment for psychotic depression? *Prog. Neuropsychopharmacol. Biol. Psychiatry*, **15**, 765–70.

Khan, A., Warner, H. A., and Brown, W. A. (2000). Symptom reduction and suicide risk in patients treated with placebo in antidepressant clinical trials: an analysis of the Food and Drug Administration database. *Arch. Gen. Psychiatry*, **57**, 311–17.

Khan, A., Detke, M., Khan, S. R. F., and Mallinckrodt, C. (2003a). Placebo response and antidepressant clinical trial outcome. *J. Nerv. Ment. Dis.*, **191**, 211–18.

Khan, A., Khan, S., Kolts, R., and Brown, W. A. (2003b). Suicide rates in clinical trials of SSRIs, other antidepressants, and placebo: analysis of FDA reports. *Am. J. Psychiatry*, **160**, 790–2.

Khan, A., Kolts, R., Thase, M. E., Kishnan, K. R., and Brown, W. (2004). Research design features and patient characteristics associated with the outcome of antidepressant clinical trials. *Am. J. Psychiatry*, **161**, 2045–9.

Kho, K. H., van Vreeswijk, M. F., Simpson, S., and Zwinderman, A. H. (2003). A meta-analysis of electroconvulsive therapy efficacy in depression. *J. ECT*, **19**, 139–47.

Kilzieh, N. and Akiskal, H. S. (1999). Rapid-cycling bipolar disorder. An overview of research and clinical experience. *Psychiatr. Clin. North Am.*, **22**, 585–607.

Kimmel, P. L. (2002). Depression in patients with chronic renal disease: what we know and what we need to know. *J. Psychosom. Res.*, **53**, 951–6.

King, D. A., Conwell, Y., Cox, C., *et al.* (2000). A neuropsychological comparison of depressed suicide attempters and nonattempters. *J. Neuropsychiatry Clin. Neurosci.*, **12**, 64–70.

King, R. A., Riddle, M. A., Chappell, P. B., *et al.* (1991). Emergence of self-destructive phenomena in children and adolescents during fluoxetine treatment. *J. Am. Acad. Child Adolesc. Psychiatry*, **30**, 179–86.

Kirkwood, S. C., SU, J. L., Conneally, M., and Foroud, T. (2001). Progression of symptoms in the early and middle stages of Huntington disease. *Arch. Neurol.*, **58**, 273–8.

Kirli, S. and Caliskan, M. (1998). A comparative study of sertraline versus imipramine in postpsychotic depressive disorder or schizophrenia. *Schizophr. Res.*, **7**, 103–11.

Kirsch, I., Moore, T. J., Scoboria, A., and Nicholls, S. S. (2002). The emperor's new drugs: an analysis of antidepressant medication data, submitted to the U. S. Food and Drug Administration. *Prevent. Treat*, **5**, 1–11.

Kirschbaum, C. and Hellhammer, D. H. (1994). Salivary cortisol in psychoneuroendocrine research: recent developments and applications. *Psychoneuroendocrinology*, **19**, 313–33.

Kizilbash, A. H., Vanderploeg, R. D., and Curtiss, G. (2002). The effects of depression and anxiety on memory performance. *Arch. Clin. Neuropsychol.*, **17**, 57–67.

Klaassen, T., Verhey, F. R. J., Sneijders, G. H. J. M., *et al.* (1995). Treatment of depression in Parkinson's disease: a meta-analysis. *J. Neuropsychiatry Clin. Neurosci.*, **7**, 281–6.

Klaiber, E. L., Broverman, D. M., Vogel, W., and Kobayashi, Y. (1979). Estrogen therapy for severe persistent depressions in women. *Arch. Gen. Psychiatry*, **36**, 550–4.

Klee, S. H. and Garfinkel, B. D. (1984). Identification of depression in children and adolescents: the role of the dexamethasone suppression test. *J. Am. Acad. Child. Psychiatry*, **23**, 410–15.

Klein, D. F. (1964). Delineation of two-drug-responsive anxiety syndromes. *Psychopharmacologia*, **5**, 397–408.

(1967). Importance of psychiatric diagnosis in prediction of clinical drug effects. *Arch. Gen. Psychiatry*, **16**, 118–26.

(1974). Endogenomorphic depression. *Arch. Gen. Psychiatry*, **31**, 447–54.

Klein, D. F. and Fink, M. (1962a). Psychiatric reaction patterns to imipramine. *Am. J. Psychiatry*, **119**, 432–8.

(1962b). Behavioral reaction patterns with phenothiazines. *Arch. Gen. Psychiatry*, **7**, 449–59.

Klein, D. F. and Liebowitz, M. R. (1982). Hysteroid dysphoria (letter). *Am. J. Psychiatry*, **139**, 1520–1.

Klein, D. N. and Riso, L. P. (1993). Psychiatric disorders: problems of boundaries and comorbidity. In Costello, C. G. (ed). *Basic Issues in Psychopathology.* New York, NY: Guilford Press, pp. 19–66.

Klein, D. N., Clark, C., Dansky, L., and Margolis, E. T. (1988). Dysthymia in the offspring of parents with primary unipolar affective disorder. *J. Abnorm. Psychol.*, **97**, 265–74.

Klein, D. N., Riso, L. P., Donaldson, S. K., *et al.* (1995). Family study of early-onset dysthymia: mood and personality disorders in relatives of outpatients with dysthymia and episodic major depression and normal controls. *Arch. Gen. Psychiatry*, **52**, 487–96.

Klein, D. N., Kocsis, J. H., McCullough, J. P., *et al.* (1996). Symptomatology in dysthymic and major depressive disorder. *Psychiatr. Clin. North Am.*, **19**, 41–53.

Klein, D. N., Lewinsohn, P. M., Seeley, J. R., and Rohde, P. (2001). A family study of major depressive disorder in a community sample of adolescents. *Arch. Gen. Psychiatry*, **589**, 13–20.

Klein, E., Kreinin, I., Christyakov, A., *et al.* (1999). Therapeutic efficacy of right prefrontal slow repetitive transcranial magnetic stimulation in major depression. A double-blind controlled study. *Arch. Gen. Psychiatry*, **56**, 315–20.

Kleindienst, N. and Greil, W. (2003). Lithium in the long-term treatment of bipolar disorders. *Eur. Arch. Psychiatry Clin. Neurosci.*, **253**, 120–5.

Kleinman, A. and Good, B. (eds) (1985). *Culture and Depression: Studies in Antrhopology and Cross-cultural Psychiatry of Affect and Disorder (Culture and Depression).* Berkeley, CA: University of California Press.

Kleitman, N. (1939). *Sleep and Wakefulness.* Chicago, IL: University of Chicago Press.

Klerman, G. L. (1971). Clinical research in depression. *Arch. Gen. Psychiatry*, **24**, 305–19.

Klimek, V., Schenck, J. E., Han, H., Stockmeier, C. A., and Ordway, G. A. (2002). Dopaminergic abnormalities in amygdaloid nuclei in major depression: a postmortem study. *Biol. Psychiatry*, **52**, 740–8.

Kling, M. A., Roy, A., Doran, A. R., *et al.* (1991). Cerebrospinal fluid immunoreactive corticotropin-releasing hormone and adrenocorticotropin secretion in Cushing's disease and major depression: potential clinical implications. *J. Clin. Endocrinol. Metab.*, **72**, 260–71.

Klompenhouwer, J. L. and van Hulst, A. M. (1991). Classification of postpartum psychosis: a study of 250 mother and baby admissions in the Netherlands. *Acta Psychiatr. Scand.*, **84**, 255–61.

Knott, V. and Lapierre, Y. D. (1987). Computerized EEG correlates of depression and antidepressant treatment. *Prog. Neuro-psychopharmacol. Biol. Psychiatry*, **11**, 213–21.

Knott, V., Mahoney, C., Kennedy, S., and Evans, K. (2001). EEG power, frequency, asymmetry and coherence in male depression. *Psychiatry Res. Neuroimaging*, **106**, 123–40.

Kochar, D. K., Rawat, N., Agrawal, R. P., *et al.* (2004). Sodium valproate for painful diabetic neuropathy: a randomized double-blind placebo-controlled study. *Q. J. Med.*, **97**, 33–8.

Kocsis, J. H. (1997). Chronic depression: the efficacy of pharmacotherapy. In Akiskal, H. S. and Cassano, G. B. (eds) *Dysthymia and the Spectrum of Chronic Depressions.* New York: Guilford Press, pp. 66–74.

Kocsis, J. H., Frances, A. J., Voss, C., *et al.* (1988). Imipramine treatment for chronic depression. *Arch. Gen. Psychiatry*, **45**, 253–7.

Kocsis, J. H., Friedman, R. A., Markowitz, J. C., *et al.* (1996). Maintenance therapy for chronic depression. A controlled clinical trial of desipramine. *Arch. Gen. Psychiatry*, **53**, 769–74.

Kocsis, J. H., Schatzberg, A., Rush, A. J., *et al.* (2002). Psychosocial outcomes following long-term, double-blind treatment of chronic depression with sertraline vs placebo. *Arch. Gen. Psychiatry,* **59**, 723–8.

Kocsis, J. H., Rush, A. J., Markowitz, J. C., *et al.* (2003). Continuation treatment of chronic depression: a comparison of nefazodone, cognitive behavioral analysis system of psychotherapy, and their combination. *Psychopharmacol. Bull.*, **37**, 73–87.

Koenig, H. G., Meador, K. G., Cohen, J. H., and Blazer, D. G. (1992). Screening for depression in hospitalized elderly medical patients: taking a closer look. *J. Am. Geriatr. Soc.*, **40**, 1013–17.

Koike, A. K., Unutzer, J., and Wells, K. B. (2002). Improving the care for depression in patients with comorbid medical illness: *Am. J. Psychiatry,* **159**, 1738–45.

Koller, E. A. and Doraiswamy, P. M. (2002). Olanzapine-associated diabetes mellitus. *Pharmacotherapy,* **22**, 841–52.

Kolvin, I., Barrett, M. L., Bhate, S. R., *et al.* (1991). The Newcastle Child Depression Project diagnosis and classification of depression. *Br. J. Psychiatry,* **159** (suppl. 11), 9–21.

Kondro, W. (2004). Drug company experts advised staff to withhold data about SSRI use in children. *C. M. A. J.*, **170**, 783.

Kooi, K. A. (1971). *Fundamentals of Electroencephalography.* New York: Harper & Row.

Koorengevel, K. M., Gordijn, M. C., Beersma, D. G., *et al.* (2001). Extraocular light therapy in winter depression: a double-blind placebo-controlled study. *Biol. Psychiatry,* **50**, 691–8.

Koper, J. W., Stolk, R. P., de Lange, P., *et al.* (1997). Lack of association between five polymorphisms in the human glucocorticoid receptor gene and glucocorticoid resistance. *Hum. Genet.*, **99**, 663–8.

Koran, L. M., Gelenberg, A. J., Kornstein, S. G., *et al.* (2001). Sertraline versus imipramine to prevent relapse in chronic depression. *J. Affect. Disord.*, **65**, 27–36.

Koren, G., Pasturszak, A., and Ito, S. (1998). Drugs in pregnancy. *N. Engl. J. Med.*, **338**, 1128–37.

Koren, G., Cohn, T., Chitayat, D., *et al.* (2002). Use of atypical antipsychotics during pregnancy and the risk of neural tube defects in infants. *Am. J. Psychiatry,* **159**, 136–7.

Korzekwa, M. I., Lamont, J. A., and Steiner, M. (1996). Late luteal phase dysphoric disorder and the thyroid axis revisited. *J. Clin. Endocrinol. Metab.*, **81**, 2280–4.

Kornstein, S. G. and Schneider, R. K. (2001). Clinical features of treatment-resistant depression. *J. Clin. Psychiatry,* **62** (suppl. 16), 18–25.

Kosaten, T. R., Jacobs, S., and Mason, J. W. (1984). The dexamethasone suppression test during bereavement. *J. Nerv. Ment. Dis.*, **172**, 359–60.

Kosel, M., Frick, C., Lisanby, S. H., Fisch, H.-U., and Schlaepfer, T. E. (2003). Magnetic seizure therapy improves mood in refractory major depression. *Neuropsychopharm.*, **28**, 2045–8.

Kostic, V. S., Covickovic-Sternic, N., Beslac-Bumbasirevic, L., *et al.* (1990). Dexamethasone suppression test in patients with Parkinson's disease. *Move. Disord.*, **5**, 23–6.

Kovacs, M., Beck, A. T., and Weissman, A. (1976). The communication of suicidal intent. A reexamination. *Arch. Gen. Psychiatry,* **33**, 198–201.

Kovacs, M., Akiskal, H. S., Gatsonis, C., and Parrone, P. L. (1994). Childhood-onset dysthymic disorder. Clinical features and prospective naturalistic outcome. *Arch. Gen. Psychiatry,* **51**, 365–74.

Kovacs, M., Devlin, B., Pollock, M., Richards, C., and Mukerji, P. (1997). A controlled family history study of childhood-onset depressive disorder. *Arch. Gen. Psychiatry,* **54**, 613–23.

Kraemer, A. D. and Feiguine, R. J. (1981). Clinical effects of amitriptyline in adolescent depression. *J. Am. Acad. Child Psychiatry*, **20**, 636–44.

Kraepelin, E. (1896). *Psychiatrie: ein Lehrbuch für Studierende und Ärzte*, 6th edn. Leipzig: J Ambrosius Barth. Abstracted and reprinted (1902). *Clinical Psychiatry: A Textbook for Students and Physicians*. New York: Macmillan.

(1913). *Lectures on Clinical Psychiatry*. London: Bailhère, Tindall & Cox.

(1918). *Hundert Jahre Psychiatrie; ein Beitrag zur Geschichte menschlicher Gesittung*. Berlin: Springer. Translated: *One Hundred Years of Psychiatry*. New York: Philosophical Library (1962).

(1921). *Manic-Depressive Insanity and Paranoia*. Translated by Barclay, R. M. edited by Robertson, G. M. Edinburgh: E&S Livingstone. Reprinted New York: Arno Press (1976).

Kramer, B. (1982). Poor response to electroconvulsive therapy in patients with a combined diagnosis of major depression and borderline personality disorder. *Lancet*, **2**, 1048.

Kramer, B. A. (1985). Use of ECT in California, 1977–1983. *Am. J. Psychiatry*, **142**, 1190–2.

(1999). Use of ECT in California. Revisited: 1984–1994. *J. ECT*, **15**, 245–51.

Kramp, P. and Bolwig, T. G. (1981). Electroconvulsive therapy in acute delirious states. *Compr. Psychiatry*, **22**, 368–71.

Kranzler, H. R. and Van Kirk, J. (2001). Efficacy of naltrexone and acamprosate for alcoholism treatment: a meta-analysis. *Alcohol Clin. Exp. Res.*, **25**, 1335–41.

Kranzler, H. R., Burleson, J. A., Korner, P., *et al.* (1995). Placebo-controlled trial of fluoxetine as an adjunct to relapse prevention in alcoholics. *Am. J. Psychiatry*, **152**, 391–7.

Kreutzer, J. S. W., Seel, R. T., and Gourley, E. (2001). The prevalence and symptom rates of depression after traumatic brain injury: a comprehensive examination. *Brain Inj.*, **15**, 563–76.

Krishnan, K. R. (2002). Biological risk factors in late life depression. *Biol. Psychiatry*, **52**, 185–92.

(2003). Comorbidity and depression treatment. *Biol. Psychiatry*, **53**, 701–6.

Krishnan, K. R., Hays, J. C., George, L. K., and Blazer, D. G. (1998). Six-month outcomes for MRI-related vascular depression. *Depress. Anxiety*, **8**, 142–6.

Krishnan, K. R., Doraiswamy, P. M., and Clary, C. M. (2001). Clinical and treatment response characteristics of late-life depression associated with vascular disease: a pooled analysis of two multicenter trials with sertraline. *Prog. Neuropsychopharmacol. Biol. Psychiatry*, **25**, 347–61.

Krishnan, R. R., Maltbie, A. A., and Davidson, J. R. (1983). Abnormal cortisol suppression in bipolar patients with simultaneous manic and depressive symptoms. *Am. J. Psychiatry*, **140**, 203–5.

Kroes, M., Kalff, A. C., Kessels, A. G., *et al.* (2001). Child psychiatric diagnoses in a population of Dutch school children aged 6 to 8 years. *J. Am. Acad. Child Adolesc. Psychiatry*, **40**, 1401–9.

Kroessler, D. (1985). Relative efficacy rates for therapies of delusional depression. *Convuls. Ther.*, **1**, 173–82.

Kronfeld, A. (1939). Die Schockbehandlung des manischdepressiven Irreseins. *Allg. Z. Psychiatr.*, **112**, 436–45.

Kronfol, Z. and House, J. D. (1989). Lymphocyte mitogenesis, immunoglobulin and complement levels in depressed patients and normal controls. *Acta Psychiatr. Scand.*, **80**, 142–67.

Kronfol, Z. and Remick, D. G. (2000). Cytokines and the brain: implications for clinical psychiatry. *Am. J. Psychiatry*, **157**, 683–94.

Kronfol, Z., Singh, V. J., and Zhang, Q. (1995). Plasma cytokines, acute phase proteins and cortisol in major depression (abstract). *Biol. Psychiatry*, **37** (suppl.), 609A.

Kronig, M. H. and Gold, M. S. (1986). Thyroid testing in psychiatric patients. In Gold, M. S. and Pottash, A. L. C. (eds) *Diagnostic and Laboratory Testing in Psychiatry*, vol. 5. New York: Plenum Medical Book Publishing, pp. 47–58.

Krueger, J. M. and Majde, J. A. (1994). Microbial products and cytokines in sleep and fever regulation. *CRC Crit. Rev. Immunol.*, **14**, 355–79.

Kryger, M. H., Roth, T., and Dement, W. C. (2000). *Principles and Practice of Sleep Medicine*, 3rd edn. Philadelphia: Saunders.

Kryzhanovskaya, L. and Canterbury, R. (2001). Suicidal behavior inpatients with adjustment disorders. *Crisis*, **22**, 125–31.

Kubera, M., Kenis, G., Bosmans, E., *et al.* (2004). Stimulatory effect of antidepressants on the production of IL-6. *Int. Immunopharmacol.*, **4**, 185–92.

Kugaya, A., Epperson, C. N., Zoghbi, S., *et al.* (2003). Increase in prefrontal cortex serotonin$_{2A}$ receptors following estrogen treatment in postmenopausal women. *Am. J. Psychiatry*, **160**, 1522–4.

Kulin, N. A., Pastuszak, A., Sage, S. R., *et al.* (1998). Pregnancy outcome following maternal use of the new selective serotonin reuptake inhibitors: a prospective controlled multicenter study. *J. A. M. A.*, **279**, 609–10.

Kumar, A., Alcser, K., Grunhaus, L., and Greden, J. F. (1986). Relationships of the dexamethasone suppression test to clinical severity and degree of melancholia. *Biol. Psychiatry*, **21**, 436–44.

Kumar, C., McIvor, R. J., Davies, T., *et al.* (2003). Estrogen administration does not reduce the rate of recurrence of affective psychosis after childbirth. *J. Clin. Psychiatry*, **64**, 112–18.

Kunugi, H., Urushibara, T., and Nanko, S. (2004). Combined DEX/CRH test among Japanese patients with major depression. *J. Psychiatr. Res.*, **38**, 123–8.

Kuny, S. and Stassen, H. H. (1995). Cognitive performance in patients recovering from depression. *Psychopathology*, **28**, 190–207.

Künzel, H. E., Binder, E. B., Nickel, T., *et al.* (2003a). Pharmacological and nonpharmacological factors influencing hypothalamic–pituitary–adrenocortical axis reactivity in acutely depressed psychiatric in-patients, measured by the Dex-CRH test. *Neuropsychopharmacology*, **28**, 2169–78.

Künzel, H. E., Zobel, A. W., Nickel, T., *et al.* (2003b). Treatment of depression with the CRH-1-receptor antagonist R121919: endocrine changes and side effects. *J. Psychiatr. Res.*, **37**, 525–33.

Kupfer, D. J. and Reynolds, C. F III (1992). Sleep and affective disorders. In Paykel, E. S. (ed). *Handbook of Affective Disorders, 2nd ed.* Edinburgh: Churchill Livingstone, pp. 311–23.

Kupfer, D. J., Foster, F. G., Coble, P., McPartland, R. J., and Ulrich, R. F. (1978). The application of EEG sleep for the differential diagnosis of affective disorders. *Am. J. Psychiatry*, **135**, 69–74.

Kupfer, D. J., Reynolds, C. F. 3rd, Grochocinski, V. J., Ulrich, R. F., and McEachran, A. (1986). Aspects of short REM latency in affective states: a revisit. *Psychiatry Res.*, **17**, 49–59.

Kupfer, D. J., Carpenter, L. L., and Frank, E. (1988). Possible role of antidepressants in precipitating mania and hypomania in recurrent depression. *Am. J. Psychiatry*, **145**, 804–8.

Kupfer, D. J., Frank, E., and Perel, J. M. (1989). The advantage of early treatment intervention in recurrent depression. *Arch. Gen. Psychiatry*, **46**, 771–5.

Kupfer, D. J., First, M. B., and Regier, D. A. (eds) (2002). *A Research Agenda for DSM-V.* Washington, DC: American Psychiatric Press.

Küppers, E. (1939). Die Stockbehandlung des manisch-depressiven Irreseins. *Allg. Z. Psychiatry*, **112**, 436–45.

Kurki, T., Hiilesmaa, V., Raitasalo, R., Mattila, H., and Ylikorkala, O. (2000). Depression and anxiety in early pregnancy and risk for preeclampsia. *Obstet. Gynecol.*, **95**, 487–90.

Kurstjens, S. and Wolke, D. (2001). Effects of maternal depression on cognitive development of children over the first 7 years of life. *J. Child Psychol. Psychiatry*, **42**, 623–36.

Kusumakar, V. and Yatham, L. N. (1997). An open study of lamotrigine in refractory bipolar depression. *Psychiatry Res.*, **72**, 145–8.

Kutcher, S. and Marton, P. (1991). Affective disorders in first-degree relatives of adolescent onset bipolars, unipolars, and normal controls. *J. Am. Acad. Child Adolesc. Psychiatry*, **30**, 75–8.

Kutcher, S. and Robertson, H. A. (1995). Electroconvulsive therapy in treatment-resistant bipolar youth. *J. Child Adolesc. Psychopharm.*, **5**, 167–75.

Kutcher, S., Boulos, C., Ward, B., *et al.* (1994). Response to desipramine treatment in adolescent depression: a fixed-dose, placebo-controlled trial. *J. Am. Acad. Child Adolesc. Psychiatry*, **33**, 686–94.

Kwon, J., Youn, T., and Jung, H. (1996). Right hemisphere abnormalities in major depression: quantitative electroencephalographic findings before and after treatment. *J. Affect. Disord.*, **40**, 169–73.

Kye, C. and Ryan, N. (1995). Pharmacologic treatment of child and adolescent depression. *Child Adolesc. Psychiatr. Clin North. Am.*, **4**, 261–81.

Kye, C. H., Waterman, G. S., Ryan, N. D., *et al.* (1996). A randomized, controlled trial of amitriptyline in the acute treatment of adolescent major depression. *J. Am. Acad. Child Adolesc. Psychiatry*, **35**, 1139–44.

Ladd, C., Owens, K. M., and Nemeroff, C. (1996). Persistent changes in CRF neuronal systems induced by maternal deprivation. *Endocrinology*, **137**, 1212–27.

Laghrissi-Thode, F., Pollock, B. G., Miller, M., *et al.* (1995). Comparative effects of sertraline and nortriptyline on body sway in older depressed patients. *Am. J. Geriatr. Psychiatry*, **3**, 217–28.

Lai, I. C., Hong, C. J., and Tsai, S. J. (2001). Association study of nicotinic-receptor variants and major depressive disorder. *J. Affect. Disord.*, **66**, 79–82.

Laifenfeld, D., Klein, E., and Ben-Shachar, D. (2002). Norepinephrine alters the expression of genes involved in neuronal sprouting and differentiation: relevance for major depression and antidepressant mechanisms. *J. Neurochem.*, **83**, 1054–64.

Laine, K., Heikkinen, T., Ekblad, U., and Kero, P., (2003). Effects of exposure to selective serotonin reuptake inhibitors during pregnancy on serotonergic symptoms in newborns and cord blood monoamine and prolactin concentrations. *Arch. Gen. Psychiatry*, **60**, 720–6.

Lam, R. W. and Levitt, A. J. (eds) (1999). *Canadian Consensus Guidelines for the Treatment of Seasonal Affective Disorder.* Vancouver, BC: Canada, Clinical & Academic Publishing.

Lam, R. W. and Stewart, N. J. (1996). The validity of atypical depression in DSM-IV. *Compr. Psychiatry*, **37**, 375–83.

Lam, R. W., Buchanan, A., Mador, J. A., Corral, M. R., and Remick, R. A. (1992). The effects of ultraviolet A wavelengths in light therapy for seasonal depression. *J. Affect. Disord.*, **24**, 237–43.

Lam, R. W., Carter, D., Misri, S., *et al.* (1999). A controlled study of light therapy in women with late luteal phase dysphoric disorder. *Psychiatry Res.*, **86**, 185–92.

Lam, R. W., Wan, D. D., Cohen, N. L., and Kennedy, S. H. (2002). Combining antidepressants for treatment-resistant depression: a review. *J. Clin. Psychiatry*, **63**, 685–93.

Lamberg, L. (2001). Psychiatric symptoms common in neurological disorders. *J.A.M.A*, **286**, 154–6.

Lambert, G., Reid, C., Kaye, D., Jennings, G., and Esler, M. (2003). Increased suicide rate in the middle-aged and its association with hours of sunlight. *Am. J. Psychiatry*, **160**, 793–5.

Lambert, M. T., Trutia, C., and Petty, F. (1998). Extrapyramidal adverse effects associated with sertraline. *Prog. Neuropsychopharmacol. Biol. Psychiatry*, **22**, 741–8.

Lambert, M. V. and Robertson, M. M. (1999). Depression in epilepsy: etiology, phenomenology, and treatment. *Epilepsia*, **40** (suppl. 10), S21–47.

Lammers, C. H., Garcia-Borreguero, D., Schmider, J., *et al.* (1996). Combined dexamethasone/corticotrophin-releasing hormone test in patients with schizophrenia and in normal controls: II. *Biol. Psychiatry*, **40**, 560–1.

Lapipe, M. and Rondepierre, J. (1942). *Contribution a l'ĕtude physique, physiologique et clinique de l'ĕlectro-choc.* Parts: Librairie Maloine.

Lasser, R. A. and Baldessarini, R. J. (1997). Thyroid hormones in depressive disorders: a reappraisal of clinical utility. *Harv. Rev. Psychiatry*, **4**, 291–305.

Latham, A. E. and Prigerson, H. G. (2004). Suicidality and bereavement: Complicated grief as psychiatric disorder presenting greater risk for suicidality. *Suicide Life Threat Behav.*, **34**, 350–62.

Lauritzen, L., Odgaard, K., Clemmesen, L. *et al.* (1996). Relapse prevention by means of paroxetine in ECT-treated patients with major depression: a comparison with imipramine and placebo in medium-term continuation therapy. *Acta Psychiatr. Scand.*, **94**, 241–51.

Lavretsky, H. and Kumar, A. (2002). Clinically significant non-major depression: old concepts, new insights. *Am. J. Geriatr. Psychiatry*, **10**, 239–55.

Lavretsky, H. Lesser, I. M., Wohl, M., Miller, B. L., and Mehringer, C. M. (1999). Clinical and neuroradiologic features associated with chronicity in late-life depression. *Am. J. Geriatr. Psychiatry*, **7**, 309–16.

Lawrie, T. A., Hofmeyr, G. J., De Jager, M., *et al.* (1998). A double-blind randomized placebo controlled trial of postnatal norethisterone enanthate: the effect on postnatal depression and serum hormones. *Br. J. Obstet. Gynaecol.*, **105**, 1082–90.

Lawson, J. S., Inglis, J., Delva, N. J., *et al.* (1990). Electrode placement in ECT: cognitive effects. *Psychol. Med.*, **20**, 335–44.

Leckman, J. F., Weissman, M. M., Prusoff, B. A., *et al.* (1984). Subtypes of depression. *Arch. Gen. Psychiatry*, **41**, 833.

Lecrubier, Y., Clerc, G., Didi, R., and Kieser, M. (2002). Efficacy of St. John's wort extract WS 5570 in major depression: a double-blind, placebo-controlled trial. *Am. J. Psychiatry*, **159**, 1361–6.

Le Doux, J. E. (1992). Emotion and the amygdala. In Aggleton, J. P. (ed.) *The Amygdala: Neurobiological Aspects of Emotion, Memory, and Mental Dysfunction.* New York: Wiley-Liss, pp. 339–51.

Le Doux, J. E., Thompson, M. E., Ladecola, C., Tucker, L. W., and Reis, D. J. (1983). Local cerebral blood flow increases during auditory and emotional processing in the conscious rat. *Science*, **221**, 576–8.

Lee, G. P., Loring, D. W., Dahl, J. L., and Meador, K. J. (1993). Hemispheric specialization for emotional expression. *Neuropsychiatry Neuropsychol. Behav. Neurol.*, **6**, 143–8.

Lee, G. P., Meador, K. J., Loring, D. W., *et al.* (2004). Neural substrates of emotion as revealed by functional magnetic resonance imaging. *Cogn. Behav. Neurol.*, **17**, 9–17.

Lee, H. C., Chiu, H. F., Wing, Y. K., *et al.* (1994). The Zung Self-Rating Depression Scale: screening for depression among the Hong Kong Chinese elderly. *J. Geriatr. Psychiatry Neurol.*, **7**, 216–20.

Lee, S., Wing, Y. K., and Fong, S. (1998). A controlled study of folate levels in Chinese inpatients with manic depression in Hong Kong. *J. Affect. Disord.*, **49**, 73–7.

Lee, T. W., Tsai, S. J., Yang, C. H., and Hwang, J. P. (2003). Clinical and phenomenological comparisons of delusional and non-delusional major depression in the Chinese elderly. *Int. J. Geriatr. Psychiatry*, **18**, 486–90.

Leentjens, A. F., Verhey, F. R., Lousberg, R., Sptisbergen, H., and Wilmink, F. W. (2000a). The validity of the Hamilton and Montgomery-Asberg Depression rating scales as screening and diagnostic tools for depression in Parkinson's disease. *Int. J. Geriatr. Psychiatry*, **15**, 644–9.

Leentjens, A. F., Verhey, F. R., Luijckx, G. J., and Troost, J. (2000b). The validity of the Beck Depression Inventory as a screening and diagnostic instrument for depression in patients with Parkinson's disease. *Move. Disord.*, **15**, 1221–4.

Leentjens, A. F., Marinus, J., Van Hilten, J. J., Lousberg, R., and Verhey, F. R. J. (2003). The contribution of somatic symptoms to the diagnosis of depressive disorder in Parkinson's disease: a discriminant analytic approach. *J. Neuropsychiatry Clin. Neurosci.*, **15**, 74–7.

Legg, N. and Swash, M. (1974). Clinical note: seizures and EEG activation after trimipramine. *Epilepsia*, **15**, 131–5.

Lehofer, M., Moser, M., Hoehn-Saric, R., *et al.* (1999). Influence of age on the parasympatholytic property of tricyclic antidepressants. *Psychiatry Res.*, **85**, 199–207.

Lemonde, S., Turecki, G., Bakish, D., *et al.* (2003). Impaired repression at a 5-hydroxytryptamine 1A receptor gene polymorphism associated with major depression and suicide. *J. Neurosci.*, **223**, 8788–99.

Lenze, E. J., Dew, M. A., Mazumdar, S., *et al.* (2002). Combined pharmacotherapy and psychotherapy as maintenance treatment for late-life depression: effects on social adjustment. *Am. J. Psychiatry*, **159**, 466–8.

Leo, R. J. (1996). Movement disorders associated with the serotonin selective reuptake inhibitors. *J. Clin. Psychiatry*, **57**, 449–54.

Leon, A. C., Keller, M. B., Warshaw, M. G., *et al.* (1999). Prospective study of fluoxetine treatment and suicidal behavior in affectively ill subjects. *Am. J. Psychiatry*, **156**, 195–201.

Leon, A. C., Solomon, D. A., Mueller, T. I., *et al.* (2003). A 20-year longitudinal observational study of somatic antidepressant treatment effectiveness. *Am. J. Psychiatry*, **160**, 727–33.

Leonard, B. E. (2001). The immune system, depression and the action of antidepressants. *Prog. Neuro-Psychopharm. Biol. Psychiatry*, **25**, 767–80.

Leonard, J. F., Bluet-Pajot M. T., Oliver, C., and Kordan, C. (1998). Interaction of vasoactive intestinal peptide (VIP) and growth hormone releasing factor (GRF) with corticotropin releasing factor (CRF). and corticotropin secretion in vitro. *Neuropeptides*, **12**, 131–3.

Leonhard, K. (1995). *The Classification of Endogenous Psychoses.* New York: Stuttgart: Georg Thieme Verlag.

Lerer, B. and Macciardi, F. (2002). Pharmacogenetics of antidepressant and mood-stabilizing drugs: a review of candidate-gene studies and future research directions. *Int. J. Neuropsychopharmacol.*, **5**, 255–75.

Lerer, B., Shapira, B., Calev, A., *et al.* (1995). Antidepressant and cognitive effects of twice-versus three-times-weekly ECT. *Am. J. Psychiatry*, **152**, 564–70.

Lerman, C., Shields, P. G., Wileyto, E. P., *et al.* (2002). Pharmacogenetic investigation of smoking cessation treatment. *Pharmacogenetics*, **12**, 627–34.

Lesch, K. P. (2001). Variation of serotonergic gene expression: neurodevelopment and the complexity of response to psychopharmacologic drugs. *Eur. Neuropsychopharmacol.*, **11**, 457–74.

Lester, D. (1992). The dexamethasone suppression test as an indicator of suicide: a meta-analysis. *Pharmacopsychiatry*, **25**, 265–70.

Letemendia, F. J. J., Delva, N. J., Rodenburg, M., *et al.* (1993). Therapeutic advantage of bifrontal electrode placement in ECT. *Psychol. Med.*, **23**, 349–60.

Leuchter, A. F., Cook, I. A., Witte, E. A., Morgan, M., and Abrams, M. (2002). Changes in brain function of depressed subjects during treatment with placebo. *Am. J. Psychiatry*, **159**, 122–9.

Leung, C. M., Wing, Y. K., Kwong, P. K., Lo, A., and Shum, K. (1999). Validation of the Chinese-Cantonese version of the hospital anxiety and depression scale and comparison with the Hamilton Rating Scale of Depression. *Acta Psychiatr. Scand.*, **100**, 456–61.

Levin, G. M., Grum, C., and Eisele, G. (1998). Effect of over-the-counter dosages of naproxen sodium and acetaminophen on plasma lithium concentrations in normal volunteers. *J. Clin. Psychopharmacol.*, **18**, 237–40.

Levin, H. S., Brown, S. A., Song, J. X., *et al.* (2001). Depression and posttraumatic stress disorder at three months after mild to moderate traumatic brain injury. *J. Clin. Exp. Neuropsychol.*, **23**, 754–69.

Levinson, D. F., Zubenko, G. S., Crowe, R. R., *et al.* (2003). Genetics of recurrent early-onset depression (GenRED): design and preliminary clinical characteristics of a repository sample for genetic linkage studies. *Am. J. Med. Genetics*, **119B**, 118–30.

Levitan, R. D., Lesage, A., Parikh, S. V., Goering, P., and Kennedy, S. H. (1997). Reversed neurovegetative symptoms of depression: a community study of Ontario. *Am. J. Psychiatry*, **154**, 934–40.

Levitt, A. J., Lam, R. W., and Levitan, R. (2002). A comparison of open treatment of seasonal major and minor depression with light therapy. *J. Affect. Disord.*, **71**, 243–8.

Levkovitz, Y., Caftori, R., Avital, A., and Reichter-Levin, G. (2002). The SSRI drug fluoxetine, but not the noradrenergic tricyclic drug desipramine, improves memory performance during acute major depression. *Brain Res. Bull.*, **58**, 345–50.

Levy, M. L., Cummings, J. L., Fairbanks, L. A., *et al.* (1998). Apathy is not depression. *J. Neuropsychiatry Clin. Neurosci.*, **10**, 314–19.

Lewinsohn, P. M., Rohde, P., Klein, D. N., and Seeley, J. R. (1999). Natural course of adolescent major depressive disorder: I. Continuity into young adulthood. *J. Am. Acad. Child Adolesc. Psychiatry*, **38**, 56–63.

Lewinsohn, P. M., Joiner, T. E. Jr., and Rohde, P. (2001a). Evaluation of cognitive diathesis-stress models in predicting major depressive disorders in adolescents. *J. Abnorm. Psychol.*, **110**, 203–15.

Lewinsohn, P. M., Rohde, P., Seeley, J. R., and Baldwin, C. L. (2001b). Gender differences in suicide attempts from adolescence to young adulthood. *J. Am. Acad. Child Adolesc. Psychiatry*, **40**, 427–34.

Lewinsohn, P. M., Pettit, J. W., Joiner, T. E. Jr., and Seeley, J. R. (2003). The symptomatic expression of major depressive disorder in adolescents and young adults. *J. Abnorm. Psychol.*, **112**, 244–52.

Lewis, A. J. (1934a). Melancholia: a historical review. *J. Ment. Sci.*, **80**, 1–42.

(1934b). Melancholia: a clinical survey of depressive states. *J. Ment. Sci.*, **80**, 277–8.

Lewis, J. L. and Winokur, G. (1982). The induction of mania. A natural history study with controls. *Arch. Gen. Psychiatry*, **39**, 303–6.

Lewis, R. W. B. (1991). *The Jameses: A Family Narrative.* New York: Farrar, Strauss Giroux.

Lian, J. (1997). Nefazodone treatment of depression requires less use of concomitant anxiolytic and sedative/hypnotic drugs. Annual Meeting of the American Psychiatric Association. San Diego, 1997; APA New Research program and Abstracts (vol NR397), p. 175.

Licinio, J. and Wong, M. L. (1999). The role of inflammatory mediators in the biology of major depression: cerebral nervous system cytokines modulate the biological substrate of depressive symptoms, regulate stress responsive systems, and contribute to neurotoxicity and neuroprotection. *Mol. Psychiatry*, **4**, 317–27.

Lieb, R., Isensee, B., Hofler, M., Pfister, H., and Wittchen, H.-U. (2002). Parental major depression and the risk of depression and other mental disorders in offspring. A prospective-longitudinal community study. *Arch. Gen. Psychiatry*, **59**, 365–74.

Lieber, A. and Newbury, N. (1988). Diagnosis and subtyping of depressive disorders by quantitative electroencephalography: III. Discriminating unipolar and bipolar depressives. *Hillside J. Clin. Psychiatry*, **10**, 165–72.

Lieberman, J. A., Kane, J. M., Sarantakos, S., *et al.* (1985). Dexamethasone suppression tests in patients with obsessive-compulsive disorder. *Am. J. Psychiatry*, **142**, 747.

Lieberman, J. A., Stroup, T. S., McEvoy, J. P., *et al.* (2005). Effectiveness of antipsychotic drugs in patients with chronic schizophrenia. *N. Engl. J. Med.*, **353**, 1209–23.

Lima, M. S., Reisser, A. A., Soares, B. G., and Farrell, M. (2001). Antidepressants for cocaine dependence. *Cochrane Database Syst. Rev.*, CD002950.

Lin, P. Y. and Tsai, G. (2004). Association between serotonin transporter gene promoter polymorphism and suicide: results of a meta-analysis. *Biol. Psychiatry*, **55**, 1023–30.

Linde, K., Ramirez, G., Mulrow, C. D., *et al.* (1996). St. John's Wort for depression. An overview of meta-analysis of randomized clinical trials. *Br. Med. J.*, **313**, 253–8.

Linde, K., Berner, M., Egger, M., and Mulrow, C. (2005). St. John's wort for depression: meta-analysis of randomised controlled trials. *Br. J. Psychiatry*, **186**, 99–107.

Linden, M., Borchelt, M., Barnow, S., and Geiselmann, B. (1995). The impact of somatic morbidity on the Hamilton Depression Rating Scale in the very old. *Acta Psychiatr. Scand.*, **92**, 150–4.

Lindley, S. E. and Schatzberg, A. F. (2003). Historical roots of psychoneuroendocrinology. In Wolkowitz, O. M. and Rothschild, A. J. (eds) *Psychoneuroendocrinology: The Scientific Basis of Clinical Practice*, vol. 2. Washington, DC: American Psychiatric Publishing, pp. 9–28.

Linkowski, P., Brauman, H., and Mendlewicz, J. (1981). Thyrotrophin response to thyrotrophin-releasing hormone in unipolar and bipolar affective illness. *J. Affect. Disord.*, **3**, 9–16.

Linkowski, P., Kerkhofs, M., Van Onderbergen, A., *et al.* (1994). The 24-hour profiles of cortisol, prolactin, and growth hormone secretion in mania. *Arch. Gen. Psychiatry*, **51**, 616–24.

Lisanby, S. H. (2002). Update on magnetic seizure therapy: a novel form of convulsive therapy. *J. ECT*, **18**, 182–8.

Lisanby, S. H. (ed.) (2004). *Brain Stimulation in Psychiatric Treatment.* Washington, DC: American Psychiatric Press.

Lisanby, S. H., Luber, B., Schlaepfer, T. E., and Sackeim, H. A. (2003). Safety and feasibility of magnetic seizure therapy (MST) in major depression: randomized within-subject comparison with electroconvulsive therapy. *Neuropsychopharm*, **28**, 1852–65.

Liscombe, M. P., Hoffmann, R. F., Trivedi, M. H., *et al.* (2002). Quantitative EEG amplitude across REM sleep periods in depression: preliminary report. *J. Psychiatry Neurosci.*, **27**, 40–6.

Lithner, F. (2000). Venlafaxine in treatment of severe painful peripheral diabetic neuropathy. *Diabetes Care*, **23**, 1710–11.

Litman, R. E. (1982). Hospital suicides: lawsuits and standards. *Suicide Life Threat. Behav.*, **12**, 212–20.

Little, J. D., Munday, J., Lyall, G., *et al.* (2003). Right unilateral electroconvulsive therapy at six times seizure threshold. *Aust. NZ J. Psychiatry*, **37**, 715–19.

Little, J. D., Munday, J., Atkins, M. R., and Khalid, A. (2004). Does electrode placement predict time to re-hospitalization? *J. ECT*, **20**, 213–18.

Livesley, W. J., Jang, K. L., Jackson, D. N., and Vernon, P. A. (1993). Genetic and environmental contributions to dimensions of personality disorder. *Am. J. Psychiatry*, **150**, 1826–31.

Livingston, R., Nugent, H., Rader, L., and Smith, G. R. (1985). Family histories of depressed and severely anxious children. *Am. J. Psychiatry*, **142**, 1497–9.

Lockwood, K. A., Alexopoulos, G. S., and van Gorp, W. G. (2002). Executive dysfunction in geriatric depression. *Am. J. Psychiatry*, **159**, 1119–26.

Loehlin, J. C. (1992). *Genes and Environment in Personality Development.* Beverly Hills, CA: Sage.

Lohmann, T., Nishimura, K., Sabri, O., and Klosterkotter, J. (1996). Successful electroconvulsive therapy of Cotard syndrome with bitemporal hypoperfusion. *Nervenarzt*, **67**, 400–3.

Loo, C., Mitchell, P., Sachdev, P., *et al.* (1999). Double-blind controlled investigation of transcranial magnetic stimulation for the treatment of resistant major depression. *Am. J. Psychiatry*, **156**, 946–8.

Loosen, P. (1987). The TRH stimulation test in psychiatric disorders: a review. In Nemeroff, C. B. and Loosen, P. T. (eds) *Handbook of Clinical Psychoneuroendocrinology*, vol. 15. New York: Guilford Press, pp. 336–60.

Loosen, P. T. (1985). The TRH-induced TSH response in psychiatric patients: a possible neuroendocrine marker. *Psychoneuroendocrinology*, **10**, 237–60.

Lopez, J. F., Chalmers, D. T., Little, K. Y., and Watson, S. J. (1998). Regulation of serotonin 1A, glucorticoid, and mineralocorticoid receptor in rat and human hippocampus: implications for the neurobiology of depression. *Biol. Psychiatry*, **43**, 547–73.

López-Ibor, J. J. (1950). *La angustia vital, patología general psicosomática*. Madrid: paz Montalvo.

López-Ibor, J. J. Jr. (1992). Serotonin and psychiatric disorders. *Int. Clin. Psychopharmacol.*, **7** (suppl. 2), 5–11.

López-Ibor, J. J., Saiz-Ruiz, J., and Pereze de los Cobos, J. C. (1985). Biological correlations of suicide and aggressivity in major depressions (with melancholia): 5-hydroxyindoleacetic acid and cortisol in cerebral spinal fluid, dexamethasone suppression test and therapeutic response to 5-hydroxytryptophan. *Neuropsychobiology*, **14**, 67–74.

Loving, R. T., Kripke, D. F., and Shuchter, S. R. (2002). Bright light augments antidepressant effects of medication and wake therapy. *Depress. Anxiety*, **16**, 1–3.

Lowy, M. T., Reder, A. T., Gormley, G. J., and Meltzer, H. Y. (1988). Comparison of in vivo and in vitro glucocorticoid sensitivity in depression: relationship to the dexamethasone suppression test. *Biol. Psychiatry*, **24**, 619–30.

Lu, R. B., Ho, S. L., Huang, H. C., and Lin, Y. T. (1988). The specificity of the dexamethasone suppression test in endogenous depressive patients. *Neuropsychopharmacology*, **1**, 157–62.

Lublin, F. D., Whitaker, J. N., Eidelman, B. H., *et al.* (1996). Management of patients receiving interferon beta-1b for multiple sclerosis: report of a consensus conference. *Neurology*, **46**, 12–18.

Luby, J. L., Heffelfinger, A. K., Mrakotsky, C., *et al.* (2002). Preschool major depressive disorder: preliminary validation for developmentally modified DSM-IV criteria. *J. Am. Acad. Child Adolesc. Psychiatry*, **41**, 928–37.

(2003a). Alterations in stress cortisol reactivity in depressed preschoolers relative to psychiatric and no-disorder comparison groups. *Arch. Gen. Psychiatry*, **60**, 1248–55.

(2003b). The clinical picture of depression in preschool children. *J. Am. Acad. Child Adolesc. Psychiatry*, **42**, 340–8.

Luby, J. L., Mrakotsky, C., Heffelfinger, A., *et al.* (2003c). Modification of DSM-IV criteria for depressed preschool children. *Am. J. Psychiatry*, **160**, 1169–72.

Luby, J. L., Mrakotsky, C., Heffelfinger, A., Brown, K., and Spitznagel, E. (2004). Characteristics of depressed preschoolers with and without anhedonia: evidence for a melancholic depressive subtype in young children. *Am. J. Psychiatry*, **161**, 1998–2004.

Lucas, R. J. and Foster, R. G. (1999). Photoentrainment in mammals: a role for cryptochrome? *J. Biol. Rhythms*, **14**, 4–10.

Lumley, J. and Austin, M. P. (2001). What interventions may reduce postpartum depression?. *Curr. Opin. Obstet. Gynecol.*, **13**, 605–11.

Lundberg, J. M., Modin, A., and Malmstrom, R. E. (1996). Recent developments with neuropeptide Y receptor antagonists. *Trends Pharmacol. Sci.*, **17**, 301–4.

Luoma, J. B., Martin, C. E., and Pearson, J. L. (2002). Contact with mental health and primary care providers before suicide: a review of the evidence. *Am. J. Psychiatry*, **159**, 909–16.

Lustman, P. J. and Clouse, R. E. (2002). Treatment of depression in diabetes. Impact on mood and medical outcome. *J. Psychosom. Res.*, **53**, 917–24.

Lustman, P. J., Freedland, K. E., Griffith, L. S., and Clouse, R. E. (1997a). Fluoxetine for depression in diabetes. *Gen. Hosp. Psychiatry*, **19**, 138–43.

Lustman, P. J., Griffith, L. S., Clouse, R. E., *et al.* (1997b). Effects of nortriptyline on depression and glycemic control in diabetes: results of a double-blind, placebo-controlled trial. *Psychosom. Med.*, **59**, 241–50.

Lustman, P. J., Anderson, R. J., Freedland, K. E., de Groot, M., and Carney, R. M. (2000). Depression and poor glycemic control: a meta-analytic review of the literature. *Diabetes Care*, **23**, 434–42.

Lyketsos, C. G. and Olin, J. (2002). Depression in Alzheimer's disease: overview and treatment. *Biol. Psychiatry*, **52**, 243–52.

Lyketsos, C. G., Tune, L. E., Pearlson, G., and Steele, C. (1996). Major depression in Alzheimer's disease: an interaction between gender and family history. *Psychosomatics*, **37**, 380–9.

Lykouras, L., Gournellis, R., Fortos, A., Oulis, P., and Christodoulou, G. N. (2002). Psychotic (delusional) major depression in the elderly and suicidal behaviour. *J. Affect. Disord.*, **69**, 225–9.

Lynch, M. E. (2001). Antidepressants as analgesics: a review of randomized controlled trials. *J. Psychiatry Neurosci.*, **26**, 30–6.

Lyness, J. M., Caine, E. D., King, D. A., *et al.* (1999). Cerebrovascular risk factors and depression in older primary care patients. Testing a vascular brain disease model of depression. *Am. J. Geriatr. Psychiatry*, **7**, 252–8.

Lyons, M. J., Eisen, S. A., Goldberg, J., *et al.* (1998). A registry-based twin study of depression in men. *Arch. Gen. Psychiatry*, **55**, 468–72.

Lyons, W. E., Mamounas, L. A., Ricaurte, G. A., *et al.* (1999). Brain-derived neurotrophic factor-deficient mice develop aggressiveness and hyperphagia in conjunction with brain serotonergic abnormalities. *Proc. Natl. Acad. Sci. USA*, **96**, 15239–44.

Lyons-Ruth, K., Wolfe, R., Lyubchik, A., and Steingard, R. (2002). Depressive symptoms in parents of children under three: sociodemographic predictors, current correlates and associated parenting behaviors. In Halfon, N., Schuster, M., and Taaffe Young, K. (eds) *Child-Rearing in America: Challenges Facing Parents with Young Children.* New York: Cambridge University Press, pp. 217–62.

Macalpine, I. and Hunter, R. (1974). The pathography of the past. *Times Literary Suppl.*, March 15, 256–257.

Macdonald, H., Rutter, M., Howlin, P., *et al.* (1989). Recognition and expression of emotional cues by autistic and normal adults. *J. Child Psychol. Psychiatry*, **30**, 865–78.

MacEwan, G. W. and Remick, R. A. (1988). Treatment resistant depression: a clinical perspective. *Can. J. Psychiatry*, **33**, 788–92.

MacFadyen, H. W. (1975a). The classification of depressive disorders. I. A review of statistically based classification studies. *J. Clin. Psychol.*, **31**, 380–94.

(1975b). The classification of depressive disorders. II. A review of historical and physiological classification studies. *J. Clin. Psychol.*, **31**, 394–401.

MacFall, J. R., Payne, M. E., Provenzale, J. E., and Krishnan, K. R. (2001). Medial orbital frontal lesions in late-onset depression. *Biol. Psychiatry*, **49**, 803–6.

MacGillivray, S., Arrol, B., Hatcher, S., *et al.* (2003). Efficacy and tolerability of selective serotonin reuptake inhibitors compared with tricyclic antidepressants in depression treated in primary care: systematic review and meta-analysis. *Br. Med. J.*, **326**, 1014.

MacHale, S. M., Lawrie, S. M., Cavanagh, J. T. O., *et al.* (2000). Cerebral perfusion in chronic fatigue syndrome and depression. *Br. J. Psychiatry*, **176**, 550–6.

MacQueen, G. M. and Joffe, R. T. (2002). A review of gender differences in studies of thyroid function and major depression. *Psychiatr. Ann.*, **32**, 477–82.

MacQueen, G. M., Trevor Young, L., Marriott, M., *et al.* (2002). Previous mood state predicts response and switch rates inpatients with bipolar depression. *Acta Psychiatr. Scand.*, **105**, 414–18.

MacQueen, G. M., Campbell, S., McEwen, B. S., *et al.* (2003). Course of illness, hippocampal function, and hippocampal volume in major depression. *Neuroscience*, **100**, 1387–92.

Macritchie, K. A. N., Geddes, J. R., Scott, J. (2002). Valproic acid, valproate and valproex in the maintenance treatment of bipolar disorder Cochrane Database Syst Rev 3: CD003196.

Madeira, M. D., Andrade, J. P., Lieberman, A. R., *et al.* (1997). Chronic alcohol consumption and withdrawal do not induce cell death in the suprachiasmatic nucleus, but lead to irreversible depression of peptide immunoreactivity and mRNA levels. *J. Neurosci.*, **17**, 1302–19.

Mader, A. (1938). Unsere Erfahrungen mit der Cardiozolbehandlung unter besonderer Berücksichtung depressiver Zustände. *Psychiatr. Neurol. Wochenschr.*, **40**, 331–8.

Madsen, T. M., Treschow, A., Bengzon, J., *et al.* (2000). Increased neurogenesis in a model of electroconvulsive therapy. *Biol. Psychiatry*, **47**, 1043–9.

Maes, M. and Smith, R. S. (1998). Fatty acids, cytokines, and major depression. *Biol. Psychiatry*, **43**, 313–14.

Maes, M., Cosyns, P., Maes, L., D'Hondt, P., and Schotte, C. (1990a). Clinical subtypes of unipolar depression: part I. A validation of the vital and nonvital clusters. *Psychiatry Res.*, **34**, 29–41.

Maes, M., Schotte, C., Maes, L., and Cosyns, P. (1990b). Clinical subtypes of unipolar depression: part II. Quantitative and qualitative clinical differences between the vital and nonvital depression groups. *Psychiatry Res.*, **34**, 43–57.

Maes, M., Dierckx, R., Meltzer, H. Y., *et al.* (1993a). Regional cerebral blood flow in unipolar depression measured with Tc-99m-HMPAO single photon emission computed tomography: negative findings. *Psychiatry Res.*, **50**, 77–88.

Maes, M., Bosmans, E., Meltzer, H. Y., Scharpe, S., and Suy, E. (1993b). Interleukin-1b: a putative mediator of HPA axis hyperactivity in major depression? *Am. J. Psychiatry*, **150**, 1189–93.

Maes, M., Meltzer, H. Y., Cosyns, P., and Schotte, C. (1994). Evidence for the existence of major depression with and without anxiety features. *Psychopathology*, **27**, 1–13.

Maes, M., Meltzer, H., Bosmans, E., *et al.* (1995). Increased plasma concentrations of interleukin-6, soluble interleukin-6 receptor, soluble interleukin-2 receptor and transferring receptor in major depression. *J. Affect. Disord.*, **34**, 301–9.

Maes, M., Delange, J., Ranjan, R., *et al.* (1997). Acute phase proteins in schizophrenia, mania and major depression: modulation by psychotropic drugs. *Psychiatry Res.*, **66**, 1–11.

Maes, M., Song, C., Lin, A., *et al.* (1998). The effects of psychological stress on humans: increased production of pro-inflammatory cytokines and a Th^1-like response in stress-induced anxiety. *Cytokine*, **10**, 313–18.

Magiakou, M. A., Mastorakos, G., Rabin, D., *et al.* (1996). Hypothalamic corticotropin-releasing hormone suppression during the postpartum period: implications for the increase in psychiatric manifestations at this time. *J. Clin. Endocrinol. Metab.*, **81**, 1912–17.

Magnusson, A. and Boivin, D. (2003). Seasonal affective disorder: an overview. *Chronobiol. Int.*, **20**, 189–207.

Maher, B. S., Marazita, M. L., Zubenko, W. N., Kaplan, B. B., and Zubenko, G. S. (2002). Genetic segregation analysis of alcohol and other substance-use disorders in families with recurrent, early-onset major depression. *Am. J. Drug Alcohol Abuse*, **28**, 711–31.

Mahgoub, N. A. and Hossein, A. (2004). Cotard's syndrome and electroconvulsive therapy. *Psychiatric Serv.*, **55**, 1319.

Maier, W., Lichtermann, D., Minges, J., and Heun, R. (1992a). Personality traits in subjects at risk for unipolar major depression: a family study perspective. *J. Affect. Disord.*, **24**, 153–63.

(1992b). The familial relation of personality disorders (DSM-III-R) to unipolar major depression. *J. Affect. Disord.*, **26**, 151–6.

Maj, M. (2003). The effect of lithium in bipolar disorder: a review of recent research evidence. *Bipolar Disord.*, **5**, 180–8.

Maj, M., Magliano, L., Priozzi, R., Marasco, C., and Guarneri, M. (1994). Validity of rapid cycling as a course specifier for bipolar disorder. *Am. J. Psychiatry*, **151**, 1015–19.

Maj, M., Pirozzi, R., Magliano, L., and Bartoli, L. (2003). Agitated depression in bipolar I disorder: prevalence, phenomenology, and outcome. *Am. J. Psychiatry*, **160**, 2134–40.

Malberg, J. E., Eisch, A. J., Nestler, E. J., and Duman, R. S. (2000). Chronic antidepressant treatment increases neurogenesis in adult rat hippocampus. *J. Neurosci.*, **20**, 9104–10.

Malhi, G. S., Mitchell, P. B., and Salim, S. (2003). Bipolar depression: management options. *CNS Drugs*, **17**, 9–25.

Malhi, G. S., Parker, G. B., Crawford, J., Wilhelm, K., and Mitchell, P. B. (2005). Treatment-resistant depression: resistant to definition? *Acta Psychiatr. Scand.*, **112**, 302–9.

Mallinckrodt, C. H., Watkin, J. G., Liu, C., Wohlreich, M. M., and Raskin, J. (2005). Duloxetine in the treatment of major depressive disorder: a comparison of efficacy in patients with and without melancholic features. *BMC Psychiatry*, **5**, 1.

Malone, K. M. (1997). Pharmacotherapy of affectively ill suicidal patients. *Psychiatr. Clin. North Am.*, **20**, 613–24.

Malone, K. M., Haas, G. L., Sweeney, J. A., and Mann, J. J. (1995). Major depression and the risk of attempted suicide. *J. Affect. Disord.*, **34**, 173–85.

Malur, C., Fink, M., and Francis, A. (2000). Can delirium relieve psychosis? *Compr. Psychiatry*, **41**, 450–3.

Malzberg, B. (1937). Mortality among patients with involuticn [sic] melancholia. *Am. J. Psychiatry*, **93**, 1231–8.

Mandkoki, M. W., Tapia, M. R., Tapia, M. A., Sumner, G. S., and Parker, J. L. (1997). Venlafaxine in the treatment of children and adolescents with major depression. *Psychopharmacol. Bull.*, **33**, 149–54.

Maneeton, N. and Srisurapanont, M. (2000). Tricyclic antidepressants for depressive disorders in children and adolescents: a meta-analysis of randomized-controlled trials. *J. Med. Assoc. Thai.*, **83**, 1367–74.

Manji, H. K., Drevets, W. C., and Charney, D. S. (2001). The cellular neurobiology of depression. *Nat. Med.*, **7**, 541–7.

Manji, H. K., Quiroz, J. A., Sporn, J., *et al.* (2003). Enhancing neuronal plasticity and cellular resilience to develop novel, improved therapeutics for difficult-to-treat depression. *Biol. Psychiatry*, **53**, 707–42.

Mann, J. J. and Kapur, S. (1991). The emergence of suicidal ideation and behavior during antidepressant pharmacotherapy. *Arch. Gen. Psychiatry*, **48**, 1027–33.

Mann, S. C., Caroff, S. N., Bleier, H. R., Antelo, E., and Un, H (1990). Electroconvulsive therapy of the lethal catatonia syndrome. *Convuls. Ther.*, **6**, 239–47.

Mann, J. J., Oquendo, M., Underwood, M. D., and Arango, V. (1999). The neurobiology of suicide risk: a review for the clinician. *J. Clin. Psychiatry*, **60** (suppl. 2), 7–11.

Mann, J. J., Brent, D. A., and Arango, V. (2001a). The neurobiology and genetics of suicide and attempted suicide: a focus on the serotonergic system. *Neuropsychopharm.*, **24**, 467–77.

Mann, S. C., Caroff, S. N., Bleier, H. R., *et al.* (1986). Lethal catatonia. *Am. J. Psychiatry*, **143**, 1374–81.

Mann, S. C., Auriocombe, M., Macfadden, W., *et al.* (2001b). La catatonie léthale: aspects cliniques et conduite thérapeutique. Une revue de la littérature. *L'Encéphale*, **27**, 213–16.

Manning, M. (1994). *Undercurrents, A Life Beneath the Surface.* San Francisco: Harper.

Mapother, E. (1926). Manic-depressive psychosis. *Br. Med. J.*, **2**, 872–7.

Marangell, L. B. (2001). Switching antidepressants for treatment-resistant major depression. *J. Clin. Psychiatry*, **62** (suppl. 18), 12–17.

Marangell, L. B., Rush, A. J., George, M. S., *et al.* (2002). Vagus nerve stimulation (VNS) for major depressive episodes: one year outcomes. *Biol. Psychiatry*, **51**, 280–7.

March, J., Silva, S., *et al.* (2004). Fluoxetine, cognitive-behavioral therapy, and their combination for adolescents with depression: Treatment for Adolescents with Depression Study (TADS) randomized controlled trial. *J.A.M.A*, **292**, 861–3.

Marchesi, C., Silvestrini, C., Ponari, O., *et al.* (1996). Unreliability of TRH test but not dexamethasone suppression test as a marker of depression in chronic vasculopathic patients. *Biol. Psychiatry*, **40**, 637–41.

Marco, E. J., Wolkowitz, O. M., Vinogradov, S., *et al.* (2002). Double-blind antiglucocorticoid treatment in schizophrenia and schizoaffective disorder: a pilot study. *World J. Biol. Psychiatry*, **3**, 156–61.

Margolese, H. C. (2000). The male menopause and mood: testosterone decline and depression in the aging male – is there a link? *J. Geriatr. Psychiatry Neurol.*, **13**, 93–101.

Marijnissen, G., Tuinier, S., Sijben, A. E., and Verhoeven, W. M. (2002). The temperament and character inventory in major depression. *J. Affect. Disord.*, **70**, 219–23.

Marin, R. S. (1991). Apathy: a neuropsychiatric syndrome. *J. Neuropsychiatry Clin. Neurosci.*, **3**, 243–54.

Maris, R. W. (1981). *Pathways to Suicide.* Baltimore, MD: Johns Hopkins University Press.

(2002). Suicide. *Lancet*, **360**, 319–26.

Markowitz, J. (1996). Psychotherapy for dysthymic disorder. *Psychiatr. Clin. North Am.*, **19**, 133–50.

Martin, A., Kaufman, J., and Charney, D. (2000). Pharmacotherapy of early-onset depression. *Psychopharm.*, **9**, 135–57.

Martin, J. L., Barbanoj, M. J., Schlaepfer, T. E., *et al.* (2002). Transcranial magnetic stimulation for treating depression. *Cochrane Database Syst. Rev.*, CD003493.

Martin, J. L., Barbanoj, M. J., Schlaepfer, T. E., *et al.* (2003). Repetitive transcranial magnetic stimulation for the treatment of depression. Systematic review and meta-analysis. *Br. J. Psychiatry*, **182**, 480–91.

Martinez Perez, B., Gonzalez Goizueta, E., and Mauri, J. A. (2002). Depression and epilepsy. *Rev. Neurol.*, **35**, 580–6.

Martinot, J.-L., Hardy, P., Feline, A., *et al.* (1990). Left prefrontal glucose hypometabolism in the depressed state: a confirmation. *Am. J. Psychiatry*, **147**, 1313–17.

Martinovic, Z., Jovanovic, V., and Ristanovic, D. (1998). EEG power spectra of normal preadolescent twins. Gender differences of quantitative EEG maturation. *Neuropsychol. Clin.*, **28**, 231–48.

Martis, B., Alam, D., Dowd, S. M., *et al.* (2003). Neurocognitive effects of repetitive transcranial magnetic stimulation in severe major depression. *Clin. Neurophysiol.*, **114**, 1125–32.

Masi, G., Favilla, L., Mucci, M., Poli, P., and Romano, R. (2001). Depressive symptoms in children and adolescents with dysthymic disorder. *Psychopathology*, **34**, 29–35.

Mason, B., Kocis, J., Ritvo, E., and Cutler, R. (1996). A double-blind, placebo-controlled trial of desipramine for primary alcohol dependence stratified on the presence or absence of major depression. *J.A.M.A*, **275**, 761–7.

Mason, W. A., Kosterman, R., Hawkins, J. D., *et al.* (2004). Predicting depression, social phobia, and violence in early adulthood from childhood behavior problems. *J. Am. Acad. Child Adolesc. Psychiatry*, **43**, 307–15.

Mathet, F., Martin-Guelhl, C., Maurice-Tison, S., and Bouvard, M. P. (2003). Prevalence of depressive disorders in children and adolescents attending primary care. A survey with the Aquitaine Sentinelle Network. *Encephale*, **29**, 391–400.

Mathew, S. J., Coplan, J. D., Goetz, R. R., *et al.* (2003). Differentiating depressed adolescent 24h cortisol secretion in light of their adult clinical outcome. *Neuropsychopharmacology*, **28**, 1336–43.

Mathews, C. A. and Reus, V. I. (2001). Assortative mating in the affective disorders: a systematic review and meta-analysis. *Compr. Psychiatry*, **42**, 257–62.

Matousek, M. (1991). EEG patterns in various subgroups of endogenous depression. *Int. J. Psychophysiol.*, **10**, 239–43.

Matsunaga, H. and Sarai, M. (2000). Low-dose (p.5 mg) DST in manic and major depressive episodes: in relation to the severity of symptoms. *Seishin Shinkeigaku Zasshi*, **102**, 367–98.

Matussek, P., Soldner, M., and Nagel, D. (1981). Identification of the endogenous depressive syndrome based on the symptoms and the characteristics of the course. *Br. J. Psychiatry*, **138**, 361–72.

Mayberg, H. S. (1994). Frontal lobe dysfunction in secondary depression. *J. Neuropsychiatry Clin. Neurosci.*, **6**, 428–42.

(1997). Limbic-cortical dysregulation: a proposed model of depression. *J. Neuropsychiatry*, **9**, 471–81.

(2003). Modulating dysfunctional limbic-cortical circuits in depression: towards development of brain-based algorithms for diagnosis and optimized treatment. *Br. Med. Bull.*, **65**, 193–207.

Mayberg, H. S., Liotti, M., Brannan, S. K., *et al.* (1999). Reciprocal limbic-cortical function and negative mood: converging PET findings in depression and normal sadness. *Am. J. Psychiatry*, **156**, 675–82.

Mayberg, H. S., Silva, A., Brannan, S. K., *et al.* (2002). The functional neuroanatomy of the placebo effect. *Am. J. Psychiatry*, **159**, 728–37.

Mayberg, H. S., Lozano, A. M., Voon, V., *et al.* (2005). Deep brain stimulation for treatment-resistant depression. *Neuron*, **45**, 651–60.

Mazeh, D., Melamed, Y., and Elizur, A. (1999). Venlafaxine in the treatment of resistant postpsychotic depressive symptoms of schizophrenia. *J. Clin. Psychopharmacol.*, **19**, 284–5.

Mbaya, P. (2002). Safety and efficacy of high dose of venlafaxine XL in treatment resistant major depression. *Hum. Psychopharmacol.*, **17**, 335–9.

McBride, W. J., Lovinger, D. M., Machu, T., *et al.* (2004). Serotonin-3 receptors in the actions of alcohol, alcohol reinforcement, and alcoholism. *Alcohol Clin. Exp. Res.*, **28**, 257–67.

McCall, W. V. (2001). Electroconvulsive therapy in the era of modern psychopharmacology. *Int. J. Neuropsychopharm.*, **4**, 315–24.

McCall, W. V., Reboussin, D. M., Weiner, R. D., and Sackeim, H. A. (2000). Titrated moderately suprathreshold vs fixed high-dose right unilateral electroconvulsive therapy. *Arch. Gen. Psychiatry*, **57**, 438–44.

McCauley, J., Kern, D. E., Kolodner, K., *et al.* (1997). Clinical characteristics of women with a history of childhood abuse. *J.A.M.A*, **277**, 1362–8.

McClure, G. M. G. (2001). Suicide in children and adolescents in England and Wales 1970–1998. *Br. J. Psychiatry*, **178**, 469–74.

McCombs, J. S., Stimmel, G. L., Hui, R. L., and White, T. J. (2001). The economic impact of treatment non-response in major depressive disorders. In Amsterdam, J. D., Hornig, M., and Nierenberg, A. A. (eds) *Treatment-Resistant Mood Disorders*. Cambridge UK: Cambridge University Press, pp. 491–516.

McDowell, D. M. and Clodfelter, R. C. Jr. (2001). Depression and substance abuse: considerations of etiology, comorbidity, evaluation, and treatment. *Psychiatr. Ann.*, **31**, 244–51.

McDowell, D. M., Levin, F. R., Seracini, A. M., and Nunes, E. V. (2000). Venlafaxine treatment of cocaine abusers with depressive disorders. *Am. J. Drug Alcohol Abuse*, **26**, 25–31.

McElhatton, P. R., Garbis, H. M., Elefant, E., *et al.* (1996). The outcome of pregnancy in 689 women exposed to therapeutic doses of antidepressants: a collaborative study of the European Network of Teratology Information Services (ENTIS). *Reprod. Toxicol.*, **10**, 285–94.

McElroy, S. L., Zarate, C. A., Cookson, J., *et al.* (2004). A 52-week, open-label continuation study of lamotrigine in the treatment of bipolar depression. *J. Clin. Psychiatry*, **65**, 204–10.

McGinn, L. K., Asnis, G. M., and Rubinson, E. (1996). Biological and clinical validation of atypical depression. *Psychiatry Res.*, **60**, 191–8.

McGrath, P., Nunes, E., Stewart, J., *et al.* (1996). Imipramine treatment of alcoholics with primary depression: a placebo controlled trial. *Arch. Gen. Psychiatry*, **53**, 232–40.

McGrath, P. J., Stewart, J. W., Harrison, W. M., *et al.* (1992). Predictive value of symptoms of atypical depression for differential drug treatment outcome. *J. Clin. Psychopharm.*, **12**, 197–202.

McGue, M. and Lykken, D. T. (1992). Genetic influence on risk of divorce. *Psychol. Sci.*, **3**, 368–73.

McGuffin, P. and Katz, R. (1989). The genetics of depression and manic-depressive disorder. *Br. J. Psychiatry*, **155**, 294–304.

McGuffin, P., Rijsdijk, F., Andrew, M., *et al.* (2003). The heritability of bipolar affective disorder and the genetic relationship to unipolar depression. *Arch. Gen. Psychiatry*, **60**, 497–502.

McHolm, A. E., MacMillan, H. L., and Jamieson, E. (2003). The relationship between childhood physical abuse and suicidality among depressed women: results from a community sample. *Am. J. Psychiatry*, **160**, 933–8.

McHugh, P. R. and Slavney, P. R. (1982). Methods of reasoning in psychopathology: conflict and resolution. *Compr. Psychiatry*, **23**, 197–215.

McIntyre, R. S., Mancini, D. A., McCann, S., *et al.* (2002). Topiramate versus bupropion SR when added to mood stabilizer therapy for the depressive phase of bipolar disorder: a preliminary single-blind study. *Bipolar Disord.*, **4**, 207–13.

McKittrick, C. R., Magarinos, A. M., Blanchard, D. C., *et al.* (2000). Chronic social stress reduces dendritic arbors in CA3 of hippocampus and decreases binding to serotonin transporter sites. *Synapse*, **36**, 85–94.

McNamara, B., Ray, J. L., Arthurs, O. J., and Boniface, S. (2001). Transcranial magnetic stimulation for depression and other psychiatric disorders. *Psychol. Med.*, **31**, 1141–6.

McPherson, H., Walsh, A., and Silverstone, T. (2003).Growth hormone and prolactin response to apomorphine in bipolar and unipolar depression. *J. Affect. Disord.*, **76**, 121–5.

McQuillan, C. T. and Rodriguez, J. (2000). Adolescent suicide: a review of the literature. *Bol. Asoc. Med. P. R.*, **92**, 30–8.

Medawar, C. and Hardon, A. (2004). *Medicines out of Control? Antidepressants and the Conspiracy of Goodwill.* Amsterdam: Aksant.

Medical Research Council (1965). Clinical trial of the treatment of depressive illness. *Br. Med. J.*, **1**, 881–6.

Meduna, L. (1935). Versuche über die biologische Beeinflussung des Ablaufes der Schizophrenie: Camphor und Cardiozolkrampfe. *Z. Ges. Neurol. Psychiatr.*, **152**, 235–62.

(1937a). Die Bedeutung des epileptischen Anfalls in der Insulin- und Cardiozolbehandlung der Schizophrenie. *Psychiatrisch-Neurolog. Wochenschr.*, **30**, 1–11.

(1937b). *Die Konvulsionstherapie der Schizophrenie.* Halle: Karl Marhold.

(1950). *Oneirophrenia.* Urbana, IL: University of Illinois Press.

(1985). Autobiography. *Convuls. Ther.*, **1**, 43–57, 121–38.

Meier, A. (1979). The research diagnostic criteria: historical background, development, validity, and reliability. *Can. J. Psychiatry*, **24**, 167–78.

Meijer, O. C. and de Kloet, E. R. (1998). Corticosterone and serotonergic neurotransmission in the hippocampus: functional implications of central corticosteroid receptor diversity. *Crit. Rev. Neurobiol.*, **12**, 1–20.

Meijer, W. E. E., Bouvy, M. L., Heerdink, E. R., Urquhart, J., and Leufkens, H. G. M. (2001). Spontaneous lapses in dosing during chronic treatment with selective serotonin reuptake inhibitors. *Br. J. Psychiatry*, **179**, 519–22.

Melander, H., Ahlqvist-Rastad, J., Meijer, G., and Berermann, B (2003). Evidence biased medicine – selective reporting from studies sponsored by pharmaceutical industry: review of studies in new drug applications. *Br. Med. J.*, **326**, 1171–3.

Meldrum, B. S. (1994). Lamotrigine – a novel approach. *Seizure*, **3** (suppl. A), 41–5.

Mendels, J. (1965). Electroconvulsive therapy and depression. II. Significance of endogenous and reactive syndromes. *Br. J. Psychiatry*, **111**, 682–6.

Mendels, J. (1967). The prediction of response to electroconvulsive therapy, *Am. J. Psychiatry*, **124**, 153–9.

Mendelson, W. B. (1987). *Human Sleep*. New York: Plenum Medical Books.

Menna-Barreto, L., Isola, A., Louzada, F., Benedito-Silva, A. A., and Mello, L. (1996). Becoming circadian — a one-year study of the development of the sleep–wake cycle in children. *Braz. J. Med. Biol. Res.*, **29**, 125–9.

Menting, J. E., Honig, A., Verhey, F. R., *et al.* (1996). Selective serotonin reuptake inhibitors (SSRIs) in the treatment of elderly depressed patients: a qualitative analysis of the literature on their efficacy and side-effects. *Int. Clin. Psychopharmacol.*, **11**, 165–75.

Merikangas, K. R., Prusoff, B. A., and Weissman, M. M. (1988a). Parental concordance for affective disorders: psychopathology in offspring. *J. Affect. Disord.*, **15**, 279–90.

Merikangas, K. R., Weissman, M. M., Prusoff, B. A., and John, K. (1988b). Assortative mating and affective disorders: psychopathology in offspring. *Psychiatry*, **51**, 48–57.

Merikangas, K. R., Chakravarti, A., Moldin, S. O., *et al.* (2002). Future of genetics of mood disorders research. *Biol. Psychiatry*, **52**, 457–77.

Mesulam, M. M. (1999). Neuroplasticity failure in Alzheimer's disease: bridging the gap between plaques and tangles. *Neuron*, **24**, 521–9.

Meyer, S. E., Chrousos, G. P., and Gold, P. W. (2001). Major depression and the stress system: a life span perspective. *Dev. Psychopathol.*, **13**, 565–80.

Meyer, W. J. D., Richards, G. E., Cavallo, A., *et al.* (1991). Depression and growth hormone [letter, comment]. *J. Am. Acad. Child Adolesc. Psychiatry*, **30**, 335.

Meyers, B. S., Klimstra, S. A., Gabriele, M., *et al.* (2001). Continuation treatment of delusional depression in older adults. *Am. J. Geriatr. Psychiatry*, **9**, 415–22.

Michael, N., Erfurth, A., Ohrmann, P., *et al.* (2003). Metabolic changes within the left dorsolateral prefrontal cortex occurring with electroconvulsive therapy in patients with treatment resistant unipolar depression. *Psychol. Med.*, **33**, 1277–84.

Michell, P. B. and Malhi, G. S.. (2004). Bipolar depression: phenomenological overview and clinical characteristics. *Bipolar Disord.*, **6**, 530–9.

Miklowitz, D., Simoneau, T., George, E., *et al.* (2000). Family-focused treatment of bipolar disorder: 1-year effects of a psychoeducational program in conjunction with pharmacotherapy. *Biol. Psychiatry*, **48**, 582–92.

Milberger, S., Biederman, J., Faraone, S. V., Chen, L., and Jones, J. (1996). Is maternal smoking during pregnancy a risk factor for attention deficit hyperactivity disorder in children? *Am. J. Psychiatry*, **153**, 1138–42.

Miles, P. (1977). Conditions predisposing to suicide: a review. *J. Nerv. Ment. Dis.*, **164**, 231–46.

Miller, A., Fox, N. A., Cohn, J. F., *et al.* (2002a). Regional patterns of brain activity in adults with a history of childhood-onset depression: gender differences and clinical variability. *Am. J. Psychiatry*, **159**, 934–40.

Miller, F. T. and Chabrier, L. A. (1988). Suicide attempts correlate with delusional content in major depression. *Psychopathology*, **21**, 34–7.

Miller, F. T. and Freilicher, J. (1995). Comparison of TCAs and SSRIs in the treatment of major depression in hospitalized geriatric patients. *J. Geriatr. Psychiatry Neurol.*, **8**, 173–6.

Miller, G. E., Cohen, S., and Herbert, T. B. (1999). Pathways linking major depression and immunity in ambulatory female patients. *Psychosom. Med.*, **61**, 850–60.

Miller, K. B. and Nelson, J. C. (1987). Does the dexamethasone suppression test relate to subtypes, factors, symptoms, or severity? *Arch. Gen. Psychiatry*, **44**, 769–74.

Miller, L. J. (1994). Use of electroconvulsive therapy during pregnancy. *Hosp. Commun. Psychiatry*, **45**, 444–50.

(2002). Postpartum depression. *J.A.M.A*, **287**, 762–5.

Miller L. J, Rukstalis M: Beyond the "blues": hypotheses about postpartum reactivity. In Miller, LJ., *Postpartum Mood Disorders*. Washington, DC, American Psychiatric Press, 1999, pp. 3–19.

Miller, M. C., Jacobs, D. G., and Gutheil, T. G. (1998). Talisman or taboo: the controversy of the suicide-prevention contract. *Harv. Rev. Psychiatry*, **6**, 78–87.

Miller, M. D., Lenze, E. J., Dew, M. A., *et al.* (2002b). Effect of cerebrovascular risk factors on depression treatment outcome in later life. *Am. J. Geriatr. Psychiatry*, **10**, 592–8.

Miller, N. S., Summers, G. L., and Gold, M. S. (1993). Cocaine dependence: alcohol and other drug dependence and withdrawal characteristics. *J. Addict. Dis.*, **12**, 25–35.

Millman, R. P., Fogel, B. S., McNamara, M. E., and Carlisle, C. C.(1989). Depression as a manifestation of obstructive sleep apnea: reversal with nasal continuous positive airway pressure. *J. Clin. Psychiatry*, **50**, 348–51.

Minov, C., Baghai, T. C., Schule, C., *et al.* (2001). Serotonin-2A-receptor and -transporter polymorphisms: lack of association in patients with major depression. *Neurosci. Lett.*, **303**, 119–22.

Mirmiran, M. (1995). The function of fetal/neonatal rapid eye movement sleep. *Behav. Brain Res.*, **69**, 13–22.

Mirmiran, M. and Van Someran, E. (1993). Symposium: normal and abnormal REM sleep regulation. The importance of REM sleep for brain maturation. *J. Sleep. Res.*, 188–92.

Mirmiran, M., Maas, Y. G. H., and Ariagno, R. L. (2003). Development of fetal and neonatal sleep and circadian rhythms. *Sleep Med. Rev.*, **7**, 321–34.

Mitchell, A. J. (2004). Antidepressants and suicide (letter). *Br. Med. J.*, **329**, 461.

Mitchell, P. B. and Malhi, G. S. (2004). Bipolar depression: phenomenological overview and clinical characteristics. *Bipolar Disord.*, **6**, 530–9.

Mitchell, J., McCauley, E., Burke, P., Calderon, R., and Schloredt, K. (1989). Psychopathology in parents of depressed children and adolescents. *J. Am. Acad. Child Adolesc. Psychiatry*, **28**, 352–7.

Mittmann, N., Herrmann, N., Einarson, T. R., *et al.* (1997). The efficacy, safety and tolerability of antidepressants in late life depression: a meta-analysis. *J. Affect. Disord.*, **46**, 191–217.

Moberg, P. J., Lazarus, L. W., Mesholam, R. I., *et al.* (2001). Comparison of the standard and structured interview guide for the Hamilton Depression Rating Scale in depressed geriatric inpatients. *Am. J. Geriatr. Psychiatry*, **9**, 35–40.

Modell, S., Lauer, C. J., Schreiber, W., *et al.* (1998). Hormonal response pattern in the combined DEX-CRH test is stable over time in subjects at high familiar risk for affective disorder. *Neuropsychopharmacology*, **18**, 253–62.

Modestin, J. and Schwartzenbach, F. (1992). Effect of psychopharmacotherapy on suicide risk in discharged psychiatric inpatients. *Acta Psychiatr. Scand.*, **85**, 173–5.

Moffoot, A. P. R., O'Carroll, R. E., Bennie, J., *et al.* (1994). Diurnal variation of mood and neuropsychological function in major depression with melancholia. *J. Affect. Disord.*, **32**, 257–69.

Moise, F. N. and Petrides, G. (1996). Case study: Electroconvulsive therapy in adolescents. *J. Am. Acad. Child Adolesc. Psychiatry*, **35**, 312–18.

Molcho, A. and Stanley, M. (1992). Antidepressants and suicide risk: issues of chemical and behavioral toxicity. *J. Clin. Psychopharmacol.*, **12**, 13S–18S.

Moldin, S. O., Reich, T., and Rice, J. P. (1991). Current perspectives on the genetics of unipolar depression. *Behav. Genet.*, **21**, 211–42.

Möller, H. J. (1992). Attempted suicide: efficacy of different aftercare strategies. *Int. Clin. Psychopharm.*, **6** (suppl. 6), 58–69.

Möller, H. J., Bottlender, R., Grunze, H., Strauss, A., and Wittman, J. (2001). Are antidepressants less effective in the acute treatment of bipolar 1 compared to unipolar depression? *J. Affect. Disord.*, **67**, 141–6.

Mollica, R. F., Henderson, D. C., and Tor, S. (2002). Psychiatric effects of traumatic brain injury events in Cambodian survivors of mass violence. *Br. J. Psychiatry*, **181**, 339–47.

Monk, C. (2001). Stress and mood disorders during pregnancy: implications for child development. *Psychiatr. Q.*, **72**, 347–57.

Monteiro, W., Marks, I. M., Noshirvani, H., and Checkley, S. (1986). Normal dexamethasone suppression test in obsessive-compulsive disorder. *Br. J. Psychiatry*, **148**, 326.

Monteleone, P., Piccolo, A., Martino, M., and Maj, M. (1994). Seasonal variation in the dexamethasone suppression test: a longitudinal study in chronic schizophrenics and in healthy subjects. *Neuropsychobiology*, **30**, 61–5.

Montes, J., Ferrando, L., and Saiz-Ruiz, J. (2004). Remission in major depression with two antidepressant mechanisms: results from a naturalistic study. *J. Affect. Disord.*, **79**, 229–34.

Montgomery, D. B., Roberts, A., Green, M., *et al.* (1994). Lack of efficacy of fluoxetine in recurrent brief depression and suicidal attempts. *Eur. Arch. Psychiatry Clin. Neurosci.*, **244**, 211–15.

Montgomery, S., Cronholm, B., Asberg, M., and Montgomery, D. B. (1978). Differential effects on suicidal ideation of mianserin, maprotiline and amitriptyline. *Br. J. Clin. Pharmacol.*, **5**(suppl. 1), 77S–80S.

Montgomery, S. A. (1996). Efficacy in long-term treatment of depression. *J. Clin. Psychiatry*, **57**(suppl. 2), 24–30.

(1997). Suicide and antidepressants. *Ann. NY Acad. Sci.*, **836**, 329–38.

Montgomery, S. A. and Asberg, M. (1979). A new depression scale designed to be sensitive to change. *Br. J. Psychiatry*, **134**, 382–9.

Montgomery, S. A., Entsuah, R., Hackett, D., Kunz, N. R., and Rudolph, R. L. (2004). Venlafaxine 335 study group: venlafaxine versus placebo in the preventive treatment of recurrent major depression. *J. Clin. Psychiatry*, **65**, 328–36.

Morag, I., Batash, D., Keidar, R., Bulkowstein, M., and Heyman, E. (2004). Paroxetine use throughout pregnancy: does it pose any risk to the neonate? *J. Toxicol. Clin. Toxicol.*, **42**, 97–100.

Morehouse, R. L., Kusumakar, V., Kutcher, S. P., LeBlanc, J., and Armitage, R. (2002). Temporal coherence in ultradian sleep EEG rhythms in a never-depressed, high-risk cohort of female adolescents. *Biol. Psychiatry*, **51**, 446–56.

Moreno, E. M., Munoz, J. M., Valderrabanos, J. S., and Gutierrez, T. V. (1998). Electroconvulsive therapy in the first trimester of pregnancy. *J. ECT*, **14**, 251–4.

Morishita, S. and Aóki, S. (2002). Clonazepam augmentation of antidepressants: does it distinguish unipolar from bipolar depression? *J. Affect. Disord.*, **71**, 217–20.

Morris, P. L. P., Robinson, R. G., Raphael, B., and Hopwood, M. J. (1996). Lesion location and post-stroke depression. *J. Neuropsychiatry Clin. Neurosci.*, **8**, 399–403.

Morselli, P. L. (1980). Clinical pharmacokinetics in newborns and infants. *Clin. Pharmacokinet.*, **5**, 485–527.

Mortola, J. F., Brunswick, D. J., and Amsterdam, J. D. (2002). Premenstrual syndrome: cyclic symptoms in women of reproductive age. *Psychiatr. Ann.*, **32**, 452–62.

Moscicki, E. K. (1997). Identification of suicide risk factors using epidemiologic studies. *Psychiatr. Clin. North Am.*, **20**, 499–517.

Moser, M., Lehofer, M., Hoehn-Saric, R., *et al.* (1998). Increased heart rate in depressed subjects in spite of unchanged autonomic balance? *J. Affect. Disord.*, **48**, 115–24.

Mottram, P., Wilson, K., and Copeland, J. (2000). Validation of the Hamilton Depression Rating Scale and Montgomery and Asberg Rating Scales in terms of AGECAT depression cases. *Int. J. Geriatr. Psychiatry*, **15**, 1113–19.

Mouchabac, S., Ferreri, M., Cabanac, F., and Bitton, M. (2003). Residual symptoms after a treated major depressive disorder: in practice ambulatory observatory carried out of city. *Encephale*, **29**, 438–44.

Mountjoy, C. Q. and Roth, M. (1982). Studies in the relationship between depressive disorders and anxiety states. Part 2. Clinical items. *J. Affect. Disord.*, **4**, 149–61.

Moynihan, R. (2003). Cochrane plans to allay fears over industry influence. *Br. Med. J.*, **327**, 1005.

Mu, Q., Bohning, D. E., Nahas, Z., *et al.* (2004). Acute vagus nerve stimulation using different pulse widths produces varying brain effects. *Biol. Psychiatry*, **55**, 816–25.

Mueller, T. I., Leon, A. C., Keller, M. B., *et al.* (1999). Recurrence after recovery from major depressive disorder during 15 years of observational follow-up. *Am. J. Psychiatry*, **156**, 1000–6.

Muijsers, R. B., Plosker, G. L., and Noble, S. (2002). Sertraline: a review of its use in the management of major depressive disorder in elderly patients. *Drugs Aging*, **19**, 377–92.

Mukherjee, S., Sackeim, H. A., and Schnur, D. B. (1994). Electroconvulsive therapy of acute manic episodes: A review of 50 years' experience. *Am. J. Psychiatry*, **151**, 169–76.

Mula, M. and Monaco, F. (2002). Antiepileptic–antipsychotic drug interactions: a critical review of the evidence. *Clin. Neuropharmacol.*, **25**, 280–9.

Mullaney, J. A. (1984).The relationship between anxiety and depression. A review of some principal component analytic studies. *J. Affect. Disord.*, **7**, 139–48.

Muller, A. F., Drexhage, H. A., and Berhout, A. (2001). Postpartum thyroiditis and autoimmune thyroiditis in women of childbearing age: recent insights and consequences for antenatal and postnatal care. *Endocr. Rev.*, **22**, 605–30.

Muller, M. J., Szegedi, A., Wetzel, H., and Benkert, O. (2000). Moderate and severe depression. Gradations for the Montgomery-Asberg Depression Rating Scale. *J. Affect. Disord.*, **60**, 137–40.

Muller, U., Murai, T., Bauer-Wittmund, T., and von Cramon, D. Y. (1999). Paroxetine versus citalopram treatment of pathological crying after brain injury. *Brain Inj.*, **13**, 805–11.

Muller-Oerlinghausen, B., Muser-Causemann, B., and Volk, J. (1992). Suicides and parasuicides in a high-risk patient group on and off lithium long-term medication. *J. Affect. Disord.*, **225**, 261–70.

Muller-Siecheneder, F., Muller, M. J., Hillert, A., *et al.* (1998). Risperidone versus haloperidol and amitriptyline in the treatment of patients with a combined psychotic and depressive syndrome. *J. Clin. Psychopharmacol.*, **18**, 111–20.

Mullins, U. L., Gianutsos, G., and Eison, A. S. (1999). Effects of antidepressants on 5-HT7 receptor regulation in the rat hypothalamus. *Neuropsychopharmacology*, **21**, 352–67.

Mulsant, B. H., Haskett, R. F., Prudic, J., *et al.* (1997). Low use of neuroleptic drugs in the treatment of psychotic major depression. *Am. J. Psychiatry*, **154**, 559–61.

Mulsant, B. H., Pollock, B. G., Nebes, R. D., *et al.* (1999). A double-blind randomized comparison of nortriptyline and paroxetine in the treatment of late-life depression: 6-week outcome. *J. Clin. Psychiatry*, **60** (suppl. 20), 16–20.

Mulsant, B. H., Sweet, R. A., Rosen, J., *et al.* (2001). A double-blind randomized comparison of nortriptyline plus perphenazine versus nortriptyline plus placebo in the treatment of psychotic depression in late life. *J. Clin. Psychiatry*, **62**, 597–604.

Mulsant, B. H., Kastango, K. B., Rosen, J., *et al.* (2002) Interrater reliability in clinical trials of depressive disorder. *Am. J. Psychiatry*, **159**, 1598–1600.

Murata, T., Suzuki, R., Higuchi, T., and Oshima, A. (2000). Regional cerebral blood flow in the patients with depressive disorders. *Keio J. Med.*, **49** (suppl. 1), A112–13.

Murphy, B. E. (1997). Antiglucocortoid therapies in major depression: a review. *Psychoneuroendocrinology*, **22**, S125–32.

Murphy, B. E., Filipini, D., and Ghadivian, A. M. (1993). Possible use of glucocorticoid receptor antagonists in the treatment of major depression: preliminary results using RU 486. *J. Psychiatry Neurosci.*, **18**, 209–13.

Murphy, E. A. (1964). One cause? Many causes? The argument from a bimodal distribution. *J. Chron. Dis.*, **17**, 301–24.

Murphy, F. C., Sahakian, B. J., Rubinsztein, J. S., *et al.* (1999). Emotional bias and inhibitory control processes in mania and depression. *Psychol., Med.*, **29**, 1307–21.

Murphy, F. C., Michael, A., Robbins, T. W., and Sahakian, B. J. (2003a). Neuropsychological impairment in patients with major depressive disorder: the effects of feedback on task performance. *Psychol. Med.*, **33**, 455–567.

Murphy, G. E. and Wetzel, R. D. (1982). Family history of suicidal behavior among suicide attempters. *J. Nerv. Ment. Dis.*, **170**, 86–90.

Murphy, G. E., Simons, A. D., Wetzel, R. D., and Lustman, P. J. (1984). Cognitive therapy and pharmacotherapy. Singly and together in the treatment of depression. *Psychiatry*, **41**, 33–41.

Murphy, G. E., Wetzel, R. D., Robins, E., and McEvoy, L. (1992). Multiple risk factors predict suicide in alcoholism. *Arch. Gen. Psychiatry*, **49**, 459–63.

Murphy, G. M. Jr, Kremer, C., Rodrigues, H. E., and Schatzberg, A. F. (2003b). Pharmacogenetics of antidepressant medication intolerance. *Am. J. Psychiatry*, **160**, 1830–5.

Murphy, G. M. Jr, Hollander, S. B., Rodriques, H. E., Kremer, C., and Schatzberg, A. F. (2004). Effects of the serotonin transporter gene promoter polymorphism on mirtazapine and paroxetine efficacy and adverse events in geriatric major depression. *Arch. Gen. Psychiatry*, **61**, 1163–9.

Murphy, S. L. (2000). *Deaths: Final Data for 1998. National Vital Statistics Report*, 48(11). DHHS publication no. (PHS) 2000–1120, p. 86, Table 26. Hyattsville, MD: National Center for Health Statistics.

Murray, C. J. L. and Lopez, A. D. (eds) (1996). *The Global Burden of Disease*, vol. 1. Cambridge, MA: Harvard School of Public Health (on behalf of the World Health Organization and the World Bank).

Murray, G. B., Shea, V., and Conn, D. R. (1986). Electroconvulsive therapy for poststroke depression. *J. Clin. Psychiatry*, **47**, 258–60.

Murray, L., Hipwell, A., Hooper, R., Stein, A., and Cooper, P. (1996a). The cognitive development of 5-year-old children of postnatally depressed mothers. *J. Child Psychol. Psychiatry*, **37**, 927–35.

Murray, L., Fiori-Cowley, A., Hooper, R., and Cooper, P. (1996b). The impact of postnatal depression and associated adversity on early mother–infant interactions and later infant outcome. *Child Dev.*, **67**, 2512–26.

Murray, L., Cooper, P. J., Wilson, A., and Romaniuk, H. (2003). Controlled trial of the short- and long-term effect of psychological treatment of post-partum depression. 2. Impact on the mother–child relationship and child outcome. *Br. J. Psychiatry*, **182**, 420–7.

Murray, K. T. and Sines, J. O. (1996). Parsing the genetic and nongenetic variance in children's depressive behavior. *J. Affect. Disord.*, **36**, 23–34.

Musselman, D. L. and Nemeroff, C. B. (1993). The role of corticotropin-releasing factor in the pathophysiology of psychiatric disorders. *Psychiatry Ann.*, **23**, 676–81.

Musselman, D. L., Marzec, U. M., Manatunga, A., *et al.* (2000). Platelet reactivity in depressed patients treated with paroxetine: preliminary findings. *Arch. Gen. Psychiatry*, **57**, 875–82.

Musselman, D. L., Lawson, D. H., Gumnick, J. F., *et al.* (2001a).Paroxetine for the prevention of depression induced by high-dose interferon alfa. *N. Engl. J. Med.*, **344**, 961–6.

Musselman, D. L., Miller, A. H., Porter, M. R., *et al.* (2001b). Higher than normal plasma interleukin-6 concentrations in cancer patients with depression: preliminary findings. *Am. J. Psychiatry*, **158**, 1252–7.

Myers, J. E. and Thase, M. E. (2001). Risperidone: review of its therapeutic utility in depression. *Psychopharmacol. Bull.*, **35**, 109–29.

Myerson, A. (1944). Prolonged cases of grief reaction treated by electric shock. *N. Engl. J. Med.*, **230**, 255–6.

Myint, A. M. and Kim, Y. K. (2003). Cytokine–serotonin interaction through IDO: a neurodegeneration hypothesis of depression. *Med. Hypotheses*, **61**, 519–25.

Nadeau, S. E., McCoy, K. J., Crucian, G. P., *et al.* (2002). Cerebral blood flow changes in depressed patients after treatment with repetitive transcranial magnetic stimulation: evidence of individual variability. *Neuropsychiatry Neuropsychol. Behav. Neurol.*, **15**, 159–75.

Nahshoni, E., Aravot, D., Aizenberg, D., *et al.* (2004). Heart rate variability in patients with major depression. *Psychosom.*, **45**, 129–34.

Nappi, R. E., Petraglia, F., Luisi, S., *et al.* (2001). Serum allopregnanolone in women with postpartum "blues." *Obstet. Gynecol.*, **97**, 77–80.

Naranjo, C. A., Tremblay, L. K., and Busto, U. E. (2001). The role of the brain reward system in depression. *Prog. Neuro-Psychopharm. Biol. Psychiatry*, **25**, 781–823.

Narushima, K., Kosier, J. T., and Robinson, R. G. (2003). A reappraisal of poststroke depression, intra- and inter-hemispheric lesion location using meta-analysis. *J. Neuropsychiatry Clin. Neurosci.*, **15**, 422–30.

National Institute for Clinical Excellence (2003). *Guidance on the Use of Electroconvulsive Therapy.* London: NICE.

Navarro, V., Gasto, C., Torres, X., Marcos, T., and Pintor, L. (2001). Citalopram versus nortriptyline in late-life depression: a 12-week randomized single-blind study. *Acta Psychiatr. Scand.*, **103**, 435–40.

Navarro, V., Gasto, C., Lomena, F., *et al.* (2002). Normalization of frontal cerebral perfusion in remitted elderly major depression: a 12-month follow-up SPECT study. *Neuroimage*, **16**, 781–7.

(2004). Frontal cerebral perfusion after antidepressant drug treatment versus ECT in elderly patients with major depression: a 12-month follow-up control study. *J. Clin. Psychiatry*, **65**, 656–61.

Ndosi, N. K. and Mtawali, M. L. (2002). The nature of puerperal psychosis at Muhimbili National Hospital: its physical co-morbidity, associated main obstetric and social factors. *Afr. J. Reprod. Health*, **6**, 41–9.

Nebes, R. D., Vora, I. J., Meltzer, C. C., *et al.* (2001). Relationship of deep white matter hyperintensities and apolipoprotein E genotype to depressive symptoms in older adults without clinical depression. *Am. J. Psychiatry*, **158**, 878–84.

Neiswanger, K., Zubenko, G. S., Giles, D. E., *et al.* (1998). Linkage and association analysis of chromosomal regions containing genes related to neuroendocrine or serotonin function in families with early-onset, recurrent major depression. *Am. J. Med. Gen. (Neuropsychiatr. Gen.)*, **81**, 443–9.

Nelsen, M. R. and Dunner, D. L. (1995). Clinical and differential diagnostic aspects of treatment-resistant depression. *J. Psychiatr. Res.*, **29**, 43–50.

Nelson, J. C. and Charney, D. S. (1981). The symptoms of major depressive illness. *Am. J. Psychiatry*, **138**, 1–13.

Nelson, J. C. and Davis, J. M. (1997). DST studies in psychotic depression: a meta-analysis. *Am. J. Psychiatry*, **154**, 1497–503.

Nelson, J. C. Charney, D. D. S., and Vingiano, A. W. (1978). False-positive diagnosis with primary-affective-disorder criteria. *Lancet*, **2**, 1252–3.

Nelson, J. C., Charney, D. S., and Quinlan, D. M. (1980). Characteristics of autonomous depression. *J. Nerv. Ment. Dis.*, **168**, 637–43.

Nelson, J. C., Mazure, C. M., and Jatlow, P. I. (1990). Does melancholia predict response in major depression? *J. Affect. Disord.*, **18**, 157–65.

(1994). Characteristics of desipramine-refractory depression. *J. Clin. Psychiatry*, **55**, 12–19.

Nelson, J. C., Kennedy, J. S., Pollock, B. G., *et al.* (1999). Treatment of major depression with nortriptyline and paroxetine in patients with ischemic heart disease. *Am. J. Psychiatry*, **156**, 1024–8.

Nemeroff, C. B. (2002a). New directions in the development of antidepressants: the interface of neurobiology and psychiatry. *Hum. Psychopharmacol.*, **17** (suppl. 1), S13–16.

(2002b). Recent advances in the neurobiology of depression. *Psychopharm. Bull.*, **36** (suppl. 2), 6–23.

Nemeroff, C. B. and Evans, D. L. (1988). Correlation between the dexamethasone suppression test in depressed patients and clinical response. *Am. J. Psychiatry*, **141**, 247–9.

Nemeroff, C. B. and Loosen, P. T. (eds) (1987). *Handbook of Clinical Psychoneuroendocrinology.* New York: Guilford Press.

Nemeroff, C. B., DeVane, L., and Pollock, B. G. (1996). Newer antidepressants and the cytochrome P450 system. *Am. J. Psychiatry*, **153**, 311–20.

Nemeroff, C. B., Compton, M. T., and Berger, J. (2001a). The depressed suicidal patient. *Ann. NY Acad. Sci.*, **932**, 1–23.

Nemeroff, C. B., Evans, D. L., Gyulai, L., *et al.* (2001b). Double-blind, placebo-controlled comparison of imipramine and paroxetine in the treatment of bipolar depression. *Am. J. Psychiatry*, **158**, 906–12.

Nemets, B., Stahl, Z., and Belmaker, R. (2002). Addition of omega-3 fatty acid to maintenance medication treatment for recurrent unipolar depressive disorder. *Am. J. Psychiatry*, **159**, 477–9.

Nestler, E. J., McMahon, A., Sabban, E. L., Tallman, J. F., and Duman, R. S. (1990). Chronic antidepressant administration decreases the expression of tyrosine hydroxylase in rat locus ceruleus. *Proc. Natl Acad. Sci.*, **87**, 7522–6.

Nestler, E. J., Barrot, M., DiLeone, R. J., *et al.* (2002). Neurobiology of depression. *Neuron*, **34**, 13–25.

Neugebauer, V., Zinebi, F., Russell, R., Gallagher, J. P., and Shinnick-Gallagher, P. (2000). Cocaine and kindling alter the sensitivity of group II and III metabotropic glutamate receptors in the central amygdala. *J. Neurophysiol.*, **84**, 759–70.

Neuman, R., Geller, B., Rice, J. P., and Todd, R. (1997). Increased prevalence and earlier onset of mood disorders among relatives of prepubertal versus adult probands. *J. Am. Acad. Child Adolesc. Psychiatry*, **36**, 466–73.

Neumeister, A., Nugent, A. C., Waldeck, T., *et al.* (2004). Neural and behavioral responses to tryptophan depletion in unmedicated patients with remitted major depressive disorder and controls. *Arch. Gen. Psychiatry*, **61**, 765–73.

Newburn, G., Edwards, R., Thomas, H., *et al.* (1999). Moclobemide in the treatment of major depressive disorder (DSM-3) following traumatic brain injury. *Brain Inj.*, **13**, 637–42.

Newcomer, J. W., Craft, S., Hershey, T., Askins, K., and Bardgett, M. E. (1994). Glucocorticoid-induced impairment in declarative memory performance in adult humans. *J. Neurosci.*, **14**, 2047–53.

Newcomer, J. W., Selke, G., Melson, A. K., *et al.* (1999). Decreased memory performance in healthy humans induced by stress-level cortisol treatment. *Arch. Gen. Psychiatry*, **56**, 527–33.

Ney, P. G., Tam, W. W., and Maurice, W. L. (1990). Factors that determine medical student interest in psychiatry. *Aust. NZ J. Psychiatry*, **24**, 65–76.

Nia, R., Spring, B., Borrelli, B., *et al.* (2002). Multicenter trial of fluoxetine as an adjunct to behavioral smoking cessation treatment. *J. Consult. Clin. Psychol.*, **70**, 887–96.

Nibuya, M., Morinobu, S., and Duman, R. S. (1995). Regulation of BDNF and trkB mRNA in rat brain by chronic electroconvulsive seizure and antidepressant drug treatments. *J. Neurosci.*, **15**, 7539–47.

Nibuya, M., Nestler, E. J., and Duman, R. S. (1996). Chronic antidepressant administration increases the expression of cAMP response element binding protein (CREB) in rat hippocampus. *J. Neurosci.*, **16**, 2365–72.

Nieber, D. and Schlegel, S. (1992). Relationship between psychomotor retardation and EEG power spectrum in major depression. *Neuropsychobiology*, **25**, 20–3.

Nierenberg, A. A. and Amsterdam, J. D. (1990). Treatment-resistant depression: definition and treatment approaches. *J. Clin. Psychiatry*, **51** (suppl. 6), 39–47.

Nierenberg, A. A., Feighner, J. P., Rudolph, R., Cole, J. O., and Sullivan, J. (1994). Venlafaxine for treatment-resistant unipolar depression. *J. Clin. Psychopharmacol.*, **14**, 419–23.

Nierenberg, A. A., Papakostas, G. I., Petersen, T., *et al.* (2003). Nortriptyline for treatment-resistant depression. *J. Clin. Psychiatry*, **64**, 35–9.

Niethammer, R., Keller, A., and Weisbrod, M. (2000). Delirium syndrome as a side-effect of lithium in normal lithium levels (in German). *Psychiatr. Prax.*, **27**, 296–7.

Nilsson, F. M. and Kessing, L. V. (2004). Increased risk of developing stroke for patients with major affective disorder. A registry study. *Eur. Arch. Psychiatry Clin. Neurosci.*, **254**, 387–91.

Nilsson, F. M., Kessing, L. V., Sorensen, T. M., Andersen, P. K., and Bolwig, T. G. (2002). Enduring increased risk of developing depression and mania in patients with dementia. *J. Neurol. Neurosurg. Psychiatry*, **73**, 40–4.

Nobler, M. S. and Roose, S. P. (1998). Differential response to antidepressants in melancholic and severe depression. *Psychiatr. Ann.*, **28**, 84–8.

Nobler, M. S., Sackeim, H. A., Prohovnik, I., *et al.* (1994). Regional cerebral blood flow in mood disorders, III. Treatment and clinical response. *Arch. Gen. Psychiatry*, **51**, 884–97.

Nofzinger, E. A., Keshavan, M. S., Buysse, D. J., *et al.* (1999a). Neurobiology of sleep in relation to mental illness. In Charney, D. S., Nestler, E. J., and Bunney, B. S. (eds) *Neurobiology of Mental Illness*. New York: Oxford University Press, pp. 915–29.

Nofzinger, E. A., Nichols, T. E., Meltzer, C. C., *et al.* (1999b). Changes in forebrain function from waking to REM sleep in depression: preliminary analyses of [^{18}F]FDG PET studies. *Psychiatry Res. Neuroimag.*, **91**, 59–78.

Nofzinger, E. A., Price, J. C., Meltzer, C. C., *et al.* (2000). Towards a neurobiology of dysfunctional arousal in depression: the relationship between beta EEG power and regional cerebral glucose metabolism during NREM sleep. *Psychiatry Res. Neuroimag.*, **98**, 71–91.

Nolen, W. A. and Bloemkolk, D. (2000). Treatment of bipolar depression, a review of the literature and a suggestion for an algorithm. *Neuropsychobiology*, **42** (suppl. 1), 11–17.

Norman, S., Troster, A. I., Fields, J. A., and Brooks, R. (2002). Effects of depression and Parkinson's disease on cognitive functioning. *J. Neuropsychiatry Clin. Neurosci.*, **14**, 31–6.

Norman, W. H., Brown, W. A., Miller, I. W., Keitner, G. I., and Overholser, J. C. (1990). The dexamethasone suppression test and completed suicide. *Acta Psychiatr. Scand.*, **81**, 120–5.

Norris, E. J. (2001). Double-blinded, single-blinded, or just blind? *Anesth. Analg.*, **93**, 1361.

Nowak, G., Ordway, G. A., and Paul, I. A. (1995). Alterations in the *N*-methyl-D-aspartate (NMDA) receptor complex in the frontal cortex of suicide victims. *Brain Res.*, **675**, 157–64.

Nuland, S. B. (2003). *Lost in America. A Journey with My Father.* New York: Alfred A. Knopf.

Nulman, I., Rovet, J., Stewart, D. E., *et al.* (2002). Child development following exposure to tricyclic antidepressants or fluoxetine throughout fetal life: a prospective, controlled study. *Am. J. Psychiatry*, **159**, 1889–95.

Nunes, E. V., McGrath, P. J., Quitkin, F. M., *et al.* (1995). Imipramine treatment of cocaine abuse: possible boundaries of efficacy. *Drug Alcohol Depend.*, **39**, 185–95.

Nurcombe, B., Seifer, R., Scioli, A., *et al.* (1989). Is major depressive disorder in adolescence a distint diagnostic entity? *J. Am. Acad. Child Adolesc. Psychiatry*, **28**, 333–42.

Nurnberger, J. I. Jr, Foroud, T., Flury, L., *et al.* (2001). Evidence for a locus on chromosome 1 that influences vulnerability to alcoholism and affective disorder. *Am. J. Psychiatry*, **158**, 718–24.

Nuttall, G. A., Bowersox, M. R., Douglass, S. B., *et al.* (2004). Morbidity and mortality in the use of electroconvulsive therapy. *J. ECT*, **20**, 237–41.

O'Brien, J., Ames, D., Chiu, E., *et al.* (1998). Severe deep white-matter lesions and outcome in elderly patients with major depressive disorder: follow-up study. *Br. Med. J.*, **317**, 982–4.

O'Brien, J., Thomas, A., Ballard, C., *et al.* (2001). Cognitive impairment in depression is not associated with neuropathologic evidence of increased vascular or Alzheimer-type pathology. *Biol. Psychiatry*, **49**, 130–6.

O'Brien, J. T., Desmond, P., Ames, D., *et al.* (1997). Temporal lobe magnetic resonance imaging can differentiate Alzheimer's disease from normal aging, depression, vascular dementia and other causes of cognitive impairment. *Psychol. Med.*, **27**, 1267–75.

O'Brien, J. T., Metcalfe, S., Swann, A., *et al.* (2000). Medial temporal lobe width on CT scanning in Alzheimer's disease: comparison with vascular dementia, depression and dementia with Lewy bodies. *Dement. Geriatr. Cogn. Disord.*, **11**, 114–18.

O'Connor, D., Gwirtsman, H., and Loosen, P. T. (2003a). Thyroid function in psychiatric disorders. In Wolkowitz, O. W. and Rothschild, A. J. (eds) *Psychoneuroendocrinology: The Scientific Basis of Clinical Practice*, vol. 14. Washington, DC: American Psychiatric Publishing, pp. 361–418.

O'Connor, M., Brenninkmeyer, C., Morgan, A., *et al.* (2003b). Relative effects of repetitive transcranial magnetic stimulation and electroconvulsive therapy on mood and memory: a neurocognitive risk–benefit analysis. *Cog. Behav. Neurol.*, **16**, 118–27.

O'Connor, M. K., Knapp, R., Husain, M., *et al.* (2001). The influence of age on the response of patients with major depression to electroconvulsive therapy. *Am. J. Geriatr. Psychiatry*, **9**, 382–90.

O'Connor, T., Hetherington, E. M., Reiss, D., and Plomin, R. (1995). A twin-sibling study of observed parent-adolescent interactions. *Child Dev.*, **66**, 812–29.

O'Connor, T. G., Heron, J., Golding, J., Beveridge, M., and Glover, V. (2002). Maternal antenatal anxiety and children's behavioural/emotional problems at 4 years. Report from the Avon Longitudinal Study of Parents and Children. *Br. J. Psychiatry*, **180**, 502–8.

Ohaeri, J. U. and Otote, D. I. (2002). Family history, life events and the factorial structure of depression in a Nigerian sample of inpatients. *Psychopathology*, **35**, 210–19.

O'Hara, M. W., Schlecte, J. A., Lewis, D. A., and Varner, M. W. (1991). Controlled prospective study of postpartum mood disorder: psychological, environmental, and hormonal variables. *J. Abnorm. Psychol.*, **100**, 63–73.

Ohayon, M. M. and Schatzberg, A. F. (2002). Prevalence of depressive episodes with psychotic features in the general population. *Am. J. Psychiatry*, **159**, 1855–61.

Okun, M. S., Green, J., Saben, R., *et al.* (2003). Mood changes with deep brain stimulation of STN and GPi: results of a pilot study. *J. Neurol. Neurosurg. Psychiatry*, **74**, 1584–6.

O'Leary, D., Paykel, E., Todd, C., and Vardulaki, K. (2001). Suicide in primary affective disorders revisited: a systematic review by treatment era. *J. Clin. Psychiatry*, **62**, 804–11.

Olfson, M., Marcus, S., Sackeim, H. A., Thompson, J., and Pincus, H. A. (1998). Use of ECT for the inpatient treatment of recurrent major depression. *Am. J. Psychiatry*, **155**, 22–9.

Olfson, M., Shaffer, D., Marcus, S. C., and Greenberg, T. (2003). Relationship between antidepressant medication treatment and suicide in adolescents. *Arch. Gen. Psychiatry*, **60**, 978–82.

Olie, J. P., Elomari, F., Spadone, C., and Lepine, J. P. (2002). Antidepressants consumption in the global population in France. *Encephale.*, **28**, 411–17.

Olin, S. C. S., Mednick, S. A., Cannon, T., *et al.* (1998). School teacher ratings predictive of psychiatric outcome 25 years later. *Br. J. Psychiatry*, **172** (suppl. 33), 7–13.

Olsson, G. I. and von Knorring, A. L. (1999). Adolescent depression: prevalence in Swedish high-school students. *Acta Psychiatr. Scand.*, **99**, 324–31.

O'Malley, P. G., Balden, E., Tomkins, G., *et al.* (2000). Treatment of fibromyalgia with antidepressants: a meta-analysis. *J. Gen. Intern. Med.*, **15**, 659–66.

O'Malley, S. (2004). *Are You There Alone?* New York: Simon & Schuster.

Ongur, D., Drevets, W. C., and Price, J. L. (1998). Glial reduction in the subgenual prefrontal cortex in mood disorders. *Proc. Natl Acad. Sci. USA*, **95**, 13290–5.

Ono, Y., Ando, J., Onoda, N., *et al.* (2002). Dimensions of temperament as vulnerability factors in depression. *Mol. Psychiatry*, **7**, 948–53.

Opdyke, K. S., Reynolds, C. F. 3rd, Frank, E., *et al.* (1996–97). Effect of continuation treatment on residual symptoms in late-life depression: how well is "well"? *Depress. Anxiety*, **4**, 312–19.

Oquendo, M. A., Malone, K. M., Ellis, S. P., Sackeim, H. A., and Mann, J. J. (1999). Inadequacy of antidepressant treatment for patients with major depression who are at risk for suicidal behavior. *Am. J. Psychiatry*, **156**, 190–4.

Oquendo, M. A., Waternaux, C., Brodsky, B., *et al.* (2000). Suicidal behavior in bipolar mood disorder: clinical characteristics of attempters and nonattempters. *J. Affect. Disord.*, **59**, 107–17.

Oquendo, M. A., Ellis, S. P., Greenwald, S., *et al.* (2001). Ethnic and sex differences in suicide rates relative to major depression in the United States. *Am. J. Psychiatry*, **158**, 1652–8.

Oquendo, M. A., Kamali, M., Ellis, S. P., *et al.* (2002). Adequacy of antidepressant treatment after discharge and the occurrence of suicidal acts in major depression: a prospective study. *Am. J. Psychiatry*, **159**, 1746–51.

Oquendo, M. A., Placidi, G. P., Malone, K. M., *et al.* (2003). Positron emission tomography of regional brain metabolic responses to a serotonergic challenge and lethality of suicide attempts in major depression. *Arch. Gen. Psychiatry*, **60**, 14–22.

Oquendo, M. A., Galfalvy, H., Russo, S., *et al.* (2004). Prospective study of clinical predictors of suicidal acts after a major depressive episode in patients with major depressive disorder or bipolar disorder. *Am. J. Psychiatry*, **161**, 1433–41.

Ordway, G. A. (1997). Pathophysiology of the locus ceruleus in suicide. *Ann. NY Acad. Sci.*, **836**, 233–52.

Ordway, G. A., Gambarana, C., Tejani-Butt, S. M., *et al.* (1991). Preferential reduction of binding of ^{125}I-iodopindolol to beta-1 adrenoceptors in the amygdala of rats after antidepressant treatments. *J. Pharmacol. Exp. Ther.*, **257**, 681–90.

O'Reardon, J. P. and Amsterdam, J. D. (2001). Medical disorders and treatment-resistant depression. In Amsterdam, J. D., Hornig, M., and Nierenberg, A. A. (eds) *Treatment-Resistant Mood Disorders.* Cambridge, UK: Cambridge University Press, pp. 405–29.

O'Reilly, R. L., Bogue, L., and Singh, S. M. (1994). Pharmacogenetic response to antidepressants in a multicase family with affective disorder. *Biol. Psychiatry*, **36**, 467–71.

Oren, D. A., Wisner, K. L., Spinelli, M., *et al.* (2002). An open trial of morning light therapy for treatment of antepartum depression. *Am. J. Psychiatry*, **159**, 666–9.

Orvaschel, H., Walsh-Allis, G., and Ye, W. (1988). Psychopathology in children of parents with recurrent depression. *J. Abnorm. Child Psychol.*, **16**, 17–28.

Oslin, D. W., Katz, I. R., Edell, W. S., and Ten Have, T. R. (2000). Effects of alcohol consumption on the treatment of depression among elderly patients. *Am. J. Geriatr. Psychiatry*, **8**, 215–20.

Osvath, P. and Fekete, S. (2001). Suicidal behavior in the elderly. Review of results at the Pecs Center of the WHO/EURO Multicenter Study on Suicide. *Orv. Hetil.*, **142**, 1161–4.

Oswald, I. (1962). *Sleeping and Waking.* Amsterdam: Elsevier.

Othmer, S. C., Othmer, E., Preskorn, S. H., and Mac, D. (1988). Differential effect of amitriptyline and bupropion on primary and secondary depression: a pilot study. *J. Clin. Psychiatry*, **49**, 310–12.

O'Toole, S. M., Sekula, L. K., and Rubin, R. T. (1997). Pituitary–adrenal cortical axis measures as predictors of sustained remission in major depression. *Biol. Psychiatry*, **42**, 85–9.

Otto, M. W., Reilly-Harrington, N., and Sachs, G. S. (2003). Psychoeducational and cognitive-behavioral strategies in the management of bipolar disorder. *J. Affect. Disord.*, **73**, 171–81.

Ottosson, J.-O. and Fink, M. (2004). *Ethics in Electroconvulsive Therapy.* New York: Brunner-Routledge.

Overall, J. E. and Hollister, L. E. (1979). Comparative evaluation of research diagnostic criteria for schizophrenia. *Arch. Gen. Psychiatry*, **36**, 1198–205.

(1980). Phenomenological classification of depressive disorders. *J. Clin. Psychol.*, **367**, 372–7.

Owens, M. J. (1997). Molecular and cellular mechanisms of antidepressant drugs. *Depress. Anxiety*, **41**, 53–9.

Oyebola, D. D. and Adewoye, O. E. (1998). Preference of preclinical medical students for medical specialties and the basic medical sciences. *Afr. J. Med. Med. Sci.*, **27**, 209–12.

Ozaki, S. and Wada, K. (2001). Amotivational syndrome in organic solvent abusers. *Nippon Yakurigaku Zasshi*, **117**, 42–8.

Padberg, F. and Möller, H. J. (2003). Repetitive transcranial magnetic stimulation: does it have potential in the treatment of depression? *CNS Drugs*, **17**, 383–403.

Padberg, F., Zwanzger, P., Thoma, H., *et al.* (1999). Repetitive transcranial magnetic stimulation (rTMS) in pharmacotherapy-refractory major depression: comparative study of fast, slow and sham rTMS. *Psychiatry Res.*, **88**, 163–71.

Padberg, F., Zwanzger, P., Keck, M., *et al.* (2002). Repetitive transcranial magnetic stimulation (rTMS) in major depression. Relation between efficacy and stimulation intensity. *Neuropsychopharmacology*, **27**, 638.

Paffenberger, R. S. (1982). Epidemiological aspects of mental illness associated with childbearing. In Brockington, I. F. and Kumar, R. (eds) *Motherhood and Mental Illness, vol. 2.* London: Academic Press, pp. 19–36.

Paffenberger, R. S. and McCabe, L. J. (1966). The effect of obstetric and perinatal events on risk of mental illness in women of childbearing age. *Am. J. Public Health*, **56**, 400–7.

Pagnin, D., deQueiroz, V. Pini, S., and Cassano, G. B. (2004). Efficacy of ECT in depression: a meta-analysis review. *J. ECT*, **20**, 13–20.

Pancheri, P., Picardi, A., Pasquini, M., Gaetano, P., and Biondi, M. (2002). Psychopathological dimensions of depression: a factor study of the 17-item Hamilton depression rating scale in unipolar depressed outpatients. *J. Affect. Disord.*, **68**, 41–7.

Pande, A. C. and Sayler, M. E. (1993). Severity of depression and response to fluoxetine. *Int. Clin. Psychopharamcol.*, **8**, 243–5.

Pande, A. C., Haskett, R. F., and Greden, J. F. (1992). Seasonality in atypical depression. *Biol. Psychiatry*, **31**, 965–7.

Pandey, S. C., Zhang, D., Mittal, N., and Nayyar, D. (1999). Potential role of the gene transcription factor cyclic AMP-responsive element binding protein in ethanol withdrawal-related anxiety. *J. Exp. Ther.*, **288**, 866–78.

Papakostas, G. I., Petersen, T. J., Farabaugh, A. H., *et al.* (2003). Psychiatric comorbidity as a predictor of clinical response to nortriptyline in treatment-resistant major depressive disorder. *J. Clin. Psychiatry*, **64**, 1357–61.

Papakostas, Y., Fink, M., Lee, J., Irwin, P., and Johnson, L. (1980). Neuroendocrine measures in psychiatric patients: Course and outcome with ECT. *Psychiatry Res.*, **4**, 55–64.

Paradiso, S., Lamberty, G. J., Garvey, M. J., and Robinson, R. G. (1997). Cognitive impairment in the euthymic phase of chronic unipolar depression. *J. Nerv. Ment. Dis.*, **185**, 748–54.

Parianti, C. M. and Miller, A. H. (2001). Glucocorticoid receptors in major depression: relevance to pathophysiology and treatment. *Biol. Psychiatry*, **49**, 391–404.

Parianti, C. M., Pearce, B. D., Pisell, T. L., Owens, M. J., and Miller, A. H. (1997). Steroid-independent translocation of the glucocorticoid receptor by the antidepressant desipramine. *Mol. Pharmacol.*, **52**, 571–81.

Parikh, R. M., Lipsey, J. R., Robinson, R. G., and Price, T. R. (1987). Two-year longitudinal study of post-stroke mood disorders: dynamic changes in correlates of depression at one and two years. *Stroke*, **18**, 579–84.

Parker, G. (2000). Classifying depression: should paradigms lost be regained? *Am. J. Psychiatry*, **157**, 1195–203.

(2004). Evaluating treatments for the mood disorders: time for the evidence to get real. *Aust. NZ J. Psychiatry*, **38**, 408–14.

Parker, G. and Hadzi-Pavlovic, D. (1993). Old data, new interpretation: a re-analysis of Sir Aubrey Lewis' M. D. thesis. *Psychol. Med.*, **23**, 859–70.

(1996). *Melancholia: A Disorder of Movement and Mood.* Cambridge, UK: Cambridge University Press.

Parker, G. and Parker, K. (2003). Which antidepressants flick the switch? *Aust. NZ. J. Psychiatry*, **37**, 464–8.

Parker, G., Hadzi-Pavlovic, D., Hickie, I., *et al.* (1991). Distinguishing psychotic and non-psychotic melancholia. *J. Affect. Disord.*, **22**, 135–48.

Parker, G., Roy, K., Hadzi-Pavlovic, D., and Pedic, F. (1992). Psychotic (delusional) depression: a meta-analysis of physical treatments. *J. Affect. Disord.*, **24**, 17–24.

Parker, G., Hadzi-Pavlovic, D., Brodaty, H., *et al.* (1993). Psychomotor disturbance in depression: defining the constructs. *J. Affect. Disord.*, **27**, 255–65.

Parker, G., Hadzi-Pavlovic, D., Wilhelm, K., *et al.* (1994). Defining melancholia: properties of a refined sign-based measure. *Br. J. Psychiatry*, **164**, 316–26.

Parker, G., Hadzi-Pavlovic, D., Austin, M. P., *et al.* (1995a). Sub-typing depression. I. Is psychomotor disturbance necessary and sufficient to the definition of melancholia? *Psychol. Med.*, **25**, 815–23.

Parker, G., Hadzi-Pavlovic, D., Brodaty, H., *et al.* (1995b). Sub-typing depression, II. Clinical distinction of psychotic depression and non-psychotic melancholia. *Psychol. Med.*, **25**, 825–32.

Parker, G., Roy, K., Hadzi-Pavlovic, D., Greenwald, S., and Weissman, M. (1995c). Low parental care as a risk factor to lifetime depression in a community sample. *J. Affect. Disord.*, **33**, 173–80.

Parker, G., Gladstone, G., Wilhelm, K., *et al.* (1997). Dysfunctional parenting: over-representation in non-melancholic depression and capacity of such specificity to refine sub-typing depression measures. *Psychiatry Res.*, **73**, 57–71.

Parker, G., Gladstone, G., Roussos, J., *et al.* (1998a). Qualitative and quantitative analysis of a "lock and key" hypothesis of depression. *Psychol. Med.*, **28**, 1263–73.

Parker, G., Hadzi-Pavlovic, D., Roussos, J., *et al.* (1998b). Non-melancholic depression: the contribution of personality, anxiety and life. *Psychol. Med.*, **28**, 1209–19.

Parker, G., Roy, K., *et al.* (1999a). Sub-grouping non-melancholic depression from manifest clinic features. *J. Affect. Disord.*, **53**, 1–13.

Parker, G., Wilhelm, K., Mitchell, P., Roy, K., and Hadzi-Pavlovic, D. (1999b). Subtyping depression: testing algorithms and identification of a tiered model. *J. Nerv. Ment. Dis.*, **187**, 610–17.

Parker, G., Mitchell, P., Wilhelm, K., *et al.* (1999c). Are the newer antidepressant drugs as effective as established physical treatments? Results from an Australasian clinical pan review. *Aust. NZ J. Psychiatry*, **33**, 874–81.

Parker, G., Roy, K., Hadzi-Pavlovic, D., *et al.* (2000a). Subtyping depression by clinical features: the Australasian database. *Acta Psychiatr. Scand.*, **101**, 21–8.

Parker, G., Roy, K., Wilhelm, K., Mitchell, P., and Hadzi-Pavlovic, D. (2000b). The nature of bipolar depression: implications for the definition of melancholia. *J. Affect. Disord.*, **59**, 217–24.

Parker, G., Roy, K., Hadzi-Pavlovic, D., Wilhelm, K., and Mitchell, P. (2001). The differential impact of age on the phenomenology of melancholia. *Psychol. Med.*, **31**, 1231–6.

Parker, G., Roy, K., Mitchell Ph., *et al.* (2002). Atypical depression: a reappraisal. *Am. J. Psychiatry*, **159**, 1470–9.

Parker, G., Roy, K., and Eyers, K. (2003). Cognitive behavior therapy for depression? Choose horses for courses. *Am. J. Psychiatry*, **160**, 825–34.

Parry, B. L., Javeed, S., Laughlin, G. A., Hauger, R., and Clopton, P. (2000). Cortisol circadian rhythms during the menstrual cycle and with sleep deprivation in premenstrual dysphoric disorder and normal control subjects. *Biol. Psychiatry*, **48**, 920–31.

Pasic, J., Levy, W. C., and Sullivan, M. D. (2003). Cytokines in depression and heart failure. *Psychosom. Med.*, **65**, 181–93.

Passik, S. D., Lundberg, J. C., Rosenfeld, B., *et al.* (2000). Factor analysis of the Zung Self-Rating Depression Scale in a large ambulatory oncology sample. *Psychosom.*, **41**, 121–7.

Pastuszak, A., Schick-Boschetto, B., Zuber, C., *et al.* (1993). Pregnancy outcome following first-trimester exposure to fluoxetine (Prozac). *J. A. M. A.*, **269**, 2246–8.

Patchev, V. K. and Almeida, O. F. X. (1996). Gonadal steroids exert facilitating and buffering effects on glucocorticoid-mediated transcriptional regulation of corticotrophin-releasing hormone and corticosteroid receptor genes in rat brain. *J. Neurosci.*, **21**, 7077–84.

Patten, C. A., Martin, J. E., Myers, M. G., Calfas, K. J., and Williams, C. D. (1998). Effectiveness of cognitive-behavioral therapy for smokers with histories of alcohol dependence and depression. *J. Stud. Alcohol*, **59**, 327–35.

Patton, G. C., Coffey, C., Carlin, J. B., *et al.* (2002). cohort study. Cannabis use and mental health in young patients: cohort study. *Br. Med. J.*, **325**, 1195–8.

Paykel, E. S. (1971). Classification of depressed patients: a cluster-analysis derived grouping. *Br. J. Psychiatry*, **118**, 275–88.

(1975). Environmental variables in the etiology of depression. In Flach, F. F. and Draghi, S. C. (eds) *The Nature and Treatment of Depression*. New York: John Wiley, pp. 57–72.

(1994). Epidemiology of refractory depression. In Nolen, W. A., Zohar, J., Roose, J. P., and Amsterdam, J. D. (eds) *Refractory Depression: Current Strategies and Future Directions*. Chichester, UK: John Wiley, pp. 3–17.

(2001a). Stress and affective disorders in humans. *Semin. Clin. Neuropsychiatry*, **6**, 4–11.

(2001b). Continuation and maintenance therapy in depression. *Br. Med. Bull.*, **57**, 145–59.

(2002). Mood disorders: review of current diagnostic systems. *Psychopathology*, **35**, 94–9.

Paykel, E. S. and Henderson, A. J. (1997). Application of cluster analysis in the classification of depression. *Neuropsychobiology*, 1977, **3**, 111–19.

Paykel, E. S., Prusoff, B. A., Klerman, G. L., Haskell, D., and diMascio, A. (1973). Clinical response to amitriptyline among depressed women. *J. Nerv. Ment. Dis.*, **156**, 149–65.

Paykel, E. S., Parker, R. R., Rowan, P. R., Rao, B. M., and Taylor, C. N. (1983). Nosology of atypical depression. *Psychol. Med.*, **13**, 131–9.

Paykel, E. S., Ramana, R., Cooper, Z., *et al.* (1995). Residual symptoms after partial remission: an important outcome in depression. *Psychol. Med.*, **25**, 1171–80.

Paykel, E. S., Cooper, Z., Ramana, R., and Hayhurst, H. (1996). Life events, social support and marital relationships in the outcome of severe depression. *Psychol. Med.*, **26**, 121–33.

Paykel, E. S., Scott, J., Teasdale, J. D., *et al.* (1999). Prevention of relapse in residual depression by cognitive therapy. A controlled trial. *Arch. Gen. Psychiatry*, **56**, 829–35.

Pearce, J., Hawton, K., Blake, F., *et al.* (1997). Psychological effects of continuation versus discontinuation of hormone replacement therapy by estrogen implants: a placebo-controlled study. *J. Psychosom. Res.*, **42**, 177–86.

Pearlman, C. A. (1986). Neuroleptic malignant syndrome: a review of the literature. *J. Clin. Psychopharm.*, **6**, 257–73.

Peck, A. W., Stern, W. C., and Watkinson, C. (1983). Incidence of seizures during treatment with tricyclic antidepressant drugs and bupropion. *J. Clin. Psychiatry*, **44**, 197–201.

Peet, M. (1994). Induction of mania with selective serotonin reuptake inhibitors and tricyclic antidepressants. *Br. J. Psychiatry*, **164**, 549–50.

Peeters, B. W. M. M., Van Der Heijden, R., Gubbels, D. G., and Vanderheyden, P. M. L. (1994). Effects of chronic antidepressant treatment on the hypothalamic–pituitary–adrenal axis of Wistar rats. *Ann. NY Acad. Sci.*, **746**, 449–52.

Peirano, P., Algarin, C., and Uauy, R. (2003). Sleep–wake states and their regulatory mechanisms throughout early human development. *J. Pediatr.*, **143** (suppl. 1), 70–9.

Pendse, B. P., Engstrom, G., and Traskman-Bendz, L. (2004). Psychopathology of seasonal affective disorder patients in comparison with major depression patients who have attempted suicide. *J. Clin. Psychiatry*, **65**, 322–7.

Penninx, B. W., Beekman, A. T., Honig, A., *et al.* (2001). Depression and cardiac mortality. Results from a community-based longitudinal study. *Arch. Gen. Psychiatry*, **58**, 221–7.

Pepin, M.-C., Govindan, M. V., and Barden, N. (1992a). Increased glucocorticoid receptor gene promoter activity after antidepressant treatment. *Mol. Pharmacol.*, **41**, 1016–22.

Pepin, M.-C., Pothier, F., and Barden, N. (1992b). Antidepressant drug action in a transgenic mouse model of the endocrine changes seen in depression. *Mol. Pharmacol.*, **42**, 991–5.

Pepper, C. M., Klein, D. N., Anderson, R. L., *et al.* (1995). DSM-III-R axis II comorbidity in dysthymia and major depression. *Am. J. Psychiatry*, **152**, 239–47.

Pepper, G. M. and Krieger D. T. (1984). Hypothalamic–pituitary–adrenal abnormalities in depression: their possible relation to central mechanisms regulating ACTH release. In Post, R. M. and Ballenger, J. C. (eds) *Neurobiology of Mood Disorders*. Baltimore, MD: Williams & Wilkins, pp. 245–70.

Perkonigg, A., Yonkers, K. A., Pfister, H., Lieb, R., and Wittchen, H. U. (2004). Risk factors for premenstrual dysphoric disorder in a community sample of young women: the role of traumatic events and posttraumatic stress disorder. *J. Clin. Psychiatry*, **65**, 1314–22.

Perlis, R. H., Nierenberg, A. A., Alpert, J. E., *et al.* (2002). Effects of adding cognitive therapy to fluoxetine dose increase on risk of relapse and residual depressive symptoms in continuation treatment of major depressive disorder. *J. Clin. Psychopharmacol.*, **22**, 474–80.

Perlis, R. H., Mischoulon, D., Smoller, J. W., *et al.* (2003). Serotonin transporter polymorphism and adverse effects with fluoxetine treatment. *Biol. Psychiatry*, **54**, 879–83.

Perris, C. (1966). A study of bipolar (manic-depressive) and unipolar recurrent depressive psychoses. Introduction. *Acta Psychiatr. Scand. Suppl.*, **194**, 9–14.

(1969). The separation of bipolar (manic-depressive) from unipolar recurrent depressive psychoses. *Behav. Neuropsychiatry*, **1**, 17–24.

(1992). The distinction between unipolar and bipolar mood disorders. A 25-years perspective. *Encephale*, **18** (spec. no. 1), 9–13.

Perry, A., Tarrier, N., Morriss, R., McCarthy, E., and Limb, K. (1999). Randomised controlled trial of efficacy of teaching patients with bipolar disorder to identify early symptoms of relapse and obtain treatment. *Br. Med. J.*, **318**, 149–53.

Perry, E. B., Berman, R. M., Sanacora, G., *et al.* (2004). Pindolol augmentation in depressed patients resistant to selective serotonin reuptake inhibitors: a double-blind, randomized, controlled study. *J. Clin. Psychiatry*, **65**, 238–43.

Perry, P. J. (1996). Pharmacotherapy for major depression with melancholic features: relative efficacy of tricyclic versus selective serotonin reuptake inhibitor antidepressants. *J. Affect. Disord.*, **20**, 1–396.

Perry, P. J., Alexander, B., and Liskow, B. I. (1997). *Psychotropic Drug Handbook*, 7th edn. Washington, DC: APA Press, p. 131.

Persinger, M. A. (2000). Subjective improvement following treatment with carbamazepine (Tegretol) for a subpopulation of patients with traumatic brain injuries. *Percept. Motor Skills*, **90**, 37–40.

Perugi, G., Akiskal, H. S., Lattanzi, L., *et al.* (1998). The high prevalence of "soft" bipolar (II) features in atypical depression. *Compr. Psychiatry*, **39**, 63–71.

Pesola, GR. and Avasarala, J. (2002). Bupropion seizure proportion among new-onset generalized seizures and drug related seizures presenting to an emergency department. *J. Emerg. Med.*, **22**, 235–9.

Peteranderl, C., Antonijevic, I. A., Steiger, A., *et al.* (2002). Nocturnal secretion of TSH and ACTH in male patients with depression and healthy controls. *J. Psychiatr. Res.*, **36**, 189–96.

Petersen, T., Gordon, J. A., Kant, A., *et al.* (2001). Treatment-resistant depression and axis I comorbidity. *Psychol. Med.*, **31**, 1223–9.

Petersen, T., Hughes, M., Papakostas, G. I., *et al.* (2002a). Treatment-resistant depression and axis II comorbidity. *Psychother. Psychosom.*, **71**, 269–74.

Petersen, T., Papakostas, G. I., Bottonari, K., *et al.* (2002b). NEO-FFI factor scores as predictors of clinical response to fluoxetine in depressed outpatients. *Psychiatry Res.*, **109**, 9–16.

Petho, B. (1986). An intrinsic way of multiclassification of endogenous psychoses. A follow-through investigation/Budapest 2000/based upon Leonhard's classification. *Psychiatr. Neurol. Med. Psychol. Beih.*, **33**, 67–83.

Petrakis, I., Carroll, K. M., Nich, C., *et al.* (1998). Fluoxetine treatment of depressive disorders in methadone-maintained opioid addicts. *Drug Alcohol Depend.*, **50**, 221–6.

Petrides, G. and Fink, M. (1996). The "half-age" stimulation strategy for ECT dosing. *Convuls. Ther.*, 1996 **12**, 138–46.

Petrides, G., Dhosshe, D., Fink, M.. and Francis, A. (1994). Continuation ECT: relapse prevention in affective disorders. *Convuls. Ther.*, **10**, 189–94.

Petrides, G., Fink, M., Husain, M. M., *et al.* (2001). ECT remission rates in psychotic versus nonpsychotic depressed patients: a report from CORE. *J. ECT* **17**, 244–53.

Petrov, T., Krukoff, T. L., and Jhamandas, J. H. (1993). Branching projections of catecholaminergic brainstem neurons to the paraventricular hypothalamic nucleus and the central nucleus of the amygdala in the rat. *Brain Res.*, **609**, 81–92.

Petti, T. A. and Law, W. III (1982). Imipramine treatment of depressed children double-blind pilot study. *J. Clin. Psychopharm.*, **2**, 107–10.

Pettigrew, J. D. and Miller, S. M. (1998). A 'sticky' interhemispheric switch in bipolar disorder? *Proc. R. Soc. Lond. B*, **265**, 2141–8.

Pezawas, L., Wittchen, H.-U., Pfister, H., *et al.* (2003). Recurrent brief depressive disorder reinvestigated: a community sample of adolescents and young adults. *Psychol. Med.*, **33**, 407–18.

Pfeffer, C. R., Stokes, P., and Shindledecker, R. (1991). Suicidal behavior and hypothalamic–pituitary–adrenocortical axis indices in child psychiatric inpatients. *Biol. Psychiatry*, **29**, 909–17.

Pfeffer, C. R., Normandin, L., and Tatsuyuki, K. (1994). Suicidal children grow-up: suicidal behavior and psychiatric disorders among relatives. *J. Am. Acad. Child Psychiatry*, **33**, 1087–97.

Pfefferbaum, A., Eenegrat, B. G., Ford, J. M., Roth, W. T., and Kopell, B. S. (1984). Clinical application of the P3 component of event-related potentials. II. Dementia, depression and schizophrenia. *Electroencephalogr. Clin. Neurophysiol.*, **59**, 104–24.

Pfennig, A., Kunzel, H. E., Kern, N., *et al.* (2005). Hypothalamus–pituitary–adrenal system regulation and suicidal behavior in depression. *Biol. Psychiatry*, **57**, 336–42.

Pfohl, B., Satangl, D., and Zimmerman, M. (1984). The implications of DSM-III personality disorders for patients with major depression. *J. Affect. Disord.*, **7**, 309–18.

Pfuhlmann, B., Stober, G., Franzek, E., and Beckmann, H. (1998). Cycloid psychoses predominate in severe postpartum psychiatric disorders. *J. Affect. Disord.*, **50**, 125–34.

Pfuhlmann, B., Stober, G., and Beckmann, H. (2002). Postpartum psychoses: prognosis, risk factors, and treatment. *Curr. Psychiatry Rep.*, **4**, 185–90.

Philbrick, K. L. and Rummans, T. A. (1994). Malignant catatonia. *J. Neuropsychiatry Clin. Neurosci.*, **6**, 1–13.

Philibert, R., Caspers, K., Langbehn, D., *et al.* (2002). The association of a HOPA polymorphism with major depression and phobia. *Compr. Psychiatry*, **43**, 404–10.

Phillips, M. L., Drevets, W. C., Rauch, L. S., and Lane, R. (2003a). Neurobiology of emotion perception I: the neural basis of normal emotion perception. *Biol. Psychiatry*, **54**, 504–14.

Phillips, M. L., Drevets, W. C., Rauch, L. S., and Lane, R. (2003b). Neurobiology of emotion perception II: implications for major psychiatric disorders. *Biol. Psychiatry*, **54**, 515–28.

Piccinelli, M. and Wilkinson, G. (2000). Gender differences in depression. Critical review. *Br. J. Psychiatry*, **177**, 486–92.

Pichot, W., Reggers, J., Pinto, E., Hansenne, M., and Ansseau, M. (2003). Catecholamine and HPA axis dysfunction in depression: relationship with suicidal behavior. *Neuropsychobiology*, **47**, 152–7.

Pieri-Balandraud, N., Hugueny, P., Henry, J. F., Tournebise, H., and Dupont, C. (2001). Hyperparathyroidism induced by lithium. A new case. *Rev. Med. Interne*, **22**, 460–6.

Pies, R. (2002). Have we undersold lithium for bipolar disorder? *J. Clin. Psychopharmacol.*, **22**, 445–9.

Pinel, P. (1806). *A Treatise on Insanity.* Translated by Davis D. D. Sheffield: W. Todd.

Pini, S., de Queiroz, V., Dell'Osso, L., *et al.* (2004). Cross-sectional similarities and differences between schizophrenia, schizoaffective disorder and mania or mixed mania with mood-incongruent psychotic features. *Eur. Psychiatry*, **19**, 8–14.

Pintor, L., Gasto, C., Navarro, V., Torres, X., and Fananas, L. (2003). Relapse of major depression after complete and partial remission during a 2-year follow-up. *J. Affect. Disord.*, **73**, 237–44.

Pirl, W. F., Siegel, G. I., Goode, M. J., and Smith, M. R. (2002). Depression in men receiving androgen deprivation therapy for prostate cancer: a pilot study. *Psychooncology*, **11**, 518–23.

Pizzagalli, D., Pascual-Marqui, R. D., Nitschke, J. B., *et al.* (2001). Anterior cingulate activity as a predictor of degree of treatment response in major depression: evidence from brain electrical tomography analysis. *Am. J. Psychiatry*, **158**, 405–15.

Pizzagalli, D. A., Nitschke, J. B., Oakes, T. R., *et al.* (2002). Brain electrical tomography in depression: the importance of symptom severity, anxiety, and melancholic features. *Biol. Psychiatry*, **52**, 73–85.

Pizzagalli, D. A., Oakes, T. R., Fox, A. S., *et al.* (2004). Functional but not structural subgenual prefrontal cortex abnormalities in melancholia. *Mol. Psychiatry*, **9**, 393–405.

Pjrek, E., Winkler, D., Stastny, J., *et al.* (2004). Bright light therapy in seasonal affective disorder – does it suffice? *Eur. Neuropsychopharmacol.*, **14**, 347–51.

Plocka-Lewandowska, M., Araszkiewicz, A., and Rybakowski, J. K. (2001). Dexamethasone suppression test and suicide attempts in schizophrenic patients. *Eur. Psychiatry*, **16**, 428–31.

Plomin, R., Reiss, D., Hetherington, E. M., and Howe, G. (1994). Nature and nurture: genetic contributions to measures of the family environment. *Dev. Psychol.*, **30**, 32–43.

Podewils, L. J. and Lyketsos, C. G. (2002). Tricyclic antidepressants and cognitive decline. *Psychosom.*, **43**, 31–5.

Poewe, W. and Seppi, K. (2001). Treatment options for depression and psychosis in Parkinson's disease. *J. Neurol.*, **248** (suppl. 3), 12–21.

Poirier, M. F. and Boyer, P. (1999). Venlafaxine and paroxetine in treatment-resistant depression. Double-blind, randomised comparison. *Br. J. Psychiatry*, **175**, 12–16.

Poirier, M. F., Loo, H., Galinowski, A., *et al.* (1995). Sensitive assay of thyroid stimulating hormone in depressed patients. *Psychiatry Res.*, **57**, 41–8.

Pokorny, A. D. (1993). Suicide prediction revisited. *Suicide Life Threat. Behav.*, **23**, 1–10.

Polewka, A., Groszek, B., Trela, F., *et al.* (2002). The completed and attempted suicide in Krakow: similarities and differences. *Przegl Lek.*, **59**, 298–303.

Pollack, M., Klein D. F, Willner, A., Blumberg A. G., and Fink, M. (1965). Imipramine-induced behavioral disorganization in schizophrenic patients: physiological and psychological correlates. In Wortis, J. (ed.) *Biological Psychiatry*, vol. 7. New York: Plenum Press, 53–61.

Pollock, V. E. and Schneider, L. S. (1990). Quantitative, waking EEG research on depression. *Biol. Psychiatry*, **27**, 757–80.

Pope, H. G., Gruber, A. J., Hudson, J. I., Huestis, M. A., and Yurgelun-Todd, D. (2001). Neuropsychological performance in long-term cannabis users. *Arch. Gen. Psychiatry*, **58**, 909–15.

Pope, H. G., Cohane, G. H., Kanayama, G., Siegel, A. J., and Hudson, J. I. (2003). Testosterone gel supplementation for men with refractory depression: a randomized, placebo-controlled trial. *Am. J. Psychiatry*, **160**, 105–11.

Porges, S. W., Doussard-Roosevelt, J. A., and Maiti, A. K. (1994). Vagal tone and the physiological regulation of emotion. *Monogr. Soc. Res. Child Dev.*, **59**, 167–86.

Portales, A. L., Doussard-Roosevelt, J. A., Lee, H. B., and Porges, S. W. (1992). Infant vagal tone predicts 3-year child behavior problems. *Infant Behav. Dev.*, **15**, 363.

Porter, R. (2002). *Madness: A Brief History.* New York: Oxford University Press.

Posener, J. A., DeBattista, C., Williams, G. H., *et al.* (2000). 24-hour monitoring of cortisol and corticotropin secretion in psychotic and nonpsychotic major depression. *Arch. Gen. Psychiatry*, **57**, 755–60.

Posener, J. A., DeBattista, C., Veldhuis, J. D., *et al.* (2004). Process irregularity of cortisol and adrenocorticotropin secretion in men with major depressive disorder. *Psychoneuroendocrinology*, **29**, 1129–37.

Post, R. M. (1988). Time course of clinical effects of carbamazepine: implications for mechanism of action. *J. Clin. Psychiatry*, **49** (suppl.), 35–48.

Post, R. M., Uhde, T. W., Roy-Byrne, P. P., and Joffe, R. T. (1986). Antidepressant effects of carbamazepine. *Am. J. Psychiatry*, **143**, 29–34.

Post, R. M. and Weiss, S. R. B. (1989). Kindling and manic-depressive illness. In Bolwig, T. G. and Trimble, M. (eds) *The Clinical Relevance of Kindling*, vol. 14. Chichester, UK: John Wiley, pp. 209–30.

Post, R. M. and Weiss, S. R. B. (1997). Kindling and stress sensitization. In Young, L. T. and Joffe, R. T. (eds) *Bipolar Disorder: Biological Models and Their Clinical Application.* New York: Marcel Dekker, pp. 93–126.

Post, R. M., Altshuler, L. L., Frye, M. A., *et al.* (2001). Rate of switch in bipolar patients prospectively treated with second-generation antidepressants as augmentation to mood stabilizers. *Bipolar Disord.*, **3**, 259–65.

Post, R. M., Leverich, G. S., Nolen, W. A., *et al.* (2003). A re-evaluation of the role of antidepressants in the treatment of bipolar depression: data from the Stanley Foundation Bipolar Network. *Bipolar Disord.*, **5**, 396–406.

Posternak, M. A. and Zimmerman, M. (2001). Switching versus augmentation: a prospective, naturalistic comparison in depressed, treatment-resistant patients. *J. Clin. Psychiatry*, **62**, 135–42.

Posternak, M. A. and Zimmerman, M. (2002a). The prevalence of atypical features across mood, anxiety, and personality disorders. *Compr. Psychiatry*, **43**, 253–62.

Posternak, M. A. and Zimmerman, M.. (2002b). Lack of association between seasonality and psychopathology in psychiatric outpatients. *Psychiatry Res.*, **112**, 187–94.

Posternak, M. A. and Zimmerman, M. (2005). Is there a delay in the antidepressant effect? A meta-analysis. *J. Clin. Psychiatry*, **66**, 148–58.

Potter, W. Z., Rudorfer, M. V., and Manji, H. (1991). The pharmacologic treatment of depression. *N. Engl. J. Med.*, **325**, 633–42.

Powell, J. C., Silviera, W. R., and Lindsay, R. (1988). Pre-pubertal depressive stupor: a case report. *Br. J. Psychiatry*, **153**, 689–92.

Prange, A. J. (1974). *The Thyroid Axis, Drugs and Behavior.* New York: Raven Press.

Prasko, J., Horacek, J., Klaschka, J., *et al.* (2002). Bright light therapy and/or imipramine for inpatients with recurrent non-seasonal depression. *Neuroendocrinol. Lett.*, **23**, 109–13.

Preisig, M., Fenton, B. T., Stevens, D. E., and Merikangas, K. R. (2001). Familial relationship between mood disorders and alcoholism. *Compr. Psychiatry*, **42**, 87–95.

Prescott, C. A., Aggen, S. H., and Kendler, K. S. (2000). Sex-specific genetic influences on the comorbidity of alcoholism and major depression in a population-based sample of US twins. *Arch. Gen. Psychiatry*, **57**, 803–11.

Preskorn, S. H. (1997). Clinically relevant pharmacology of selective serotonin reuptake inhibitors. *Clin. Pharmacokinet.*, **32** (suppl. 1), 1–21.

Preskorn, S. H. and Burke, M. (1992). Somatic therapy for major depressive disorder: selection of an antidepressant. *J. Clin. Psychiatry*, **53** (suppl.), 5–18.

Preskorn, S. H. and Fast, G. A. (1991). Therapeutic drug monitoring for antidepressants: efficacy, safety, and cost effectiveness. *J. Clin. Psychiatry*, **52** (suppl.), 23–33.

(1993). Tricyclic antidepressant-induced seizures and plasma drug concentration. *J. Clin. Psychiatry*, **54**, 201–2.

Preskorn, S. H., Weller, E. B., and Weller, R. A. (1982). Depression in children: relationship between plasma imipramine levels and response. *J. Clin. Psychiatry*, **43**, 450–3.

Preskorn, S. H., Weller, E. B., Hughes, C. W., Weller, R. A., and Bolte, K. (1987). Depression in prepubertal children: dexamethasone nonsuppression predicts differential response to imipramine vs. placebo. *Psychopharm. Bull.*, **23**, 128–33.

Pressman, J. D. (1998). *Last Resort: Psychosurgery and the Limits of Medicine.* Cambridge, UK: Cambridge University Press.

Preuss, U. W., Schuckit, M. A., Smith, T. L., *et al.* (2003). Predictors and correlates of suicide attempts over 5 years in 1237 alcohol-dependent men and women. *Am. J. Psychiatry*, **160**, 56–63.

Price, J. L. (1999). Networks within the orbital and medial prefrontal cortex. *Neurocase*, **5**, 231–41.

Price, J. S. (1978). Chronic depressive illness. *Br. Med. J.*, **1**, 1200–1.

Price, L. H. and Heninger, G. R. (1994). Lithium in the treatment of mood disorders. *N. Engl. J. Med.*, **331**, 591–8.

Price, L. H., Nelson, J. C., Charney, D. S., and Quinlan, D. M. (1984). Family history in delusional depression. *J. Affect. Disord.*, **6**, 109.

Price, L. H., Carpenter, L. L., and Rasmussen, S. A. (2001). Drug combination strategies. In Amsterdam, J. D., Hornig, M., and Nierenberg, A. A. (eds) *Treatment-Resistant Mood Disorders.* Cambridge, UK, Cambridge University Press, pp. 194–222.

Pridmore, S., Bruno, R., Turnier-Shea, Y., Reid, P., and Rybak, M. (2000). Comparison of unlimited numbers of rapid transcranial magnetic stimulation (rTMS) and ECT treatment sessions in major depressive episode. *Int. J. Neuropsychopharmacol.*, **3**, 129–34.

Prien, R. F., Kupfer, D. J., Mansky, P. A., *et al.* (1984). Drug therapy in the prevention of recurrences in unipolar and bipolar affective disorders. Report of the NIMH Collaborative Study Group comparing lithium carbonate, imipramine, and a lithium carbonate–imipramine combination. *Arch. Gen. Psychiatry*, **41**, 1096–104.

Protheroe, C. (1969). Puerperal psychoses: a long term study 1927–1961. *Br. J. Psychiatry*, **115**, 9–30.

Prudic, J. and Sackeim, H. A. (1999). Electroconvulsive therapy and suicide risk. *J. Clin. Psychiatry*, **60** (suppl. 2), 104–10.

Prudic, J., Sackeim, H. A., and Devanand, D. P. (1990). Medication resistance and clinical response to electroconvulsive therapy. *Psychiatry Res.*, **31**, 287–96.

Prudic, J., Haskett, R. F., Mulsant, B., *et al.* (1996). Resistance to antidepressant medications and short-term clinical response to ECT. *Am. J. Psychiatry*, **153**, 985–92.

Prudic, J., Olfson, M., and Sackeim, H. A. (2001). Electro-convulsive therapy practices in the community. *Psychol. Med.*, **31**, 929–34.

Prudic, J., Olfson, M., Marcus, S. C., Fuller, R. B., and Sackeim, H. A. (2004). Effectiveness of electroconvulsive therapy in community settings. *Biol. Psychiatry.*, **55**, 301–12.

Pruessner, J. C., Gaab, J., Hellhammer, D. H., *et al.* (1997). Increasing correlations between personality traits and cortisol stress responses obtained by data aggregation. *Psychoneuroendocrinology*, **22**, 615–25.

Prusoff, B. A. and Paykel, E. S. (1977). Typological prediction of response to amitriptyline: a replication study. *Int. Pharmacopsychiatry*, **12**, 153–9.

Puig-Antich, J., Perel, J. M., Lupatkin, W., *et al.* (1979). Plasma levels of imipramine (IMI) and desmethylimipramine (DMI) and clinical response in prepubertal major depressive disorder. *J. Am. Acad. Child Psychiatry*, **18**, 616–27.

Puig-Antich, J., Perel, J. M., Lupatkin, W., *et al.* (1987). Imipramine in prepubertal major depressive disorders. *Arch. Gen. Psychiatry*, **44**, 81–9.

Puig-Antich, J., Goetz, D., Davies, M., *et al.* (1989). A controlled family history study of prepubertal major depressive disorder. *Arch. Gen. Psychiatry*, **46**, 406–18.

Pullar, I. A., Carney, S. L., Colvin, E. M., *et al.* (2000). LY367265, an inhibitor of the 5-hydroxytryptamine transporter and 5-hydroxytryptamine (2A) receptor antagonist: a comparison with the antidepressant, nefazodone. *Eur. J. Pharmacol.*, **407**, 39–46.

Puri, B. K., Counsell, S. J., Richardson, A. J., and Horrobin, D. F. (2002). Eicosapentaenoic acid in treatment resistant depression (letter). *Arch. Gen. Psychiatry*, **59**, 91–2.

Qin, P., Agerbo, E., and Mortensen, P. B. (2003). Suicide risk in relation to socioeconomic, demographic, psychiatric, and familial factors: a national register-based study of all suicides in Denmark, 1981–1997. *Am. J. Psychiatry*, **160**, 765–72.

Queneau, P., Asmar, R., and Safar, M. (2002). Placebo effect on diastolic, systolic and pulsed arterial pressure. *Presse Med.*, **31**, 1220–3.

Quitkin, F. M. (1985). The importance of dosage in prescribing antidepressants. *Br. J. Psychiatry*, **147**, 593–7.

Quitkin, F., Rabkin, J., Ross, D., and McGrath, P. J. (1984). Duration of antidepressant treatment. What is an adequate trial? *Arch. Gen. Psychiatry*, **41**, 238–45.

Quitkin, F. M., McGrath, P. J., Stewart, J. W., *et al.* (1989). Phenelzine and imipramine in mood reactive depressives. Further delineation of the syndrome of atypical depression. *Arch. Gen. Psychiatry*, **46**, 787–93.

Quitkin, F. M., Harrison, W., Stewart, J. W., *et al.* (1991). Response to phenelzine and imipramine in placebo nonresponders with atypical depression. A new application of the crossover design. *Arch. Gen. Psychiatry*, **48**, 319–23.

Quitkin, F. M., Stewart, J. W., McGrath, P. J., *et al.* (1993). Columbia atypical depression. A subgroup of depressives with better response to MAOI than to tricyclic antidepressants or placebo. *Br. J. Psychiatry*, **21** (suppl.), 30–4.

Raadsheer, F. C., van Heerikhuize, J. J., Lucassen, P. J., *et al.* (1995). Corticotropin-releasing hormone mRNA levels in the paraventricular nucleus of patients with Alzheimer's disease and depression. *Am. J. Psychiatry*, **152**, 1372–6.

Rabey, J. M., Scharf, M., Oberman, Z., Zohar, M., and Graff, E. (1990). Cortisol, ACTH, and beta-endorphin after dexamethasone administration in Parkinson's dementia. *Biol. Psychiatry*, **27**, 581–91.

Rabheru, K. and Persad, E. (1997). A review of continuation and maintenance electroconvulsive therapy. *Can. J. Psychiatry*, **42**, 476–84.

Rabiner, E. A., Bhagwagar, Z., Gunn, R. N., *et al.* (2001). Pindolol augmentation of selective serotonin reuptake inhibitors: PET evidence that the dose used in clinical trials is too low. *Am. J. Psychiatry*, **158**, 2080–2.

Rabkin, J. G., Stewart, J. W., McGrath, P. J., *et al.* (1987). Baseline characteristics of 10-day placebo washout responders in antidepressant trials. *Psychiatry Res.*, **21**, 9–22.

Rabkin, J. G., Stewart, J. W., Quitkin, F. M., *et al.* (1996). Should atypical depression be included in DSM-IV? In Widiger, T. A. (ed.) *Should Atypical Depression be included in DSM-IV?* Washington, DC: American Psychiatric Press, pp. 239–60.

Radden, J. (2000). *The Nature of Melancholy. From Aristotle to Kristeve.* New York: Oxford University Press.

Radke, A. Q. (1999). The last taboo. Talking to patients about suicide. *Minn. Med.*, **82**, 42–4.

Radke-Yarrow, M., Nottelmann, E., Marttinez, P., Fox, M. B., and Belmont, B. (1992). Young children of affectively ill parents: a longitudinal study of psychosocial development. *J. Am. Acad. Child Adolesc. Psychiatry*, **31**, 68–77.

Rahman, A., Iqbal, Z., Bunn, J., Lovel, H., and Harrington, R. (2004). Impact of maternal depression on infant nutritional status and illness: a cohort study. *Arch. Gen. Psychiatry*, **61**, 946–52.

Rahmann, S., Li, P. P., Young, L. T., *et al.* (1997). Reduced [^{3}H] cyclic AMP binding in postmortem brain from subjects with bipolar affective disorder. *J. Neurochem.*, **68**, 297–304.

Rajkowska, G., Miguel-Hidalgo, J. J., Jinrong, W., *et al.* (1999). Morphometric evidence for neuronal and glial prefrontal cell pathology in major depression. *Biol. Psychiatry*, **45**, 1085–98.

Ramklint, M. and Ekselius, L. (2003). Personality traits and personality disorders in early onset versus late onset major depression. *J. Affect. Disord.*, **75**, 35–42.

Ramos Platon, M. J. and Espinar Sierra, J. (1992). Changes in psychopathological symptoms in sleep apnea patients after treatment with nasal continuous positive airway pressure. *Int. J. Neurosci.*, **62**, 173–95.

Rampello, L., Chiechio, S., Raffaele, R., Vecchio, I., and Nicoletti, F. (2002). The SSRI, citalopram, improves bradykinesia in patients with Parkinson's disease treated with L-dopa. *Clin. Neuropharmacol.*, **25**, 21–4.

Ranen, N. G., Peyser, C. E., and Folstein, S. E. (1994). ECT as a treatment for depression in Huntington's disease. *J. Neuropsychiatry Clin. Neurosci.*, **6**, 154–9.

Rao, V. and Lyketsos, C. G. (2000). The benefits and risks of ECT for patients with degenerative dementia who also suffer from depression. *Int. J. Geriatr. Psychiatry*, **15**, 729–35.

Rao, M. L., Ruhrmann, S., Retey, B., *et al.* (1996a). Low plasma thyroid indices of depressed patients are attenuated by antidepressant drugs and influence treatment outcome. *Pharmacopsychiatry*, **29**, 180–6.

Rao, U., Weissman, M. M., Martin, J. A., and Hammond, R. W. (1993). Childhood depression and risk of suicide: a preliminary report of a longitudinal study. *J. Am. Acad. Child Adolesc. Psychiatry*, **32**, 21–7.

Rao, U., Dahl, R. E., Ryan, N. D., *et al.* (1996b). The relationship between longitudinal clinical course and sleep and cortisol changes in adolescent depression. *Biol. Psychiatry*, **40**, 474–84.

Rao, U., Dahl, R. E., Ryan, N. D., *et al.* (2002). Heterogeneity in EEG sleep findings in adolescent depression: unipolar versus bipolar clinical course. *J. Affect. Disord.*, **70**, 273–80.

Rao, U., Lin, K. M., Schramm, P., and Poland, R. E. (2004). REM sleep and cortisol responses to scopolamine during depression and remission in women. *Int. J. Neuropsychopharmacol.*, **7**, 265–74.

Rapaport, M. H., Judd, L. L., Schjettler, P. J., *et al.* (2002). A descriptive analysis of minor depression. *Am. J. Psychiatry*, **159**, 637–43.

Rasmussen, K. G., Snyder, K. A., Knapp, R. G., *et al.* (2004). Relationship between somatization and remission with ECT. *Psychiatry Res.*, **129**, 293–5.

Rasmussen, S. L., Overo, K. F., and Tanghoj, P. (1999). Cardiac safety of citalopram: prospective trials and retrospective analyses. *J. Clin. Psychopharmacol.*, **19**, 407–15.

Rauch, S. L., Jenike, M. A., Alpert, N. M., *et al.* (1994). Regional cerebral blood flow measured during symptom provocation in obsessive-compulsive disorder using oxygen 15-labeled carbon dioxide and positron emission tomography. *Arch. Gen. Psychiatry*, **51**, 62–70.

Ravindran, A. V. and Lapierre, Y. D. (1997). Primary dysthymia: predictors of treatment response. In Akiskal, H. S. and Cassano, G. B. (eds), *Dysthymia and the Spectrum of Chronic Depressions*. New York: Guilford Press, pp. 44–53.

Ray, W. A., Meredith, S., Thapa, P. B., Hall, K., and Murray, K. T. (2004). Cyclic antidepressants and the risk of sudden cardiac death. *Clin. Pharmacol. Ther.*, **75**, 234–41.

Read, C. F. (1940). Consequences of metrazol shock therapy. *Am. J. Psychiatry*, **97**, 667–76.

Read, C. F., Steinberg, L., Liebert, E., and Finkelman, I. (1939). Use of metrazol in the functional psychoses. *Am. J. Psychiatry*, **95**, 781–6.

Reagen, L. and McEwen, B. (1997). Controversies surrounding glucocorticoid-mediated cell death in the hippocampus. *J. Chem. Neuroanat.*, **13**, 149–58.

Reed, P., Sermin, N., Appleby, L., and Faragher, B. (1999). A comparison of clinical response to electroconvulsive therapy in puerperal and non-puerperal psychoses. *J. Affect. Disord.*, **54**, 255–60.

Reeves, R. R., Pinkofsky, H. B., and Stevens, L. (1998). Medicolegal errors in the ED related to the involuntary confinement of psychiatry patients. *Am. J. Emerg. Med.*, **16**, 631–3.

Regenold, W. T., Weintraub, D., and Taller, A. (1998). Electroconvulsive therapy for epilepsy and major depression. *Am. J. Geriatr. Psychiatry*, **6**, 180–3.

Reich, L. H., Davies, R. K., and Himmelhoch, J. M. (1974). Excessive alcohol use in manic-depressive illness. *Am. J. Psychiatry*, **131**, 83–5.

Reid, D., Duke, L., and Allen, J. (1998). Resting frontal electroencephalographic asymmetry in depression: inconsistencies suggest the need to identify mediating factors. *Psychophysiology*, **35**, 389–404.

Reimherr, F. W., Amsterdam, J. D., Quitkin, F. M., *et al.* (1998). Optimal length of continuation therapy in depression: a prospective assessment during long-term fluoxetine treatment. *Am. J. Psychiatry*, **155**, 1247–53.

Reisner, A. D. (2003). The electroconvulsive therapy controversy: evidence and ethics. *Neuropsychol. Rev.*, **13**, 199–219.

Rende, R. D., Plomin, R., Reiss, D., and Hetherington, E. M. (1993). Genetic and environmental influences on depressive symptomatology in adolescence: individual differences and extreme scores. *J. Child Psychol. Psychiatry*, **34**, 1387–98.

Rennie, T. A. C. (1943). Prognosis in manic-depressive and schizophrenic conditions following shock treatment. *Psychiatr. Q.*, **17**, 642–54.

Repke, J. T. and Berger, N. G. (1984). Electroconvulsive therapy in pregnancy. *Obstet. Gynecol.*, **63**, 39S–41S.

Ressler, K. J. and Nemeroff, C. B. (1999). The role of norepinephrine in the pathophysiology and treatment of mood disorders. *Biol. Psychiatry*, **46**, 1219–33.

Ressler, K. J. and Nemeroff, C. B. (2000). Role of serotonergic and noradrenergic systems in the pathophysiology of depression and anxiety disorders. *Depress. Anxiety*, **12** (suppl. 1), 2–19.

Rey, J. M. and Walter, G. (1997). Half a century of ECT use in young people. *Am. J. Psychiatry*, **154**, 595–602.

Reynolds, C. F. 3rd, Frank, E., Perel, J. M., *et al.* (1996). High relapse rate after discontinuation of adjunctive medication for elderly patients with recurrent major depression. *Am. J. Psychiatry*, **153**, 1418–22.

Reynolds, C. F. III, Frank, E., Dew, M. A., *et al.* (1999). Treatment of 70+-year-olds with recurrent major depression. *Am. J. Geriatr. Psychiatry*, **7**, 64–9.

Reza, A., Mercy, J. A., and Krug, E. (2001). Epidemiology of violent deaths in the world. *Inj. Prev.*, **7**, 104–11.

Reznik, I., Rosen, Y., and Rosen, B. (1999). An acute ischaemic event associated with the use of venlafaxine: a case report and proposed pathophysiological mechanisms. *J. Psychopharmacol.*, **13**, 193–5.

Ribiero, S. C. M., Tandon, R., Grunhaus, L., and Greden, J. F. (1993). The DST as a predictor of outcome in depression: a meta-analysis. *Am. J. Psychiatry*, **150**, 1618–29.

Rice, J. P., Goate, A., Williams, J. T., *et al.* (1997). Initial genome scan of the NIMH genetics initiative bipolar pedigrees: chromosomes 1, 6, 8, 10 and 12. *Am. J. Med. Genet. Neuropsychiatry Gene.*, **74**, 247–53.

Richard, I. H. (2000). Depression in Parkinson's disease. *Curr. Treat. Options Neurol.*, **2**, 263–73.

Richard, I. H. and Kurlan, R. (1997). A survey of antidepressant drug use in Parkinson's disease. *Neurology*, **49**, 1168–70.

Rifkin, A. (1988). ECT versus tricyclic antidepressants in depression: a review of the evidence. *J. Clin. Psychiatry*, **49**, 3–7.

(2003). Comparing depression treatments (letter and reply). *Am. J. Psychiatry*, **160**, 1186–8.

Rigaud, A. S., Latour, F., Moulin, F., *et al.* (2002). Apolipoprotein E episilon4 allele and clinically defined vascular depression. *Arch. Gen. Psychiatry*, **59**, 290–1.

Rihmer, Z. and Kiss, K. (2002). Bipolar disorders and suicidal behaviour. *Bipolar Disord.*, **4** (suppl. 1), 21–5.

Rihmer, Z. and Pestality, P. (1999). Bipolar II disorder and suicidal behavior. *Psychiatr. Clin. North Am.*, **22**, 667–73.

Rihmer, Z., Arato, M., Szadoczky, E., *et al.* (1984). The dexamethasone suppression test in psychotic versus non-psychotic endogenous depression. *Br. J. Psychiatry*, **145**, 508–11.

Rihmer, Z., Barsi, J., Arato, M., and Demeter, E. (1990a). Suicide in subtypes of primary major depression. *J. Affect. Disord.*, **18**, 221–5.

Rihmer, Z., Barsi, J., Veg, K., and Katona, C. L. E. (1990b). Suicide rates in Hungary correlate negatively with reported rates of depression. *J. Affect. Disord.*, **20**, 87–91.

Rinaldi, P., Mecocci, P., Benedetti, C., *et al.* (2003). Validation of the five-item geriatric depression scale in elderly subjects in three different settings. *J. Am. Geriatr. Soc.*, **51**, 694–8.

Ring, H. A., Bench, C. J., Trimble, M. R., *et al.* (1994). Depression in Parkinson's disease. A positron emission study. *Br. J. Psychiatry*, **165**, 333–9.

Rivest, S. and Rivier, C. (1993). Centrally injected interleukin-1b inhibits the hypothalamic LHRH secretion and circulating LH levels via prostaglandins in rats. *J. Neuroendocrinol.*, **5**, 445–50.

Rivier, C. (1993). Neuroendocrine effects of cytokines in the rat. *Rev. Neurosci.*, **4**, 223–37.

Robbins, D. R., Alessi, N. E., Yanchyshyn, G. W., and Colfer, M. V. (1983). The dexamethasone suppression test in psychiatrically hospitalized adolescents. *J. Am. Acad. Child Psychiatry*, **22**, 467–9.

Robertson, H. A., Lam, R. W., Stewart, J. N., *et al.* (1996). Atypical depressive symptoms and clusters in unipolar and bipolar depression. *Acta Psychiatr. Scand.*, **94**, 421–7.

Robins, E. (1981). *The Final Months.* New York: Oxford University Press.

Robins, E. and Guze, S. B. (1972). Classification of affective disorders; the primary–secondary, the endogenous–reactive, and the neurotic–psychotic concepts. In Williams, T. A., Katz, M. M., and Shield, J. A. (eds) *Recent Advances in Psychobiology of the Affective Illnesses.* Washington, DC: US Government Printing Office.

Robins, L. N. and Barrett, J. E. (1989). (eds): *The Validity of Psychiatric Diagnosis.* New York, Raven Press.

Robinson, D. S. (2002). Monoamine oxidase inhibitors: a new generation. *Psychopharmacol. Bull.*, **36**, 124–38.

Robinson, R. G. (1998). Relation of depression to lesion location. In Robinson, R. G. (ed.) *The Clinical Neuropsychiatry of Stroke.* Cambridge, UK: Cambridge University Press, pp. 93–124.

Robinson, R. G., Kubos, K. L., Starr, L. B., Rao, K., and Price, T. R. (1983). Mood changes in stroke patients: relationship to lesion location. *Compr. Psychiatry*, **24**, 555–66.

Robinson, R. G., Schultz, S. K., Castillo, C., *et al.* (2000). Nortriptyline versus fluoxetine in the treatment of depression and in short-term recovery after stroke: a placebo-controlled, double-blind study. *Am. J. Psychiatry*, **157**, 351–9.

Robling, S. A., Paykel, E. S., Dunn, V. J., Abbott, R., and Katona, C. (2000). Long-term outcome of severe puerperal psychiatric illness. *Psychol. Med.*, **30**, 1263–71.

Rogers, M. A., Bradshaw, J. L., Phillips, J. G., *et al.* (2000). Parkinsonian motor characteristics in unipolar major depression. *J. Clin. Exp. Neuropsychol.*, **22**, 232–44.

Rohan, K. J., Lindsey, K. T., Roecklein, K. A., and Lacy, T. J. (2004). Cognitive-behavioral therapy, light therapy, and their combination in treating seasonal affective disorder. *J. Affect. Disord.*, **80**, 273–83.

Romney, D. M. and Candido, C. L. (2001). Anhedonia in depression and schizophrenia: a reexamination. *J. Nerv. Ment. Dis.*, **189**, 735–40.

Roose, S. P., Glassman, A. H., Walsh, B. T., Woodring, S., and Vital-Herne, J. (1983). Depression, delusions, and suicide. *Am. J. Psychiatry*, **140**, 1159–62.

Roose, S. P., Dalack, G. W., Glassman, A. H., *et al.* (1991). Cardiovascular effects of bupropion in depressed patients with heart disease. *Am. J. Psychiatry*, **148**, 512–16.

Roose, S. P., Glassman, A. H., Attia, E., and Woodring, S. (1994). Comparative efficacy of selective serotonin reuptake inhibitors and tricyclics in the treatment of melancholia. *Am. J. Psychiatry*, **151**, 1735–9.

Roose, S. P., Laghrissi-Thode, F., Kennedy, J. S., *et al.* (1998). Comparison of paroxetine and nortriptyline in depressed patients with ischemic heart disease. *J.A.M.A.*, **279**, 287–91.

Roose, S. P., Sackeim, H. A., Krishnan, E. R., *et al.* (2004). Antidepressant pharmacotherapy in the treatment of depression in the very old: a randomized, placebo-controlled trial. *Am. J. Psychiatry*, **161**, 2050–9.

Rorsman, B., Grasbeck, A., Hagnell, O., *et al.* (1990). A prospective study of first-incidence depression. The Lundby Study, 1957–72. *Br. J. Psychiatry*, **156**, 336–42.

Rosche, J., Uhlmann, C., and Froscher, W. (2003). Low serum folate levels as a risk factor for depressive mood in patients with chronic epilepsy. *J. Neuropsychiatry Clin. Neurosci.*, **15**, 64–6.

Roschke, J. and Mann, K. (2002). The sleep EEG's microstructure in depression: alterations of the phase relations between EEG rhythms during REM and NREM sleep. *Sleep Med.*, **3**, 501–5.

Rosen, C. (2005). The anatomy lesson. *NY Rev. Books*, **52**, 55–9.

Rosenberg, D. R. and Lewis, D. A. (1995). Postnatal maturation of the dopaminergic innervation of monkey prefrontal and motor cortices: a tyrosine hydroxylase immunohistochemical analysis. *J. Comp. Neurol.*, **358**, 383–400.

Rosenberg, D. R., Macmaster, F. P., Mirza, Y., *et al.* (2005). Reduced anterior cingulate glutamate in pediatric major depression: a magnetic resonance spectroscopy study. *Biol. Psychiatry*, **58**: 700–04.

Rosenberg, L. E. (2002). Brainsick: a physician's journey to the brink. *Cerebrum*, **4**, 2–10.

Rosenblatt, A. and Leroi, I. (2000). Neuropsychiatry of Huntington's disease and other basal ganglia disorders. *Psychosom.*, **41**, 24–30.

Rosenfeld, J. A. and Everett, K. (1996). Factors related to planned and unplanned pregnancies. *J. Fam. Prac.*, **43**, 161–6.

Rosenstein, D. L., Nelson, J. C., and Jacobs, S. C. (1993). Seizures associated with antidepressants: a review. *J. Clin. Psychiatry*, **54**, 289–99.

Rosenthal, N. E., Sack, D. A., Gillin, J. C. *et al.* (1984). Seasonal affective disorder. A description of the syndrome and preliminary findings with light therapy. *Arch. Gen. Psychiatry*, 41, 72–80.

Rosenthal, N. E., Moul, D. E., Hellekson, C. J., *et al.* (1993). A multicenter study of the light visor for seasonal affective disorder. No differences in efficacy found between two different intensities. *Neuropsychopharmacol.*, **8**, 151–60.

Rosenzweig, A., Prigerson, H., Miller, M. D., and Reynolds, C. F. III (1997). Bereavement and late-life depression: grief and its complications in the elderly. *Annu. Rev. Med.*, **48**, 421–8.

Rossby, S. P., Liang, S., Manier, D. H., *et al.* (2000). Molecular psychopharmacology as a prelude to a molecular psychopathology of affective disorders. The significance of differential display methodology to study programs of gene expression. In Briley, M. and Sulser, F. (eds) *Molecular Genetics of Mental Disorders.* London: Martin Dunitz, pp. 31–46.

Rossi, A., Daneluzzo, E., Arduini, L., *et al.* (2001). A factor analysis of signs and symptoms of the manic episode with Bech-Rafaelsen Mania and Melancholia Scales. *J. Affect. Disord.*, **64**, 267–70.

Rothermundt, M., Arolt, V., Fenker, J., *et al.* (2001a). Different immune patterns in melancholic and non-melancholic major depression. *Eur. Arch. Psychiatry Clin. Neurosci.*, **251**, 90–7.

Rothermundt, M., Arolt, V., Peters, M., *et al.* (2001b). Inflammatory markers in major depression and melancholia. *J. Affect. Disord.*, **63**, 93–102.

Rothschild, A. J. (2003a). Challenges in the treatment of depression with psychotic features. *Biol. Psychiatry*, **53**, 680–90.

Rothschild, A. J. (2003b). The hypothalamic–pituitary–adrenal axis and psychiatric illness. In Wolkowitz, O. M. and Rothschild, A. J. (eds) *Psychoneuroendocrinology: The Scientific Basis of Clinical Practice*, vol. 6. Washington, DC: American Psychiatric Publishing, pp. 139–63.

Rothschild, A. J., Schatzberg, A. F., Rosenbaum, A. H., Stahl, J. B., and Cole, J. O. (1982). The dexamethasone suppression test as a discriminator among subtypes of psychotic patients. *Br. J. Psychiatry*, **141**, 471–474.

Rothschild, A. J., Benes, F., Hebben, N., *et al.* (1989). Relationships between brain CT scan findings and cortisol in psychotic and nonpsychotic depressed patients. *Biol. Psychiatry*, **6**, 565–75.

Rothschild, A. J., Samson, J. A., Bessette, M. P., and Carter-Campbell, J. T. (1993). Efficacy of the combination of fluoxetine and perphenazine in the treatment of psychotic depression. *J. Clin. Psychiatry*, **54**, 338–42.

Rothschild, A. J., Bates, K. S., Boehringer, K. L., and Syed, A. (1999). Olanzapine response in psychotic depression. *J. Clin. Psychiatry*, **60**, 116–18.

Roubicek, J. (1946). *Šokové Léčeni Duševnich Chorob.* Prague: Nǎkladem Lékarského Knihkupectvi A Nakladatelstvi.

Roueché, B. (1974). As empty as eve. *N. Yorker*, Sept. 9, 84–100.

Rowe, P. C., Bou-Holaigah, I., Kan, J. S., and Calkins, H. (1995). Is neurally mediated hypotension an unrecognized cause of chronic fatigue? *Lancet*, **345**, 623–4.

Roy, A. (1992). Hypothalamic–pituitary–adrenal axis function and suicidal behavior in depression. *Biol. Psychiatry*, **32**, 812–16.

(2001). Characteristics of cocaine-dependent patients who attempt suicide. *Am. J. Psychiatry*, **158**, 1215–19.

Roy, A., Segal, N. L., Centerwall, B, S., and Robinette, C. D. (1991). Suicide in twins. *Arch. Gen. Psychiatry*, **48**, 29–32.

Roy-Byrne, P., Afari, N., Ashton, S., *et al.* (2002). Chronic fatigue and anxiety/depression: a twin study. *Br. J. Psychiatry*, **180**, 29–34.

Roy-Byrne, P. P., Pages, K. P., Russo, J. E., *et al.* (2000). Nefazodone treatment of major depression in alcoholic-dependent patients: a double-blind, placebo-controlled trial. *J. Clin. Psychopharmacol.*, **20**, 129–36.

Royall, D. R. (1999). Frontal systems impairment in major depression. *Semin. Clin. Neuropsychiatry*, **4**, 13–23.

Rubin, E., Sackeim, H. A., Nobler, M. S., and Moeller, J. R. (1994). Brain imaging studies of antidepressant treatments. *Psychiatr. Ann.*, **24**, 653–8.

Rubin, E., Sackeim, H. A., Prohovnik, I., *et al.* (1995). Regional cerebral blood flow in mood disorders: IV. Comparison of mania and depression. *Psychiatry Res. Neuroimaging*, **61**, 1–10.

Rubinow, D. R. (1992). The premenstrual syndrome: new views. *J.A.M.A.*, **268**, 1908–12.

Rubio, A., Vestner, A. L., Stewart, J. M., *et al.* (2001). Suicide and Alzheimer's pathology in the elderly: a case-control study. *Biol. Psychiatry*, **49**, 137–45.

Rucci, P., Frank, E., Kostelnik, B., *et al.* (2002). Suicide attempts in patients with bipolar I disorder during acute and maintenance phases of intensive treatment with pharmacotherapy and adjunctive psychotherapy. *Am. J. Psychiatry*, **159**, 1160–4.

Rudolph, R. L. (2002). Achieving remission from depression with venlafaxine and venlafaxine extended release: a literature review of comparative studies with selective serotonin reuptake inhibitors. *Acta Psychiatr. Scand.*, **415**, (suppl.) 24–30.

Ruedrich, S. L., Chu, C. C., and Moore, S. L. (1983). ECT for major depression in a patient with acute brain trauma. *Am. J. Psychiatry*, **140**, 928–9.

Runeson, B. and Asberg, M. (2003). Family history of suicide among suicide victims. *Am. J. Psychiatry*, **160**, 1525–6.

Runeson, B. S., Beskow, J., and Waern, M. (1996). The suicidal process in suicides among young people. *Acta Psychiatr. Scand.*, **93**, 35–42.

Rupniak, N. M. and Kramer, M. S. (1999). Discovery of the antidepressant and anti-emetic efficacy of substance P receptor (NK1) antagonists. *Trends Pharmacol. Sci.*, **20**, 485–90.

Rush, A. (1998). Cognitive approaches to adherence. In Frances, A. and Hales, R. (eds) *Review of Psychiatry*, vol. 8. Washington, DC: APA Press.

Rush, A. J. and Weissenburger, J. E. (1994). Melancholic symptom features and DSM-IV. *Am. J. Psychiatry*, **151**, 489–98.

Rush, A. J., Giles, D. E., Schlesser, M. A., *et al.* (1996). The dexamethasone suppression test in patients with mood disorders. *J. Clin. Psychiatry*, **57**, 470–84.

Rush, A. J., Giles, D. E., Schlesser, M. A., *et al.* (1997). Dexamethasone response, thyrotropin-releasing hormone stimulation, rapid eye movement latency, and subtypes of depression. *Biol. Psychiatry*, **41**, 915–28.

Rush, A. J., George, M. S., Sackeim, H. A., *et al.* (2000). Vagus nerve stimulation (VNS) for treatment-resistant depressions: a multicenter study. *Biol. Psychiatry*, **47**, 276–86.

Russo-Neustadt, A., Beard, R. C., and Cotman, C. W. (1999). Exercise, antidepressant medications, and enhanced brain derived neurotrophic factor expression. *Neuropsychopharm.*, **21**, 679–82.

Rutkowski, N. J., Fitch, C. A., Yeiser, E. C., *et al.* (1999). Regulation of neuropeptide Y mRNA and peptide concentrations by copper in rat olfactory bulb. *Brain Res. Mol. Brain Res.*, **65**, 80–6.

Rutz, W., Von Knorring, L., and Walinder, J. (1992). Long-term effects of an educational program for general practitioners given by the Swedish Committee for the Prevention and Treatment of Depression. *Acta Psychiatr. Scand.*, **85**, 83–8.

Ryan, N. D. (1992). The pharmacologic treatment of child and adolescent depression. *Psychiatr. Clin. North Am.*, **15**, 29–40.

(2003). Medication treatment for depression in children and adolescents. *CNS Spectrums*, **8**, 283–7.

Ryan, N. D., Puig-Antich, J., Ambrosini, P., *et al.* (1987). The clinical picture of major depression in children and adolescents. *Arch. Gen. Psychiatry*, **44**, 854–61.

Ryan, N. D., Puig-Antich, J., Rabinovich, H., *et al.* (1988a). MAOIs in adolescent major depression unresponsive to tricyclic antidepressants. *J. Am. Acad. Child Adolesc. Psychiatry*, **27**, 755–8.

Ryan, N. D., Meyer, V., Dachille, S., Mazzie, D., and Puig-Antich, J. (1988b). Lithium antidepressant augmentation in TCA-refractory depression in adolescents. *J. Am. Acad. Child Adolesc. Psychiatry*, **27**, 371–6.

Rybakowski, J. and Plocka, M. (1992). Seasonal variations of the dexamethasone suppression test in depression compared with schizophrenia: a gender effect. *J. Affect. Disord.*, **24**, 87–91.

Rybakowski, J. K. and Twardowska, K. (1999). The dexamethasone/corticotropin-releasing hormone test in depression in bipolar and unipolar affective illness. *J. Psychiatry Res.*, **33**, 363–70.

Sachar, E. J. (ed). (1976). *Hormones, Behavior and Psychopathology*. New York: Raven Press.

Sachs, G. S. (2004). Strategies for improving treatment of bipolar disorder: integration of measurement and management. *Acta Psychiatr. Scand.*, **422** (suppl.), 7–17.

Sachs, G. S., Lafer, B., Stoll, A. L., *et al.* (1994). A double-blind trial of bupropion versus desipramine for bipolar depression. *J. Clin. Psychiatry*, **55**, 391–3.

Sachs, G. S., Printz, D. J., Kahn, D. A., Carpenter, D., and Docherty, J. P. (2000). Medication treatment of bipolar disorder 2000. *Postgrad. Med. Special Rep.*, 1–104.

Sachs, G. S., Thase, M. E., Otto, M. W., *et al.* (2003). Rationale, design, and methods of the systematic treatment enhancement program for bipolar disorder (STEP-BD). *Biol. Psychiatry*, **53**, 1028–42.

Sackeim, H. A. (1994). Continuation therapy following ECT: directions for future research. *Psychopharm. Bull.*, **30**, 501–21.

Sackeim, H. A. and Mukherjee, S. (1986). Neurophysiologic variability in the effects of the ECT stimulus. *Convuls. Ther.*, **2**, 267–76.

Sackeim, H. A., Greenberg, M. S., Weiman, A. L., *et al.* (1982). Hemispheric asymmetry in the expression of positive and negative emotions. *Arch. Neurol.*, **39**, 210–18.

Sackeim, H. A., Decina, P., Portnoy, S., Neeley, P., and Malitz, S. (1987). Studies of dosage, seizure threshold, and seizure duration in ECT. *Biol. Psychiatry*, **22**, 249–68.

Sackeim, H. A., Devanand, D. P., and Prudic, J. (1991). Stimulus intensity, seizure threshold, and seizure duration: impact on efficacy and safety of electroconvulsive therapy. *Psychiatr. Clin. North Am.*, **14**, 803–43.

Sackeim, H. A., Prudic, J., Devanand, D., *et al.* (1993). Effects of stimulus intensity and electrode placement on the efficacy and cognitive effects of electroconvulsive therapy. *N. Engl. J. Med.*, **328**, 839–46.

Sackeim, H. A., Luber, B., Katzman, G. P., *et al.* (1996). The effects of electroconvulsive therapy on quantitative electroencephalograms. *Arch. Gen. Psychiatry*, **53**, 814–24.

Sackeim, H. A., Prudic, J., Devanand, D. P., *et al.* (2000). A prospective, randomized, double-blind comparison of bilateral and right unilateral electroconvulsive therapy at different stimulus intensities. *Arch. Gen. Psychiatry*, **57**, 425–34.

Sackeim, H. A., Haskett, R. F., Mulsant, B. H., *et al.* (2001a). Continuation pharmacotherapy in the prevention of relapse following electroconvulsive therapy: a randomized controlled trial. *J.A.M.A.*, **285**, 1299–307.

Sackeim, H. A., Rush, A. J., George, M. S., *et al.* (2001b). Vagus nerve stimulation (VNS) for treatment-resistant depression: efficacy, side effects, and predictors of outcome. *Neuropsychopharmacology*, **25**, 713–28.

Sadler, J. Z., Wiggins, O. P., and Schwartz, M. A. (eds) (1994). *Philosophical Perspectives on Psychiatric Diagnostic Classification.* Baltimore, MD: Johns Hopkins University Press.

Safer, D. (2002). Design and reporting modifications in industry-sponsored comparative psychopharmacology trials. *J. Nerv. Ment. Dis.*, **190**, 583–92.

Saiz-Ruiz, J., Ibanez, A., Diaz-Marsa, M., *et al.* (2002). Efficacy of venlafaxine in major depression resistant to selective serotonin reuptake inhibitors. *Prog. Neuropsychopharmacol. Biol. Psychiatry*, **26**, 1129–34.

Sajatovic, M., Mullen, J. A., and Sweitzer, D. E. (2002). Efficacy of quetiapine and risperidone against depressive symptoms in outpatients with psychosis. *J. Clin. Psychiatry*, **63**, 1156–63.

Sakel, M. (1938). *The Pharmacological Shock Treatment of Schizophrenia.* Translated by Wortis, J. New York: Nervous and Mental Disease Publishing.

Salzman, C., Wong, E., and Wright, B. C. (2002). Drug and ECT treatment of depression in the elderly, 1996–2001: a literature review. *Biol. Psychiatry*, **52**, 265–84.

Sanchez, A. I., Buela-Casal, G., Bermudez, M. P., and Casas-Maldanado, F. (2001). The effects of continuous positive air pressure treatment on anxiety and depression levels in apnea patients. *Psychiatry Clin. Neurosci.*, **55**, 641–6.

Sanchez, M. M., Aguado, F., Sanchez-Toscano, F., and Saphier, D. (1998). Neuroendocrine and immunocytochemical demonstrations of decreased hypothalamo–pituitary–adrenal axis responsiveness to restraint stress after long-term social isolation. *Endocrinology*, **139**, 579–87.

Sanders, A. R, Detera-Wadleigh S. D., and Gershon E. S. (1999). Molecular genetics of mood disorders. In Charney, D. S., Nestler, E. J., and Bunney, B. S. (eds) *Neurobiology of Mental Illness.* New York: Oxford University Press.

Sandifer, M. G., Hordern, A., Timbury, G. C., and Green, L. M. (1969). Similarities and differences in patient evaluation by U.S. and U.K. psychiatrists. *Am. J. Psychiatry*, **126**, 206–12.

Santosh, P. J., Malhotra, S., Raghunathan, M., and Mehra, Y. N. (1994). A study of P300 in melancholic depression – correlation with psychotic features. *Biol. Psychiatry*, **35**, 474–9.

Sapolsky, R. (1996). Stress, glucocorticoids, and damage to the nervous system: the current state of confusion. *Stress*, **1**, 1–11.

Sapolsky, R. M. (2000). Glucocorticoids and hippocampal atrophy in neuropsychiatric disorders. *Arch. Gen. Psychiatry*, **57**, 925–35.

Sareen, J., Enns, M. W., and Guertin, J. E.. (2000). The impact of clinically diagnosed personality disorders on acute one year outcomes of electroconvulsive therapy. *J. ECT*, **16**, 43–51.

Sargant, W. and Slater, E. (1946). *An introduction to Physical Methods of Treatment in Psychiatry.* Edinburgh: E&S Livingston.

Sargent, P. A., Kjaer, K. H., Bench, C. J., *et al.* (2000). Brain Serotonin 1A receptor finding measured by positron emission tomography. with [11c]WAY-100635: effects of depression and antidepressant treatment. *Arch. Gen. Psychiatry*, **57**, 174–80.

Sarwer-Foner, G. J. (1988). The course of manic-depressive (bipolar) illness. In Georgotas, A. and Cancro, R. (eds) *Depression and Mania*, vol. 4. New York: Elsevier, pp. 55–75.

Sassi, R. B., Nicoletti, M., Brambilla, P., *et al.* (2001). Decreased pituitary volume in patients with bipolar disorder. *Biol. Psychiatry*, **50**, 271–80.

Sato, T., Narita, T., Hirano, S., *et al.* (2001). Factor validity of the temperament and character inventory in patients with major depression. *Compr. Psychiatry*, **42**, 337–41.

Sauer, W. H., Berlin, J. A., and Kimmel, S. E. (2001). Selective serotonin reuptake inhibitors and myocardial infarction. *Circulation*, **104**, 1894–8.

Saxena, S., Brody, A. L., Ho, M. L., *et al.* (2001). Cerebral metabolism in major depression and obsessive-compulsive disorder occurring separately and concurrently. *Biol. Psychiatry*, **50**, 159–70.

Saxena, S., Brody, A. L., Ho, M. L., *et al.* (2002). Differential cerebral metabolic changes with paroxetine treatment of obsessive-compulsive disorder vs. major depression. *Arch. Gen. Psychiatry*, **59**, 250–61.

Schafer, W. R. (1999). How do antidepressants work? Prospects for genetic analysis of drug mechanisms. *Cell*, **98**, 551–4.

Schatzberg, A. F. (1998). Noradrenergic versus serotonergic antidepressants: predictors of treatment response. *J. Clin. Psychiatry*, **59** (suppl. 14), 15–18.

Schatzberg, A. F. (2003). New approaches to managing psychotic depression. *J. Clin. Psychiatry*, **64** (suppl. 1), 19–23.

Schatzberg, A. F. and Nemeroff, C. B. (eds) (1988). *The Hypothalamic–Pituitary–Adrenal Axis.* New York: Raven Press.

Schatzberg, A. F. and Rothschild, A. J. (1986). Psychotic (delusional) major depression: should it be included as a distinct syndrome in DSM-IV? In Widiger, T. A., Frances, A. J., Pincus, H. A., *et al.* (eds) *DSM-IV Sourcebook*, vol. 2. Washington, DC: American Psychiatric Association, pp. 127–80.

Schatzberg, A. F. and Rothschild, A. J. (1992). Psychotic (delusional) major depression: should it be included as a distinct syndrome in DSM-IV? *Am. J. Psychiatry*, **149**, 733–45.

Schatzberg, A. F., Rothschild, A. J., Stahl, J. B., *et al.* (1983). The dexamethasone suppression test: identification of subtypes of depression. *Am. J. Psychiatry*, **140**, 88–91.

Schatzberg, A. F., Rothschild, A. J., Bond, T. C., and Cole, J. O. (1984). The DST in psychotic depression: diagnostic and pathophysiologic implications. *Psychopharmacol. Bull.*, **20**, 362–4.

Schatzberg, A. F., Posener, J. A., DeBattista, C., *et al.* (2000). Neuropsychological deficits in psychotic versus nonpsychotic major depression and no mental illness. *Am. J. Psychiatry*, **157**, 1095–100.

Schelde, J. T. (1998a). Major depression: behavioral markers of depression and recovery. *J. Nerv. Ment. Dis.*, **186**, 133–40.

(1998b). Major depression: behavioral parameters of depression and recovery. *J. Nerv. Ment. Dis.*, **186**, 141–9.

Schelfout, K., Van Goethem, M., Kersschot, E., *et al.* (2004). Contrast-enhanced MR imaging of breast lesions and effect on treatment. *Eur. J. Surg. Oncol.*, **30**, 501–7.

Schiffer, R. B. (2002). Neuropsychiatric problems in patients with multiple sclerosis. *Psychiatr. Ann.*, **32**, 128–32.

Schiffer, R. B. and Wineman, N. M. (1990). Antidepressant pharmacotherapy of depression associated with multiple sclerosis. *Am. J. Psychiatry*, **147**, 1493–7.

Schiffer, R. B., Herndon, R. M., and Rudick, R. A. (1985). Treatment of pathologic laughing and weeping with amitriptyline. *N. Engl. J. Med.*, **312**, 1480–2.

Schildkraut, J., Green, A., and Mooney, J. (1989). Mood disorders: biochemical aspects. In Kaplan, H. and Sadock, B. (eds) *Comprehensive Textbook of Psychiatry*, vol. 1, Baltimore, MD: Williams & Wilkins.

Schlegel, S., Nieber, D., Herrmann, C., and Bakauski, E. (1991). Latencies of the P300 component of the auditory event-related potential in depression are related to the Bech-Rafaelsen Melancholia Scale but not to the Hamilton Rating Scale for Depression. *Acta Psychiatr. Scand.*, **83**, 438–40.

Schlesser, M. A., Winokur, G., and Sherman, B. M. (1980). Hypothalamic–pituitary–adrenal axis activity in depressive illness: its relationship to classification. *Arch. Gen. Psychiatry*, **37**, 737.

Schlienger, R. G., Klink, M. H., Eggenberger, C., and Drewe, J. (2000). Seizures associated with therapeutic doses of venlafaxine and trimipramine. *Ann. Pharmacother.*, **34**, 1402–5.

Schmider, J., Lammers, C. H., Gotthardt, U., *et al.* (1995). Combined dexamethasone/corticotropin-releasing hormone test in acute and remitted manic patients, in acute depression, and in normal controls: I. *Biol. Psychiatry*, **38**, 797–802.

Schmidt-Degenhard, M. (1983). *Melancholie und Depression.* Stuttgart: Verlag W. Kohlhammer.

Schmidtke, A., Fleckenstein, P., and Beckmann, H. (1989). The dexamethasone suppression test and suicide attempts. *Acta Psychiatr. Scand.*, **79**, 276–82.

Schmitz, J. M., Stotts, A. L., Averill, P., Rothfleisch, J., and Bailey, S. (2000). Cocaine dependence with and without comorbid depression: a comparison of patient characteristics. *Drug Alcohol Depend.*, **60**, 189–98.

Schmitz, J. M., Averill, P., Stotts, A. L., *et al.* (2001). Fluoxetine treatment of cocaine-dependent patients with major depressive disorder. *Drug Alcohol Depend.*, **63**, 207–14.

Schneekloth, T. D., Rummans, T. A., and Logan, K. M. (1993). Electroconvulsive therapy in adolescents. *Convuls. Ther.*, **9**, 158–66.

Schneider, B., Philipp, M., and Muller, M. J. (2001b). Psychopathological predictors of suicide in patients with major depression during a 5-year follow-up. *Eur. Psychiatry*, **16**, 283–8.

Schneider, F., Gur, R. E., Mozley, L. H., *et al.* (1995). Mood effects on limbic blood flow correlate with emotional self-rating: a PET study with oxygen-15 labeled water. *Psychiatry Res.*, **61**, 265–83.

Schneider, L. S., Small, G. W., Hamilton, S. H., *et al.* (1997). Estrogen replacement and response to fluoxetine in a multicenter geriatric depression trial. Fluoxetine Collaborative Study Group. *Am. J. Geriatr. Psychiatry*, **5**, 97–106.

Schneider, L. S., Nelson, J. C., Clary, C. M., *et al.* (2003). An 8-week multicenter, parallel-group, double-blind, placebo-controlled study of sertraline in elderly outpatients with major depression. *Am. J. Psychiatry*, **160**, 1277–85.

Schotte, C. K., Maes, M., Cluydts, R., De Doncker, D., and Cosyns, P. (1997a). Construct validity of the Beck Depression Inventory in a depressive population. *J. Affect. Disord.*, **46**, 115–25.

Schotte, C. K., Maes, M., Cluydts, R., and Cosyns, P. (1997b). Cluster analytic validation of the DSM melancholic depression. The threshold model: integration of quantitative and qualitative distinctions between unipolar depressive subtypes. *Psychiatry Res.*, **71**, 181–95.

Schou, M. (1998). Treating recurrent affective disorders during and after pregnancy. What can be taken safely? *Drug Safety*, **18**, 143–52.

Schrader, G. D. (1995). An attempt to validate Akiskal's classification of chronic depression using cluster analysis. *Compr. Psychiatry* **36**, 344–52.

Schreiber, W., Lauer, C. J., Drumrey, K., Holsboer, F., and Krieg, J. C. (1996). Dysregulation of the hypothalamic–pituitary–adrenocortical system in panic disorder. *Neuropsychopharmacology*, **15**, 7–15.

Schuld, A., Kraus, T., Haack, M., *et al.* (2001). Effects of dexamethasone on cytokine plasma levels and white blood cell counts in depressed patients. *Psychoneuroendocrinology*, **26**, 65–76.

Schuld, A., Schmid, D. A., Haack, M., *et al.* (2003). Hypothalamo–pituitary–adrenal function in patients with depressive disorders is correlated with baseline cytokine levels, but not with cytokine responses to hydrocortisone. *J. Psychiatr. Res.*, **37**, 463–70.

Schulsinger, F., Kety, S. S., Rosenthal, D., and Wender, P. H. (1979). A family study of suicide. In Schou, M. and Stromgren, E. (eds) *Origin, Prevention and Treatment of Affective Disorders*. London: Academic Press, pp. 277–87.

Schweitzer, I. and Tuckwell, V. (1998). Risk of adverse events with the use of augmentation therapy for the treatment of treatment resistant depression. *Drug Experience*, **19**, 455–64.

Schwenk, T. L. (2002). Diagnosis of late life depression: the view form primary care. *Biol. Psychiatry*, **52**, 157–63.

Sclar, D. A., Robinson, L. M., Skaer, T. L., and Galin, R. S. (1998). Trends in the prescribing of antidepressant pharmacotherapy: office-based visits, 1990–1995. *Clin. Ther.*, **20**, 871–84.

Scott, D. (1976). *Understanding EEG*. London: Duckworth.

Scott, J. (1992). Are there different subtypes of chronic primary major depression? A preliminary report. *Adv. Affect. Disord.*, **7**, 6–7.

Scott, J. (1995a). Psychological treatments of depression: an update. *Br. J. Psychiatry*, **167**, 289–92.

Scott, J. (1995b). Predictors of non-response to antidepressants. In Nolen, W. A., Zohar, J., and Roose, S. P., Amsterdam, J. D. (eds) *Refractory Depression: Current Strategies and Future Directions.* Chichester, UK: John Wiley, pp. 19–28.

Secunda, S. K., Cross, C. K., Koslow, S., *et al.* (1986). Biochemistry and suicidal behavior in depressed patients. *Biol. Psychiatry,* **21**, 756–67.

Sedler, M. (1983). Falret's discovery: the origin of the concept of bipolar illness. *Am. J. Psychiatry,* **140**, 1127–33.

Seel, R. T., Kreutzer, J. S., Rosenthal, M., *et al.* (2003). Depression after traumatic brain injury: a National Institute on Disability and Rehabilitation Research Model Systems multicenter investigation. *Arch. Phys. Med. Rehab.*, **84**, 177–84.

Seeman, M. V. (1997). Psychopathology in women and men: focus on female hormones. *Am. J. Psychiatry,* **154**, 1641–7.

Segal, Z., Vincent, P., and Levitt, A. (2002). Efficacy of combined, sequential, and cross-over psychotherapy and pharmacotherapy in improving outcomes in depression. *J. Psychiatry Neurosci.*, **27**, 281–90.

Segurado, R., Detera-Wadleigh, S. D., Levinson, D. F., *et al.* (2003). Genome scan meta-analysis of schizophrenia and bipolar disorder, part III: bipolar disorder. *Am. J. Hum. Genet,* **73**, 49–62.

Seidman, S. N. (2003). The aging male: androgens, erectile dysfunction, and depression. *J. Clin. Psychiatry,* **64** (suppl. 10), 31–7.

Seidman, S. N. and Rabkin, J. G. (1998). Testosterone replacement therapy for hypogonadal men with SSRI-refractory depression. *J. Affect. Disord.*, **48**, 157–61.

Seidman, S. N., Spatz, E., Rizzo, C., and Roose, S. P. (2001). Testosterone replacement therapy for hypogonadal men with major depressive disorder: a randomized, placebo-controlled clinical trial. *J. Clin. Psychiatry,* **62**, 406–12.

Seidman, S. N., Araujo, A. B., Roose, S. P., *et al.* (2002). Low testosterone levels in elderly men with dysthymic disorder. *Am. J. Psychiatry,* **159**, 456–9.

Seifer, R., Sameroff, A. J., Dickstein, S., Hayden, L., and Schiller, M. (1996). Parental psychopathology and sleep variation in children. *Child Psychiatr. Clin. North Am.*, **5**, 715–27.

Seifritz, E. (2001). Contribution of sleep physiology to depressive pathophysiology, *Neuropsychopharmacology,* **25**, S85–8.

Seligman, M. E. P. (1997). Learned helplessness as a model of depression. Comment and integration. *J. Abnorm. Psychol.*, **87**, 165–79.

Selye, H. (1950). *The Physiology and Pathology of Exposure to Stress.* Montreal: Acta.

Selye, H. and Stone, H. (1950) *On the Experimental Morphology of the Adrenal Cortex.* Springfield, IL: CC Thomas.

Sen, S., Nesse, R. M., Stoltenberg, S. F., *et al.* (2003). A BDNF coding variant is associated with the NEO personality inventory domain neuroticism, a risk factor for depression. *Neuropsychopharmacology,* **28**, 397–401.

Senge, P. (1990). *The Fifth Discipline.* New York: Doubleday.

Senra, C. (1996). Evaluation and monitoring of symptom severity and change in depressed outpatients. *J. Clin. Psychol.*, **52**, 317–24.

Senra Rivera, C., Rancano Perez, C., Sanchez Cao, E., and Barba Sixto, S. (2000). Use of three depression scales for evaluation of pretreatment severity and of improvement after treatment. *Psychol. Rep.*, **87**, 389–94.

Serra, M., Pisul, M. G., Dazzi, L., Purdy, R. H., and Biggio, G. (2002). Prevention of the stress-induced increase in the concentration of neuroactive steroids in rat brain by long-term administration of mirtazapine but not of fluoxetine. *J. Psychopharmacol.*, **16**, 133–8.

Serretti, A., Franchini, L., Gasperini, M., Rampoldi, R., and Smeraldi, E. (1998a). Mode to inheritance in mood disorders families according to fluvoxamine response. *Acta Psychiatr. Scand.*, **98**, 443–50.

Serretti, A., Lattuada, E., Cusin, C., Macciardi, F., and Smeraldi, E. (1998b). Analysis of depressive symptomatology in mood disorders. *Depress. Anxiety*, **8**, 80–5.

Serretti, A., Lattuada, E., Franchini, L., and Smeraldi, E. (2000a). Melancholic features and response to lithium prophylaxis in mood disorders. *Depress. Anxiety*, **11**, 73–9.

Serretti, A., Macciardi, F., Cusin, C., *et al.* (2000b). Linkage of mood disorders with D2, D3 and TH genes: a multicenter study. *J. Affect. Disord.*, **58**, 51–61.

Serretti, A., Zanardi, R., Cusin, C., *et al.* (2001a). Tryptophan hydroxylase gene associated with paroxetine antidepressant activity. *Eur. Neuropsychopharmacol.*, **11**, 375–80.

Serretti, A., Zanardi, R., Rossini, D., *et al.* (2001b). Influence of tryptophan hydroxylase and serotonin transporter genes on fluvoxamine antidepressant activity. *Mol. Psychiatry*, **6**, 586–92.

Serretti, A., Lilli, R., and Smeraldi, E. (2002). Pharmacogenetics in affective disorders. *Eur. J. Pharmacol.*, **438**, 117–28.

Settle, E. C. (1998). Antidepressant drugs: disturbing and potentially dangerous adverse effects. *J. Clin. Psychiatry*, **59** (suppl. 16), 25–30.

Severinó, S. K. and Yonkers, K. A. (1993). A literature review of psychotic symptoms associated with the premenstrum. *Psychosomatics*, **34**, 299–306.

Seyfried, L. S. and Marcus, S. M. (2003). Postpartum mood disorders. *Int. Rev. Psychiatry* **15**, 231–242.

Shabetai, R. (2002). Depression and heart failure. *Psychosom. Med.*, **64**, 13–14.

Shagass, C. (1954). The sedation threshold. A method for estimating tension in psychiatric patients. *EEG Clin. Neurophysiol.*, **8**, 221–33.

(1957). A measurable neurophysiological factor of psychiatric significance. *EEG Clin. Neurophysiol.*, **9**, 101–8.

(1972). *Evoked Potentials in Psychiatry.* New York: Plenum Press.

(1983). Evoked potentials in adult psychiatry. In Hughes, J. R. and Willson, W. P. (eds) *EEG and Evoked Potentials in Psychiatry and Behavioral Neurology*, vol. 9. Woburn, MA: Butterworth, pp. 169–210.

Shah, P. J., Ebmeier, K. P., Glabus, M. F., and Goodwin, G. M. (1998). Cortical grey matter reductions associated with treatment-resistant chronic unipolar depression: controlled magnetic resonance imaging study. *Br. J. Psychiatry*, **172**, 527–32.

Shankman, S. A. and Klein, D. N. (2002). Dimensional diagnosis of depression: adding the dimension of course to severity, and comparison to the DSM. *Compr. Psychiatry*, **43**, 420–6.

Shapira, B., Oppenhiem, G., Zohar, J., *et al.* (1985). Lack of efficacy of estrogen supplementation to imipramine in resistant female depressives. *Biol. Psychiatry*, **20**, 576–9.

Sharma, V. (1999). Retrospective controlled study of inpatient ECT: does it prevent suicide? *J. Affect. Disord.*, **56**, 183–7.

Sharp, D., Hay, D. F., Pawlby, S., Schmucker, G., Allen, H., and Kumar, R. (1995). The impact of postnatal depression on boys' intellectual development. *J. Child. Psychol. Psychiatry*, **36**, 1315–36.

Shearman, L. P., Zylka, M. J., Weaver, D. R., *et al.* (1997). Two period homologs: circadian expression and photic regulation in the suprachiasmatic nuclei. *Neuron*, **19**, 1261–9.

Sheehan, D., Dunbar, G. C., and Fuell, D. L. (1992). The effect of paroxetine on anxiety and agitation associated with depression. *Psychopharmacol. Bull.*, **28**, 139–43.

Sheline, Y. I., Wang, P. W., Gado, M. H., Csernansky, J. G., and Vannier, M. W. (1996). Hippocampal atrophy in recurrent major depression. *Proc. Natl Acad. Sci*, **93**, 908–13.

Sheline, Y. I., Sanghavi, M., Mintun, M. A., and Gado, M. H. (1999). Depression duration but not age predicts hippocampal volume loss in medically healthy women with recurrent major depression. *J. Neurosci.*, **19**, 5034–43.

Sheline, Y. I., Gado, M. H., and Kraemer, H. C. (2003). Untreated depression and hippocampal volume loss. *Am. J. Psychiatry*, **160**, 1515–18.

Shelton, C. I. (2004). Long-term management of major depressive disorder: are differences among antidepressant treatments meaningful? *J. Clin. Psychiatry*, **65** (suppl. 17), 29–33.

Shelton, R. C., Manier, D. H., and Sulser, F. (1996). Cyclic AMP-dependent protein kinase activity in major depression. *Am. J. Psychiatry*, **153**, 1037–42.

Shelton, R. C., Davidson, J., Yonkers, K. A., *et al.* (1997). The undertreatment of dysthymia. *J. Clin. Psychiatry*, **58**, 59–65.

Shelton, R. C., Manier, D. H., Ellis, T., Peterson Ch. S, and Sulser, F. (1999). Cyclic AMP dependent protein kinase in subtypes of major depression and normal volunteers. *Int. J. Neuropsychopharmacol.*, **3**, 187–92.

Sheng, Z., Yanai, A., Fujinaga, R., *et al.* (2003). Gonadal and adrenal effects on the glucocorticoid receptor in the rat hippocampus, with special reference to regulation by estrogen from an immunohistochemical view-point. *Neurosci. Res.*, **46**, 205–18.

Sher, L., Oquendo, M. A., Li, S., *et al.* (2003). Prolactin response to fenfluramine administration in patients with unipolar and bipolar depression and healthy controls. *Psychoneuroendocrinology*, **28**, 559–73.

Shneidman, E. S. (1981). The psychological autopsy. *Suicide Life Threat. Behav.*, **11**, 325–40.

Shores, M. M., Pascualy, M., and Veith, R. C. (1998). Major depression and heart disease: treatment trials. *Semin. Clin. Neuropsychiatry*, **3**, 87–101.

Shors, T. J. and Leuner, B. (2003). Estrogen-mediated effects on depression and memory formation in females. *J. Affect. Disord.*, **74**, 85–96.

Shorter, E. (1992). *From Paralysis to Fatigue: A History of Psychosomatic Illness in the Modern Era*. New York: Free Press.

(1997). *A History of Psychiatry*. New York: John Wiley.

(2005). *Historical Dictionary of Psychiatry*. New York: Oxford university press.

Shorter, E. and Healy, D. *Sometimes you need a Big Deal: A History of Shock Therapy*. In preparation.

Shuchter, S. R., Zisook, C., Kirkorowicz, C., and Risch, C., (1986). The dexamethasone suppression test in acute grief. *Am. J. Psychiatary*, **143**, 879–81.

Shulz, K. (2004). Did antidepressants depress Japan? *N. York Times Magazine*, August 22, 39–41.

Shumake, J., Edwards, E., and Gonzalez-Lima, F. (2001). Hypermetabolism of paraventricular hypothalamus in the congenitally helpless rat. *Neurosci. Lett.*, **311**, 45–8.

Sienaert, P., Filip, B., Willy, M., and Joseph, P. (2005). Electroconvulsive therapy in Belgium: a questionnaire on the practice of electroconvulsive therapy in Flanders and the Brussels Capital region. *J. ECT*, **21**, 3–6.

Silva, S. M., Madeira, M. D., Ruela, C., and Paula-Barbosa, M. M. (2002). Prolonged alcohol intake leads to irreversible loss of vasopressin and oxytocin neurons in the paraventricular nucleus of the hypothalamus. *Brain Res.*, **925**, 76–88.

Silver, J. M. and Yudofsky, S. C. (1992). Drug treatment of depression in Parkinson's disease. In Huber, S. J. and Cummings, J. L. (eds) *Parkinson's Disease: Neurobehavioral Aspects*. New York: Oxford University Press, 240–54.

Silver, J. M., Yudofsky, S. C., and Hales, R. E. (1994). *Neuropsychiatry of Traumatic Brain Injury*. Washington, DC: American Psychiatric Press.

Silverman, C. (1968). The epidemiology of depression. A review. *Am. J. Psychiatry*, **124**, 883–91.

Silverstone, T. (2001). Moclobemide vs. imipramine in bipolar depression: a multicentre double-blind clinical trial. *Acta Psychiatr. Scand.*, **104**, 104–9.

Silverstone, P. H. and Silverstone, T. (2004). A review of acute treatments for bipolar depression. *Int. Clin. Psychopharmacol.*, **19**, 113–24.

Simeon, J. G., Dinicola, V. F., Ferguson, H. B., and Copping, W. (1990). Adolescent depression: a placebo-controlled fluoxetine treatment study and follow-up. *Prog. Neuropsychopharmacol. Biol. Psychiatry*, **14**, 791–5.

Simon, G. E., Cunningham, M. L., and Davis, R. L. (2002). Outcomes of prenatal antidepressant exposure. *Am. J. Psychiatry*, **159**, 2055–61.

Simon, N. M., Otto, M. W., Weiss, R. D., *et al.* (2004). Pharmacotherapy for bipolar and comorbid conditions: baseline data from STEP-BD. *J. Clin. Psychopharmacol.*, **24**, 512–20.

Simon, R. I. (1999). The suicide prevention contract: clinical, legal, and risk management issues. *J. Am. Acad. Psychiatry Law*, **27**, 445–50.

Simpson, G. M., El Sheshai, A., Rady, A., Kingsbury, S. J., and Fayek, M. (2003). Sertraline as monotherapy in the treatment of psychotic and nonpsychotic depression. *J. Clin. Psychiatry*, **64**, 959–65.

Simpson, H. B., Nee, J. C., and Endicott, J. (1997). First-episode major depression. *Arch. Gen. Psychiatry*, **54**, 633–9.

Simpson, S., Baldwin, R. C., Jackson, A., and Burns, H. S. (1998). Is subcortical disease associated with a poor response to antidepressants? Neurological, neuropsychological, and neuroradiological findings in late-life depression. *Psychol. Med.*, **28**, 1015–26.

Simpson, S., Baldwin, R. C., Jackson, A., Burns, A., and Thomas, P. (2000). Is the clinical expression of late-life depression influenced by brain changes? MRI subcortical neuroanatomical correlates of depressive symptoms. *Int. Psychogeriatr.*, **12**, 425–34.

Sinclair, D. and Murray, L. (1998). Effects of postnatal depression on children's adjustment to school: teacher's reports. *Br. J. Psychiatry*, **172**, 58–63.

Sindrup, S. H., Brosen, K., Gram, L. F., *et al.* (1992). The relationship between paroxetine and the sparteine oxidation polymorphism. *Clin. Pharmacol. Ther.*, **51**, 278–87.

Singareddy, R. K. and Balon, R. (2001). Sleep and suicide in psychiatric patients. *Ann. Clin. Psychiatry*, **13**, 93–101.

Siris, S. G., Rifkin, A. E., and Reardon, G. T. (1982). Response of postpsychotic depression to adjunctive imipramine or amitriptyline. *J. Clin. Psychiatry*, **43**, 485–6.

Sitland-Marken, P. A., Wells, B. G., Froemming, J. H., Chu, C.-C., and Brown, C. S. (1990). Psychiatric applications of bromocriptine therapy. *J. Clin. Psychiatry*, **51**, 68–82.

Siuciak, J. A., Lewis, D. R., Wiegand, S. J., and Lindsay, R. M. (1997). Antidepressant-like effect of brain-derived neurotrophic factor (BDNF). *Pharmacol. Biochem. Behav.*, **56**, 131–7.

Skop, B. P. and Brown, T. M. (1996). Potential vascular and bleeding complications of treatment with selective serotonin reuptake inhibitors. *Psychosomatics*, **37**, 12–16.

Slaughter, J. R., Martens, M. P., and Slaughter, K. A. (2001a). Depression and Huntington's disease: prevalence, clinical manifestations, etiology, and treatment. *CNS Spectrums*, **6**, 306–26.

Slaughter, J. R., Slaughter, K. A., Nichols, D., Holmes, S. E., and Martens, M. P. (2001b). Prevalence, clinical manifestations, etiology, and treatment of depression in Parkinson's disease. *J. Neuropsychiatry Clin. Neurosci.*, **13**, 187–96.

Slavney, P. R. (1999). Diagnosing demoralization in consultation psychiatry. *Psychosom.*, **40**, 325–9.

Sleath, B. and Shih, Y. C. (2003). Sociological influences on antidepressant prescribing. *Soc. Sci. Med.*, **56**, 1335–44.

Slimmer, L. M., Lyness, J. M., and Caine, E. D. (2001). Stress, medical illness, and depression. *Semin. Clin. Neuropsychiatry*, **6**, 12–26.

Small, J. G. (1990). Anticonvulsants in affective disorders. *Psychopharmacol. Bull.*, **26**, 25–36.

Small, J. G., Klapper, M. H., Kellams, J. J., *et al.* (1988). Electroconvulsive therapy compared with lithium in the management of manic states. *Arch. Gen. Psychiatry*, **45**, 727–32.

Smith, D., Dempster, C., Glanville, J., Freemantle, N., and Anderson, I. (2002a). The efficacy and tolerability of venlafaxine compared with selective serotonin reuptake inhibitors and other antidepressants: a meta-analysis. *Br. J. Psychiatry*, **180**, 396–404.

Smith, G. S., Reynolds, C. F. III, Houck, P. R., *et al.* (2002b). Glucose metabolic response to total sleep deprivation, recovery sleep, and acute antidepressant treatment as functional neuroanatomic correlates of treatment outcome in geriatric depression. *Am. J. Geriatr. Psychiatry*, **10**, 561–7.

Smith, M. A., Makino, S., Kim, S. Y., and Kvetnansky, R. (1995a). Stress increases brain-derived neurotrophic factor messenger ribonucleic acid in the hypothalamus and pituitary. *Endocrinology*, **136**, 3743–50.

Smith, R., Cubis, J., Brinsmead, M., *et al.* (1990). Mood changes, obstetric experience and alterations in plasma cortisol, beta-endorphin and corticotrophin releasing hormone during pregnancy and the puerperium. *J. Psychosom. Res.*, **34**, 53–69.

Smith, R. N., Studd, J. W., Zamblera, D., and Holland, E. F. (1995b). A randomized comparison over 8 months of 100 micrograms and 200 micrograms twice weekly doses of transdermal oestradiol in the treatment of severe premenstrual syndrome. *Br. J. Obstet. Gynaecol.*, **102**, 475–84.

Snowdon, J. and Baume, P. (2002). A study of suicides of older people in Sydney. *Int. J. Geriatr. Psychiatry*, **17**, 261–9.

Soares, J. C. and Mann, J. J. (1997). The functional neuroanatomy of mood disorders. *J. Psychiatr. Res.*, **31**, 393–432.

Soares, C. N., Almeida, O. P., Joffe, H., and Cohen, L. S. (2001). Efficacy of estradiol for the treatment of depressive disorders in perimenopausal women. A double-blind, randomized, placebo-controlled trial. *Arch. Gen. Psychiatry*, **58**, 529–34.

Sobczak, S., Honig, A., van Duinen, M. A., and Riedel, W. J. (2002). Serotonergic dysregulation in bipolar disorders: a literature review of serotonergic challenge studies. *Bipolar Disord.*, **4**, 347–56.

Sofuoglu, M., Dudish-Poulsen, S., Brown, S,. B., and Hatsukami, D. K. (2003). Association of cocaine withdrawal symptoms with more severe dependence and enhanced subjective response to cocaine. *Drug Alcohol Depend.*, **69**, 273–82.

Sokolski, K. N., Chicz-Demet, A., and Demet, E. M. (2004). Selective serotonin reuptake inhibitor-related extrapyramidal symptoms in autistic children: a case series. *J. Child Adolesc. Psychopharmacol.*, **14**, 143–7.

Solai, L. K., Pollock, B. G., Mulsant, B. H., *et al.* (2002). Effect of nortriptyline and paroxetine on CYP2D6 activity in depressed elderly patients. *J. Clin. Psychopharmacol.*, **22**, 481–6.

Solomon, A., Haaga, D. A. F., and Arnow, B. A. (2001). Is clinical depression distinct from subthreshold depressive symptoms? A review of the continuity issue in depression research. *J. Nerv. Ment. Dis.*, **180**, 498–506.

Solomon, D. A., Keller, M. B., Leon, A. C., *et al.* (2000). Multiple recurrences of major depressive disorder. *Am. J. Psychiatry*, **157**, 229–33.

Somnath, C. P., Janardhan Reddy, Y. C., and Jain, S. (2002). Is there a familial overlap between schizophrenia and bipolar disorder? *J. Affect. Disord.*, **72**, 243–7.

Sotsky, S. M. and Simmens, S. J. (1999). Pharmacotherapy response and diagnostic validity in atypical depression. *J. Affect. Disord.*, **54**, 237–47.

Souetre, E., Pringuey, D., Salvati, E., Robert, P., and Darcourt, G. (1985). Circadian rhythms of the central temperature and blood cortisol in endogenous depression. *Encephale*, **11**, 185–98.

Soultanian, C., Perisse, D., Revah-Levy, A., *et al.* (2005). Cotard's syndrome in adolescents and young adults: a possible onset of bipolar disorder requiring a mood stabilizer. *J. Child. Adolesc. Psychopharmacol.*, **15**, 706–11.

Spalletta, G. and Caltagirone, G. (2003). Sertraline treatment of post-stroke major depression: an open study in patients with moderate to severe symptoms. *Funct. Neurol.*, **18**, 227–32.

Spiker, D. G., Stein, J., and Rich, C. L. (1985). Delusional depression and electroconvulsive therapy: one year later. *Convuls. Ther.*, **1**, 167–72.

Spiker, D. G., Perel, J. M., Hanin, I., *et al.* (1986). The pharmacological treatment of delusional depression: part II. *J. Clin. Psychopharmacol.*, **6**, 339–42.

Spinelli, M. (ed). (2003). *Infanticide: Psychosocial and Legal Perspectives on Mothers Who Kill.* Washington, DC: American Psychiatric Press.

Spinelli, M. G. (1997). Interpersonal psychotherapy for depressed antepartum women: a pilot study. *Am. J. Psychiatry*, **154**, 1028–30.

Spinelli, M. G. (2004). Maternal infanticide associated with mental illness: prevention and the promise of saved lives. *Am. J. Psychiatry*, **161**, 1548–57.

Spinelli, M. G. and Endicott, J. (2003). Controlled clinical trial of interpersonal psychotherapy versus parenting education program for depressed pregnant women. *Am. J. Psychiatry*, **160**, 555–62.

Spitzer, R. L. and Fleiss, J. L. (1974). A re-analysis of the reliability of psychiatric diagnosis. *Br. J. Psychiatry*, **125**, 341–7.

Spitzer, R. L. and Klein, D. F. (eds) (1968). *Critical Issues in Psychiatric Diagnosis*. New York: Raven Press.

Spitzer, R. L. and Williams, J. B. (1982). Hysteroid dysphoria: an unsuccessful attempt to demonstrate its syndromal validity. *Am. J. Psychiatry*, **139**, 1286–91.

Spitzer, R. L., Endicott, J., and Robins, E. (1975). Research diagnostic criteria (RDC). *Psychopharm. Bull.*, **11**, 22–4.

Spitzer, R. L., Endicott, J., and Robins, E. (1978). Research diagnostic criteria: rationale and reliability. *Arch. Gen. Psychiatry*, **35**, 773–82.

Spitzer, R. L., First, M. B., Gibbons, M., and Williams, J. B. W. (2004). *Treatment Companion to the DSM-IV-TR Casebook*. Washington, DC: American Psychiatric Press, p. 112.

Sporn, J. and Sachs, G. (1997). The anticonvulsant lamotrigine in treatment-resistant manic-depressive illness. *J. Clin. Psychopharmacol.*, **17**, 185–9.

Spreux-Varoquaux, O., Alvarez, J. C., Berlin, I., *et al.* (2001). Differential abnormalities in plasma 5-HIAA and platelet serotonin concentrations in violent suicide attempters: relationships with impulsivity and depression. *Life Sci.*, **69**, 647–57.

Squitieri, F., Cannella, M., Piorcellini, A., *et al.* (2001). Short-term effects of olanzapine in Huntington disease. *Neuropsychiatry Neuropsychol. Behav. Neurol.*, **14**, 69–72.

Srisurapanont, M., Yatham, L. N., and Zis, A. P. (1995). Treatment of acute bipolar depression: a review of the literature. *Can. J. Psychiatry*, **40**, 533–44.

Staab, J. P. and Evans, D. L. (2000). Efficacy of venlafaxine in geriatric depression. *Depress. Anxiety*, **12** (suppl. 1), 63–8.

Stage, K. B., Bech, P., Gram, L. F., *et al.* (1998). Are in-patient depressives more often of the melancholic subtype? Danish University Antidepressant Group. *Acta Psychiatr. Scand.*, **98**, 432–6.

Stahl, S. M. (1998). Mechanism of action of selective serotonin reuptake inhibitors. Serotonin receptors and pathways mediate therapeutic effects and side effects. *J. Affect. Disord.*, **51**, 215–35.

(2000). *Essential Psychopharmacology: Neuroscientific Basis and Practical Applications, 2nd* edn. Cambridge, UK: Cambridge University Press.

Stahl, S. M., Entsuah, R., and Rudolph, R. L. (2002). Comparative efficacy between venlafaxine and SSRIs: a pooled analysis of patients with depression. *Biol. Psychiatry*, **52**, 1166–74.

Stampfer, H. G. (1998). The relationship between psychiatric illness and the circadian pattern of heart rate. *Aust. NZ J. Psychiatry*, **32**, 187–98.

Staner, L., Linkowski, P., and Mendlewicz, J. (1994). Biological markers as classifiers for depression: a multivariate study. *Prog. Neuropsychopharmacol. Biol. Psychiatry*, **18**, 899–914.

Staner, L., Duval, F., Calvi-Gries, F., *et al.* (2001). Morning and evening TSH response to TRH and sleep EEG disturbances in major depressive disorder. *Prog. Neuropsychopharmacol. Biol. Psychiatry*, **25**, 535–47.

Staner, L., Duval, F., Haba, J., Mokrani, M. C., and Macher, J. P. (2003). Disturbances in hypothalamo-pituitary-adrenal and thyroid axis identify different sleep EEG patterns in major depressed patients. *J. Psychiatr. Res.*, **37**, 1–8.

Starkstein, S. E. and Manes, F. (2000). Apathy and depression following stroke. *CNS Spectrums*, **5**, 43–50.

Starkstein, S. E., Robinson, R. G., and Price, T. R. (1987). Comparison of cortical and subcortical lesions in the production of post-stroke mood disorders. *Brain*, **110**, 1045–59.

Starkstein, S. E., Robinson, R. G., Berthier, M. L., Parikh, R. M., and Price, T. R. (1988). Differential mood changes following basal ganglia versus thalamic lesions. *Arch. Neurol.*, **45**, 725–30.

Statham, D. J., Heath, A. C., Madden, P. A., *et al.* (1998). Suicidal behaviour: an epidemiological and genetic study. *Psychol. Med.*, **28**, 839–55.

Stefanis, N. C., Delespaul, P., Henquet, C., *et al.* (2004). Early adolescent cannabis exposure and positive and negative dimensions of psychosis. *Addiction*, **99**, 1333–41.

Steffens, D. C., Bosworth, H. B., Provenzale, J. M., and MacFall, J. R. (2002). Subcortical white matter lesions and functional impairment in geriatric depression. *Depress. Anxiety*, **15**, 23–8.

Steffens, D. C., Norton, M. C., Hart, A. D., *et al.* (2003). Apolipoprotein E genotype and major depression in a community of older adults. The Cache County Study. *Psychol. Med.*, **33**, 541–7.

Stefos, G., Staner, L., Kerkhofs, M., *et al.* (1998). Shortened REM latency as a psychobiological marker for psychotic depression? An age-, gender-, and polarity-controlled study. *Biol. Psychiatry*, **44**, 1314–20.

Steimer, W., Zopf, K., von Amelunxen, S., *et al.* (2004). Amitriptyline or not, that is the question: Pharmacogenetic testing of CYP2D6 and CYP2C19 identifies patients with low and high risk for side effects in amitriptyline therapy. *Clin. Chem.*, **51**, 375–85.

Stein, D., Kurtsman, L., Stier, S., *et al.* (2004). Electroconvulsive therapy in adolescent and adult psychiatric inpatients – a retrospective chart design. *J. Affect. Disord.*, **82**, 335–42.

Stein, G. (1982). The maternity blues. In vol. 5. Brockington, I. F. and Kumar, R. (eds) *Motherhood and Mental Illness*, London: Academic Press, pp. 119–54.

Stein, G. (1992). Drug treatment of the personality disorders. *Br. J. Psychiatry*, **161**, 167–84.

Steiner, M. and Born, L. (2000). Diagnosis and treatment of premenstrual dysphoric disorder: an update. *Int. Clin. Psychopharmacol.*, **15** (suppl. 3), S5–17.

Steiner, M. and Pearlstein, T. (2000). Premenstrual dysphoria and the serotonin system: pathophysiology and treatment. *J. Clin. Psychiatry*, **61** (suppl. 12), 17–21.

Steiner, M. and Tam, W. Y. K. (1999). Postpartum depression in relation to other psychiatric disorders. In Miller, L. J. (ed.) *Postpartum Mood Disorders*. Washington, DC: American Psychiatric Press, pp. 47–63.

Stern, W. C., Harto-Truax, N., and Bauer, N. (1983). Efficacy of bupropion in tricyclic-resistant or intolerant patients. *J. Clin. Psychiatry*, **44**, 148–52.

Sternbach, H. (1988). Age-associated testosterone decline in men: clinical issues for psychiatry. *Am. J. Psychiatry*, **155**, 1310–18.

Stewart, J. W., Quitkin, F. M., Terman, M., and Terman, J. S. (1990). Is seasonal affective disorder a variant of atypical depression? Differential response to light therapy. *Psychiatry Res.*, **33**, 121–8.

Stewart, J. W., McGrath, P. J., Rabkin, J. G., and Quitkin, F. M. (1993). Atypical depression. A valid clinical entity? *Psychiatr. Clin. North Am.*, **16**, 479–95.

Stewart, J. W., Tricamo, E., McGrath, P., and Quitkin, F. M. (1997). Prophylactic efficacy of phenelzine and imipramine in chronic atypical depression: likelihood of recurrence on discontinuation after 6 months' remission. *Am. J. Psychiatry*, **154**, 31–6.

Stewart, R., Prince, M., Mann, A., Richards, M., and Brayne, C. (2001). Stroke, vascular risk factors and depression. Cross-sectional study in a UK Caribbean-born population. *Br. J. Psychiatry*, **178**, 23–8.

Stillinger, J. (ed.) (1978/1982). *John Keats, Complete Poems*. Cambridge, MA: Belknap Press of Harvard University Press, pp. 283–4.

Stimpson, N., Agrawal, N., and Lewis, G. (2002). Randomised controlled trials investigating pharmacological and psychological interventions for treatment-refractory depression. *Br. J. Psychiatry*, **181**, 284–94.

Stockmeier, C. A. (1997). Neurobiology of serotonin in depression and suicide. *Ann. NY Acad. Sci.*, **836**, 220–32.

Stoll, A. L., Severus, W. E., Freeman, M. P., *et al.* (1999). Omega 3 fatty acids in bipolar disorder. A preliminary double-blind, placebo-controlled trial. *Arch. Gen. Psychiatry*, **56**, 407–12.

Stone, E. A. and Platt, J. E. (1982). Brain adrenergic receptors and resistance to stress. *Brain Res.*, **237**, 405–14.

Stone-Harris, R. (2000). Avoiding the legal pitfalls in mental health commitments. *Tex. Med.*, **96**, 56–63.

Stout, S. C., Owens, M. J., and Nemeroff, C. B. (2002). Regulation of corticotropin-releasing factor neuronal systems and hypothalamic–pituitary–adrenal axis activity by stress and chronic antidepressant treatment. *Pharmacol.*, **300**, 1085–92.

Strain, J. J., Smith, G. C., Hammer, J. S. *et al.* (1998). Adjustment disorder: a multisite study of its utilization and interventions in the consultation-liaison psychiatry setting. *Gen. Hosp. Psychiatry*, **20**, 139–49.

Strakowski, S. M., DelBello, M. P., Adler, C., Cecil, K. M., and Sax, K. W. (2000a). Neuroimaging in bipolar disorder. *Bipolar Disord.*, **2**, 148–64.

Strakowski, S. M., McElroy, S. L., and Keck, P. E, (2000b). Clinical efficacy of valproate in bipolar illness: comparisons and contrasts with lithium. In Halbreich, U. and Montgomery, S. A. (eds) *Pharmacotherapy for Mood, Anxiety, and Cognitive Disorders*. Washington, DC: American Psychiatric Press, pp. 143–57.

Strauss, H., Ostow, M., and Greenstein, L. (1952). *Diagnostic Electroencephalography*. New York: Grune & Stratton.

Strik, J. J., Honig, A., Lousberg, R., *et al.* (2000). Efficacy and safety of fluoxetine in the treatment of patients with major depression after first myocardial infarction: findings from a double-blind, placebo-controlled trial. *Psychosom. Med.*, **62**, 783–9.

Strik, J. J., Honig, A., Lousberg, R., *et al.* (2001). Clinical correlates of depression following myocardial infarction. *Int. J. Psychiatry Med.*, **31**, 255–64.

Strober, M., Lampert, C., Schmidt, S., and Morrell, W. (1993). The course of major depressive disorder in adolescents: I. Recovery and risk of manic switching in a follow-up of psychotic and nonpsychotic subtypes. *J. Am. Acad. Child Adolesc. Psychiatry*, **32**, 34–42.

Strober, M., Rao, U., DeAntonio, M., *et al.* (1998). Effects of ECT in adolescents with severe endogenous depression resistant to pharmacotherapy. *Biol. Psychiatry*, **43**, 335–8.

Strömgren, L. S. (1997). ECT in acute delirium and related clinical states. *Convuls. Ther.*, **13**, 10–17.

Styra, R., Joffe, R., and Singer, W. (1991). Hyperthyroxinemia in major affective disorders. *Acta Psychiatr. Scand.*, **83**, 61–3.

Styron, W. (1990). *Darkness Visible: A Memoir of Madness.* New York: Random House.

Sullivan, P. F., Kessler, R. C., and Kendler, K. S. (1998). Latent class analysis of lifetime depressive symptoms in the national comorbidity survey. *Am. J. Psychiatry*, **155**, 1398–406.

Sullivan, P. F., Neale, M. C., and Kendler, K. S. (2000). Genetic epidemiology of major depression: review and meta-analysis. *Am. J. Psychiatry*, **157**, 1552–62.

Sullivan, P. F., Prescott, C. A., and Kendler, K. S. (2002). The subtypes of major depression in a twin registry. *J. Affect. Disord.*, **68**, 273–84.

Sulser, F. (2002). The role of CREB and other transcription factors in the pharmacotherapy and etiology of depression. *Ann. Med.*, **34**, 348–56.

Sunderland, T., Cohen, R. M., Molchan, S., *et al.* (1994). High-dose selegiline in treatment-resistant older depressive patients. *Arch. Gen. Psychiatry*, **51**, 607–15.

Suominen, K., Isometsa, E., Heila, H., Lonnqvist, J., and Henriksson, M. (2002). General hospital suicides–a psychological study in Finland. *Gen. Hosp. Psychiatry*, **24**, 412–16.

Suominen, K. H., Isometsa, E. T., Henriksson, M. M., *et al.* (1998). Inadequate treatment for major depression both before and after attempted suicide. *Am. J. Psychiatry*, **155**, 1778–80.

Suri, R., Stowe, Z. N., Hendrick, V., *et al.* (2002). Estimates of nursing infant daily dose of fluoxetine through breast milk. *Biol. Psychiatry*, **52**, 446–51.

Sutor, B., Rummans, T. A., Jowsey, S. G., *et al.* (1998). Major depression in medically ill patients. *Mayo Clin. Proc.*, **73**, 329–37.

Suzuki, K., Awata, S., and Matsuoka, H. (2003). Short-term effect of ECT in middle-aged and elderly patients with intractable catatonic schizophrenia. *J. ECT*, **19**, 73–80.

Svanborg, P. and Asberg, M. (2001). A comparison between the Beck Depression Inventory (BDI) and the self-rating version of the Montgomery-Asberg Depression Rating Scale (MADRS). *J. Affect. Disord.*, **64**, 203–16.

Swann, A. C., Stokes, P. E., Caspar, R., *et al.* (1992). Hypothalamic–pituitary–adrenocortical function in mixed and pure mania. *Acta Psychiatr. Scand.*, **85**, 270–4.

Swann, A. C., Bowden, C. L., Morris, D., *et al.* (1997). Depression during mania. Treatment response to lithium or divalproex. *Arch. Gen. Psychiatry*, **54**, 37–42.

Swartz, C. M. (1984). The time course of post-ECT prolactin levels after bilateral and unilateral ECT. *Br. J. Psychiatry*, **144**, 643–5.

(1985). The time course of post-ECT prolactin levels. *Convuls. Ther.*, **1**, 81–8.

(1992). Electroconvulsive therapy-induced cortisol release after dexamethasone in depression. *Neuropsychobiology*, **25**, 130–3.

(2000). Physiological response to ECT stimulus dose. *Psychiatr. Res.*, **97**, 229–35.

Swartz, C. M. and Abrams, R. (1984). Prolactin levels after bilateral and unilateral ECT. *Br. J. Psychiatry*, **144**, 643–5.

Swartz, C. M. and Chen, J. J. (1985). Electroconvulsive therapy-induced cortisol release: Changes in depressive state. *Convuls. Ther.*, **1**, 15–21.

Swartz, C. M. and Guadagno, G. (1998). Melancholia with onset during treatment with SSRIs. *Ann. Clin. Psychiatry*, **10**, 177–9.

Swartz, C. M. and Larson, G. (1989). ECT stimulus duration and its efficacy. *Ann. Clin. Psychiatry*, **1**, 147–52.

Swartz, C. M. and Mehta, R. (1986). Double electroconvulsive therapy for resistant depression. *Convuls. Ther.*, **2**, 55–7.

Swift, R. M. (2000). Opioid antagonists and alcoholism treatment. *CNS Spectrums*, **5**, 49–57.

Szanto, K., Mulsant, B. H., Houck, P. R., *et al.* (2001). Treatment outcome in suicidal vs. non-suicidal elderly patients. *Am. J. Geriatr. Psychiatry*, **9**, 261–8.

Szegedi, A., Kohnen, R., Dienel, A., and Kieser, M. (2005). Acute treatment of moderate to severe depression with hypericum extract WS 5570 (St John's wort): randomized controlled double blind non-inferiority trial versus paroxetine. *Br. Med. J.*, **330**, 503.

Szuba, M. P., Guze, B. H., and Baxter, L. R. Jr. (1997). Electroconvulsive therapy increases circadian amplitude and lowers core body temperature in depressed subjects. *Biol. Psychiatry*, **42**, 1130–7.

Szuba, M. P., Fernando, A. T., and Groh-Szuba, G. (2001). Sleep abnormalities in treatment-resistant mood disorders. In Amsterdam, J. D., Hornig, M., and Nierenberg, A. A. (eds) *Treatment-Resistant Mood Disorders.* Cambridge, UK: Cambridge University Press, pp. 96–110.

Szymanska, A., Rabe-Jablonska, J., and Karasek, M.. (2001). Diurnal profile of melatonin concentrations in patients with major depression: relationship to the clinical manifestation and antidepressant treatment. *Neuro. Endocrinol. Lett.*, **22**, 192–8.

Tabbane, K., Charfi, F., Dellabi, L., Guizani, L., and Boukadida, L. (1999). [Acute postpartum psychoses.] *Encephale*, **25** (spec. no. 3), 12–17.

TADS. (2005). The Treatment for Adolescents with Depression Study (TADS) (2000). demographic and clinical characteristics. *J. Am. Acad. Child Adolesc. Psychiatry*, 44, 28–40.

Taieb, O., Flament, M., Chevret, S., *et al.* (2002). Clinical relevance of electroconvulsive therapy (ECT) in adolescents with severe mood disorder: evidence from a follow-up study. *Eur. Psychiatry*, **17**, 206–12.

Takeshita, J., Masaki, K., Ahmed, I., *et al.* (2002). Are depressive symptoms a risk factor for mortality in Elderly Japanese American men? The Honolulu–Asia aging study. *Am. J. Psychiatry*, **159**, 1127–32.

Tam, E. M., Lam, R. W., Robertson, H. A., *et al.* (1997). Atypical depressive symptoms in seasonal and nonseasonal mood disorders. *J. Affect. Disord.*, **44**, 39–44.

Tamminga, C. A., Nemeroff, C. B., Blakely, R. D., *et al.* (2002). Developing novel treatments for mood disorders: accelerating discovery. *Biol. Psychiatry*, **52**, 539–609.

Tancer, M. E. and Evans, D. L. (1989). Electroconvulsive therapy in geriatric patients undergoing anticoagulant therapy. *Convuls. Ther.*, **5**, 102–9.

Tandon, R., Mazzara, C., DeQuardo, J., *et al.* (1991). Dexamethasone suppression test in schizophrenia: relationship to symptomatology, ventricular enlargement, and outcome. *Biol. Psychiatry*, **29**, 953–64.

Tandon, R., Lewis, C., Taylor, S. F., *et al.* (1996). Relationship between DST nonsuppression and shortened REM latency in schizophrenia. *Biol. Psychiatry*, **40**, 660–3.

Tannenbaum, B. and Anisman, H. (2003). Impact of chronic intermittent challenges in stressor-susceptible and resilient strains of mice. *Biol. Psychiatry*, **53**, 292–303.

Tanney, B. L. (1986). Electroconvulsive therapy and suicide. *Suicide Life Threat. Behav.*, **16**, 116–40.

Tantam, D. (1988). Asperger's syndrome. *J. Child Psychol. Psychiatry*, **29**, 245–53.

Targum, S. D., Rosen, L., and Capodanno, A. E. (1983). The dexamethasone suppression test in suicidal patients with unipolar depression. *Am. J. Psychiatry*, **140**, 877–9.

Taylor, C. B., Young-Blood, M. E., Cateuier, D., *et al.* (2005). Effects of antidepressant medication on morbidity and mortality in depressed patients after myocardial infarction. *Arch. Gen. Psychiatry*, **62**, 792–8.

Taylor, M. A. (1984). Schizo-affective and allied disorders. In Post, R. M. and Ballenger, J. C. (eds) *The Neurobiology of Manic-Depressive Illness.* Baltimore, MD: Williams and Wilkins, pp. 136–56.

(1986). The validity of schizo-affective disorders. Treatment and prevention studies. In Maneros, A. and Tsuang, M. T. (eds) *Schizo-Affective Psychoses.* Berlin/Heidelberg: Springer Verlag, 94–113.

Taylor, M. A. (1992). Are schizophrenia and affective disorder related? A selective literature review. *Am. J. Psychiatry*, **149**, 22–32.

(1999). *The Fundamentals of Clinical Neuropsychiatry.* New York: Oxford University Press.

Taylor, M. A. and Abrams, R. (1973). The phenomenology of mania: a new look at some old patients. *Arch. Gen. Psychiatry*, **29**, 520–2.

(1980). Reassessing the bipolar–unipolar dichotomy. *J. Affect. Disord.*, **2**, 195–217.

Taylor, M. A. and Fink, M. (2003). Catatonia in psychiatric classification: a home of its own. *Am. J. Psychiatry*, **160**, 1233–41.

Taylor M. A., Abrams R., and Hayman M. (1980). The classification of affective disorder: A reassessment of the bipolar-unipolar dichotomy; Part 1: A clinical, laboratory and family study. *J. Affective Disord.*, **2**, 95–109.

Taylor, W. D. and Doraiswamy, P. M. (2004). A systematic review of antidepressant placebo-controlled trials for geriatric depression: limitations of current data and directions for the future. *Neuropsychopharmacology*, **29**, 2285–99.

Tedlow, J., Smith, M., Neault, N., *et al.* (2002). Melancholia and axis II comorbidity. *Compr. Psychiatry*, **43**, 331–5.

Teicher, M. H., Glod, C. A., Harper, D., *et al.* (1993). Locomotor activity in depressed children and adolescents: I. Circadian dysregulation. *J. Am. Acad. Child Adolesc. Psychiatry*, **32**, 760–9.

Teicher, M. H., Glod, C. A., Magnus, E., *et al.* (1997). Circadian rest–activity disturbances in seasonal affective disorder. *Arch. Gen. Psychiatry*, **54**, 124–30.

Terman, M., Terman, J. S., and Ross, D. C. (1998). A controlled trial of timed bright light and negative air ionization for treatment of winter depression. *Arch. Gen. Psychiatry*, **55**, 875–82.

Teufel-Mayer, R. and Gleitz, J. (1997). Effects of long-term administration of hypericum extracts on the affinity and density of the central serotonergic 5-HT1 A and 5-HT2 A receptors. *Pharmacopsychiatry*, **30** (suppl. 2), 113–16.

Thase, M. E. (1998). Effects of venlafaxine on blood pressure: a meta-analysis of original data from 3744 depressed patients. *J. Clin. Psychiatry*, **59**, 502–8.

(2002). What role do atypical antipsychotic drugs have in treatment resistant depression? *J. Clin. Psychiatry*, **63**, 95–103.

(2003). Effectiveness of antidepressants: comparative remission rates. *J. Clin. Psychiatry*, **64** (suppl. 2), 3–7.

Thase, M. E., Kupfer, D. J., and Ulrich, R. F. (1986). Electroencephalographic sleep in psychotic depression. A valid subtype? *Arch. Gen. Psychiatry*, **43**, 886–93

Thase, M. E., Carpenter, L., Kupfer, D. J., and Frank, E. (1991a). Clinical significance of reversed vegetative subtypes of recurrent major depression. *Psychopharmacol. Bull.*, **27**, 17–22.

Thase, M. E., Simons, A. D., Cahalane, J., McGeary, J., and Harden, T. (1991b). Severity of depression and response to cognitive behavior therapy. *Am. J. Psychiatry*, **148**, 784–9.

Thase, M. E., Greenhouse, J. B., Frank, E., *et al.* (1997b). Treatment of major depression with psychotherapy or psychotherapy–pharmacotherapy combinations. *Arch. Gen. Psychiatry*, **54**, 1009–15.

Thase, M. E., Kupfer, D. J., Fasiczka, A. J., *et al.* (1997c). Identifying an abnormal electroencephalographic sleep profile to characterize major depressive disorder. *Biol. Psychiatry*, **41**, 964–73.

Thase, M. E. and Sachs, G. S. (2000). Bipolar depression: pharmacotherapy and related therapeutic strategies. *Biol. Psychiatry*, **48**, 558–72.

Thase, M. E., Entsuah, A. R., and Rudolph, R. L. (2001a). Remission rates during treatment with venlafaxine or selective serotonin reuptake inhibitors. *Br. J. Psychiatry*, **178**, 234–41.

Thase, M. E., Nierenberg, A. A., Keller, M. B., *et al.* (2001b). Efficacy of mirtazapine for prevention of depressive relapse: a placebo-controlled double-blind trial of recently remitted high-risk patients. *J. Clin. Psychiatry*, **62**, 782–8.

Thase, M. E., Rush, A. J., Howland, R. H., *et al.* (2002). Double-blind switch study of imipramine or sertraline treatment of antidepressant-resistant chronic depression. *Arch. Gen. Psychiatry*, **59**, 233–9.

Thase, M. E., Haught, B. R., Richard, N., *et al.* (2005). Remission rates following antidepressant therapy with bupropion or selective reuptake inhibitors: a meta-analysis of original data from 7 nonrandomized controlled trails. *J. Clin. Psychiatry*, **66**, 974–81.

Thies-Flechtner, K., Muller-Oerlinghausen, B., Seibert, W., Walther, A., and Greil, W. (1996). Effect of prophylactic treatment on suicide risk in patients with major affective disorders: data from a randomized prospective trial. *Pharmacopsychiatry*, **29**, 103–7.

Thoenen, H. (1995). Neurotrophins and neuronal plasticity. *Science*, **270**, 593–8.

Thomas, A. J., Ferrier, I. N., Kalaria, R. N., *et al.* (2001). A neuropathological study of vascular factors in late-life depression. *J. Neurol. Neurosurg. Psychiatry*, **70**, 83–7.

Thomas, A. J., Perry, R., Kalaria, R. N., *et al.* (2003). Neuropathological evidence for ischemia in the white matter of the dorsolateral prefrontal cortex in late-life depression. *Int. J. Geriatr. Psychiatry*, **18**, 7–13.

Thomas, A. M. and Forehand, R. (1991). The relationship between paternal depressive mood and early adolescent functioning. *J. Fam. Psychol.*, **4**, 260–71.

Thompson, C., Roden, L., and Birtwhistle, J. (1999). Light therapy for seasonal and nonseasonal affective disorder: a Cochrane meta-analysis. *Soc. Light Treat. Biolo. Rhythms* (abstracts), **11**, 11.

Thompson, J. K. (1985). Right brain, left brain; left face, right face: hemisphericity and the expression of facial emotion. *Cortex*, **21**, 281–99.

Thorsteinsson, H. S., Gillin, J. C., Patten, C. A., *et al.* (2001). The effects of transdermal nicotine therapy for smoking cessation on depressive symptoms in patients with major depression. *Neuropsychopharmacol.*, **24**, 350–8.

Thurber, S., Snow, M., and Honts, C. R. (2002). The Zung Self-Rating Depression Scale: convergent validity and diagnostic discrimination. *Assessment*, **9**, 401–5.

Tillotson, K. J. and Sulzbach, W. (1944). A comparative study and evaluation of electric shock therapy in depressive states. *Am. J. Psychiatry*, **101**, 455–9.

Timbremont, B., Braet, C., and Dreessen, L. (2004). Assessing depression in youth: relation between the Children's Depression Inventory and a structured interview. *J. Clin. Child Adolesc. Psychol.*, **33**, 149–57.

Todd, R., Geller, B., Neuman, R., Fox, L. W., and Hickok, J. (1996). Increased prevalence of alcoholism in relatives of depressed and bipolar children. *J. Am. Acad. Child Adolesc. Psychiatry*, **35**, 716–24.

Todd, R. D., Neuman, R., Geller, B., Fox, L. W., and Hickok, J. (1993). Genetic studies of affective disorders: should we be starting with childhood onset probands? *J. Am. Acad. Child Adolesc. Psychiatry*, **32**, 1164–71.

Tohen, M., Vieta, E., Calabrese, J., *et al.* (2003). Efficacy of olanzapine and olanzapine–fluoxetine combination in the treatment of bipolar I depression. *Arch. Gen. Psychiatry*, **60**, 1079–88.

Tohen, M., Chengappa, K. N. R., Suppes, T., *et al.* (2004). Relapse prevention in bipolar I disorder: 18-month comparison of olanzapine plus mood stabilizer v. mood stabilizer alone. *Br. J. Psychiatry*, **184**, 337–45.

Tokuyama, M., Nakao, K., Seto, M., Watanabe, A., and Takeda, M. (2003). Predictors of first-onset major depressive episodes among white-collar workers. *Psychiatry Clin. Neurosci.*, **57**, 523–31.

Tollefson, G. D. (1993). Adverse drug reactions/interactions in maintenance therapy. *J. Clin. Psychiatry*, **54** (suppl. 8), 48–58.

Tollefson, G. D., Greist, J. H., Jefferson, J. W., *et al.* (1994a). Is baseline agitation a relative contraindication for a selective serotonin reuptake inhibitor: a comparative trial of fluoxetine versus imipramine. *J. Clin. Psychopharmacol.*, **14**, 385–91.

Tollefson, G. D., Rampey, A. H. Jr., Beasley, C. M. Jr., Enas, C. G., and Potvin, J. H. (1994b). Absence of a relationship between adverse events and suicidality during pharmacotherapy for depression. *J. Clin. Psychopharmacol.*, **14**, 163–9.

Tollefson, G. D. and Rosenbaum, J. F. (1998). Selective serotonin reuptake inhibitors. In Schatzberg, A. F. and Nemeroff, C. B. (eds) *The American Psychiatric Press Textbook of Psychopharmacology.* Washington, DC: APA Press, pp. 219–38.

Tombaugh, T. N. and McIntyre, N. J. (1992). The Mini-Mental State Examination: a comprehensive review. *J. Am. Geriatr. Soc.*, **40**, 922–35.

Tondo, L. and Baldessarini, R. J. (2000). Reduced suicide risk during lithium maintenance treatment. *J. Clin. Psychiatry*, **61**, 97–104.

Tondo, L., Baldessarini, R. J., Hennen, J., *et al.* (1998). Lithium treatment and risk of suicidal behavior in bipolar disorder patients. *J. Clin. Psychiatry*, **59**, 405–14.

Tondo, L., Hennen, J., and Baldessarini, R. J. (2001). Lower suicide risk with long-term lithium treatment in major effective illness: a meta-analysis. *Acta Psychiatr. Scand.*, **104**, 163–72.

Tonstad, S. (2002). Use of sustained-release bupropion in specific patient populations for smoking cessation. *Drugs*, **62** (suppl. 2), 37–43.

Torgersen, S. (1986). Genetic factors in moderately severe and mild affective disorders. *Arch. Gen. Psychiatry*, **43**, 222.

Tranter, R., O'Donovan, C., Chandarana, P., and Kennedy, S. (2002). Prevalence and outcome of partial remission in depression. *J. Psychiatry Neurosci.*, **27**, 241–7.

Trimble, M. (1978). Serum prolactin in epilepsy and hysteria. *Br. Med. J.*, **2**, 1682.

Trimble, M. (2004). *Somatoform Disorders: A Medicolegal Guide.* Cambridge, UK: Cambridge University Press.

Trivedi, M. H. (2003). Treatment-resistant depression: new therapies on the horizon. *Ann. Clin. Psychiatry*, **15**, 59–70.

Troller, J. N. and Sachdev, P. S. (1999). Electroconvulsive treatment of neuroleptic malignant syndrome: a review and report of cases. *Aust. NZ J. Psychiatry*, **33**, 650–9.

Tse, W. S. and Bond, A. J. (2001). Serotonergic involvement in the psychosocial dimension of personality. *J. Psychopharmacol.*, **15**, 195–8.

Tsoh, J. Y., Humfleet, G. L., Munoz, R. F., *et al*, (2000). Development of major depression after treatment for smoking cessation. *Am. J. Psychiatry*, **157**, 368–74.

Tsuang, M. T. and Faraone, S. V. (1990). *The Genetics of Mood Disorders.* Baltimore, MD: Johns Hopkins University Press.

Tsuang, M. T., Faraone, S. V., and Fleming, J. A. (1985). Familial transmission of major affective disorders: is there evidence supporting the distinction between unipolar and bipolar disorders? *Br. J. Psychiatry*, **146**, 268.

Tsuang, M. T., Faraone, S. V., and Green, R. R. (1994). Genetic epidemiology of mood disorders. In Papolos, D. F. and Lachman, H. M. (eds) *Genetic Studies in Affective Disorders.* New York: Wiley, pp. 3–27.

Tsuang, M. T., Bar, J. L., Harley, R. M., and Lyons, M. J. (2001). The Harvard Twin Study of Substance Abuse: What we have learned. *Harv. Rev. Psychiatry*, **9**, 267–79.

Tupler, L. A., Krishnan, K. R. R., McDonald, W. M., *et al.* (2002). Anatomic location and laterality of MRI signal hyperintensities in late-life depression. *J. Psychosom. Res.*, **53**, 665–76.

Turecki, G. (2001). Suicidal behavior: is there a genetic predisposition? *Bipolar Disord.*, **3**, 335–49.

Tylee, A., Gastpar, M., Lepine, J. P., and Mendlewicz, J. (1999). Identification of depressed patient types in the community and their treatment needs: findings from the DEPRES II (Depression Research in European Society II) survey. DEPRES Steering Committee. *Int. Clin. Psychopharmacol.*, **14**, 153–65.

Uebelhack, R., Gruenwald, J., Graubaum, H. J., and Busch, R. (2004). Efficacy and tolerability of hypericum extract STW 3-VI in patients with moderate depression: a double-blind, randomized, placebo-controlled clinical trial. *Adv. Ther.*, **21**, 265–75.

Uhlenhuth, E. H., Balter, M. B., Ban, T. A., and Yang, K. (1999). International study of expert judgment on therapeutic use of benzodiazepines and other psychotherapeutic medications: IV. Therapeutic dose dependence and abuse liability of benzodiazepines in the long-term treatment of anxiety disorders. *J. Clin. Psychopharm.*, **19** (suppl. 2), 23S–29S.

UK ECT Review Group, Geddes, J. (2003). Efficacy and safety of electroconvulsive therapy in depressive disorders: systematic review and meta-analysis. *Lancet*, 361, 799–808.

Uncapher, H. and Arean, P. A. (2000). Physicians are less willing to treat suicidal ideation in older patients. *J. Am. Geriatr. Soc.*, **48**, 188–92.

Unden, F. and Aperia, B. (1994). Major affective disorders – prospective clinical course during a 5-year to 7-year follow-up in relation to neuroendocrine function tests. *Nord. Jrl Psychiatry*, **48**, 131–7.

Unutzer, J. (2002). Diagnosis and treatment of older adults with depression in primary care. *Biol. Psychiatry*, **52**, 285–92.

Urcelay-Zaldua, I., Hansenne, M., and Ansseau, M. (1995). The influence of suicide risk and despondency on the amplitude of P300 in major depression. *Neurophysiol. Clin.*, **25**, 291–6.

Uston, T. B., Ayuso-Mateos, J. L., Chatterji, S., Mathers, C., and Murray, C. J. L. (2004). Global burden of depressive illness in the year 2000. *Br. J. Psychiatry*, **184**, 386–92.

Valentino, R. J., Curtis, A. L., Parris, D. G., and Webby, R. G. (1990). Antidepressant actions on brain noradrenergic neurons. *J. Pharmacol. Exp. Ther.*, **253**, 833–40.

Valuck, R. J., Libby, A. M., Sills, M. R., Giese, A. A., and Allen, R. R. (2004). Antidepressant treatment and risk of suicide attempt by adolescents with major depressive disorder: a propensity-adjusted retrospective cohort study. *CNS Drugs*, **18**, 1119–32.

Van de Kar, L. D. and Blair, M. L. (1999). Forebrain pathways mediating stress-induced hormone secretion. *Front. Neuroendocrinol.*, **20**, 1–48.

Van den Berg, M. D., Oldehinkel, A. J., Bouhuys, A. L., *et al.* (2001). Depression in later life: three etiologically different subgroups. *J. Affect. Disord.*, **65**, 19–26.

van der Hart, M. G., Czeh, B., de Biurrun, G., *et al.* (2002). Substance P receptor antagonist and clomipramine prevent stress induced alterations in cerebral metabolites, cytogenesis in the dentate gyrus and hippocampal volume. *Mol. Psychiatry*, **7**, 933–41.

Van der Lely, A. J., Foeken, K., van der Mast, R. C., and Lamberts, S. W. J. (1991). Rapid reversal of acute psychosis in the Cushing syndrome with cortisol-receptor antagonist mifepristone (RU 486). *Ann. Intern. Med.*, **114**, 143–4.

Van Der Meer, Y. G., Loendersloot, E. W., and Van Loenen, A. C. (1984). Postpartum blues syndrome. *J. Psychosom. Obstet. Gynaecol.*, **3**, 67–8.

Vandoolaeghe, E., van Hunsel, F., Nuyten, D., and Maes, M. (1998). Auditory event related potentials in major depression: prolonged P300 latency and increased P200 amplitude. *J. Affect. Disord.*, **48**, 105–13.

van Eck, M., Berkhof, H., Nicolson, N., and Sulon, J. (1996). The effects of perceived stress, traits, mood states, and stressful daily events on salivary cortisol. *Psychosom. Med.*, **58**, 447–58.

van Laar, M. W., van Willigenburg, A. P. P., and Volkerts, E. R. (1995). Acute and subchronic effects of nefazodone and imipramine on highway driving, cognitive functions, and daytime sleepiness in healthy adult and elderly subjects. *J. Clin. Psychopharmacol.*, **15**, 30–40.

Van Renynghe de Voxvrie, G. (1993). [Reactualization of the concept of unitary psychoies introduced by Joseph Guislain (in French).] *Acta Psychiatr. Belg.*, **93**, 203–19.

van West, D. and Maes, M. (1999). Activation of the inflammatory response system: a new look at the etiopathogenesis of major depression. *Neuroendocrinol. Lett.*, **20**, 11–17.

Vataja, R., Pohjasvaara, T., Leppavuori, A., *et al.* (2001). Magnetic resonance imaging correlates of depression after ischemic stroke. *Arch. Gen. Psychiatry*, **58**, 925–31.

Veenema, A. H., Meijer, O. C., de Kloet, E. R., and Koolhaas, J. M. (2003). Genetic selection for coping style predicts stressor susceptibility. *J. Neuroendocrinol.*, **15**, 256–67.

Veijola, J., Maki, P., Joukamaa, M., *et al.* (2004). Parental separation at birth and depression in adulthood: a long-term follow-up of the Finnish Christmas Seal Home Children. *Psychol. Med.*, **34**, 357–62.

Vega, J. A. W., Mortimer, A. M., and Tyson, P. J. (2000). Somatic treatment of psychotic depression: Review and recommendations for practice. *J. Clin. Psychopharm.*, **20**, 504–19.

Veith, R. C., Lewis, N., Linares, O. A., *et al.* (1994). Sympathetic nervous system activity in major depression. *Arch. Gen. Psychiatry*, **51**, 411–22.

Velazquez, C., Carlson, A., Stokes, K. A., and Leikin, J. B. (2001). Relative safety of mirtazapine overdose. *Vet. Hum. Toxicol.*, **43**, 342–4.

Ventura, R., Cabib, S., and Puglisi-Allegra, S. (2002). Genetic susceptibility of mesocortical dopamine to stress determines liability to inhibition of mesoaccumbens dopamine and to behavioral 'despair' in a mouse model of depression. *Neuroscience*, **115**, 999–1007.

Vercoulen, J. H., Swanink, C. M., Zitman, F. G., *et al.* (1996). Randomised, double-blind, placebo-controlled study of fluoxetine in chronic fatigue syndrome. *Lancet*, **347**, 858–61.

Verdoux, H., Sutter, A. L., Glatigny-Dallay, E., and Minisini, A. (2002). Obstetrical complications and the development of postpartum depressive symptoms: a prospective survey of the MATQUID cohort. *Acta. Psychiatr. Scand.*, **106**, 212–19.

Verkes, R. J., Van der Mast, R. C., Hengeveld, M. W., *et al.* (1998). Reduction by paroxetine of suicidal behavior in patients with repeated suicide attempts but not major depression. *Am. J. Psychiatry*, **155**, 543–7.

Versiani, M. and Nardi, A. E. (1997). Dysthymia: clinical picture, comorbidity, and outcome. In Akiskal, H. S. and Cassano, G. B. (eds) *Dysthymia and the Spectrum of Chronic Depressions.* New York: Guilford Press, pp. 35–43.

Vestergaard, P., Gram, L. F., Kragh-Sorensen, P., *et al.* (1993). Therapeutic potentials of recently introduced antidepressants. Danish University Antidepressant Group. *Psychopharmacol. Ser.*, **10**, 190–8.

Vickers, K. and McNally, R. J. (2004). Is premenstrual dysphoria a variant of panic disorder? A review. *Clin. Psychol. Rev.*, **24**, 933–56.

Victoroff, J. I., Benson, F., Grafton, S. T., Engel, J. Jr., and Mazziotta, J. C. (1994). Depression in complex partial seizures. Electroencephalography and cerebral metabolic correlates. *Arch. Neurol.*, **51**, 155–63.

Videbech, P. and Ravnkilde, B. (2004). Hippocampal volume and depression: a meta-analysis of MRI studies. *Am. J. Psychiatry*, **161**, 1957–66.

Vieta, E. and Colom, F. (2004). Psychological interventions in bipolar disorder: from wishful thinking to an evidence-based approach. *Acta Psychiatr. Scand.*, **110** (suppl. 422), 34–8.

Vieta, E., Gasto, C., Otero, O., Nieto, E., and Vallejo, J. (1997). Differential features between bipolar I and bipolar II disorder. *Compr. Psychiatry*, **38**, 98–101.

Vieta, E., Martinez-Aran, A., Goikolea, J. M, *et al.* (2002). A randomized trial comparing paroxetine and venlafaxine in the treatment of bipolar depressed patients taking mood stabilizers. *J. Clin. Psychiatry*, **63**, 508–12.

Viguera, A. C., Baldessarini, R. J., and Tondo, L. (2001). Response to lithium maintenance treatment in bipolar disorders: comparison of women and men. *Bipolar Disord.*, **3**, 245–52.

Viinamaki, H., Tanskanen, A., Honkalampi, K., *et al.* (2004). Is the Beck Depression Inventory suitable for screening major depression in different phases of the disease? *Nord. J. Psychiatry*, **58**, 49–53.

Vitiello, B. and Swedo, S. (2004). Antidepressant medications in children. *N. Engl. J. Med.*, **350**, 1489–91.

Voderholzer, U., Valerius, G., Schaerer, L., *et al.* (2003). Is the antidepressive effect of sleep deprivation stabilized by three day phase advance of the sleep period? A pilot study. *Eur. Arch. Psychiatry Clin. Neurosci.*, **253**, 68–72.

Voirol, P., Hodel, P. F., Zullino, D., and Baumann, P. (2000). Serotonin syndrome after small doses of citalopram or sertraline. *J. Clin. Psychopharmacol.*, **20**, 713–14.

Volavka, J., Feldstein, S., Abrams, R., Dornbush, R., and Fink, M. (1972). EEG and clinical change after bilateral and unilateral electroconvulsive therapy. *EEG Clin. Neurophysiol.*, **32**, 631–9.

Volz, H.-P. (1997). Controlled clinical trials of hypericum extracts in depressed patients: an overview. *Pharmacopsychiatry*, **30**, 72–6.

von Baeyer, W. R. (1951). *Die Moderne Psychiatrische Schockbehandlung.* Stuttgart: Georg Thieme Verlag.

von Braunmühl, A. (1947). *Insulinshock und Heilkrampf in der Psychiatrie.* Stuttgart: Wissenschaftliche Verlagsgesellschaft.

von Gunten, A., Fox, N. C., Cipolotti, L., and Ron, M. A. (2000). A volumetric study of hippocampus and amygdala in depressed patients with subjective memory problems. *J. Neuropsychiatry Clin. Neurosci.*, **12**, 493–8.

Vorstman, J., Lahuis, B., and Buitelaar, J. K. (2001). SSRIs associated with behavioral activation and suicidal ideation. *J. Am. Acad. Child Adolesc. Psychiatry*, **40**, 1364–5.

Vythilingam, M., Chen, J., Bremner, J. D., *et al.* (2003). Psychotic depression and mortality. *Am. J. Psychiatry*, **160**, 574–6.

Wadhwa, P. D. Sandman, C. A., Porto, M.,. Dunkel-Schetter, C., and Garite, T. J. (1993). The association between prenatal stress and infant birth weight and gestational age at birth: a prospective investigation. *Am. J. Obstet. Gynecol.*, **169**, 858–65.

Waern, M., Runeson, B., Allebeck, P., *et al.* (2002a). Mental disorder in elderly suicides. *Am. J. Psychiatry*, **159**, 450–5.

Waern, M., Spak, F., and Sundh, V. (2002b). Suicidal ideation in a female population sample. Relationship with depression, anxiety disorder and alcohol dependence/abuse. *Eur. Arch. Psychiatry Clin. Neurosci.*, **252**, 81–5.

Wagner, K. D. and Ambrosini, P. J. (2001). Childhood depression: pharmacological therapy/ treatment (pharmacotherapy of childhood depression). *J. Clin. Child Psychol.*, **30**, 88–97.

Wagner, K. D. Ambrosini, P., Rynn, M., *et al.* (2003). Efficacy of sertraline in the treatment of children and adolescents with major depressive disorder: two randomized controlled trials. *J.A.M.A.*, **290**, 1033–41.

Wagner, K. D., Robb, A. S., Findling, R. L., *et al.* (2004). A randomized, placebo-controlled trial of citalopram for the treatment of major depression in children and adolescents. *Am. J. Psychiatry*, **161**, 1079–83.

Walker, R. and Swartz, C. M. (1994). Electroconvulsive therapy during high-risk pregnancy. *Gen. Hosp. Psychiatry*, **16**, 348–53.

Wallace, D. M., Magnuson, D. J., and Gray, T. S. (1992). Organization of amygdaloid projections to brainstem dopaminergic, noradrenergic, and adrenergic cell groups in the rat. *Brain Res. Bull.*, **28**, 447–54.

Wallace, E. R. (1994). Psychiatry and its nosology: a historico-philosophical overview. In Sadler, J. Z., Wiggins, O. P., and Schwartz, M. A. (eds) *Philosophical Perspectives on Psychiatric Diagnostic Classification*. Baltimore, MD: Johns Hopkins Press, pp. 16–88.

Walsh, B. T., Seidman, S. N., Sysko, R., and Gould M. (2002). Placebo response in studies of major depression: variable, substantial, and growing. *J.A.M.A*, **287**, 1840–7.

Walsh, N. (2002). Herbal anxiolytic pulled from European markets. *Clin. Psychiatry News*, **30**, 1–2.

Walter, G. and Rey, J. M. (1997). An epidemiological study of the use of ECT in adolescents. *J. Am. Acad. Child Adolesc. Psychiatry*, **36**, 809–15.

Walter, G., Rey, J. M., and Mitchell, P. B. (1999). Practitioner review: electroconvulsive therapy in adolescents. *J. Child Psychol. Psychiatry*, **40**, 325–34.

Wamboldt, M. Z., Yancey, A. G. Jr., and Roesler, T. A. (1997). Cardiovascular effects of tricyclic antidepressants in childhood asthma: a case series and review. *J. Child Adolesc. Psychopharmacol.*, **7**, 45–64.

Wang, D., Cui, L. N., and Renaud, L. P. (2003). Pre- and postsynaptic GABA(B) receptors modulate rapid neurotransmission from suprachiasmatic nucleus to parvocellular hypothalamic paraventricular nucleus neurons. *Neuroscience*, **118**, 49–58.

Wang, J. and Patten, S. B. (2001a). A prospective study of sex-specific effects of major depression on alcohol consumption. *Can. J. Psychiatry*, **46**, 422–5.

(2001b). Alcohol consumption and major depression: findings from a follow-up study. *Can. J. Psychiatry*, **46**, 632–8.

Wang, P. S., Bohn, R. L., Glynn, R. J., Mogun, k. H., and Avorn, J. (2001a). Hazardous benzodiazepine regimens in the elderly: effects of half-life, dosage, and duration on risk of hip fracture. *Am. J. Psychiatry*, **158**, 892–8.

Wang, P. S., Walker, A. M., Tsuang, M. T., *et al.* (2001b). Antidepressant use and the risk of breast cancer: a non-association. *J. Clin. Epidemiol.*, **54**, 728–34.

Warner, P., Bancroft, J., Dixson, A., and Hampson, M. (1991). The relationship between perimenstrual depressive mood and depressive illness. *J. Affect. Disord.*, **23**, 9–23.

Warner, V., Mufson, I., and Weissman, M. M. (1995). Offspring at high and low risk for depression and anxiety: mechanisms of psychiatric disorder. *J. Am. Acad. Child Adolesc. Psychiatry*, **33**, 1256–64.

Warner, V., Weissman, M. M., Mufson, L., and Wickramaratne P. (1999). Grandparents, parents and grandchildren at high risk for depression: a three-generation study. *J. Am. Acad. Child Adolesc. Psychiatry*, **38**, 289–96.

Watanabe, Y., Gould, E., Daniels, D. C., Cameron, H., and McEwen, B. S. (1992). Tianeptine attenuates stress-induced morphological changes in the hippocampus. *Eur. J. Pharmacol.*, **222**, 157–62.

Watson, D., Weber, K., Assenheimer, J. S., *et al.* (1995). Testing a tripartite model. I. Evaluating the convergent and discriminant validity of anxiety and depression symptom scales. *J. Abnorm. Psychol.*, **104**, 3–14.

Watson, J. B., Mednick, S. A., Huttunen, M., and Wang, X. (1999). Prenatal teratogens and the development of adult mental illness. *Dev. Psychopathol.*, **11**, 457–66.

Watson, S. and Young, A. H. (2002). Hypothalamic–pituitary–adrenal-axis function in bipolar disorder. *Clin. Approach Bipolar Disord.*, **1**, 57–64.

Weardon, A. J., Morris, R. K., Mullis, R., *et al.* (1998). Randomised, double-blind, placebo-controlled treatment trial of fluoxetine and graded exercise for chronic fatigue syndrome. *Br. J. Psychiatry*, **172**, 485–90.

Weaver, D. R., Rivkees, S. A., Reppert, S. M. (1992). D1-dopamine receptors activate c-*fos* expression in the fetal suprachiasmatic nuclei. *Proc. Natl. Acad. Sci.*, **89**, 9201–4.

Weddington, W. W., Brown, B. S., Haertzen, C. A., *et al.* (1991). Comparison of amantadine and desipramine combined with psychotherapy for treatment of cocaine dependence. *Am. J. Drug Alcohol Abuse*, **17**, 137–52.

Wehr, T. A. (1989). Seasonal affective disorders: a historical overview. In Rosenthal, N. E. and Blehar, M. C. (eds) *Seasonal Affective Disorders and Phototherapy*, vol. 2. New York: Guilford Press, pp. 11–32

(1996). 'A clock for all seasons' in the human brain. *Prog. Brain Res.*, **111**, 321–42.

Wehr, T. A. and Goodwin, F. K. (1987). Can antidepressants cause mania and worsen the course of affective illness? *Am. J. Psychiatry*, **144**, 1403–11.

Weinberg, M. K. and Tronick, E. Z. (1998). The impact of maternal psychiatric illness on infant development. *J. Clin. Psychiatry*, **59** (suppl. 2), 53–61.

Weiner, R. D. (1979). The psychiatric use of electrically induced seizures. *Am. J. Psychiatry*, **136**, 1507–17.

(1980). ECT and seizure threshold: effects of stimulus wave form and electrode placement. *Biol. Psychiatry*, **15**, 225–41.

(1988). The first ECT devices. *Convuls. Ther.*, **4**, 50–61.

Weinstein, E. A. and Kahn, R. L. (1955). *Denial of Illness.* Springfield, IL: CC Thomas.

Weintraub, D. (2001). Nortriptyline in geriatric depression resistant to serotonin reuptake inhibitors: case series. *J. Geriatr. Psychiatry Neurol.*, **14**, 28–32.

Weiss, R. D., Griffin, M. L., and Mirin, S. M. (1992). Drug abuse as self-medication for depression: an empirical study. *Am. J. Drug Alcohol Abuse*, **18**, 121–9.

Weissman, A. M., Levy, B. T., Hartz, A. J., *et al.* (2004). Pooled analysis of antidepressant levels in lactating mothers, breast milk, and nursing infants. *Am. J. Psychiatry*, **161**, 1066–78.

Weissman, M. M. (1988). Psychopathology in the children of depressed parents: direct interview studies. In Dunner, D. L., Gershon, E. S., and Barrett, J. B. (eds) *Relatives at Risk for Mental Disorder.* New York, NY: Raven Press, pp. 143–59.

Weissman, M. M., Gershon, E. S., Kidd, K. K., *et al.* (1984a). Psychiatric disorders in the relatives of probands with affective disorder. *Arch. Gen. Psychiatry*, **41**, 13–21.

Weissman, M. M., Prusoff, B. A., Gammon, G. D., *et al.* (1984b). Psychopathology in the children (ages 6–18) of depressed and normal parents. *J. Am. Acad. Child Psychiatry*, **23**, 78–84.

Weissman, M. M., Prusoff, B. A., and Merikangas K. R. (1984c). Is delusional depression related to bipolar disorder? *Am. J. Psychiatry*, **141**, 892.

Weissman, M. M., Gammon, D., John, K., and Merikangas, K. R. (1987). Children of depressed parents. *Arch. Gen. Psychiatry*, **44**, 847–53.

Weissman, M. M., Warner, V., Wickramaratne, P., and Prusoff, B. A. (1988). Early-onset major depression in parents and their children. *J. Affect. Disord.*, **15**, 269–77.

Weissman, M. M, Warner, V., Wickramaratne, P., Moreau, D., and Olfson, M. (1997). Offspring of depressed parents: 10 years later. *Arch. Gen. Psychiatry*, **54**, 932–40.

Weissman, M. M., Fendrich, M., Warner, V., and Wickramaratne, P. J. (1992). Incidence of psychiatric disorders in offspring at high and low risk for depression. *J. Am. Acad. Child Adolesc. Psychiatry*, **31**, 640–8.

Weissman, M. M., Wolk, S., Goldstein, R. B., *et al.* (1999). Depressed adolescents grown up. *J.A.M.A.*, **281**, 1707–13.

Weizman, R., Laor, N., Podliszewski, E., *et al.* (1994). Cytokine production in major depressed patients before and after clomipramine treatment. *Biol. Psychiatry*, **35**, 42–7.

Welch, C. A. and Drop, L. J. (1989). Cardiovascular effects of ECT. *Convuls. Ther.*, **5**, 35–43.

Weller, E. B., Weller, R. A., Fristad, M. A., and Bowes, J. M., (1990). Dexamethasone suppression test and depressive symptoms in bereaved children: a preliminary report. *J. Neuropsychiatry Clin. Neurosci.*, **2**, 418–21.

Weller, R. A. and Weller, E. B. (1986). Tricyclic antidepressants in prepubertal depressed children: review of the literature. *Hillside J. Clin. Psychiatry*, **8**, 46–55.

Weller, R. A., Kapadia, P., Weller, E. B. *et al.* (1994). Psychopathology in families of children with major depressive disorders. *J. Affect. Disord.*, **31**, 247–52.

Wengel, S. P., Burke, W. J., Pfeiffer, R. F., Roccaforte, W. H., and Page, S. R. (1998). Maintenance electroconvulsive therapy for intractable Parkinson's disease. *Am. J. Geriatr. Psychiatry*, **6**, 263–9.

Werhane, P. H. (1999). *Moral Imagination and Management Decision-Making*. New York: Oxford University Press.

Werry, J. S., Biederman, J., Thisted, R., Greenhill, L., and Ryan, N. (1995). Resolved: cardiac arrhythmias make desipramine an unacceptable choice in children. *J. Am. Acad. Child Adolesc. Psychiatry*, **34**, 1239–45.

Wesely, S. (1993). The neuropsychiatry of chronic fatigue syndrome. In Bock, G. R. and Whelan J. (eds) *Chronic Fatigue Syndrome*. Ciba Foundation Symposium 173. UK: Wiley, pp. 212–37.

West, E. D. and Dally, P. J. (1959). Effect of iproniazid in depressive syndromes. *Br. Med. J.*, **1**, 1491–4.

Westlund Tam, L. and Parry, B. L. (2003). Does estrogen enhance the antidepressant effects of fluoxetine? *J. Affect. Disord.*, **77**, 87–92.

Westrin, A., Frii, K., and Taskman-Bendz, L. (2003). The dexamethasone suppression test and DSM-III-R diagnoses in suicide attempters. *Eur. Psychiatry*, **18**, 350–5.

Wheatley, D. P., van Moffaert, M., Timmerman, L., and Kremer, C. M. (1998). Mirtazapine: efficacy and tolerability in comparison with fluoxetine in patients with moderate to severe major depressive disorder. Mirtazapine-Fluoxetine Study Group. *J. Clin. Psychiatry*, **59**, 306–12.

Wheeler Vega, J. A., Mortimer, A. M., and Tyson, P. J. (2000). Somatic treatment of psychotic depression. Review and recommendations for practice. *J. Clin. Psychopharmacol.*, **20**, 504–19.

Whiteford, H. A. and Evans, L. (1984). Agoraphobia and the dexamethasone suppression test: atypical depression? *Aust. N. Z. J. Psychiatry*, **18**, 374–7.

Whittington, C. J., Kendall, T., Fonagy, P., *et al.* (2004). Selective serotonin reuptake inhibitors in childhood depression: systematic review of published versus unpublished data. *Lancet*, **363**, 1341–5.

Whybrow, P. C. and Prange, A. J. Jr. (1981). A hypothesis of thyroid–catecholamine-receptor interaction. *Arch. Gen. Psychiatry*, **38**, 106–11.

Whyte, E. M. and Mulsant B. H. (2002). Post stroke depression: epidemiology, pathophysiology, and biological treatment. *Biol. Psychiatry*, **52**, 253–64.

Whyte, E. M., Pollock, B. G., Wagner, W. R., *et al.* (2001). Influence of serotonin-transporter-linked promoter region polymorphism on platelet activation in geriatric depression. *Am. J. Psychiatry*, **158**, 2074–6.

Whyte, I. M., Dawson, A. H., and Buckley, N. A. (2003). Relative toxicity of venlafaxine and selective serotonin reuptake inhibitors in overdose compared to tricyclic antidepressants. *Q. J. Med.*, **96**, 369–74.

Wickramaratne, P. J. and Weissman, M. M. (1998). Onset of psychopathology in offspring by developmental phase and parental depression. *J. Am. Acad. Child Adolesc. Psychiatry*, **37**, 933–42.

Wiegartz, P., Seidenberg, M., Woodard A, Gidal, B., and Hermann, B. (1999). Co-morbid psychiatric disorder in chronic epilepsy: recognition and etiology of depression. *Neurology*, **53** (suppl. 2), S3–8.

Wileman, S. M., Eagles, J. M., Andrew, J. E., *et al.* (2001). Light therapy for seasonal affective disorder in primary care: randomised controlled trial. *Br. J. Psychiatry*, **178**, 311–16.

Wilens, T. E., Biederman, J., Geist, D. E., Steingard, R., and Spencer, T. (1994). Nortriptyline in the treatment of ADHD: a chart review of 58 cases. *J. Am. Acad. Child Adolesc. Psychiatry*, **33**, 142–3.

Wilens, T. E., Biederman, J., Baldessarini, R. J., *et al.* (1996). Cardiovascular effects of therapeutic doses of tricyclic antidepressants in children and adolescents. *J. Am. Acad. Child Adolesc. Psychiatry*, **35**, 1491–501.

Wilhelm, S. M., Lee, J., and Prinz, R. A. (2004). Major depression due to primary hyperparathyroidism: a frequent and correctable disorder. *Am. Surg.*, **70**, 175–80.

Wilkinson, D., Holmes, C., Woolford, J., Stammers, S., and North, J. (2002). Prophylactic therapy with lithium in elderly patients with unipolar major depression. *Int. J. Geriatr. Psychiatry*, **17**, 619–22.

Williams, A. N. and Birmingham, L. (2002). The art of making ineffective treatments effective. *Lancet*, **359**, 1937–9.

Williamson, D. E., Ryan, N. D., Birmaher, B., *et al.* (1995). A case-control family history study of depression in adolescents. *J. Am. Acad. Child Adolesc. Psychiatry*, **34**, 1596–607.

Williamson, D. E., Coleman, K., Bacanu, S.-A., *et al.* (2003). Heritability of fearful-anxious endophenotypes in infant rhesus macaques: a preliminary report. *Biol. Psychiatry*, **53**, 284–91.

Williamson, D. E., Birmaher, B., Axelson, D. A., Ryan, N. D., and Dahl, R. E. (2004). First episode of depression in children at low and high familial risk for depression. *J. Am. Acad. Child Adolesc. Psychiatry*, **43**, 291–7.

Wilsnack, R. W., Klassen, A. D., and Wilsnack, S. C. (1986). Retrospective analysis of lifetime changes in women's drinking behavior. *Adv. Alcohol Subst. Abuse*, **5**, 9–28.

Wilsnack, S. C., Klassen, A. D., Schur, B. E., and Wilsnack, R. W. (1991). Predicting onset and chronicity of women's problem drinking: a five-year longitudinal analysis. *Am. J. Public Health*, **81**, 305–18.

Winokur, G. (1979). Unipolar depression: is it divisible into autonomous subtypes? *Arch. Gen. Psychiatry*, **36**, 47–52.

Winokur, G., Clayton, P., and Reich, T. (1969). *Manic Depressive Illness*. St. Louis, MO: CV Mosby.

Winokur, G., Coryell, W., Keller, M., Endicott, J., and Akiskal, H. (1993). A prospective follow-up of patients with bipolar and primary unipolar affective disorder. *Arch. Gen. Psychiatry*, **50**, 457–65.

Winokur, G., Monahan, P., Coryell, W., and Zimmerman, M. (1996). Schizophrenia and affective disorder – distinct entities or continuum? An analysis based on a prospective 6-year follow-up. *Compr. Psychiatry*, **37**, 77–87.

Winokur, G., Turvey, C., Akiskal, H., *et al.* (1998). Alcoholism and drug abuse in three groups – bipolar I, unipolars and their acquaintances. *J. Affect. Disord.*, **50**, 81–9.

Winsberg, M. E., DeGolia, S. G., Strong, C. M., and Ketter, T. A. (2001). Divalproex therapy in medication-naive and mood-stabilizer-naive bipolar II depression. *J. Affect. Disord.*, **67**, 207–12.

Wirz-Justice, A. (1998). Biological rhythms of mood disorders. In Bloom, F. E. and Kupfer, D. J. (eds) *Psychopharmacology, The Fourth Generation of Progress* (CD ROM). New York: Lippincott, Williams and Wilkins, Chapter 97.

Wise, M. G., Ward, S. C., Townsend-Parchman, W., *et al.* (1984). Case report of ECT during high-risk pregnancy. *Am. J. Psychiatry*, **141**, 99–101.

Wisner, K. L. and Stowe, Z. N. (1997). Psychobiology of postpartum mood disorders. *Semin. Reprod. Endocrinol.* **15**, 77–89.

Wisner, K. L., Peindl, K. P., and Hanusa, B. H. (1993). Relationship of psychiatric illness to childbearing status: a hospital-based epidemiologic study. *J. Affect. Disord.*, **28**, 39–50.

(1995). Psychiatric episodes in women with young children. *J. Affect. Disord.*, **34**, 1–11.

Wisner, K. L., Perel, J. M., and Findling, R. L. (1996). Antidepressant treatment during breast-feeding. *Am. J. Psychiatry*, **153**, 1132–7.

Wisner, K. L., Zarin, D. A., Holmboe, E. S., *et al.* (2000). Risk–benefit decision making for treatment of depression during pregnancy. *Am. J. Psychiatry*, **157**, 1933–40.

Wisner, K. L., Perel, J. M., Peindl, K. S., *et al.* (2001). Prevention of recurrent postpartum depression: a randomized clinical trial. *J. Clin. Psychiatry*, **62**, 82–6.

Wolf, A. W., De Andraca, I., and Lozoff, B. (2002). Maternal depression in three Latin American samples. *Soc. Psychiatry Psychiatr. Epidemiol.*, **37**, 169–76.

Wolfersdorf, M., Steiner, B., Keller, F., Hautzinger, M., and Hole, G. (1990). Depression and suicide: is there a difference between suicidal and non-suicidal depressed in-patients? *Eur. J. Psychiatry*, **4**, 235–52.

Wolfersdorf, M., Barg, R., Konig, F., Leibfarth, M., and Grunewald, I. (1995). Paroxetine as antidepressant in combined antidepressant-neuroleptic therapy in delusional depression: observation of clinical use. *Pharmacopsychiatry*, **28**, 56–60.

Wolf, C. T., Friedman, S. B., Hofer, M. A. and Mason, J. W. Relationship between psychological defenses and mean urinary 17-hydroxycorticosteroid excretion rates. *Psychosom. Med.* **26**, 576–609.

Wolkowitz, O. M. and Rothschild, A. J. (eds) (2003). *Psychoneuroendocrinology: The Scientific Basis of Clinical Practice.* Washington, DC: American Psychiatric Publishing.

Wolkowitz, O. M. and Reus, V. I. (1999). Treatment of depression with antiglucocorticoid drugs. *Psychosom. Med.*, **61**, 698–711.

Wolkowitz, O. M., Reus, V. I., Chan, T., *et al.* (1999). Antiglucocorticoid treatment of depression: double-blind ketoconazole. *Biol. Psychiatry*, **45**, 1070–4.

Wong, D. T. and Bymaster, F. P. (2002). Dual serotonin and noradrenaline uptake inhibitor class of antidepressants potential for greater efficacy or just hype? *Prog. Drug Res.*, **58**, 169–222.

Wong, M. L., Kling, M. A., Munson, P. J., *et al.* (2000). Pronounced and sustained central hypernoradrenergic function in major depression with melancholic features: relation to hypercortisolism and corticotropin-releasing hormone. *Proc. Natl Acad. Sci. USA*, **97**, 325–30.

Woodruff, R. A., Goodwin, D. W., and Guze, S. B. (1974). *Psychiatric Diagnosis.* New York: Oxford University Press.

Woodward, L. J. and Fergusson, D. M. (2001). Life course outcomes of young people with anxiety disorders in adolescence. *J. Am. Acad. Child Adolesc. Psychiatry*, **40**, 1086–93.

Wozniak, J., Spencer, T., Biederman, J., *et al.* (2004). The clinical characteristics of unipolar vs. bipolar major depression in ADHD youth. *J. Affect. Disord.*, **82** (suppl. 1), S59–69.

Wu, J. C., Gillin, J. C., Buchsbaum, M. S., *et al.* (1992). Effect of sleep deprivation on brain metabolism of depressed patients. *Am. J. Psychiatry*, **149**, 538–43.

Wyllie, A. M. (1940). Convulsion therapy of the psychoses. *J. Ment. Sci.*, **86**, 248–59.

Yamashita, H., Fujikawa, T., Yanai, I., Morinobu, S., and Yamawaki, S. (2001). Clinical features and treatment response of patients with major depression and silent cerebral infarction. *Neuropsychobiology*, **44**, 176–82.

Yatham, L. N., Clark, C. C., and Zis, A. P. (2000). A preliminary study of the effects of electroconvulsive therapy on regional brain glucose metabolism in patients with major depression. *J. ECT*, **16**, 171–6.

Yatham, L. N., Kusumakar, V., Calabrese, J. R., *et al.* (2002). Third generation anticonvulsants in bipolar disorder: a review of efficacy and summary of clinical recommendations. *J. Clin. Psychiatry*, **63**, 275–83.

Yehuda, R., Boisoneau, D., Mason, J. W., and Giller, E. L. (1993). Glucocorticoid receptor number and cortisol excretion in mood, anxiety and psychotic disorders. *Biol. Psychiatry*, **34**, 18–25.

Yeragani, V. K. (1990). The incidence of abnormal dexamethasone suppression in schizophrenia: a review and a meta-analytic comparison with the incidence in normal controls. *Can. J. Psychiatry*, **35**, 128–32.

Yeragani, V. K., Pesce, V., Jayaraman, A., and Roose, S. (2002). Major depression with ischemic heart disease: effects of paroxetine and nortriptyline on long-term heart rate variability measures. *Biol. Psychiatry*, **52**, 418–29.

Yerevanian, B. I., Feusner, J. D., Koek, R. J., and Mintz, J. (2004a). The dexamethasone suppression test as a predictor of suicidal behavior in unipolar depression. *J. Affect. Disord.*, **83**, 103–8.

Yerevanian, B. I., Koek, R. J., Feusner, J. D., Hwang, S., and Mintz, J. (2004b). Antidepressants and suicidal behaviour in unipolar depression. *Acta Psychiatr. Scand.*, **110**, 452–8.

Yonkers, K. A. (1997). The association between premenstrual dysphoric disorder and other mood disorders. *J. Clin. Psychiatry*, **58** (suppl. 15), 19–25.

Yoshioka, H., Ida, S., Yokota, M., *et al.* (2000). Effects of lithium on the pharmacokinetics of valproate in rats. *J. Pharm. Pharmacol.*, **52**, 97–301.

Young, A. H., Gallagher, P., Watson, S., *et al.* (2004). Improvements in neurocognitive function and mood following adjunctive treatment with mifepristone (RU-486) in bipolar disorder. *Neuropsychopharmacology*, **29**, 1538–45.

Young, A. S., Klap, R., Sherbourne, C. D., and Wells, K. B. (2001). The quality of care for depressive and anxiety disorders in the United States. *Arch. Gen. Psychiatry*, **58**, 55–61.

Young, A. W., Robertson, I. H., Hellawell, D. J., de Pauw, K. W., and Pentland, B (1992). Cotard delusion after brain injury. *Psychol. Med.*, **22**, 799–804.

Young, A. W., Leafhead, K. M., and Szulecka, T. K. (1994). The Capgras and Cotard delusions. *Psychopathology*, **27**, 226–31.

Young, E. A., Haskett, R. F., Murphy-Weinberg, V., Watson, S. J., and Akil, H. (1991). Loss of glucocorticoid fast feedback in depression. *Arch. Gen. Psychiatry*, **48**, 693–9.

Young, E. A., Akil, H., Haskett, R. F., and Watson, S. J. (1995). Evidence against changes in corticotroph CRF receptors in depressed patients. *Biol. Psychiatry*, **37**, 355–63.

Young, E. A., Lopez, J. F., Murphy-Weinberg, V., Watson, S. J., and Akil, H. (2000a). Hormonal evidence for altered responsiveness to social stress in major depression. *Neuropsychopharmacology*, **23**, 411–18.

Young, L. T., Joffe, R. T., Robb, J. C., *et al.* (2000b). Double-blind comparison of addition of a second mood stabilizer versus an antidepressant to an initial mood stabilizer for treatment of patients with bipolar depression. *Am. J. Psychiatry*, **157**, 124–7.

Young, M. A., Scheftner, W. A., Klerman, G. L., Andreasen, N. C., and Hirschfeld, R. M. A. (1986). The endogenous sub-type of depression: a study of its internal construct validity. *Br. J. Psychiatry*, **148**, 257–67.

Yuen, A. W., Land, G., Weatherley, B. C., and Peck, A. W. (1992). Sodium valproate acutely inhibits lamotrigine metabolism. *Br. J. Clin. Pharmacol.*, **33**, 511–13.

Zafonte, R. D., Cullen, N., and Lexell, J. (2002). Serotonin agents in the treatment of acquired brain injury. *J. Head Trauma Rehabil.*, **17**, 322–34.

Zalsman, G., Frisch, A., Apter, A., and Weizman, A. (2002). Genetics of suicidal behavior: candidate association genetic approach. *Isr. J. Psychiatry Relat. Sci.*, **39**, 252–61.

Zanardi, R., Franchini, L., Gasperini, M., Perez, J., and Smeraldi, E. (1996). Double-blind controlled trial of sertraline versus paroxetine in the treatment of delusional depression. *Am. J. Psychiatry*, **153**, 1631–3.

Zanardi, R., Franchini, L., Serretti, A., Perez, J., and Smeeraldi, E. (2000). Venlafaxine versus fluvoxamine in the treatment of delusional depression: a pilot double-blind controlled study. *J. Clin. Psychiatry*, **61**, 26–9.

Zarate, C. A., Kando, J. C., Tohen, M., Weiss, M. K., and Cole, J. O., (1996). Does intolerance or lack of response with fluoxetine predict the same will happen with sertraline? *J. Clin. Psychiatry*, **57**, 67–71.

Zarate, C. A. Jr., Du, J., Quiroz, J., *et al.* (2003). Regulation of cellular plasticity cascades in the pathophysiology and treatment of mood disorders: role of the glutamatergic system. *Ann. NY Acad. Sci.*, **1003**, 273–91.

Zaratiegui, R. (2002). Psychotic depression. *Vertex*, **13** (suppl. 1), 40–8.

Zelkowitz, P. and Milet, T. H. (2001). The course of postpartum psychiatric disorders in women and their partners. *J. Nerv. Ment. Dis.*, **189**, 575–82.

Zesiewicz, T. A., Gold, M., Chari, G., and Hauser, R. A. (1999). Current issues in depression in Parkinson's disease. *Am. J. Geriatr. Psychiatry*, **7**, 110–18.

Zeskind, P. S. and Stephens, L. E. (2004) Maternal selective serotonin reuptake inhibitor use during pregnancy and newborn neurobehavior. *Pediatrics*, **113**, 368–75.

Zhou, J. N., Riemersma, R. F., Unmehopa, U. A., *et al.* (2001). Alterations in arginine vasopressin neurons in the suprachiasmatic nucleus in depression. *Arch. Gen. Psychiatry*, **58**, 655–62.

Zilboorg, G. (1941). *A History of Medical Psychology*. New York: WW Norton.

Zill, P., Baghai, T. C., Zwanzger, P., *et al.* (2002). Association analysis of a polymorphism in the G-protein stimulatory α subunit in patients with major depression. *Am. J. Med. Genet.*, **114**, 530–2.

Zimmerman, M., Coryell, W., Pfohl, B., and Stangl, D. (1985) Four definitions of endogenous depression and the dexamethasone suppression test. *J. Affect. Disord.*, **8**, 37–45.

Zimmerman, M., Coryell, W., Pfohl, B., and Stangl, D. (1986a). The validity of four definitions of endogenous depression. *Arch. Gen. Psychiatry*, **43**, 234.

Zimmerman, M., Coryell, W., Pfohl, B., Corenthal, C., and Stangl, D. (1986b). ECT response in depressed patients with and without a DSM-III personality disorder. *Am. J. Psychiatry*, **143**, 1030–2.

Zimmerman, M., Coryell, W., and Pfohl, B. (1986c). The validity of the dexamethasone suppression test as a marker for endogenous depression. *Arch. Gen. Psychiatry*, **43**, 347–55.

Zimmerman, M., Lish, J. D., Lush, D. T., *et al.* (1995). Suicidal ideation among urban medical outpatients. *J. Gen. Intern. Med.*, **10**, 573–6.

Zimmerman, M., Mattia, J. I., and Posternak, M. A. (2002). Are subjects in pharmacological treatment trials of depression representative of patients in routine clinical practice? *Am. J. Psychiatry*, **159**, 469–73.

Zimmerman, M., Chelminski, I., and Posternak, M. (2004). A review of studies of the Montgomery-Asberg Depression Rating Scale in controls: implications for the definition of remission in treatment studies of depression. *Int. Clin. Psychopharmacol.*, **19**, 1–7.

Ziskind, E., Somerfeld-Ziskind, E., and Ziskind, L. (1942). Metrazol therapy in the affective psychoses. Study of a controlled series of cases. *J. Nerv. Ment. Dis.*, **95**, 460–73.

Ziskind, E., Somerfeld-Ziskind, E., and Ziskind, L. (1945). Metrazol and electric convulsive therapy of the affective psychoses. A controlled series of observations covering a period of five years. *Arch Neurol. Psychiatry*, **53**, 212–17.

Zisook, S. and Shuchter, S. R. (1993). Uncomplicated bereavement. *J. Clin. Psychiatry*, **54**, 365–72.

Zobel, A. W., Yassourides, A., Frieboes, R. M., and Holsboer, F. (1999). Prediction of medium-term outcome by cortisol response to the combined dexamethasone-CRH test in patients with remitted depression. *Am. J. Psychiatry*, **156**, 949–51.

Zobel, A. W., Nickel, T., Kunzel, H. E., *et al.* (2000). Effects of the high-affinity corticotropin-releasing hormone receptor 1 antagonist R121919 in major depression: the first 20 patients treated. *J. Psychiatr. Res.*, **34**, 171–81.

Zobel, A. W., Nickel, T., Sonntag, A., *et al.* (2001). Cortisol response in the combined dexamethasone/CRH test as predictor of relapse in patients with remitted depression, a prospective study. *J. Psychiatr. Res.*, **35**, 83–94.

Zornberg, G. L. and Pope, H. G. (1993). Treatment of depression in bipolar disorder: new directions for research. *J. Clin. Psychopharmacol.*, **13**, 397–408.

Zubenko, G. S., Maher, B., Hughes, H. B. III, *et al.* (2003a). Genome-wide linkage survey for genetic loci that influence the development of depressive disorders in families with recurrent, early-onset, major depression. *Am. J. Med. Genet. Part B: Neuropsychiatr. Genet.*, **123B**, 1–18.

Zubenko, G. S., Zubenko, W. N., McPherson, S., *et al.* (2003b). A collaborative study of the emergence and clinical features of the major depressive syndrome of Alzheimer's disease. *Am. J. Psychiatry*, **160**, 857–66.

Zuckerman, B., Bauchner, H., Parker, S., and Cabral, H. (1990). Maternal depressive symptoms during pregnancy, and newborn irritability. *J. Dev. Behav. Pediatr.*, **11**, 190–4.

Zulkifli, A. and Rogayah, J. (1997). Career preferences of male and female medical students in Malaysia. *Med. J. Malaysia*, **52**, 76–81.

Zwanzger, P., Baghai, T. C., Padberg, F., *et al* (2003). The combined dexamethasone-CRH test before and after repetitive transcranial magnetic stimulation (rTMS) in major depression. *Psychoneuroendocrinology*, **28**, 376–85.

Zylka, M. J., Shearman, L. P., Weaver, D. R., and Reppert, S. M. (1998). Three period homologs in mammals: differential light responses in the sup. *Neuron*, **20**, 1103–10.

Index

abnormal bereavement, 8, 9
  characteristics, 102
  classification issues, 347
  and cortisol levels, 36
  diagnostic criteria, 23
  diagnostic issues, 36
  and melancholia, 36–37, 46, 97
Abrams, R., 19, 27
Accreditation Council of Graduate Medical Education (ACGME) (USA), 352
ACTH *see* adrenocorticotropic hormone (ACTH)
AD *see* Alzheimer's disease (AD)
Addison's disease
  differential diagnosis, 111
  etiology, 111
adjustment disorder with depressed mood, 47, 97
  adolescents, 102
  differential diagnosis, 101–102
  and suicide risk, 102
adolescents
  adjustment disorder with depressed mood, 102
  cognitive-behavior therapy, 245
  electroconvulsive therapy, 165–70
    case studies, 168–70
    efficacy, 165–67, 244
    safety issues, 165
  manic-depressive illness, 245
  melancholia, 103–104
    comorbidity, 91–93, 103
    pharmacotherapy, 244–50
    prevalence, 103
    recommendations, 250
    sample heterogeneity, 245–46
  psychotherapy, 244–45
adrenalectomy, 62
adrenal glands
  atrophy, 62
  and stress, 62–63
adrenocorticotropic hormone (ACTH), 64
  and pregnancy, 33
  release, 64
  and stress responses, 309
adrenocorticotropin *see* adrenocorticotropic hormone (ACTH)
AEPs *see* auditory evoked potentials (AEPs)
affective disorders, convulsive therapy, 155
affective reactions, 8
African-Americans, suicide rates, 126
agitation
  with melancholia, suicide risk assessment, 135–36
  symptoms, 16
agomelatine, 290
Akiskal, H. S., 21
alcohol abuse
  and depressive mood disorders, 255, 301
  and melancholia, 108–109
    pharmacotherapy, 255–56
  and sleep, 357
  and suicide risk, 137
alcoholism, genetic factors, 255
Alzheimer's disease (AD)
  differential diagnosis, 106
  with melancholia, pharmacotherapy, 260–61
  and pseudodementia, 261
    differential diagnosis, 118, 158
American Academy of Child and Adolescent Psychiatry, 165
American College of Obstetricians and Gynecologists, 291
American Journal of Psychiatry, 200, 288
American Psychiatric Association (APA), 6, 8
  classification issues, 365
  dexamethasone suppression test assessment, 70
  suicidal patient guidelines, 143
  Task Force on ECT, 167
    recommendations, 182
  see also Diagnostic and Statistical Manual of Mental Disorders (DSM)
amines, secondary vs tertiary, 199, 211
Amish, suicide risk, 136
amitriptyline, 50
  effectiveness, 202–203
    adolescents, 247
  effects on suicide rates, 140
    studies, 141
  and electroconvulsive therapy compared, 157
  with haloperidol, 224
  melancholia treatment, 211
  studies, 54

amobarbital, electroencephalography studies, 323
amygdala
  metabolism, 318–19
  and stress responses, 308–11
Angst, J., 21
animal studies
  abnormal neuroplasticity, 314–15
  noradrenergic dysfunction, 314
  reward mechanisms, 315
  serotonin function, 312–13
  stress responses, 306, 308
anterior cingulate cortex, volume reduction, 317–18, 319
anterior insular cortex, increased metabolism, 319–20
anticonvulsants
  approved, 50
  diabetes with melancholia treatment, 264–65
  effects on seizure, 188
  efficacy, 24
  epilepsy with melancholia treatment, 260
  in mania treatment, 23
  manic-depressive illness treatment, 228–29
  neonatal issues, 242
antidepressants, 5–6
  Alzheimer's disease with melancholia treatment, 261
  with antipsychotics, 223–24
  approved, increase, 50
  comparisons
    biased, 197, 198, 199–01
    methodology issues, 200
    placebo effects, 200–201
    unfavorable, 198
  controlled studies
    bias, 198
    limitations, 197
    reviews, 199
    volunteer criteria, 198
  diabetes with melancholia treatment, 264–65
  dosing issues, 214, 247–48
  drug–drug interactions, 265
  drug-switching, 213–14, 217–18
  effects on glucocorticoid receptors, 311
  effects on suicide rates, 140–42
    meta-analyses, 140–41
    studies, 142
  efficacy, tricyclics vs SSRIs, 201–204
  fetal safety issues, 243
  and glucose metabolism, 226
  mania induction, 22–23
    incidence, 22
  and manic-depressive illness
    mood switch risk, 225–26
    treatment, 226–27
  marketing strategies, 51
  medical illness with melancholia treatment, 261–62
  meta-analyses, 197, 199–00, 201–204
  novel, and industry influences, 197–99
  overdose, lethality, 142–43
  postpartum depression treatment, 163
  prescriptions, 50, 141–42
  selection criteria, 240
  side-effects, 205
  simultaneous application, 217
  and suicide prevention, 132
  teratogenicity, 240–41
  thyroid disease with melancholia treatment, 265
  use of term, 7–8
  vs electroconvulsive therapy, 156, 157, 158, 161, 188–90
    in pregnancy, 164
    suicide risk, 159
  see also monoamine oxidase inhibitors (MAOIs); selective serotonin reuptake inhibitors (SSRIs); tricyclic antidepressants (TCAs)
antipsychotics
  with antidepressants, 223–24
  approved, 50
  drug augmentation, 217
  drug–drug interactions, 265
  fetal safety issues, 243
  indications, 223–24
  side-effects, 223, 224
  use of term, 7–8
anxiety disorders
  differential diagnosis, 109
  with melancholia, suicide risk assessment, 135–36
anxious depression, 54–55
APA *see* American Psychiatric Association (APA)
apathetic syndromes
  differential diagnosis, 109–13
  and neurologic diseases, 113–18
apathy
  associated conditions, 264
  symptoms, 112
apolipoprotein E_4 gene, and Alzheimer's disease, 106
approach–withdrawal theories, of hemisphere specialization, 322
Arateus, on melancholia, 3
Archives of General Psychiatry, 200
aripiprazole, 224
Ashby, D., 141–42
Asperger syndrome, with melancholia, 104
atypical depression, 9, 54, 97
  age of onset, 98
  comorbidity, 98
  differential diagnosis, 98–99
  prevalence, 98
  symptoms, 98, 278
  treatment, 99
  see also seasonal affective disorder (SAD)
auditory evoked potentials (AEPs), 323–24
  advantages, 324
  limitations, 324
  mood disorder studies, 324
Australia
  antidepressant studies, 202
  electroconvulsive therapy studies, 166
  suicide rates, 126, 140–41

autism
  with melancholia, 104
    treatment, 104
avolitional syndromes, differential diagnosis, 112–13

Baillarger, Jules-Gabriel-François, 4, 18
Baltimore Epidemiologic Catchment Area (USA), 252
basal ganglia disease, differential diagnosis, 291
Baxter, Richard, on melancholia, 3
BDI *see* Beck Depression Inventory (BDI)
BDNF *see* brain-derived neurotrophic factor (BDNF)
BDRS (Brief Depression Rating Scale), 94
Bech–Rafaelsen Melancholia Scale (BRMS), 94
Beck Depression Inventory (BDI), 50, 93
  applications, 94
behavior disorders, classification, 1
Benazzi, F., 21, 55
Bennett, A. E., 153
benzodiazepines
  and breast-feeding, 244
  in catatonia diagnosis, 31, 161
  effectiveness, elderly, 253
  effects on seizure, 188
  and fetal safety, 239
bereavement
  use of term, 46–47
  see also abnormal bereavement
Berger, Hans, 321, 323
beta-blockers, effects on seizure, 188
Bethlem Hospital, 4
bilateral electroconvulsive therapy (BL-ECT), 184
  energy dosing, 186
  and right unilateral electroconvulsive therapy compared, 184
biological clock, 356
bipolar depression, 8, 46
  antidepressant-induced, 22–23
  early studies, 19
  electroconvulsive therapy, 172–74
    case studies, 173–74
bipolar disorders
  Bipolar I, 8–9, 19
    studies, 21
  Bipolar II, 8–9, 19
    longitudinal studies, 20–21
    studies, 21
  case studies, 22
  diagnostic criteria, 8–9, 18
  psychopathologic studies, 20
bipolarity, lack of support for, 24
bipolar–unipolar dichotomy
  clinical studies, 20–22
  criticisms, 19, 20
  early studies, 19
  research issues, 21
  vs continuum model, 19–20
bipolar–unipolar overlap, 23
  issues, 24
  studies, 21
  twin studies, 23
BL-ECT *see* bilateral electroconvulsive therapy (BL-ECT)
borderline personality disorder, 99
BPRS (Brief Psychotic Rating Scale), 166
bradykinesia, 88
bradykinetic syndromes, differential diagnosis, 112–13
bradyphrenia, 88
brain
  feedback mechanisms, 63
  see also hemispheres
brain-derived neurotrophic factor (BDNF), 315–16
  abnormalities, 316
  and reward mechanisms, 315
brain injury
  and depressive mood disorders, 317
  see also traumatic brain injury (TBI)
brain metabolism, abnormal, in melancholia, 318–20, 332, 343
brain structure
  abnormal
    in melancholia, 317–18, 329, 346
    postmortem studies, 317–18
breast cancer, drug-induced, 224
breast-feeding
  melancholia in, pharmacotherapy, 239–44
  and psychotropic drugs, 243–44
brief depression, 46
  differential diagnosis, 101
Brief Depression Rating Scale (BDRS), applications, 94
Brief Psychotic Rating Scale (BPRS), 166
brief recurrent depression, 9
Bright, Timothy, on melancholia, 3
Britain *see* United Kingdom (UK)
British Journal of Psychiatry, 288
BRMS (Bech–Rafaelsen Melancholia Scale), 94
brofaromine, 290
bromocriptine
  drug augmentation, 216
  Parkinson's disease with melancholia
    treatment, 259
Brooklyn State Hospital (USA), 154
bupropion, 225
  effectiveness, elderly, 253
  heart disease with melancholia
    treatment, 262–63
  mania induction, 23
  in smoking cessation therapy, 256
  trials data, 350
Burke, W. J., 203
Burton, Robert, on melancholia, 3

California (USA)
  electroconvulsive therapy, adolescents, 165
  Medicaid, 270
cAMP *see* cyclic adenosine monophosphate (cAMP)

Canada, electroconvulsive therapy studies, 166
cancers
  breast cancer, 224
  and depression risk, 111
Cannon, Walter, 62–63
Capgras syndrome, and psychotic depression, 30
carbamazepine
  drug–drug interactions, 265
  in mania treatment, 23
  manic-depressive illness treatment, 229
  neonatal issues, 242
Cardiazol *see* pentylenetetrazol
cardiovascular disease
  and electroconvulsive therapy, 170
  with melancholia, pharmacotherapy, 262–64
  see also heart disease
Carroll, Bernard J., 64–65, 66, 68, 75
  on dexamethasone suppression test, 66, 69, 70–71
Carroll Rating Scale (CRS), 94
  applications, 94
catalepsy, 30
catatonia, 9, 46, 88
  antidepressant treatment, 161
  case studies, 30–31, 32
  diagnosis, 31
  diagnostic criteria, 25
  differential diagnosis, 30, 161
  electroconvulsive therapy, 161–63
    case studies, 162–63
    efficacy, 161
  malignant, 161
  and melancholia, 30, 32, 97
  pharmacotherapy, 224–25
  retarded, 162
  symptoms, 31, 161
CBT *see* cognitive-behavior therapy (CBT)
CCKs (cholecystokinins), 317
central nervous system (CNS), and hypothalamic–pituitary–adrenal axis, 64
cerebral hemispheric instability, and manic-depressive illness, 329–30
cerebrovascular disease, elderly, 105
cerebrovascular stroke, differential diagnosis, 114
CFS (chronic fatigue syndrome), 112
characterological conditions, and electroconvulsive therapy, 171–72
characterological depression, 46
Charney, D. S., 57
chemical messengers, 63
chemical neurotransmission, 62
child abuse
  identifying, 357
  stress responses, 306
Child and Adolescent Consortium (USA), electroconvulsive therapy studies, 165–66
childhood stress, and melancholia, 306
children
  cognitive-behavior therapy, 245
  of depressed mothers, 305–306
  electroconvulsive therapy, 165–70
    case studies, 168–70
    efficacy, 167, 244
  manic-depressive illness, 245
  marital conflict effects on, 306
  melancholia, 103–104
    comorbidity, 91–93, 103
    pharmacotherapy, 244–50
    prevalence, 103
    prevention, 354–58
    recommendations, 250
    sample heterogeneity, 245–46
  psychotherapy, 244–45
  temperament, 302
Children's Depression Rating Scale-Revised, 248
China, suicide rates, 125
chlordiazepoxide, effectiveness, children and adolescents, 249
chlorpromazine
  drug–drug interactions, 265
  mood disorder treatment studies, 7–8
  in postpartum depression treatment, 36
cholecystokinins (CCKs), roles, 317
chromosome 12, 362
chronic depression, differential diagnosis, 101
chronic fatigue syndrome (CFS), and melancholia, differential diagnosis, 112
chronicity, prevention, 358
chronic renal disease, and depression risk, 111
cimetidine, drug–drug interactions, 265
circadian cycles
  and CLOCK genes, 361–62
  fetus, 356
  and melancholia, 310
citalopram
  and breast-feeding, 243–44
  effectiveness, 203
    children and adolescents, 248
  effects on suicide rates, 141
  heart disease with melancholia treatment, 263, 264
  Parkinson's disease with melancholia treatment, 259
  post-stroke depression treatment, 258
clinical examination, 85–95
  cognition, 90–91
  mood, 87, 441
  personality disorders, 91
  psychomotor functioning, 88
  for psychotic features, 89–90, 441
  strategies, 86–87, 446
  for suicidal thoughts, 90
  for vegatitive signs, 88–89
CLOCK genes, 361
  ethnic and racial differences, 361
  localization, 361
  mutations, 361
clomipramine
  effectiveness, 203
    adolescents, 248
  epilepsy with melancholia treatment, 260
clonidine, in smoking cessation therapy, 256
clozapine, 223–24
  drug–drug interactions, 265
CME (continuing medical education), 352
CNS (central nervous system), 64

cocaine, and depressive mood disorders, 256
cocaine withdrawal
  comorbidity, 109
  and melancholia, differential diagnosis, 109–10
  pharmacotherapy, 256
Cochrane Collaboration, 199, 203
cognition, clinical examination, 90–91
cognitive-behavior therapy (CBT)
  in depression treatment, 218
  effectiveness
    adolescents, 245
    children, 245, 248
  in postpartum depression treatment, 243
cognitive deficits
  in melancholia, 327–28
    studies, 327–28
Colorado (USA), electroconvulsive therapy, adolescents, 165
comas, 30
  see also insulin coma
complications
  melancholic patients
    recommendations, 266–68
consent issues, electroconvulsive therapy, 162, 167
continuing medical education (CME), programs, 352
continuous positive airway pressure (CPAP), 269
convulsive therapy, 6–7
  affective disorder treatment, 155
  early studies, 153–55, 161
  fear of treatment, 183
  manic-depressive illness treatment, early studies, 153–54
  mechanisms, future studies, 353–54
  melancholia, 346
  mood disorder treatment, 154
  see also electroconvulsive therapy (ECT); pentylenetetrazol
Cook, L. C., 153
CORE study, 158, 160, 171, 189
corpus callosum
  reduced volume, 306, 317–18
    and reduced metabolism, 319
corticotropin *see* adrenocorticotropic hormone (ACTH)
corticotropin-releasing factor (CRF), 64
corticotropin-releasing factor-1 receptor antagonists, 363
corticotropin-releasing hormone (CRH)
  and pregnancy, 33
  release, 64
  and stress responses, 309–11
corticotropin-releasing hormone antagonists, 363
cortisol
  assays, 66
  inhibition, 64
  levels
    and abnormal bereavement, 15–36
    and depression, 65, 66
    and premenstrual dysphoric disorder, 102
    and stress, 302
    and pregnancy, 33
  resistance, 311
  suppression, 354
  urinary free, 67
Cotard syndrome
  case studies, 29
  diagnostic criteria, 29
  electroconvulsive therapy, 30
  and psychotic depression, 29–30
CPAP (continuous positive airway pressure), 269
CREB (cyclic AMP response element-binding protein), 362
CRF *see* corticotropin-releasing factor (CRF)
CRH *see* corticotropin-releasing hormone (CRH)
Crohn's disease, and depression, 111
CRS *see* Carroll Rating Scale (CRS)
crying, pathological, 116
Culture and Depression, 51
Cushing's syndrome, 62
  differential diagnosis, 111
  etiology, 111
  and hypercortisolemia, 64
cyclic adenosine monophosphate (cAMP), 360
  abnormalities, 311
cyclic AMP response element-binding protein (CREB), 362
cyclothymia, use of term, 18
cyclothymic disorder, 8–9
CYP2D6 gene, 359
cytokines
  abnormalities, and depression, 63
  in depressed patients, 364
  roles, 363–64

D_2-receptor genes, 362
D_3-receptor genes, 362
Danish University Antidepressant Group, 203
dawn simulation, 285
DeCarolis, V., 157
de Clérambault syndrome, and psychotic depression, 30
delirium
  case studies, 128–29
  electroencephalography, 321
delivery, and postpartum blues, 33
delusional depression
  diagnostic criteria, 25–26
  see also psychotic depression
delusions
  mood-congruent, 26–27
  nihilistic, 29
  see also mood-incongruent delusions
delusions of negation, case studies, 29
dementia
  differential diagnosis, 117–18
  electroencephalography, 321
  with melancholia, pharmacotherapy, 260–61
  see also Alzheimer's disease (AD); pseudodementia

dementia praecox, 4
  and catatonia, 161
  and manic-depressive illness compared, 18–19
  see also schizophrenia
demyelinating disease, differential
    diagnosis, 116
depressed mothers, 305–306
  studies, 354–58
depressed patients
  compliance issues, 358
  cytokines in, 364
  electroencephalography studies, 321–23
  sleep disturbances, 73, 325
  suicide rates, 125
  see also melancholic patients
depression
  anxious, 54–55
  chronic, 101
  classification, 46–51
    future trends, 346–49
    issues, 46–48
  cognitive-behavior therapy, 218
  concept of, expansion, 50
  and cortisol levels, 65, 66
  and Crohn's disease, 111
  delusional, 25–26
  diagnostic criteria, 7, 46–51
    choices, 47
    in clinical practice, 47
    cross-sectional vs longitudinal
      approaches, 55–56
    industry influences, 50–51
    limitations, 48–50
  diagnostic issues, 62
  epidemic, 50–51
  genetic risk factors, 543
  geriatric, 9
  interpersonal therapy, 218
  involutional, 9
  irritable, 54
  and Lyme disease, 111
  and mania, 4, 18
  markers, 63, 66, 77, 325
    neurobiologic, 328
  mild, 51, 54
  non-nuclear, 57
  nuclear, 57
  and pancreatic carcinoma, 111
  post-schizophrenia, 106
  prevalence, 49–50
  psychotherapies, 2
  rating scales, 91–95
  reactive, 3, 8
  relapse, 73
    risk factors, 358
  seizure-related, 117
  sleep electroencephalography studies, 73–74,
      75, 76
  subsyndromal, 46
  superimposed, 106
  and syphilis, 111
  and thyroid-stimulating hormone
      levels, 72
  and thyrotropin-releasing hormone
      levels, 72
  treatment, issues, 47
  twin studies, 49
  use of term, 15
    as buzzword, 51
    Meyer's views, 6
  and vascular disease, 106
  vital, 8
  see also atypical depression; bipolar depression;
      brief depression; depressive mood disorders;
      double depression; endogenomorphic
      depression; endogenous depression;
      major depression; manic depression;
      melancholia; minor depression; neurotic
      depression; non-melancholic depression;
      postpartum depression; post-psychotic
      depression; post-stroke depression;
      prepartum depression; psychotic
      depression; puerperal depression;
      treatment-resistant depression
      (TRD); unipolar depression;
      vascular depression
depression with catatonia or stupor, as severe
    melancholia, 30
Depression Interview and Structured
    Hamilton, 92
depression-like syndromes, and neurologic
    diseases, 113–18
depressive mood disorders, 9
  and alcohol abuse, 255, 301
  and brain injury, 317
  classification issues, 25–26, 346–49
  diagnosis, 24, 85
  differential diagnosis, 5
  elderly, 105
  family studies, 299–01
  genetic factors, 255
  genetic studies, 348
  and lupus erythematosus, 111
  melancholia as, 45, 58
  mild, 46
  misdiagnosis
    case studies, 130
    and suicide risk, 129–30
  and multiple sclerosis, 116
  and nicotine, 256
  non-melancholic, 97
    differential diagnosis, 98–03
  norepinephrine function, Table 14.3, 304
  pathophysiology, 298
  prevention, and sleep, 356–57
  as reactions, 6
  and reward mechanisms, 315
  risk factors, 111
  serotonin function, Table 14.2, 313
  and stress, 129–30
    misdiagnosis, 129
  and stroke, 317
  and substance abuse, 256
  and suicide risk, 125
  threshold model, 56
  treatment

depressive mood disorders (*cont.*)
algorithms, 47–48
issues, 8, 47
twin studies, 301, 303
under-diagnosis, 126–29
clinical ambiguities, 127
studies, 127
unrecognized
case studies, 127, 128–29
suicide risk, 126–29
see also melancholia
depressive reactions, 46
diagnostic criteria, 8
depressive spectrum disease, 19
depressive stupor
electroconvulsive therapy, 161–63
pharmacotherapy, 224–25
desipramine
comparative studies, 199–00
effectiveness, 202–203
alcoholics, 255
melancholia treatment, 211
studies, 202
dexamethasone, 64
in cortisol suppression, 65
dexamethasone/corticotropin-releasing-horm (DEX/CRH) test, 63
applications, 71
sensitivity, 71–72
dexamethasone suppression test (DST), 26
assessment studies, 69–71
children and adolescents, 245
development, 64–65
diagnostic issues, 66–67, 108
as diagnostic screening test, 68–69
and electroconvulsive therapy, 68
outcomes evaluation, 181
limitations, 62, 63, 69, 109
non-suppression, incidence, 69
and Parkinson's disease, 115
and pregnancy, 33
principles, 65–66
prognostic value, 68
re-examination, 63
rejection, 71
schizophrenia diagnosis, 107–108
with sleep electroencephalography, 75
studies, 67–69
meta-analyses, 67
and suicide risk, 68, 138–39
technical issues, 66
validation, 66
DEX/CRH test *see* dexamethasone/ corticotropin-releasing-hormone (DEX/CRH) test
dextroamphetamine, drug augmentation, 216
diabetes, with melancholia, pharmacotherapy, 264–65
Diagnostic and Statistical Manual of Mental Disorders (DSM)
classification issues, future trends, 346–49, 365
cross-sectional approach, criticisms, 55–56
depression, 46–51
choices, 47, 536
classification issues, 46–48
diagnostic criteria limitations, 48–50
future trends, 346–49
limitations, 348
validity issues, 49
melancholia, future trends, 348–49
Diagnostic and Statistical Manual of Mental Disorders (DSM-I) (1952), 6
depressive reactions, 8
Diagnostic and Statistical Manual of Mental Disorders (DSM-II) (1968), 6, 8
criticisms, 8
depression, 7
reliability issues, 8
Diagnostic and Statistical Manual of Mental Disorders (DSM-III) (1980), 8
bipolar disorder, 18
major depression, 18
melancholia, 55
mood-congruence, 26–27
mood disorders, 8
psychotic disorders, 25
Diagnostic and Statistical Manual of Mental Disorders (DSM-IIIR) (1987), 8
mood disorders, 9
Diagnostic and Statistical Manual of Mental Disorders (DSM-IV) (1994)
abnormal bereavement, 23
depressive disorders, criticisms, 103
limitations, 2, 9
mood disorders, 9
psychotic disorders, 25, 106
Diagnostic and Statistical Manual of Mental Disorders (DSM-V), proposals, 9
differential diagnosis, melancholia, 58, 97–18
diphenhydramine, drug–drug interactions, 265
Donovan, S., 141
dopamine dysfunction
and melancholia, 315
postmortem studies, 315
dopaminergic agents, 290
dorsolateral prefrontal cortex, reduced metabolism, 319
dosing issues
antidepressants, 214, 247–48
elderly, 250
double depression, 9, 100
differential diagnosis, 101
treatment resistance, 101
dramatic-emotional personality disorders, comorbidity, 109
Drevets, W. C., 312
drug abuse, and melancholia, pharmacotherapy, 255, 256
drug augmentation
limitations, 216
limitation trials, 214–15
options, 216–17
see also lithium augmentation
drug–drug interactions, 265
elderly, 250
in melancholia treatment, 265, 650

drug metabolism
  and pharmacogenetics, 359–60
  studies, 359
drug overdose, antidepressants, 142–43
drug overuse, and melancholia, differential diagnosis, 110
drug-related depressive-like states, differential diagnosis, 109–10
drugs
  in electroconvulsive therapy, 188
  mood disorder induction, 110, 655
drug-switching
  antidepressants, 213–14, 217–18
  in melancholia treatment, 221
  trials, 214–15
DSM *see Diagnostic and Statistical Manual of Mental Disorders (*DSM)
DSM-I *see Diagnostic and Statistical Manual of Mental Disorders* (DSM-I) (1952)
DSM-II *see Diagnostic and Statistical Manual of Mental Disorders* (DSM-II) (1968)
DSM-III *see Diagnostic and Statistical Manual of Mental Disorders* (DSM-III) (1980)
DSM-IIIR *see Diagnostic and Statistical Manual of Mental Disorders* (DSM-IIIR) (1987)
DSM-IV *see Diagnostic and Statistical Manual of Mental Disorders* (DSM-IV) (1994)
DSM-V *see Diagnostic and Statistical Manual of Mental Disorders* (DSM-V)
DST *see* dexamethasone suppression test (DST)
dysrhythmias, electroencephalography, 321
dysthymia, 8, 46, 97
  classification issues, 347
  diagnostic criteria, 100–101
  differential diagnosis, 100–101
  treatment, 101–10

ECT *see* electroconvulsive therapy (ECT)
ECT Review Group (UK), 156
Edinburgh Postnatal Depression Scale, 94
EEG *see* electroencephalography (EEG)
ego, 6
Einheitspsychose, 4, 35
elderly
  antidepressants, meta-analyses, 200
  cerebrovascular disease, 105
  depressive mood disorders, 105
  dosing issues, 250
  drug–drug interactions, 250
  electroconvulsive therapy, 170–71
    case studies, 170–71
  manic-depressive illness, lithium treatment, 227–28
  melancholia, 104–106
    case studies, 170–71
    comorbidity, 105
    continuation treatment, 254
    maintenance treatment, 254
    mortality rates, 250
    pharmacotherapy, 250–54
    prevalence, 104–105
    recommendations, 254
    risk factors, 105
  pharmacotherapy
    issues, 250–51
    responsiveness, 251
  suicide prevention errors, 126
  and vascular brain disease, 251
  vascular disease, 106
electroconvulsive therapy (ECT)
  adolescents, 165–70
    case studies, 168–70
    efficacy, 165–67, 244
    safety issues, 165
  advantages, 182, 224
  applicability, 156–57
  availability, recommendations, 352
  barriers to, 174
  benefits, 187
  bipolar depression treatment, 172–74
    case studies, 173–74
  and cardiovascular disease, 170
  catatonia treatment, 161–63
    case studies, 162–63
    efficacy, 161
  and characterological conditions, 171–72
  children, 165–70
    case studies, 168–70
    efficacy, 167, 244
  concurrent medications, 188
  consent issues, 162, 167
  continuation
    strategies, 188–90
    studies, 189
  contraindications, 184
  Cotard syndrome treatment, 30
  course design, 187–88
  current, AC vs square wave, 184
  depressive stupor treatment, 161–63
  and dexamethasone suppression test, 68
  early studies, 155
  effective
    achieving, 181–90
    issues, 190
  effective seizures, characterization, 185
  efficacy, 24, 202
    optimal, 354
  elderly, 170–71
    case studies, 170–71
  electrode placement, 184
    bilateral, 184
    right unilateral, 184
  electrode selection, 186
  energy dosing, 186
  epilepsy with melancholia treatment, 260
  failure to administer, and suicide risk, 134
  ineffective, studies, 187–88
  mechanisms, 353–54
    neuroendocrine hypothesis, 353
    neurohumoral theory, 353–54
    neurophysiologic hypotheses, 353
  melancholia treatment, 174, 221
    case studies, 157
    effectiveness, 155–57, 211
    issues, 174

electroconvulsive therapy (ECT) (*cont.*)
mild/moderate melancholia treatment, 230
and neurologic traits, 171–72
case studies, 171–72
outcomes, 181
characteristics, 715, 716
clinical criteria, 182
laboratory tests, 181
patient selection, 181–83
and personality disorders, 172
postpartum depression treatment, 36, 163–65
case studies, 164–65
post-stroke depression treatment, 258
and pregnancy, 163–65
psychosis studies, 25
psychotic depression treatment, 157–59, 223
case studies, 158–59
efficacy, 157, 158
relapse rates, 154, 188–89
remission rates, 181
age differences, 182
issues, 187–88
response issues, 182–83
risk factors, 183, 184
and schizophrenia treatment, 162
seizures
duration, 185
optimization, 185–86
side-effects, minimization, 101–84
stigmatization, 156, 174
and suicide prevention, 132
and suicide risk, 159–61
case studies, 160–61
technical issues, 183–90
training recommendations, 351–52
and transcranial magnetic stimulation compared, 286–87
treatment frequency, 186–87
and treatment-resistant depression, 272–73
unipolar depression treatment, 172–74
vs antidepressants, 156, 157, 158, 161, 188–90
in pregnancy, 164
suicide risk, 159
vs pentylenetetrazol, 154
see also bilateral electroconvulsive therapy (BL-ECT); right unilateral electroconvulsive therapy (RUL-ECT)
electroencephalography (EEG), 63
activated, 323–27
medication induction, 323
advantages, 320
arousal issues, 323
depressed patient studies, 321–23
drug effects, 322
early applications, 321
early studies, 321
in electroconvulsive therapy, 185–86
electrode placement issues, 322
and melancholia, 321
melancholia studies, 72–73
non-activated, 321
see also sleep electroencephalography
electrophysiologic abnormalities, in melancholia, 320–27
electrophysiologic measures, and melancholia, 72–76
emotional incontinence, 116
emotional lability, 116
emotions
expressed, 358
processing, hemispheric differences, 329
regulation, 364
empirical approach
limitations, 52
to syndromes, 52
endocrinology, historical background, 62
endocrinopathies, and melancholia, differential diagnosis, 111
endogenomorphic depression, 9
concept of, 67
endogenous depression, 8
use of term, 54
see also melancholia
endophenotype, 331–32
England and Wales, suicide rates, 126
Enhancing Recovery in Coronary Heart Disease (ENRICHD) trial, 263
environmental factors
genetically influenced, 303
interuterine, 304
in melancholia, 303–307, 332–33
and temperament, 302
epilepsy
case studies, 116–17
differential diagnosis, 116–17
electroencephalography, 321
with melancholia, pharmacotherapy, 260
epinephrine, isolation, 62
episodic memory, impairment, 327
eptapirone, 290
estrogen
effects on serotonin, 307, 313
and melancholia, 307
in melancholia treatment, 291
Euro-Americans, suicide rates, 125, 126
Europe, depression, prevalence, 50
examination (clinical) *see* clinical examination
excitatory amino acids, and melancholia, 316
exorcism, 3
expressed emotions, 358

facial expressions, and mood, 87
Falret, Jean Pierre, 18
on melancholia, 4
familial pure depressive disease, 19
family background, and suicide risk, 135–36
family studies, depressive mood disorders, 299–01
fathers, depressed, and genetic vulnerability, 305–306
Feighner criteria, 51
Feinberg, M., 75

fetus
  circadian cycles, 356
  drug safety issues, 239–40, 243
  intrauterine stress responses, 304
  malformations, 240–41
  sleep and, 356–57
Fink, Max, 7–8
Finland
  depression studies, 354–55
  electroconvulsive therapy, and suicide risk, 159–60
firearms
  access removal, 145
  and suicide, 125–26, 133, 137
    case studies, 133
fluoxetine
  and breast-feeding, 243
  drug–drug interactions, 265
  effectiveness, 202–203, 204
    adolescents, 249
    children, 248
    elderly, 253
  effects on suicide rates, 140, 141
  heart disease with melancholia treatment, 263
  neonatal issues, 241
  and placebo response, 201
  post-stroke depression treatment, 258
  side-effects, 205
  studies, 202
flupenthixol, effects on suicide rates, 140
fluvoxamine
  drug–drug interactions, 265
  effects on suicide rates, 141
folate deficiency, and depression risk, 111
folic acid, in pregnancy, 242
follow-up studies, inadequate, and suicide risk, 132–33
France
  antidepressants, prescription increases, 50
  electroconvulsive therapy studies, 166–67
Freemantle, N., 199–00
Freud, Siegmund, melancholia theories, 6
frontal lobe disease
  differential diagnosis, 113–14, 814
  symptoms, 113–14

GABAergic agents, 290
GAF (Global Assessment of Function), 202
Galen, 3
Ganser syndrome, and psychotic depression, 30
Geddes, J., 203
genetic factors
  alcoholism, 255
  and depression risk, 543
  depressive mood disorders, 255
  manic-depressive illness, 330
  melancholia, 298, 299–03, 331–32, 361
  temperament, 332
  see also heritability
genetic vulnerability, 299–01, 331–32
  depressed fathers, 305–306
  depressed mothers, 305–306
  mechanisms, 362
gepirone, 290
geriatric depression, 9
Geriatric Depression Scale, 94
Germany, St. John's wort studies, 293
Glasgow Depression Scale, 94
Global Assessment of Function (GAF), 202
glucocorticoid receptors (GRs)
  abnormal functioning, 311
  antidepressant effects, 311
  cortisol resistance, 311
  reduced, 310–11
  type I, 308
  type II, 308
glucocorticoids
  adaptive effects, 308–309
  animal studies, 308
  overexposure effects, 309
  roles, 308
  synthetic, 64
glucocorticosteroid receptor agonists, in melancholia treatment, 289–90
glucose metabolism
  and antidepressants, 226
  decrease, 319
  elevated, 318–19
  and sleep, 325
glutamate NMDA, 290
glutamate signaling modifiers, 363
Goodwin, F. K., 19–20
  on antidepressant-induced mania, 22
G-protein, 362
Greenblatt, M., 156
GRs *see* glucocorticoid receptors (GRs)
Gunnell, D., 141–42
guns *see* firearms

Hadzi-Pavlovic, D., 25–26, 53
hallucinations, 89
haloperidol, with amitriptyline, 224
HAMD *see* Hamilton Rating Scale for Depression (HRSD)
Hamilton Rating Scale for Depression (HRSD), 91–93, 137, 171
  applications, 94–95
  in electroconvulsive therapy studies, 158, 160, 165, 171
  limitations, 92
  shorter versions, 93, 847
Harris, Geoffrey, 62
Haslam, John, on melancholia, 4
HD *see* Huntington's disease (HD)
health professionals
  accreditation, 351
  education
    electroconvulsive therapy training, 351–52
    in mood disorders, 351–52
heart disease
  with melancholia
    mortality rates, 262

heart disease (*cont.*)
pharmacotherapy, 262–64
see also cardiovascular disease
heart failure, risks, 262
hemispheres
emotion-processing, 329
specialization, approach–withdrawal theories, 322
hemispheric instability, and manic-depressive illness, 329–30
hemispheric sleep phase coherence, 326
sex differences, 326
herbal remedies, for melancholia, 292–94
heritability
estimates, 300
melancholia, 346
neurogenesis, 363
and temperament, 302
see also genetic factors
Hickie, I., 202
Hill, Sir John Denis Nelson, 5–6
hippocampus, neurogenesis, 363
Hippocrates, on melancholia, 2–3
histrionic personality disorder, 98
Hoch, August, case studies, 32
homeostatic functions, perturbations, 88–89
HOPA gene, polymorphisms, 362
Hopewell-Ash, Edwin Lancelot
on melancholia, 5
Melancholia in Everyday Practice (1934), 16, 17
hormonal changes
during pregnancy, 33
and puerperal psychosis, 36
hormones
imbalance, 111
and melancholia, 306–307
in melancholia treatment, 291–92
systemic effects, 63
therapeutic replacement, 62
see also adrenocorticotropic hormone (ACTH); corticotropin-releasing hormone (CRH); thyroid-stimulating hormone (TSH); thyrotropin-releasing hormone (TRH)
hospitalization
failure
case studies, 133
and suicide risk, 133–34
suicidal melancholic patients, 143–45
guidelines, 143
indications, 143
and suicide risk, 135, 143–44
HPA axis *see* hypothalamic–pituitary–adrenal (HPA) axis
HPGH (hypothalamic–pituitary–growth hormone) system, 63
HPT axis *see* hypothalamic–pituitary–thyroid (HPT) axis
HRSD *see* Hamilton Rating Scale for Depression (HRSD)
5-HT_{1A} (5-β-hydroxytryptamine receptor 1) agonists, 290
5-HT2A receptor gene, 359–60
5-HT *see* serotonin
5-HTT gene, 303
Huntington's disease (HD)
differential diagnosis, 115–16
with melancholia, pharmacotherapy, 259–60
Huston, P. E., 155
17-hydroxycorticosteroids, and mood disorders, 64
5-hydroxytryptamine (5-HT) *see* serotonin
5-β-hydroxytryptamine receptor 1 (5-HT_{1A}) agonists, 290
5-hydroxytryptamine receptors, 5HT_{1A}, 310–11
hyperadrenalism, and insomnia, 62
hypercortisolemia, 64
as depression marker, 66, 77
hyperglycemia, 264
hypericum, in melancholia treatment, 292–93
hyperparathyroidism
differential diagnosis, 111
etiology, 111
hypnotics, and fetal safety, 239–40
hypomania, 21
hypothalamic hormones, in electroconvulsive therapy evaluation, 186
hypothalamic–pituitary–adrenal (HPA) axis, 63
abnormalities, 298
diagnostic issues, 66–67, 78
hyperactivity, 219
and melancholia, 64–72
overactivity, 364
and stress response, 307–308, 363
mechanisms, 311
suppression, 65
targeting, 363
use of term, 64
hypothalamic–pituitary–growth hormone (HPGH) system, 63
hypothalamic–pituitary–thyroid (HPT) axis, 63
evaluation, 72
functions, 72
and melancholia, 72
hypothalamus
as biological clock, 356
and stress responses, 309
hypothyroidism
comorbidity, 72
with melancholia, pharmacotherapy, 265
hysteroid dysphoria, 98–99

ICD-8 *see* International Classification of Diseases (ICD-8)
ICD-10 *see* International Classification of Diseases (ICD-10)
id, 6
imipramine, 50
drug-switching, 214
effectiveness
alcoholics, 255
children, 246, 247, 248

effects on electroconvulsive therapy, 188–89
and electroconvulsive therapy compared, 157
manic-depressive illness treatment, 227
melancholia treatment, 211
mood disorder treatment studies, 7–8
psychosis studies, 25
severe melancholia treatment, 230
immune response system, and melancholia, 363–64
implicit memory, 327
inflammatory markers
abnormalities, 63
and depression, 63
inflammatory response, 363–64
inpatient care, suicidal melancholic patients, 143–45
insanity
circular, 4
classification, 3–4
insomnia, and hyperadrenalism, 62
insulin, discovery, 62
insulin coma, 6–7
treatment, 62
International Classification of Diseases (ICD-8), 55
psychotic disorders, 106
reliability issues, 8
International Classification of Diseases (ICD-10)
limitations, 2
melancholia, 26
interpersonal therapy, in depression treatment, 218
inter-rater reliability, 200
interuterine factors, 304
involuntary commitment
and suicide risk, 133–34
case studies, 133
involutional depression, 9
iproniazid, 50
irritable depression, 54

Jamison, K. R., 19–20
on antidepressant-induced mania, 22
Japan, depression, epidemic, 50–51
Johns Hopkins Hospital (USA), Henry Phipps Psychiatric Clinic, 154–55
Journal of the American Medical Association, The, 198

Kahlbaum, Karl, 18
catatonia
case studies, 30–31
research, 30
Kalinowsky, L. B., 155
kava, side-effects, 294
Kayser–Fleischer rings, 116
Kendell, R. E., 53
on structured interviews, 85
two depression factors, 53, 54–55
Kendler, K. S., 27, 300
ketoconazole, in melancholia treatment, 290
Kirsch, I., 199
Klein, D. F., 7–8, 98–99
Kleinman, Arthur, 51
Kraepelin, Emil
on manic-depressive illness, 18–19
melancholia theories, 4–5
criticisms, 6

laboratory tests, and melancholia defined, 62–78
lamotrigine, 225, 290
manic-depressive illness treatment, 229
severe melancholia treatment, 230
late-life depression *see* vascular depression
laughing, pathological, 116
left hippocampal cortex, reduced metabolism, 319
Leonhard, Karl, 23
manic-depressive illness theories, 19
lesopitron, 290
leucotomy, 6–7
Levinson, D. F., 300
Lewis, Aubrey, on melancholia, 5
lidocaine, effects on seizure, 188
light therapy (LT), 362
dawn simulation, 285
melancholia, 284–85
Linnaeus, Carolus, 1
lithium, 50
effects on electroconvulsive therapy, 189
effects on suicide rates, 139–40
efficacy, 23, 24
in electroconvulsive therapy, 188, 189–90
manic-depressive illness treatment, 227
in melancholia treatment, 211
mild/moderate melancholia treatment, 230
neonatal issues, 242
severe melancholia treatment, 230
lithium augmentation, 215–16
dose–response characteristics, 215
effectiveness, 215–16
in melancholia treatment, 220–21
side-effects, 216
Locher, L. M., 155
Loewi, Otto, 62
London, Bethlem Hospital, 4
lorazepam
in catatonia diagnosis, 31
in catatonia treatment, 225
LT *see* light therapy (LT)
lupus erythematosus, and depressive mood disorders, 111
Lyme disease, and depression, 111

MADRS (Montgomery–Asberg Depression Rating Scale), 93
magnetic resonance imaging (MRI)
in catatonia diagnosis, 31
cerebrovascular disease studies, 105
in epilepsy studies, 117
magnetic seizure therapy (MST)
in melancholia treatment, 288
safety issues, 288

major depression, 3, 9
  case studies, 48–49
  comorbidity, 301
  diagnostic criteria, 8, 18, 48–49
  non-melancholic, 97
    differential diagnosis, 99–00
  treatment, issues, 51
major depression superimposed upon delusional disorder, 46
  see also schizophrenia
major depressive disorder, 9
  studies, 21
malarial fevers, 6–7
males, over 50 years of age, suicide risk, 136–37
malignant catatonia (MC), electroconvulsive therapy, 161
mania
  antidepressant-induced, 22–23
    incidence, 22
  classification issues, 347
  and depression, 4, 18
  early studies, 19
  and insanity, 3–4
  Kraepelin's theories, 5
  use of term, 4
manic depression, 4
  case studies, 32
  and Cotard syndrome, 29
manic-depressive illness, 18–24, 46
  adolescents, 245
  antidepressant treatment, 226–27
  and cerebral hemispheric instability, 329–30
  children, 245
  convulsive therapy, early studies, 153–54
  and dementia praecox compared, 18–19
  early studies, 173
  electroconvulsive therapy, 172–74
  genetic factors, 330
  neurobiologic markers, 328
  pharmacotherapy, 225
    mood switch risk, 225–26
  and recurrent depressive illness, 23, 301
  sensitization model, 328
  singularity, 21
  suicide in, 136
  theories
    Kraepelin's, 18–19
    Leonhard's, 19
  twin studies, 330
  see also bipolar disorders
manic episodes, in melancholia, 299, 328–30
manisch-depressive Irresein, 4
MAOIs *see* monoamine oxidase inhibitors (MAOIs)
maprotiline, epilepsy with melancholia treatment, 260
marital conflict, effects on children, 306
maternal care, 305–306
Maudsley Hospital (UK), 53
Mayo Clinic (USA), electroconvulsive therapy studies, 166
MC (malignant catatonia), 161
Mecholyl (methacholine) test, 181
Medicaid (USA), 270
medical illness
  and melancholia, 110–12
  with melancholia, pharmacotherapy, 261–65
  and suicide risk, 137–38
medical practitioners *see* health professionals
medications *see* drugs
Medline
  melancholia citations, 47
  trials data, 350
Meduna, Ladislas, 153
melancholia
  and abnormal bereavement, 36–37, 46, 97
  abnormal brain metabolism, 318–20, 332, 343
  abnormal brain structure, 317–18, 329, 346
  abnormal neurochemical functioning, 311–17
  in adolescents, 103–104
    pharmacotherapy, 244–50
    recommendations, 250
  with agitation, suicide risk assessment, 135–36
  and alcohol abuse, 108–109
    pharmacotherapy, 155–55, 256
  with anxiety, suicide risk assessment, 135–36
  with Asperger syndrome, 104
  with autism, 104
  behavioral characteristics, Table 3.4
  biological studies, issues, 299
  case studies, 16–18
    early, 16, 17
  and catatonia, 30, 32, 97
  characteristics, 15–16, 982, 346, 348
  and childhood stress, 306
  in children, 103–104
    pharmacotherapy, 244–50
    prevention, 354–58
    recommendations, 250
  and circadian cycles, 310
  classification, 16
    future trends, 346–49
    issues, 45
    simplified, 348
  clinical examination, 85–95
    strategies, 86–87, 446
  and cognition, 90–91
  cognitive deficits, 327–28
    studies, 327–28
  comorbidity
    children and adolescents, 91–93, 103
    elderly, 105
  concept of, 5
    criticisms, 53
    distinct, 51, 58
    origins, 2–9
  conceptual history, 9
  convulsive therapy, 346
  criteria, and psychotic depression, 27–29
  defined, 15–37
    by laboratory tests, 62–78
    by psychopathology, 59
    by specific event, 32–36
  definitions, 15, 97
    early, 15

as depressive disorder, 45, 58
diagnostic criteria, 62–78, 298
 future trends, 348–49
 proposals, 348–49
diagnostic issues, 155
differential diagnosis, 58, 97–18
and dopamine dysfunction, 315
and drug abuse, pharmacotherapy, 255, 256
and drug-related depressive-like states, 109–10
early studies, 5
in elderly, 104–106
 case studies, 253–54
 pharmacotherapy, 250–54
 recommendations, 254
electroconvulsive therapy, 174, 221
 case studies, 157
 effectiveness, 155–57, 211
 issues, 174
 outcomes, 181
and electroencephalography, 321
electroencephalography studies, 72–73
electrophysiologic abnormalities, 320–27
electrophysiologic measures, 72–76
environmental factors, 303–307, 332–33
 genetically influenced, 303
and estrogen, 307
and excitatory amino acids, 316
first episode, 358
future trends, 365
genetic factors, 298, 299–03, 331–32, 361
 vulnerability, 299–01
glucocorticosteroid receptor agonist treatment, 289–90
herbal remedies, 292–94
heritability, 346
historical perceptions, 45–46
histories, 2
and hormones, 306–307
hormone therapy, 291–92
and hypothalamic–pituitary–adrenal axis, 64–72
and hypothalamic–pituitary–thyroid axis, 72
and immune response system, 363–64
and insanity, 3–4
involutional, 4
light therapy, 284–85
magnetic seizure therapy, 288
manic episodes, 299, 328–30
with medical illness, 110–12
 pharmacotherapy, 261–65
Medline citations, 47
motor issues, 25–26
nature of, 56–57
neuroendocrine tests, 77–78
with neurologic diseases, pharmacotherapy, 257–61
and neuropeptides, 316–17
and neurotrophic abnormalities, 316
and noradrenergic dysfunction, 313–14
observable features, 441
and pain, 112
paradigms, 58–59
pathophysiology, 298–33
 future trends, 360–64
with personality disorders, pharmacotherapy, 265–66
and personality traits, 91
pharmacotherapy, 220–22, 346
 acute treatment, 220–21
 drug–drug interactions, 265, 650
 drug-switching, 221
 historical background, 196
 inpatient vs outpatient settings, 212
 long-term treatment, 211, 221–22
 randomized controlled trials, 196
 treatment recommendations, 229–30
pharmacotherapy literature, validity, 196–07
postmortem studies, 310, 317–18
in pregnancy
 case studies, 240
 neonatal issues, 241–42
 pharmacotherapy, 239–44
 prevention, 355–56
prevalence
 children and adolescents, 103
 elderly, 104–105
 early, 354–58
 future, 354–58
 and sleep, 356–57
and pseudodementia, 90
in psychiatric classification, 7–9
and psychomotor disturbance, 55, 57, 88
psychopathological validity, 53–56
 post-1980 literature, 54–56
 pre-1980 literature, 53–54
and psychosis, 16, 55
and psychotherapy, 218–19
and psychotic depression, 24–30, 97
with psychotic disorders, 106–108
 suicide risk assessment, 135–36
and puerperal depression, 36, 97
recognition, 348
remission, 181
 goals, 349–50
reviews, 2
and schizophrenia, differential diagnosis, 106–108
and serotonin dysfunction, 312–13
and sleep apnea, 112, 269
and sleep disturbances, 269
sleep electroencephalography studies, 73–76, 325–26
stress responses
 abnormal, 307–11
 genetically influenced, 303
 mechanisms, 311
subtypes, 97
suicide in, 125–45
as syndrome, 58
targeted neurotransmitter system agent treatment, 290
temperamental risk factors, 302
theories

melancholia (*cont.*)
    Freud's, 6
    Kraepelin's, 4–5
  transcranial magnetic stimulation, 286–88
  treatment
    algorithms, 348, 364–65
    options, 346
    proposals, 284–94
  treatment trials, recommendations, 350
  tricyclic antidepressant treatment, 206–207
  and triiodothyronine, 307
  use of term, 1, 4
    advantages, 2, 16
    historical background, 45
    Meyer's views, 6
  vagal nerve stimulation, 289
  vs psychodynamic theories, 6–7
  see also depression; endogenous depression; mild/moderate melancholia; severe melancholia
melancholia with psychosis *see* psychotic depression
melancholic patients
  cognitive deficits, 327–28
  compliance issues, 358
  memory deficits, 327
  pharmacotherapy, 211–30
    acute treatment, 211–19
    augmentation limitation, 214–15
    continuation treatment, 211, 219–20, 254
    drug-switching trials, 214–15
    issues, 211
    lithium augmentation, 215–16
    maintenance treatment, 219–20, 254
    with psychotherapy, 218–19
    rapid response, 212–14
    recommendations, 266–68
    relapse rates, 219–20
    treatment recommendations, 229–30
    treatment resistance, 212–13
  psychotherapy, with pharmacotherapy, 218–19
  see also depressed patients; suicidal melancholic patients
melancholy, definitions, 15
memory deficits, melancholic patients, 327
men, over 50 years of age, suicide risk, 136–37
Mendel, Gregor Johann, 1
mental disorders
  natural vs unnatural, 3
  and witchcraft, 3
metabolism
  stress effects on, 62–63
  see also brain metabolism; drug metabolism; glucose metabolism
methacholine test, 181
N-methyl-D-aspartate (NMDA), 363
  binding, 316
methylphenidate, drug augmentation, 216
Metrazol *see* pentylenetetrazol
Mexicans, suicide rates, 126
Meyer, Adolf, 16
  on depressive disorders, 6
mianserin, effects on suicide rates, 140
mice, stress response studies, 303
mifepristone, in melancholia treatment, 289–90
mild depression, 51, 54
mild/moderate melancholia
  electroconvulsive therapy, 230
  treatment recommendations, 229–30
Miller, F. T., 202
Mini-Mental State Examination (MMSE), 91, 252
minor depression, 46
  classification issues, 347–48
  differential diagnosis, 101
mirtazapine
  effectiveness, 204
  melancholia treatment, 211
  overdose, 142
MMSE (Mini-Mental State Examination), 91, 252
moclobemide, 290
  effectiveness, elderly, 254
  manic-depressive illness treatment, 227
monoamine deficit theory, 312
monoamine oxidase inhibitors (MAOIs)
  approved, 50
  atypical depression treatment, 99
  drug augmentation, 217
  effectiveness, 202
    children and adolescents, 249
    elderly, 254
  and electroconvulsive therapy compared, 156
  mania induction, 22
  manic-depressive illness treatment, 226
  overdose, lethality, 142–43
Montgomery–Asberg Depression Rating Scale (MADRS), 93
mood
  clinical examination, 87
  and facial expressions, 87
  screening questions, 87
  and sleep deprivation, 326–27
mood-congruence, of psychotic thoughts, 26–27
mood-congruent delusions, 26–27
mood disorder due to a general medical condition, 46
mood disorders
  classification, 1–2, 9, 18
    by treatment, 5–6
    issues, 347, 365
    simplification, 9
  convulsive therapy, 154
  diagnostic criteria, 8
  dichotomy issues, 21
  drug-induced, 655
  health professional education, 351–52
  neuroendocrine tests, 62–63
  not otherwise specified, 46
  pregnancy-related, 33–36
  psychotic, 25
  sensory evoked potentials studies, 324

treatment, early, 357–58
see also adjustment disorder with depressed mood; depressive mood disorders; puerperal mood disorders
mood-incongruent delusions, 26–27
as mood disorders, 27
reviews, 27
studies, 27
mood quality, and melancholia, 348
mood stabilizers, 23, 227–29
drug–drug interactions, 265
neonatal issues, 242–43
severe melancholia treatment, 230
mothers
psychotic, studies, 354
see also depressed mothers
MRI *see* magnetic resonance imaging (MRI)
MST *see* magnetic seizure therapy (MST)
multiple sclerosis (MS), and depressive mood disorders, 116
Myerson, A., 154
myxedema, 62

naltrexone, in alcoholism treatment, 255
National Comorbidity Survey (USA), 300
National Institute of Mental Health (NIMH) (USA)
antidepressant guidelines, 196
depression studies, 56–57
electroconvulsive therapy studies, 173
and STEP-BD algorithm, 23
NE *see* norepinephrine (NE)
NEDDI (Newcastle Endogenous Depression Diagnostic Index), 94
nefazodone
effectiveness, 205, 224
side-effects, 205–206
Nelson, J. C., 57
neonates
issues, 241–42
premature, 304
risk factors, 304
Netherlands, The, depression studies, 55
neurobiologic markers, of manic-depressive illness, 328
neurochemical functioning, abnormal, in melancholia, 311–17
neurocognitive abnormalities, 26
neuroendocrine abnormalities, 26
as markers
limitations, 63
re-examination, 63
and sleep electroencephalography studies, 63
neuroendocrine hypothesis, 353
neuroendocrine tests, 24
advantages, 77–78
as melancholia indices, 348
in mood disorders, 62–63
neuroendocrine variables, and sleep variables, 74–75
neurogenesis
heritability, 363
in hippocampus, 363
neurohumoral theory, 353–54
neuroleptic malignant syndrome (NMS)
differential diagnosis, 161–62
electroconvulsive therapy, 162
neurologic diseases
and apathetic syndromes, 113–18
and depression-like syndromes, 113–18
with melancholia, pharmacotherapy, 257–61
neurologic illness, and suicide risk, 137–38
neurologic traits
and electroconvulsive therapy, 171–72
case studies, 171–72
neuropeptides, and melancholia, 316–17
neuropeptide Y, roles, 317
neurophysiologic hypotheses, 353
neuroplasticity
abnormal, animal studies, 314–15
enhancement, 362–63
impairment, 362
neurosyphilis, 1
neurotic depression, 8
Kendell's studies, 53
neurotoxic effects
prevention, 363
reduction, 362–63
neurotrophic abnormalities, and melancholia, 316
newborn *see* neonates
Newcastle Endogenous Depression Diagnostic Index (NEDDI), 94
New England Journal of Medicine, The, 198
New Jersey Medicare (USA), 224
New York City (USA)
electroconvulsive therapy
services, 351–52
studies, 187
nicotine, and depressive mood disorders, 256
NIMH *see* National Institute of Mental Health (NIMH) (USA)
NMDA *see* *N*-methyl-D-aspartate (NMDA)
NMS *see* neuroleptic malignant syndrome (NMS)
non-melancholic depression, 54
diagnostic criteria, 25–26
differential diagnosis, 98–03
non-psychotic depression, differential diagnosis, 26
non-psychotic melancholia, diagnostic criteria, 25–26
non-tricyclic antidepressants, vs selective serotonin reuptake inhibitors, 204–206
noradrenergic agents, 290
noradrenergic dysfunction
animal studies, 314
and melancholia, 313–14
norepinephrine (NE)
dysfunction, and melancholia, 313–14
effects on glucocorticoid receptor functioning, 311
function, in depressive mood disorders, 313–14
norepinephrine–serotonin interactions, 314–15
nortriptyline
comparative studies, 199–00

nortriptyline (*cont.*)
effectiveness, 203, 204, 313
children, 246
elderly, 251, 252, 253
effects on electroconvulsive therapy, 189
in electroconvulsive therapy, 189–90
heart disease with melancholia treatment, 262–63, 264
in melancholia treatment, 211, 221
with perphenazine, 224
post-stroke depression treatment, 258
studies, 202
NREM sleep
and glucose metabolism, 325
studies, 76

obsessive-compulsive disorder (OCD), differential diagnosis, 108
olanzapine, 225
drug augmentation, 217
drug–drug interactions, 265
Huntington's disease with melancholia treatment, 260
side-effects, 223–24
olanzapine-fluoxetine, 23
omega-3 fatty acids, in melancholia treatment, 293
oneiroid states, 107
oneirophrenia, 34
orbital cortex, volume reduction, 318
organic solvent abuse, and melancholia, differential diagnosis, 110
Othello syndrome, and psychotic depression, 30
outpatients
inadequate follow-up
case studies, 133
and suicide risk, 132–33
suicidal melancholic patients, 144–45
over-the-counter drugs, and melancholia, differential diagnosis, 110

pain, and melancholia, 112
pancreatic carcinoma, and depression, 111
parenting issues, 305–306
Parker, G., 25–26, 53, 68, 199, 202
Parkinson's disease (PD)
comorbidity, 115
and dexamethasone suppression test, 115
differential diagnosis, 115
with melancholia, pharmacotherapy, 258–59
paroxetine
drug–drug interactions, 250
effectiveness, 203
adolescents, 248
children, 248
effects on electroconvulsive therapy, 188–89
effects on suicide rates, 140, 141
studies, 141
heart disease with melancholia treatment, 262–63, 264
Parkinson's disease with melancholia treatment, 259
severe melancholia treatment, 230
side-effects, 205
paternal modulation, 305–306
pathological mood, definition, 15
patient non-compliance, 220
prevention strategies, 358
patient selection, for electroconvulsive therapy, 181–83
Paxil, usage, 50–51
Paykel, E. S., 53–54
pCREB (phosphorylated cyclic AMP response element-binding protein), 360
PD *see* Parkinson's disease (PD)
PDD *see* premenstrual dysphoric disorder (PDD)
pentylenetetrazol, 153
affective disorder treatment, 155
early studies, 153–55
seizure induction, 161
vs electroconvulsive therapy, 154
perphenazine, with nortriptyline, 224
Perris, C., 23
personality disorders
borderline, 99
clinical examination, 91
and depression diagnosis, 55–56
dramatic-emotional, 109
and electroconvulsive therapy, 172
histrionic, 98
with melancholia, pharmacotherapy, 265–66
premorbid, 265–66
personality traits
and melancholia, 91
see also temperament
pharmaceutical industry
conflict-of-interest issues, 198
recommendations, 350–51
influences, and novel antidepressants, 197–99
and sponsor roles, 198
treatment efficacy standards, 199
recommendations, 350–51
pharmacogenetics, future trends, 359–60
pharmacotherapy
future research standards, 349–51
inadequate
case studies, 132
and suicide risk, 132, 141
for melancholic patients, 211–30
in complicating circumstances, 465
with psychotherapy, 218–19
pharmacotherapy literature, in melancholia, validity, 196–07
phenelzine, 50
effectiveness, children and adolescents, 249
phenytoin, drug–drug interactions, 265
phosphorylated cyclic AMP response element-binding protein (pCREB), 360
pindolol, drug augmentation, 216
pituitary gland, hypothalamic control, 62
PKA (protein kinase A), 360
Plutarch, on melancholia, 3
post-concussion syndrome, symptoms, 115
posterior orbital cortex, increased metabolism, 319–20

posterior ventrolateral prefrontal cortex, volume reduction, 318
postpartum blues, 33
postpartum depression, 9, 46
antidepressant treatment, 163
electroconvulsive therapy, 36, 163–65
case studies, 164–65
incidence, 33
light therapy, 285
and melancholia, 46
pharmacotherapy, 243
psychotherapy, 243
risk factors, 35–36
treatment outcomes, 36
postpartum non-psychotic melancholia, definition, 34
post-psychotic depression, 46
diagnostic criteria, 106
post-schizophrenia depression, diagnostic criteria, 106
post-stroke depression
pharmacotherapy, 257–58
post-traumatic stress disorder (PTSD), case studies, 130
prednisolone, 64
pregnancy
and electroconvulsive therapy, 163–65
fetal monitoring, 164
vs antidepressants, 164
hormonal changes, 33
melancholia in
case studies, 240
neonatal issues, 241–42
pharmacotherapy, 239–44
prevention, 355–56
treatment-withholding effects, 240
and mood disorders, 33–36
premature births, 304
premenstrual dysphoric disorder (PDD), 46
comorbidity, 102
differential diagnosis, 102–103
etiology, 102
inheritance, 102
treatment, 103
twin studies, 102
prepartum depression
light therapy, 285
psychotherapy, 243
risks, 240
prescription drugs, and melancholia, differential diagnosis, 110
Preskorn, S. H., 202
procylidine, mood disorder treatment studies, 7–8
progesterone
decrease, 36
effects on serotonin, 313
in melancholia treatment, 291–92
protein kinase A (PKA), responses, 360
Protheroe, C., 34
protriptyline, melancholia treatment, 211
pseudodementia
and Alzheimer's disease, 261
differential diagnosis, 118, 158
and melancholia, 90
use of term, 90
Psychiatric Annals, 2
psychiatric disorders
causes, single vs many, 4
diagnostic issues, 62
psychoactive drugs
drug–drug interactions, 265
studies, 197
psychodynamic theories, vs melancholia, 6–7
psychoeducation, 23
see also psychotherapy
psychological autopsies, 126
psychomotor disturbance
definition, 16
factors, 57
and melancholia, 55, 57, 88, 348
psychomotor functioning, clinical examination, 88
psychomotor retardation, 53, 55, 57
psychopathology
and melancholia
defined, 59
validity, 53–56
psychosis, 8
case studies, 32
detection issues, 25
diagnostic criteria 25
and melancholia, 16, 55, 348
and schizophrenia, 25
see also puerperal psychosis
psychotherapy
adolescents, 244–45
children, 244–45
effects on suicide rates, 140
and melancholia, 218–19
with pharmacotherapy, 218–19
postpartum depression, 243
prepartum depression, 243
psychoeducation, 23
psychotic depression, 8, 46, 54
antidepressant/antipsychotic treatment, 223–24
case studies, 28–29, 89–90, 223
classification issues, 347
comorbidity, 30
and Cotard syndrome, 29–30
diagnostic criteria, 25–26
differential diagnosis, 26, 97–08
electroconvulsive therapy, 157–59, 223
case studies, 158–59
efficacy, 157, 158
historical background, 24–26
Kendell's studies, 53
and melancholia, 24–30, 97
criteria, 27–29
mortality rates, 222
pharmacotherapy, 222–23
relapse rates, 26
studies, 26
suicide rates, 223
and suicide risk, 89
treatment, 108

psychotic disorders
  classification, 106
    issues, 25
  clinical examination, 89–90
  diagnostic criteria, 25
  with melancholia, 106–108
    suicide risk assessment, 135–36
  prevention, 354
psychotic mood disorder, classification issues, 25
psychotic thoughts, mood-congruence, 26–27
psychotropic drugs
  and breast-feeding, 243–44
  and fetal safety, 239–40, 243
PTSD (post-traumatic stress disorder), 243
puberty, biological differences, 245–46
puerperal depression, 33–36
  case studies, 34
  classification issues, 35, 206
  incidence, 35
  and melancholia, 36, 97
puerperal mood disorders
  and melancholia, 36
  prevention, 357
puerperal psychosis, 34
  and hormonal changes, 36
puerperal psychotic depression, diagnostic criteria, 33–34
Puerto Ricans, suicide rates, 126

quetiapine, 224
Quitkin, F. M., 98–99

R121919, 363
rapid cycling, 8–9
rating scales, 91
  applications, 94–95
  of depression, 91–95
  and diagnostic criteria, 85
  limitations, 85–86
RDC *see* Research Diagnostic Criteria (RDC)
reactive depression, 3, 8
recurrent depressive illness, and manic-depressive illness, 23, 301
remacemide, 290
REM latency, 73, 205
  as depression marker, 74, 325
  shortened, 326
  and suicide risk, 138
Research Diagnostic Criteria (RDC), 8, 51
  depression studies, 55
retardation
  and melancholia, 45–46
  psychomotor, 53, 55, 57
  symptoms, 16
reward mechanisms
  and depressive mood disorders, 315
  potentiation, 315
rheumatoid arthritis, and depression risk, 111
right unilateral electroconvulsive therapy (RUL-ECT), 184
  and bilateral electroconvulsive therapy compared, 184
  disadvantages, 184
  energy dosing, 186
risperidone
  drug augmentation, 217
  drug–drug interactions, 265
  effectiveness, 224
risperidone/fluvoxamine, 217
Rotterdam (Netherlands), 35
RU486 (mifepristone), 289–90
RUL-ECT *see* right unilateral electroconvulsive therapy (RUL-ECT)
Rush, A. J., 57

SAD *see* seasonal affective disorder (SAD)
SADHEART (Sertraline Antidepressant Heart Attack Randomized Trial), 263–64
SADS *see* Schedule for Affective Disorders and Schizophrenia (SADS)
St. John's wort
  in melancholia treatment, 292–93
  side-effects, 293
Schedule for Affective Disorders and Schizophrenia (SADS), 50
  depression studies, 55, 56–57
schizoaffective disorders, 25
schizophrenia, 46
  and dexamethasone suppression test, 107–108
  diagnostic criteria, 25
  early studies, 24–25
  and electroconvulsive therapy, 162
  and melancholia, differential diagnosis, 106–108
  and psychosis, 25
  symptoms, 106–107
  transatlantic differences, 25
  see also dementia praecox
SCN (suprachiasmatic nucleus), 356
seasonal affective disorder (SAD), 97
  comorbidity, 99
  concept of, 99–00
  diagnostic criteria, 100
  differential diagnosis, 99–00
  genetic factors, 361
  light therapy, 284–85
seasonal disorders, 9, 46
seizures
  drug effects on, 188
  electroencephalography, 321
  pentylenetetrazol-induced, 161
selective serotonin reuptake inhibitors (SSRIs), 50
  development, 312
  effectiveness, 202, 312
    children and adolescents, 244, 248–49
    elderly, 253–54
    issues, 312–13
  effects on sleep, 357
  effects on suicide rates, 140, 141
    studies, 141–42
  and electroconvulsive therapy compared, 156
  limitations, 197
  manic-depressive illness treatment, 226
  neonatal issues, 241–42
  overdose, lethality, 142–43

Parkinson's disease with melancholia treatment, 259
and placebo response, 201
vs non-tricyclic antidepressants, 204–206
vs tricyclic antidepressants, 196, 198–00, 201–204, 206–207
selegiline, Parkinson's disease with melancholia treatment, 259
Selye, Hans, 62–63
sensitization model, of manic-depressive illness, 328
sensory evoked potentials (SEPs), 323–26
mood disorder studies, 324
serotonin
dysfunction, and melancholia, 312–13
estrogen effects on, 307, 313
function
animal studies, 313–12
in depressive mood disorders, 312–13
levels, and suicide risk, 138
serotonin reuptake transporter (SERT), 359–60
sertraline
and breast-feeding, 244
drug-switching, 214
effectiveness, 204
adolescents, 248
children, 248
elderly, 251, 253
effects on suicide rates, 141
heart disease with melancholia treatment, 263–64
mania induction, 23
Parkinson's disease with melancholia treatment, 258–59
post-stroke depression treatment, 258
studies, 202
Sertraline Antidepressant Heart Attack Randomized Trial (SADHEART), 263–64
SERT (serotonin reuptake transporter), 359–60
serum prolactin, in electroconvulsive therapy evaluation, 186
severe melancholia
abnormal brain structure, 320
depression with catatonia or stupor as, 30
pharmacotherapy, 222–29
treatment recommendations, 230
sex differences
sleep electroencephalography, 76
suicide rates, 125
SFBN (Stanley Foundation Bipolar Network), 22–23
signal transduction, abnormalities, 360
single photon emission computed tomography (SPECT), 117
sleep
and fetal development, 356–57
and melancholia prevention, 356–57
sleep apnea
and melancholia, 112, 269
symptoms, 112
sleep deprivation, and mood, 326–27
sleep disturbances
depressed patients, 73, 325–27
drug-induced, 205–206
and melancholia, 269
and relapse, 73
and sleep electroencephalography, 326
and suicide risk, 138
see also hemispheric sleep phase coherence
sleep electroencephalography
advantages, 78, 320
depression studies, 73–74, 76
sex differences, 76
with dexamethasone suppression test, 75
discriminant index scores, 73
hemisphere coherence, 76
as melancholia indices, 348
melancholia studies, 73–76, 325–26
and neuroendocrine abnormalities, 63
and sleep disturbances, 326
sleep laboratory tests, 24
sleep variables, and neuroendocrine variables, 74–75
smoking cessation, strategies, 256
solvent abuse, and melancholia, differential diagnosis, 110
SPECT (single photon emission computed tomography), 117
sporadic pure depressive disease, 19
SSRIs *see* selective serotonin reuptake inhibitors (SSRIs)
Stanley Foundation Bipolar Network (SFBN), 22–23
STEP-BD algorithm, 23
stimulants
drug augmentation, 216
post-stroke depression treatment, 258
stress
childhood, 306
cycles of, 332–33
and depressive mood disorders, 129–30
misdiagnosis, 129
effects on metabolism, 62–63
stress responses
abnormal, in melancholia, 307–11
animal studies, 306, 308
child abuse, 306
genetically influenced, 303
intrauterine, 304
mechanisms, 307–11, 363
murine studies, 303
neurotoxic effects reduction, 362–63
physiologic effects, 308
and sympathetic arousal, 309
and temperament, 302
stroke
antidepressant prophylaxis, 257–58
cerebrovascular, 114
and depressive mood disorders, 317
with melancholia pharmacotherapy, 257–58
see also post-stroke depression

structured interviews
  limitations, 85
  procedures, 85
stupor
  case studies, 32
  differential diagnosis, 30
Styron, William, and melancholia, 18
sub-Saharan Africa, suicide rates, 125
substance abuse
  and depressive mood disorders, 256
  drugs, 255, 256
  solvents, 110
  and suicide risk, 137
  see also alcohol abuse
substance-induced mood disorder, 46
substance P, roles, 317
subsyndromal depression, 46
succinylcholine, 183
suicidal melancholic patients
  case studies, 125
  contact schedules, 145
  hospitalization, 143–45
    guidelines, 143
    indications, Table 7.3, 143
  inpatient care, 143–45
  management, 143–45
    case studies, 145
  outpatient care, 144–45
  removal of lethal means, 145
  supervision, 145
  symptom relief, 145
suicidal thoughts
  and alcohol use, 137
  case studies, 131
  clinical examination, 90
  communication, 131
  concealed, 131
  and decreased capacity, 127
suicide
  and firearms, 125–26, 133, 137
    case studies, 133
  in manic-depressive illness, 136
  in melancholia, 125–45
suicide prevention
  and antidepressants, 132
  errors in, 126–31
  measures for, 138
suicide rates
  age differences, 125, 126
  antidepressant treatment effects, 140–42
  depressed patients, 125
  ethnic and racial differences, 126
  global estimates, 125
  lithium treatment effects, 139–40
  psychotic depression, 223
  sex differences, 125
  and treatment type, 139–43
suicide risk
  and adjustment disorder with depressed mood, 102
  and alcohol abuse, 137
  antidepressants vs electroconvulsive therapy, 159
  case studies, 132, 133, 137
  and depressive mood disorders, 125
  and dexamethasone suppression test, 68, 138–39
  and electroconvulsive therapy, 159–61
    case studies, 160–61
  and failure to administer electroconvulsive therapy, 134
  and failure to hospitalize, 133–34
  and failure to recognize depressive mood disorders, 126–29
  familial, 135–36
  and hospitalization, 135, 143–44
    guidelines, 143
  inadequate outpatient follow-up, 132–33
  inadequate pharmacotherapy, 132, 141
    studies, 132
  and involuntary commitment, 133–34
  laboratory measures, 138–39
  males, over 50 years of age, 136–37
  and medical illness, 137–38
  and neurological illness, 137–38
  and psychotic depression, 89
  and serotonin levels, 138
  and sleep disturbances, 138
  and substance abuse, 137
  twin studies, 135–36
  under-diagnosis, 126–29
    studies, 127
suicide risk assessment, 134–36
  factors, 1298
  inadequate, 130–31
    case studies, 131
  long-term, 131
  training, 134–35
super-ego, 6
superimposed depression, diagnostic criteria, 106
suprachiasmatic nucleus (SCN), 356
Sweden, depression, prevalence, 49
Swedish Birth Registry, 241
sympathetic arousal, and stress responses, 309
syndromes
  Asperger, 104
  avolitional, 113
  bradykinetic, 113
  Capgras, 30
  de Clérambault, 30
  definitions, 51–52
    empirical, 52
    expert consensus, 51–52
  Ganser, 30
  melancholia as, 58
  Othello, 30
  post-concussion, 115
  see also apathetic syndromes; Cotard syndrome; Cushing's syndrome; neuroleptic malignant syndrome (NMS)
syphilis
  cerebral, 4
  and depression, 111
  serological identification, 62

T_3 *see* triiodothyronine (T_3)
T_4 (thyroxine), 72
tachycardia, risk factors, 262
TADS (Treatment for Adolescents with Depression Study), 249
targeted neurotransmitter system agents, in melancholia treatment, 290
Taylor, Michael Alan, 19, 27
TBI *see* traumatic brain injury (TBI)
TCAs *see* tricyclic antidepressants (TCAs)
temperament
  children, 302
  and environmental factors, 302
  genetic factors, 332
  and heritability, 302
  and melancholia risk, 302
  personality traits, 91
  and stress responses, 302
  unstable, 330
  use of term, 302
Tennessee (USA), electroconvulsive therapy, adolescents, 165
teratogenicity, antidepressants, 240–41
testosterone, in melancholia treatment, 292
Texas (USA), electroconvulsive therapy, adolescents, 165
thalamus, and stress responses, 308, 309–11
theophylline, effects on seizure, 188
thioridazine, drug–drug interactions, 265
threshold model, 56, 57
thrombosis, risk factors, 262
thyroid, functions, 72
thyroid disease
  differential diagnosis, 111
  etiology, 111
  with melancholia, pharmacotherapy, 265
thyroid dysfunction, and treatment-resistant depression, 272
thyroid function tests, 63
thyroid-stimulating hormone (TSH), 72
  levels
    and depression, 72
    and mania, 330
  and melancholia, 307
thyrotropin-releasing hormone (TRH), 72
  levels, and depression, 72
  and melancholia, 307
thyroxine (T_4), release, 72
TMS *see* transcranial magnetic stimulation (TMS)
topiramate, 290
transcranial magnetic stimulation (TMS)
  effectiveness, 287–88
  and electroconvulsive therapy compared, 286–87
  in melancholia treatment, 286–88
transcription cascades, 360
transcription factors, 360
tranylcypromine, 50
  effectiveness, children and adolescents, 249
traumatic brain injury (TBI)
  differential diagnosis, 115
  with melancholia, pharmacotherapy, 261
trazodone, side-effects, 205–206
TRD *see* treatment-resistant depression (TRD)
Treatment for Adolescents with Depression Study (TADS), 249
treatment algorithms, 47–48, 348, 364–65
  STEP-BD, 23
treatment guidelines, recommendations, 351
treatment resistance, 212–13
treatment-resistant depression (TRD)
  case studies, 270
  comorbidity, 270–72
  and electroconvulsive therapy, failure to provide, 272–73
  inadequate treatment, 270
  incorrect diagnosis 268–70
  pharmacotherapy, 268–73
  prevention, 273
  and thyroid dysfunction, 272
treatment trials, recommendations, 349–51
treatment type, and suicide rates, 139–43
TRH *see* thyrotropin-releasing hormone (TRH)
tricyclic antidepressants (TCAs)
  advantages, 197, 202
  approved, 50
  and breast-feeding, 244
  dosing issues, 247–48
  drug augmentation, 217
  effectiveness, 202
    children, 244, 246–48
    elderly, 252
  effects on suicide rates, 140
  and electroconvulsive therapy compared, 156, 157
  epilepsy with melancholia treatment, 260
  heart disease with melancholia treatment, 262–63
  mania induction, 22
  manic-depressive illness treatment, 226
  melancholia treatment, 206–207
  neonatal issues, 241, 242
  overdose, lethality, 142–43
  Parkinson's disease with melancholia treatment, 258–59
  psychosis studies, 25
  secondary vs tertiary amines, 199, 211
  side-effects, 205, 252, 260
  treatment resistance, 103
  vs selective serotonin reuptake inhibitors, 196, 198–00, 201–204, 206–207
triiodothyronine (T_3)
  drug augmentation, 216
  and melancholia, 307
  release, 72
tryptophan hydroxylase, 360
TSH *see* thyroid-stimulating hormone (TSH)
twin studies
  bipolar–unipolar overlap, 23
  depression, 49
  depressive mood disorders, 301, 303
  manic-depressive illness, 330

twin studies (*cont.*)
premenstrual dysphoric disorder, 102
suicide risk, 135–36
two depression factors, Kendell's, 53, 54–55

UFC (urinary free cortisol), 67
unipolar depression, 46
early studies, 19
electroconvulsive therapy, 172–74
recurrent, 21
subtypes, 19
unipolar disorder, psychopathologic studies, 20
unitary model, 5
United Kingdom (UK)
antidepressants
prescriptions issued, 141–42
regulations, 141
and suicide rates, 141–42
United States of America (USA)
antidepressants
studies, 142
and suicide risk, 141
electroconvulsive therapy, adolescents, 165
St. John's wort studies, 293
suicide rates, 125, 126
ethnic and racial differences, 126
suicide risk assessment, training, 134–35
University of Melbourne (Australia), 64–65
University of Michigan (USA), 64–65
electroconvulsive therapy studies, 166
urinary free cortisol (UFC), 67
urine copper assays, 116

vagal nerve stimulation (VNS)
in melancholia treatment, 289
recommendations, 289
valproic acid
drug–drug interactions, 265
manic-depressive illness treatment, 228, 229
severe melancholia treatment, 230
vascular brain disease, elderly, 251
vascular depression
age of onset, 105
use of term, 105
vascular disease, and depression, 106
vasoactive intestinal polypeptide (VIP), roles, 317
vasopressin, roles, 316–17
vegetative functions, and melancholia, 16
vegetative signs
clinical examination, 88–89
and melancholia, 348
venlafaxine
diabetes with melancholia treatment, 264–65
effectiveness, 202, 203, 205, 224
effects on suicide rates, 141
heart disease with melancholia treatment, 263
Huntington's disease with melancholia treatment, 260
mania induction, 23
melancholia treatment, 211
Parkinson's disease with melancholia treatment, 259
severe melancholia treatment, 230
side-effects, 263
toxicity, 142
ventrolateral cortex, increased metabolism, 319–20
VEPs *see* visual evoked potentials (VEPs)
Veraguth's folds, 87
verbal memory, impairment, 327
Verblödungsprocesse, 4
VIP (vasoactive intestinal polypeptide), 317
visual evoked potentials (VEPs), 323–24
mood disorder studies, 324
visual memory, impairment, 327
vital depression, 8
VNS *see* vagal nerve stimulation (VNS)

warfarin, drug–drug interactions, 265
Washington state (USA), 241
Weissenburger, J. E. 57
white matter, 116
changes, 105, 106
Wilson's disease, differential diagnosis, 116
witchcraft, and mental disorders, 3
Witzelsucht (shallow humor), 113–14
World Health Organization (WHO), depression studies, 351

ziprasidone, 224
Ziskind, E., 154, 155
Zung Self-rating Depression Scale (ZSDS), 94